Hearing Instrument Science & Fitting Practices

SECOND EDITION

Edited by
Robert E. Sandlin, Ph.D.

Published by
International Hearing Society

Library of Congress Cataloging in Publication Data — 96-067616

SANDLIN, Robert E. (Editor)
HEARING INSTRUMENT SCIENCE AND FITTING PRACTICES
(Second Edition)
Revised Printing

Published by
International Hearing Society
16880 Middlebelt Road, Livonia, MI 48154
ISBN 0-934031-06-1
ISBN 978-0-934031-06-1

Manufactured in the United States of America

LIST OF CONTRIBUTING AUTHORS

Max S. Chartrand, Ph.D	Gainesville, TX
James Curran, M.S.	Eden Prairie, MN
Linda Donaldson, M.A.	Centerville, OH
Aram Glorig, M.D.	Westminster, CA
E. Robert Libby, BC-HIS	Upper Darby, PA
Geary McCandless, Ph.D.	Salt Lake City, UT
Jay McSpaden, Ph.D.	Lebanon, OR
Robert Martin, Ph.D.	La Mesa, CA
Michael Metz, Ph.D.	Garden Grove, CA
Joel Mynders, BC-HIS	Westchester, PA
R. David Nelson, M.A.	Spencer, IA
Robert Novak, M.D.	Westminster, CA
Lisa G. Potts, M.S.	St. Louis, MO
David Preves, Ph.D.	Minneapolis, MN
Raymond Z. Rich, BC-HIS	Cleveland, OH
Robert E. Sandlin, Ph.D.	San Diego, CA
Wayne Staab, Ph.D.	Phoenix, AZ
Maureen Valente, M.A.	St. Louis, MO
Michael Valente, Ph.D.	St. Louis, MO

The International Hearing Society (IHS) and the National Institute for Hearing Instruments Studies (NIHIS) are most grateful to Dr. Robert E. Sandlin for his persistence and efforts in the completion of the second edition of *Hearing Instrument Science and Fitting Practices.* It is a difficult talk to organize and coordinate the talents of 19 outstanding professionals in our hearing health care industry. As Richard L. "Pat" Clark wrote for the first edition in 1985, the efforts put forth ". . . has resulted in a comprehensive reference book on hearing instrument dispensing." This text remains the leading reference book for hearing health care industry professionals.

No publishing effort by NIHIS can be implemented nor completed without the diligent, meticulous and hard-working efforts of

Phyllis V. Wilson, NIHIS Administrative Director and the review of each chapter by the NIHIS Publications Chair, Kathy Harvey. This text will continue to be the dominant reference for the topic of hearing instrument studies to be used by all professionals in the hearing health care arena.

Linda L. Donaldson
NIHIS Chair

Contents

XIV. LEGAL AND ETHICAL ASPECTS OF HEARING INSTRUMENT DISPENSING

Michael J. Metz

Preface

It has been over ten years since the publication of *Hearing Instruments Sciences and Fitting Practices.* During this period of time there have been a number of challenging and exciting innovations which have altered the way in which hearing instruments are selected and fitted. Simply stated, we have more knowledge of the human auditory system and its acoustic needs relative to hearing aid amplification. We have made tremendous advances in technology, which directly affect how we select and fit hearing aid devices.

In view of the many changes over the past decade, the Revised Edition incorporates new knowledge and expands upon that information presented in the first edition. Many of the original contributing authors have done a magnificent job in "updating" their individual chapters. Also, new authors and new chapter content make this textbook a most welcome one for those who contemplate hearing instrument dispensing as a profession. Further, it serves as an excellent reference source for the experienced hearing health professional.

In Chapter I, *Basic Hearing Science,* David Preves and James Curran introduce new and current information to aid the reader in understanding the importance of scientific contribution to hearing instrument fitting. They provide an overview of the human auditory system and its function. As with any new or unique information, terminology may be a challenge to the reader. However, careful reading of the most demanding sections of this chapter will have its rewards in greater understanding of hearing science.

In Chapter II, Robert Martin makes significant and important revisions in his chapter dealing with *Audiometric Assessment and*

Interpretation. The reader is provided an extensive overview of essential audiometric tests and procedures consistent with the needs of the hearing instrument dispenser. He reviews some of the pathologies affecting the way in which the auditory system performs. Of significance is his "House of Hearing" in which he delineates performance characteristics of hearing aids consistent with the needs of the hearing impaired.

In Chapter III, *Principles of Masking,* Linda Donaldson, performs a yeoman-like task of explaining the use of masking during the hearing assessment process. Masking is not a simple clinical procedure, yet one which is most significant in arriving at reliable measures of human hearing status. Not only does she explain the value of masking, but she provides a step by step procedure for obtaining reliable audiometric measures when masking is applied in the testing sequence.

Chapter IV by E. Robert Libby, *Hearing Instruments Systems Technology and Performance Standards,* represents a monumental effort to condense into a single chapter basic information regarding hearing aids and their essential components and performance characteristics. Not only are hearing instruments classified as to type, but their value and limitations are discussed. In concluding his chapter, Libby discusses alternative listening devices, which have proven to be beneficial to those with hearing loss.

Chapter V, *Human Acoustic Couplers* by Joel Mynders, has undergone a good deal of revision. Since the original text was published, there have been marked changes in hearing aid styles. No longer are BTE hearing aids, with the accompanying earmold, the most commonly dispensed. ITE, ITC and CIC instruments constitute the large majority of instruments dispensed today. Consistent with this change, Mynders emphasizes acoustic considerations as well as impression techniques to produce an "optimal" earmold or shell for the hearing aid desired.

Chapter VI, *Selecting Amplification Systems,* has been revised by Wayne Staab, yet includes essential information from Briskey's earlier work presented in the original text (Instrument Fitting Techniques). This current chapter treats such areas as hearing aid candidacy, degrees of hearing impairment, client satisfaction, hearing aid standards, factors influencing hearing aid choice and other important issues. The reader is well advised to become familiar with the content of this chapter. It is basic to one's core of knowledge relative to hearing aid amplification.

In Chapter VII, *Principles of Sound Field Audiometry.* Robert Sandlin provides an overview of sound field testing and the several clinical contributions which it offers. With the introduction of fitting formulae, in which only pure tone data is required to determine amplification needs, sound field testing has lost favor among some hearing health professionals. However, the advantages of sound field tests in the selection, fitting and verification of aided response in meeting acoustic needs of the patients are presented. It is not intended to impugn other forms of testing, but rather to recommend that sound field testing be part of the clinical assessment armamentarium.

In Chapter VIII, *Probe Microphone Measurements,* Geary McCandless reviews the rationale for and the advantages of hearing aid responses provided by real ear measurement. He carefully lists the advantages and limitations of probe microphone assessment. Additionally, he defines the various terminology which has been developed relative to the reporting of real ear measurement. Finally, he defends the value of probe microphone assessment as a very useful tool in verifying hearing aid response and whether or not certain criteria of performance have been met.

In Chapter IX, *Programmable Hearing Aid Systems,* Michael Valente and Lisa Gulledge Potts bring their considerable talent to bear on the value of programmability. They review the development of programmable hearing aid devices and their clinical application. Based on extensive, clinical experience, they list the advantages and limitations of specific instruments having programmable functions. The utility of multiprogrammable hearing aids is defended, as evidenced by the patient's immediate access to the acoustic response best suited to the environment in which listening takes place.

In Chapter X, *Post Fitting Care and Processes,* Raymond Rich and Jay MacSpaden combine their several talents to produce a definitive work which clearly identifies the responsibilities of the hearing instrument dispenser relative to patient management strategies and follow-up care. They delineate responsibilities from instrument modification to acceptance and use of amplification. This important chapter is clearly written and contains information vital to understanding hearing instrument dispensing practices.

Chapter XI, *Psycho-Social Principles: The Prospective Hearing Instrument Patient* is the contribution of Max Chartrand. He has taken the original chapter content by Reiter and expanded it to include recent thinking about the psychological status of the hearing impaired person. More emphasis is given to neurophysiological bases for those factors contributing to normal and abnormal human behaviors. He stresses the need for hearing instrument dispensers to be aware of behaviors peculiar to the hearing impaired person.

In Chapter XII, *Geriatric Considerations,* Aram Glorig combines his talents with those of Robert Novak to produce a work that clearly describes the population most susceptible to hearing impairment. Not only are the several causes of age-related hearing impairment viewed, but the behaviors of the elderly patient relative to the use and acceptance of hearing aid amplification. Cultural influences are described as they related to rehabilitation and acceptance of disability.

Dave Nelson has produced an excellent piece of work in Chapter XIII pertaining to *Management Considerations in Hearing Instrument Dispensing.* Information contained in this chapter is one with which those planning to dispense hearing aids should be very familiar. Failure to apply business management practices places in jeopardy the probability of success. Business practices range from how to set up and manage an office to the type of employee most suited to work in that professional environment.

Chapter XIV, *Legal and Ethical Aspects of Hearing Instrument Dispensing,* by Michael Metz presents a stimulating overview of legal and ethical principles underlying any professional activities. A sensitive, frank and open discussion is presented in a conscientious effort to look at hearing instrument dispensing as a recognized and developing profession. He reminds us all that we have an individual responsibility to uphold the best interests of the professional body to which we belong.

Indeed, this revised textbook should be of considerable value to those who select, fit and dispense hearing instruments.

Robert E. Sandlin, Editor

Foreword

In 1985, the first edition of Hearing Instrument Science and Fitting Practices was published by the National Hearing Aid Society. In that decade, much has happened to warrant a revised edition. Not only has the name of the National Hearing Aid Society been changed to International Hearing Society, but much more is known about the human auditory system and more is known about those criteria governing the selection and fitting of hearing aid systems.

This text is organized in a manner consistent with those basic competencies demanded of all who select and fit hearing aid devices. To that extent, it serves as a basic reference book for those entering the dispensing arena. However, its value is not limited to the novice, but can and should serve as a reference text for the experienced hearing health professional. This book is not an attempt to present an exhaustive overview of each competency area. To do so would be to extend its purpose beyond reasonable bounds. However, it does meet the academic needs and basic educational requirements of the hearing instrument dispenser.

The primary task of an Editor-in-Chief is that of selecting contributors who are knowledgeable in a specific area of concern to the hearing health professional. One feels that this has been accomplished. A secondary task is that of expediting, within reasonable bounds, the publication of the textbook itself. This has been accomplished primarily because of the untiring efforts of selected members of the National Institute for Hearing Instruments Studies (NIHIS). I wish to acknowledge the support and Herculean effort of Phyllis Wilson, without whom this text could never have become a reality.

It is with deep respect that I recognize the contribution of the International Hearing Society. Although, as a body, they have to deal with a number of issues affecting those who practice hearing instrument dispensing, they gave approval for the Revised Edition, knowing full well that it constituted a commitment requiring their time and financial resources.

As this editor noted in the Forward to the first edition: *Knowledge is a precious commodity and it is hoped that this text serves those purposes of expanding skills and increasing competencies.*

I

BASIC HEARING SCIENCE

David A. Preves Ph.D. and James R. Curran M.S.

INTRODUCTION

Each acoustic stimulus is changed into an auditory sensation having well defined dimensions as it travels through the auditory system (Figure 1). The pathways which the stimulus follows as it changes from a physical quantity to an auditory sensation, and the processes and mechanisms involved are only crudely and imperfectly understood. There is surely a physiological basis for each of the events which occurs in the auditory perceptual area. But our ability to clearly understand and explain the events which change the physical to the psychophysical world is limited.

After many years of guessing and hypothesizing, it was only fairly recently that a reliable description of the events taking place in the human cochlea was published. Scientists and researchers have always been hampered in their investigations by the virtual inaccessibility of the inner ear and higher auditory centers. With today's instrumentation, advances in understanding the auditory system are occurring. However, much has yet to be discovered. Similarly, improvements in investigational techniques happen with regularity. Old thoughts are being frequently changed by new findings and the interpretations given to them.

The description of the way in which the auditory system behaves is a blend of fact and guess. Where controversy or educated

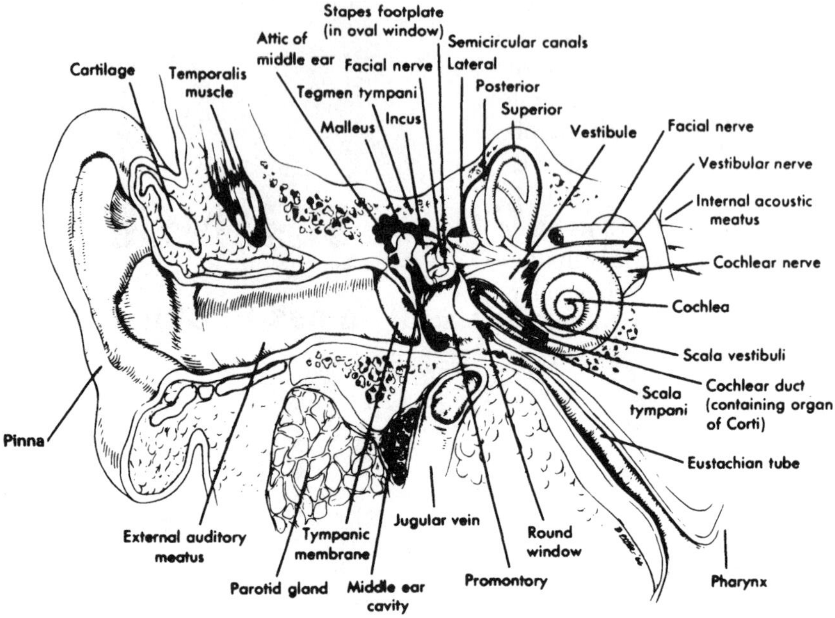

Fig. 1. Overall anatomy of the auditory system. (*Saunders, William H., Paparella, Michael M. & Miglets, Andrew W., Atlas of Ear Surgery, 3rd ed., 1980 C.V. Mosby Co.*)

guessing exists, it has been noted and sources are cited to make as clear as possible the most probable explanation.

In earlier times, before the nature of sound was really understood, a very popular philosophical question was, "If a tree falls in the forest, and no one is there to hear it, is there sound?" This was a very difficult question to answer. There was not a clear understanding of the nature of physical acoustics. But of course, we know now that the sound is there whether or not a listener is in the vicinity to "hear" it. The description of the physical events which occur in the production of sound is called acoustics, and the characteristic behavior of particles in a medium (air) goes on whether or not there is someone there to hear the sound.

It is very clear that sound can be defined both from a physical and psychological point of view. The hearing aid specialist is interested in knowing, as much as possible, all the dimensions of both aspects of sound, its generation and perception. The relationship between frequency and pitch, loudness and intensity, and the nature of the boundary between the two aspects constitutes some of the information presented in this chapter. As an example, it may be difficult to understand why a change in intensity is often not exactly equal to the change in the psychological sensation of loudness. It is a very important consideration, however. The difference between the physical stimulus and the sensation which is produced must be kept separate in one's mind, otherwise it may be assumed that a certain number of decibels increase in intensity, for example, may cause the same number of decibels increase in loudness, especially in hearing impaired listeners. Experiments have shown that this is not always a true statement. The way in which an acoustic stimulus is changed into a sensation involves a sequence of physical, physiological and psychological events which, when understood, provides a basis for better understanding the art and science of hearing aid dispensing.

CHAPTER OBJECTIVES

This chapter will acquaint the reader with basic concepts of the physics of sound and the decibel scale. After completing this chapter, the reader should understand basic anatomy of the auditory system and how sound stimuli are changed to different forms of energy as they travel through the auditory pathways. The primary purpose of this chapter is to show how basic concepts of auditory physiology and psycho-acoustics can relate to practical hearing aid fitting.

PHYSICAL CHARACTERISTICS OF SOUND

Air is a medium through which sound travels. Air consists of tiny particles (molecules) which are always in motion. This motion is random, and so slight that it is hardly possible for the human ear to detect. The particles move gently against one another, in no particularly organized manner, and this random movement is below the hearing threshold of the normal, average person. What happens, however, if a vibratory source is applied in the vicinity of the particles? The vibratory source, of course, can be of any nature: a vibrating string, the human voice or the to and fro motion of a tuning fork. Particles which are next to the source of these vibrations are set into motion, which represents the movement of the vibratory source. For example, if there is a to and fro movement of the vibratory source, the air particles nearby begin to move in that same to and fro motion.

A particle which is moved by the vibratory source will collide with other particles which are next to it, and cause them to have the identical motion. A chain of events now occurs, where successively adjacent particles collide, one with the other, each having in their own motion the same movements of as the original vibratory source. In this way sound, travels through the medium (e.g., air) from its source (vibration) towards a particular destination in a certain amount of elapsed time.

For example, when vibrations are produced by striking a tuning fork, a sound wave is produced which travels through air as shown in (Figure 2). The air molecules in the sound wave are alternately pressed more tightly together during the compression portion of the wave and are further apart during the rarefaction portion of the sound wave. The resulting sound can be described by: 1) the frequency of the vibrations or how many vibrations travel past a given point in space per second; and 2) the amplitude

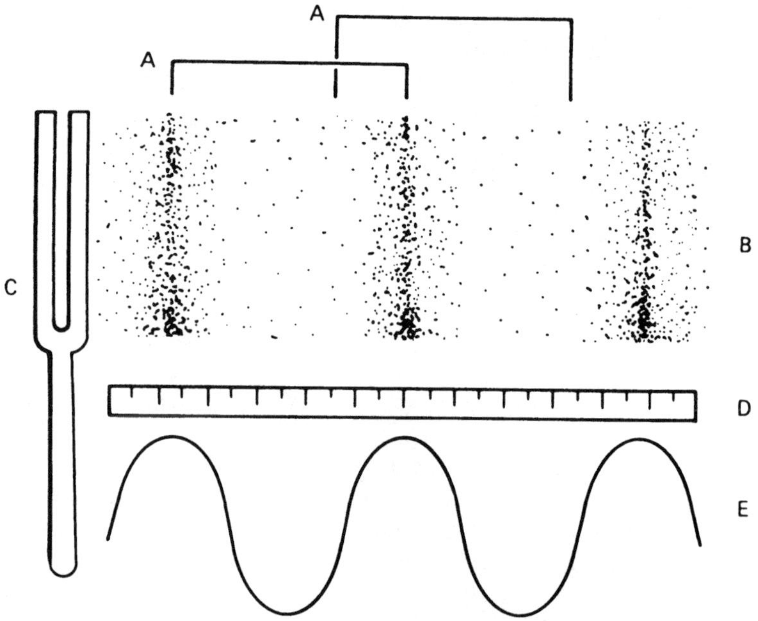

Fig. 2. Illustration of condensation and rarefaction as a sound wave travels through air. (A) is the wavelength and is measured from any point on the periodic wave to the same point on the next wave. Pressure waves (B) are formed in the air from the tuning fork vibrations (C). The sound waves form a sinusoidal waveform which moves (D) and can be displayed in time (E). (*Martin, Frederick N., Introduction to Audiology, 1975, p. 27. Reprinted by permission of Prentice-Hall, Inc., Englewood Cliffs, N.J.*)

or intensity of the vibrations—how far do the vibrations cause the air molecules to be displaced from their normal resting positions. Each of these two physical variables is directly related to a subjective sensation of sound within the human auditory system: frequency to the pitch of the sound and amplitude or intensity to the loudness of the sound. The diaphragm of a hearing aid microphone must respond accurately to the frequency and amplitude of these air molecule vibrations so that the hearing aid can faithfully amplify sound.

The amplitude or intensity of the sound produced is related to the largest air pressure changes caused by the displacement of the air molecules. The amplitude or intensity of sounds may be thought of in terms of pressure, power or energy. There is an enormous, difference between the intensity of a just detectable quiet sound at hearing threshold, and the intensity of a very loud sound at the threshold of feeling pain. The difference between intensities of these two thresholds is approximately 10 trillion. Because describing such enormous ranges of sound intensity require very large numbers, differences in sound intensities are expressed in a kind of a ratio shorthand instead.

Named after Alexander Graham Bell, this ratio method of expression is called the bel, which is defined as the logarithm to the base 10 of the ratio of two values. Instead of expressing the difference between the threshold of feeling pain via hearing and the threshold of hearing detection as a ratio of 10,000,000,000,000 times, the zeros in the number are counted and the ratio is written as 10^{13}. The ratio 10^{13} means that 10 should be multiplied by itself thirteen times. The numeral 10 refers to the "base 10". The exponent 13 refers to the result of performing the logarithm, which equals 13 bels.

However, the bel is much larger than that needed to express smaller ratios for which the decibel (dB), or 1/10th of a bel is often used. The decibel equivalent of 13 bels is $10 \times 13 = 130$ decibels (dB). Thus, the decibel scale has the advantage of being able to express large sound pressure ranges with relatively small numbers.

The intensity of a sound is usually expressed in decibels relative to a reference sound pressure. It wouldn't make any sense to say "the intensity of a sound is 80dB" because no reference sound pressure is stated. The intensity of a sound is commonly expressed in decibels of sound pressure level (dB SPL). In this case, the reference sound pressure is 20 micro Pascals (μPa). Mathematically, this looks like:

$$\text{Intensity level in dB SPL} = 20 \log_{10}(\text{sound pressure}/20\ \mu\text{Pa})$$

The peak SSPL90 (Saturation Sound pressure Level 90) measurement for a hearing aid is an example of sound intensity expressed in dB SPL. For a peak SSPL90 of 120dB SPL, the sound is one million times more intense than the reference sound pressure of 20 micro Pascals.

Another example of using a reference sound pressure is in calculating the acoustic gain of a hearing aid.

For example, if gain in a hearing aid causes a ten-fold increase in sound pressure relative to a reference input sound pressure, the result is a 20dB increase in SPL, or a 20dB gain. Correspondingly, a two-fold increase in sound pressure produced by a hearing aid results in a 6dB increase in SPL or a 6dB gain.

Mathematically, this looks like:

$$\text{Gain in dB} = 20 \log_{10}(\text{sound pressure/reference sound pressure})$$

The choice of the decibel scale to specify sound pressure level is appropriate for discussing the growth of loudness in auditory systems if the intensity of the sound increases in logarithmic steps. For example, a two-fold increase in sound intensity produces a 6 dB increase in loudness in a normal auditory system in the region around most comfortable listening level. The authors are aware that decibel notation and the concept of a logarithm are difficult for many beginning hearing aid specialists to understand. Re-reading this section several times and reviewing other descriptions of these two concepts may help. They are important to a basic understanding of hearing aids and the auditory system. For supplementary information on the decibel scale of measurement, the interested reader is referred to Small, 1978.

All complex sounds consist of a combination of pure tones. Any complex sound can be broken down into individual component frequencies by a technique known as Fourier spectral analysis. Fourier spectral analysis is a way of representing a complex sound wave in terms of energy at different frequencies. Fourier spectral analysis takes a complex waveform and converts it to a number of pure tones of different frequencies, each having a unique amplitude and phase. For example, speech from a particular speaker is often represented by a Fourier spectral analysis of the resonant frequencies of the speaker's vocal tract. Since the speaker's vocal tract changes shape during production of various sounds, the frequencies at which resonances occur also change. A graphical representation of these resonances as a function of frequency is called a spectrum. Figure 3 shows examples of the spectra over about an 80 millisecond time window for two similar sounding utterances by the same male talker - /if/ in the upper panel and /ith/ in the

Lesson 15
6-8

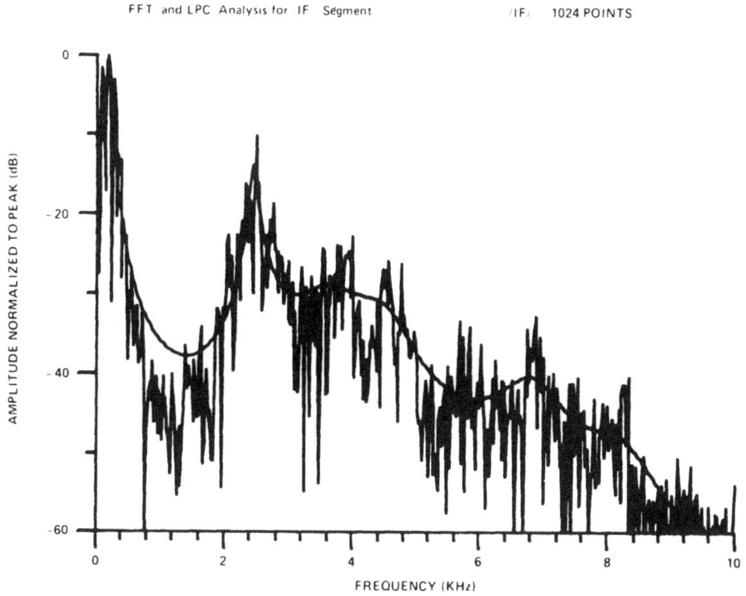

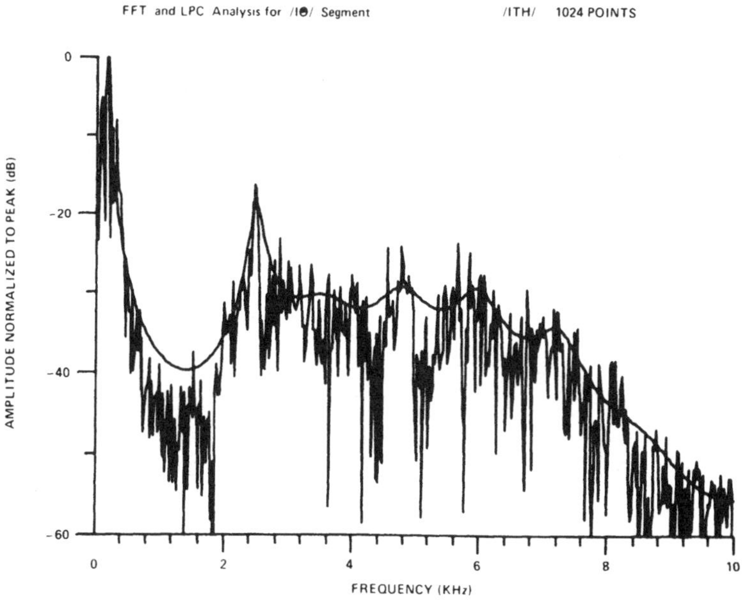

Fig. 3. Comparison of formants and high frequency energy between /ith/ and /if/.

lower panel. The jagged lines in these graphs are produced because the fundamental of the speakers vocal cords is included in the Fourier analysis of these utterances. The solid lines in these graphs represent estimates of the spectra with the vocal cord fundamental frequency component removed via Linear Predictive Coding (LPC). The resonances of these speech sounds produce peak pressures at particular frequencies in the spectrum that are called formants. For example, the second formant occurs at approximately 2500 Hz. for both utterances.

As another example, the inner ear (cochlea) performs a type of Fourier analysis on sounds entering the auditory system as it separates them into individual frequency components. The frequency response of a hearing aid may also be thought of as a Fourier spectral analysis of the hearing aid output in response to a complex input signal.

Simple to and fro motion of a particle through a complete cycle can be thought of as a sine wave, or pure tone. A rarefaction and condensation air pressure change (sinusoid) produces a pure tone sound wave. This pure tone sound has an air pressure which varies with time as shown in (Figure 4a). In this figure, sound wave in-

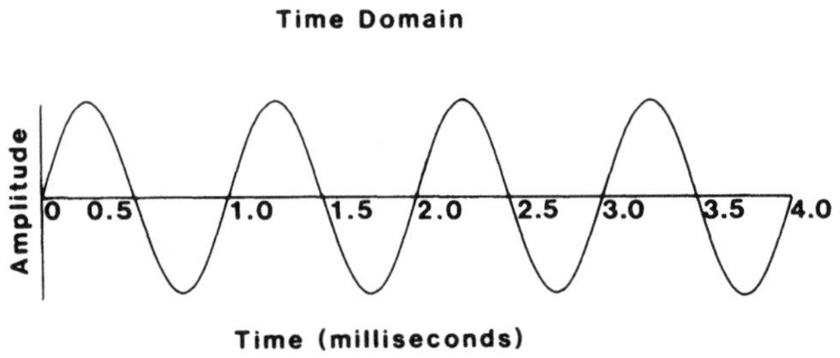

Fig. 4a. 1000 HZ - Pure tone or sine wave in time domain.

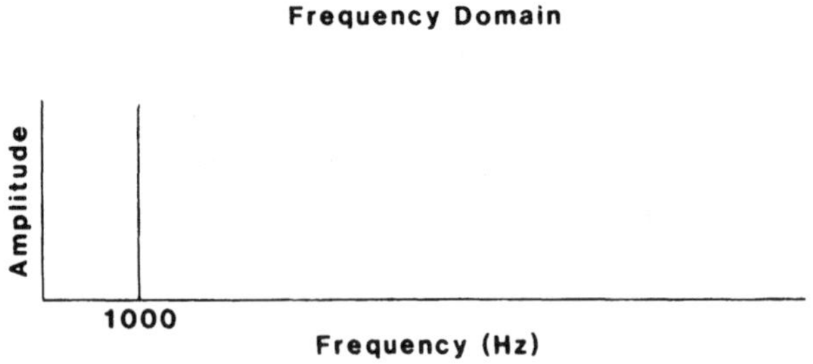

Fig. 4b. 1000 HZ - Pure tone or sinusoid (sine wave) in frequencydomain. (*Licklider in Stevens after Handbook of Experimental Psychology, John Wiley & Sons, 1960.*)

tensity is shown on the vertical scale and time is shown on the horizontal scale. Any sound can be represented in both time (called the temporal domain) as well as in frequency (called the spectral domain). The pure tone may be generated by a simple harmonic motion, produced, for example, by a pendulum swinging or a plucked violin string vibrating. A continuous 1000Hz pure tone has only one frequency component in its spectrum as shown in Figure 4b—a narrow blip whose height is directly related to the intensity of the pure tone. A somewhat more complex sound, a 1000Hz square wave, which sounds like a buzz (see time waveform in Figure 5a), contains the fundamental frequency of 1000Hz and its odd harmonics (pure tone overtones at 3, 5, 7, etc. times 1000 Hz or 3000, 5000, 7000Hz etc.) at decreasing intensities as frequency is increased. The Fourier spectral analysis of this square wave is shown in Figure 5b. A square wave is actually produced (Figure 5c) by combining pure tones of odd harmonics.

An inverse relationship often exists between the frequency range of a sound stimulus and its duration in time (Gabor, 1947).

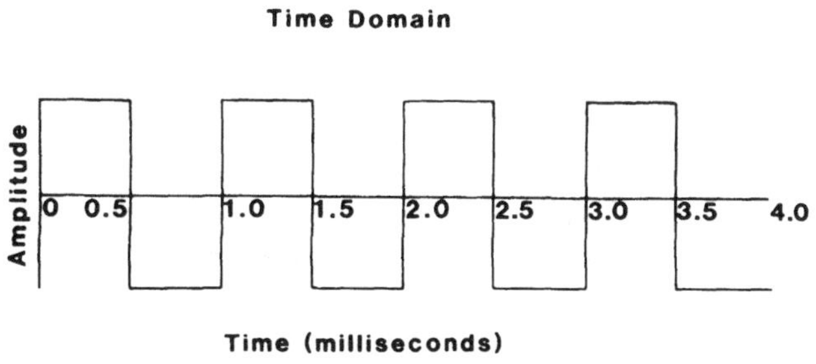

Fig. 5a. 1000 HZ - Square wave in time domain.

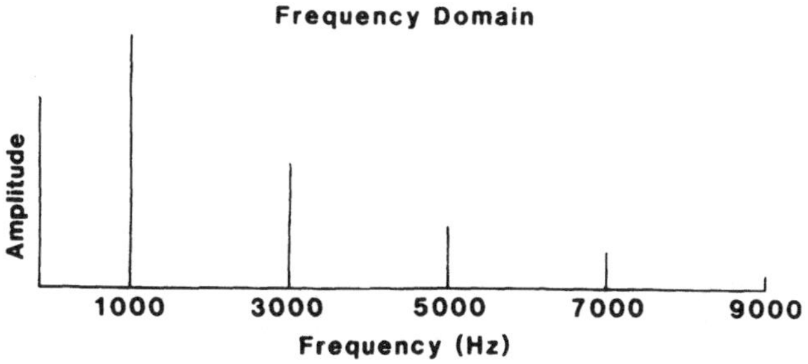

Fig. 5b. Square wave in frequency domain. (*Licklider in Stevens after Handbook of Experimental Psychology, John Wiley & Sons, 1960.*)

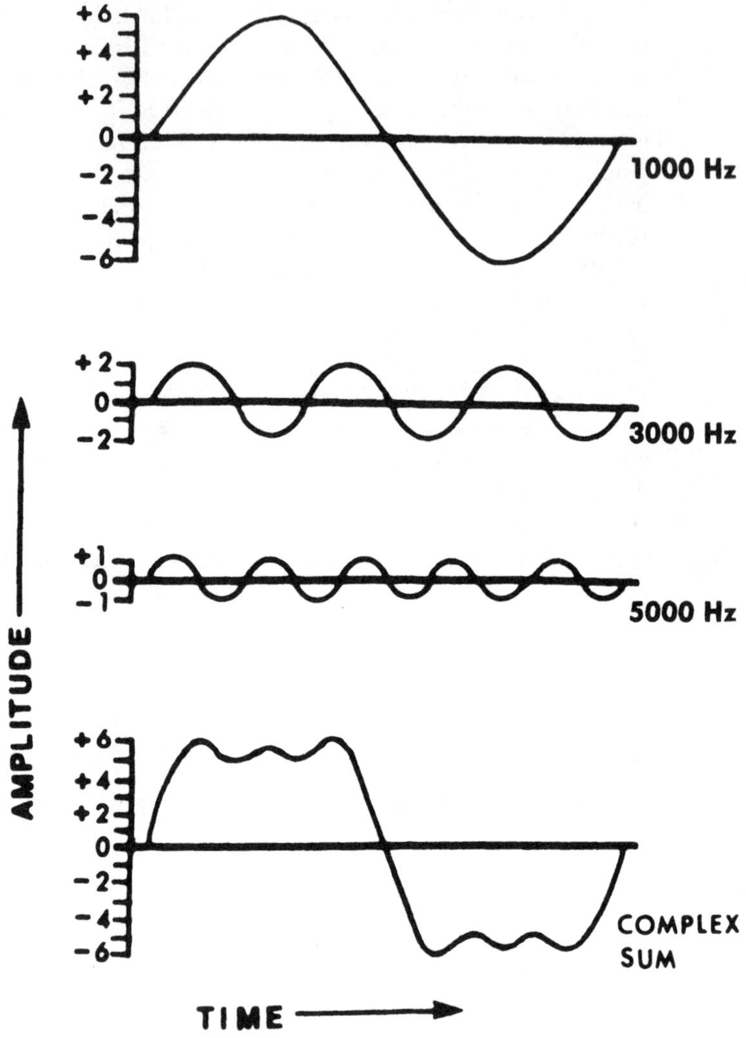

Fig. 5c. Formation of a square wave from a sum of pure tones. (*Borden and Harris, Speech Science Primer Physiology Acoustics, and Perception of Speech, after Williams and Wilkins, 1984.*)

For example, a brief click sound stimulus (Figure 6a) that is roughly similar to speech burst sounds such as /p, t, k/, has a relatively flat, broad-band spectrum in the frequency domain that is similar, at least over part of the frequency range, to the spectrum of white noise provided by an audiometer for masking. (Figure 6b).

Lesson 1 pg 11-21

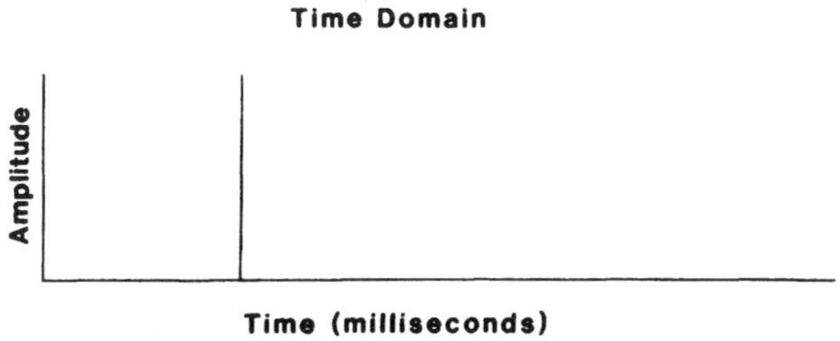

Fig. 6a. Click in time domain.

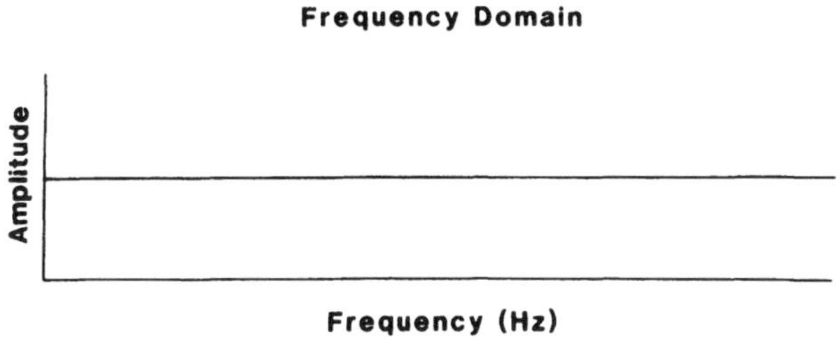

Fig. 6b. Click in frequency domain. (*Licklider in Stevens after Handbook of Experimental Psychology, John Wiley & Sons, 1960.*)

THE EXTERNAL EAR

The external ear, which consists of an external visible portion, referred to as the pinna or auricle, and the external ear canal, are anatomical features of primary importance to the hearing aid specialist. Not only must the specialist become familiar with all the anatomical landmarks (Figure 6), but certain of the parts of the external ear hold special significance for the fitting of hearing aids.

The concha, portions of the helix, and ear canal are intimately involved when an ear impression is to be taken. Good retention of an earmold or an in-the-ear hearing aid shell is often dependent upon the shape and texture of these portions of the ear. A concha that is deeply recessed below the anti-helix provides excellent potential for earmold retention; similarly, the presence of a shallow concha, a common occurrence, may signal the need for extension of the top portion of the mold or shell into the crevice underlying the helix crus (Figure 6), to hold the mold or shell in place. Since this crevice-like opening is often very narrow, the specialist must be certain that the impression is entirely accurate in this region, so that the mold is not so large that it will cause discomfort.

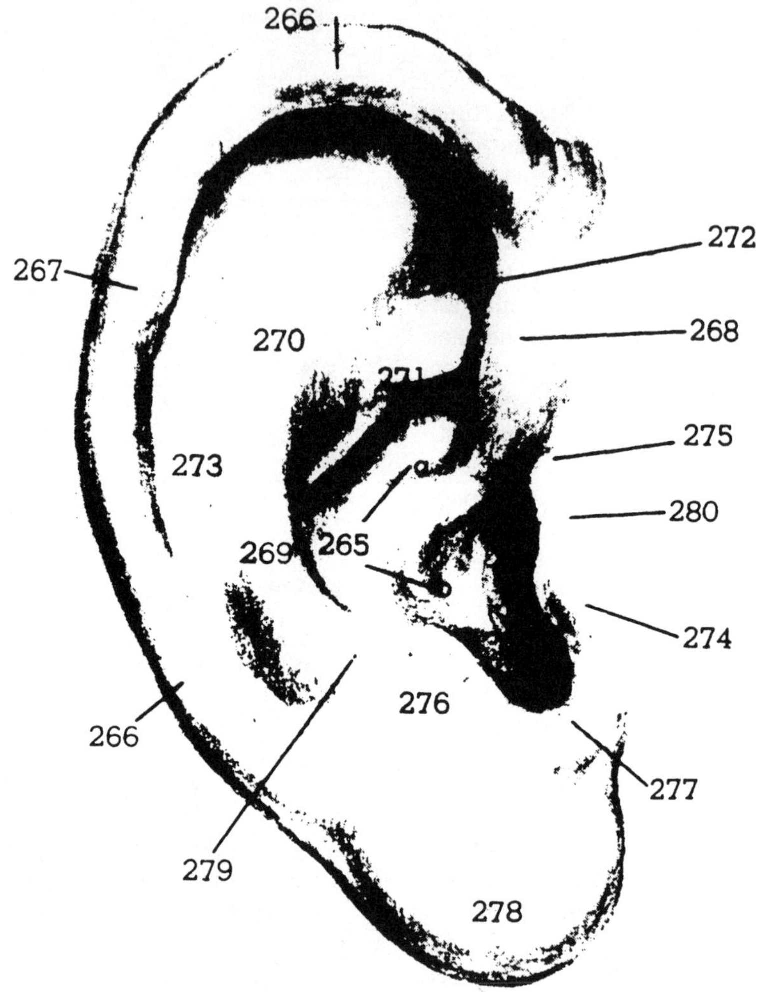

Fig. 7. Anatomical landmarks of the external ear (*Polyak, McHigh and Judd, after the Human Ear in Anatomical Transparencies, Sonotone Corporation, 1946.*) This figure shows the lateral view of the auricle; **265** concha, or "shell," of auricle (**a** "skiff", **b** "cave"); **266** helix, or "snail," **267** thickened portion of preceding, called "Darwin tubercle"; **268** crus, or "limb," or helix; **269** antihelix; **270** upper crus of anti helix; **271** lower crus of antihelix; **272** triangular fossa; **273** scaphoid, or boat-shaped, fossa; **274** tragus, or "buck"; **275** anterior notch; **276** antitragus; **277** intertragal notch; **278** lobule, or earlap; **279** posterior sulcus; **280** supratragal tubercle.

Hearing aid users having relatively straight ear canals often require earmolds and ear shells which have good retention characteristics. Otherwise the earmold or in-the-ear instrument may work out of the ear. Although the skin which covers the exterior portion of the ear (auricle) is relatively tough and resistant to normal exposure to the elements, insertion of the earmold or ear shell into the various hollows, depressions and contours of the ear can result in discomfort, minor irritations and/or increased sensitivity in some subjects.

Irritation may arise from two sources: 1) an allergic reaction to the mold or shell material, and 2) an ill fitting mold or shell. The former cause, experience suggests, is relatively rare; if an allergic reaction is suspected, it is a simple matter to tape a small piece of the suspected earmold or ear shell material to the inner surface of the ear lobe for 24 hours. If redness or eruption occurs on the skin, the material may be suspected and another should be used. But more commonly, the source of the discomfort is an ill-fitting mold. Even the slightest amount of distention or deformation of the natural contours of the ear at a critical point of contact may be sufficient to produce extreme pain, redness, swelling and/or general irritation.

The external auditory meatus, an irregularly shaped tube which varies in length from approximately 1 inch to 1-3/8 inches, is cartilaginous and is covered with thick skin for the first one third to one half of its length. The skin of the cartilaginous portion of the meatus is heavily populated with fine hairs, sebaceous (oil) and ceruminous (ear wax) glands. The latter produce cerumen, and the fine hairs in the ear canal act to gently and constantly move the dry particles of cerumen out toward the entrance of the ear canal.

The inner portion of the external canal is bony and is covered only by a thin layer of skin. The skin tissue in this deep area of the canal is extremely sensitive and prone to irritation; sometimes the gentlest rubbing or friction on the surface can result in excretions, swelling or redness. For this reason, care should be exercised when taking impressions and that the hearing aid mold or ear shell is kept clean and fits comfortably.

In the usual case, upon inspection of the ear canal with an otoscope, it will be noticed that the floor of the canal rises slightly and then slopes downward and forward toward the tympanic membrane (eardrum). In addition, the average ear tends to have a bend in its forward wall. (See Figure 8a & 8b). This combination of bends or changes in direction of the ear canal may prevent easy viewing of the eardrum, which is located at the end of the external canal. By pulling the pinna upward and back, the canal can often

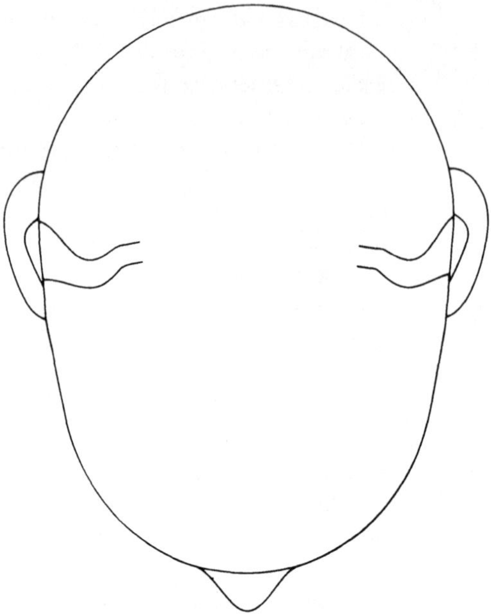

Fig. 8a. Top view of bends in ear canal.

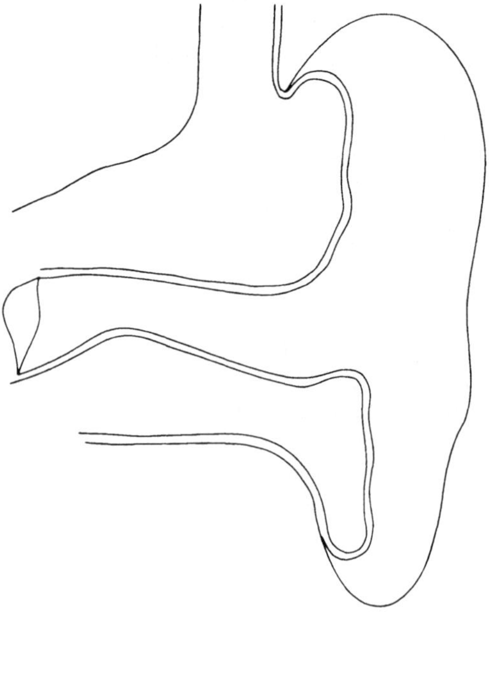

Fig. 8b. Side view of bends in ear canal. (*Martin, Principles of Audiology - A Study Guide, University Park Press, 1984.*)

be straightened out enough to permit visualization of this important anatomical feature.

The route of a branch of the Vagus nerve (tenth cranial nerve) lies on the floor of the external canal. In some persons, the deep insertion of an ear block prior to taking an ear impression will elicit a cough reflex. This reflex activity does not appear in everybody, and should not prevent the specialist from assuring that the ear block has been inserted deeply enough to take a full impression.

There is no such thing as an average normal ear canal; all vary in length, width, and directionality. But each can be pictured as a long, dark cave, or cul de sac. A specific physical configuration can have implications on the amount of sound pressure developed by a hearing aid in an individual ear canal. For example, the wider the ear canal, the sharper the dropoff in the low frequency response and the greater the risk of feedback for a hearing aid with a tube fitting. The narrower the ear canal, the greater the low frequency gain and the higher the peak gain without feedback in a tube fitting (Berland, 1975).

The objective of the hearing aid specialist during examination of the ear is to pierce the darkness of the deeply recessed ear canal cavity with the light beam of the otoscope in order to view the tympanic membrane. The normal eardrum is milky or pearly white in appearance, sometimes with a mild pinkish tinge, and in the normal instance of glint of light from the otoscope is reflected in the lower, forward part of the eardrum. Obviously, any presence of fluid, redness, swelling, perforation or foreign matter in the canal itself or at the tympanic membrane will require otological evaluation before proceeding further.

The pinna and external ear canal together provide the very special function of gathering and selectively reinforcing acoustical signals. The irregular shape of the auricle, that is, its depressions, elevations and cavities, causes increases and decreases of sound pressure to occur at different frequencies as the sound arrives at the ear. In that the pinna acts as a collector of acoustic energy, if it were absent, studies show that up to 10dB less sound energy would be delivered to the eardrum between 2000 and 5000Hz as a result. (Figure 9) The external meatus (outer ear canal), shaped as it is, forms a resonating tube, and by itself, without the concha, reinforces energy in the 3000-4000Hz frequency range by about 10dB. The average natural resonant frequency of the ear canal plus concha is approximately 2700Hz, and the amplitude of the resonant peak varies between 15 and 20dB (Wiener and Ross, 1946). The peak and range of the resonance changes according to the size, depth and shape of the ear canal (Figure 10). Therefore the ear, by its anatomical shape and

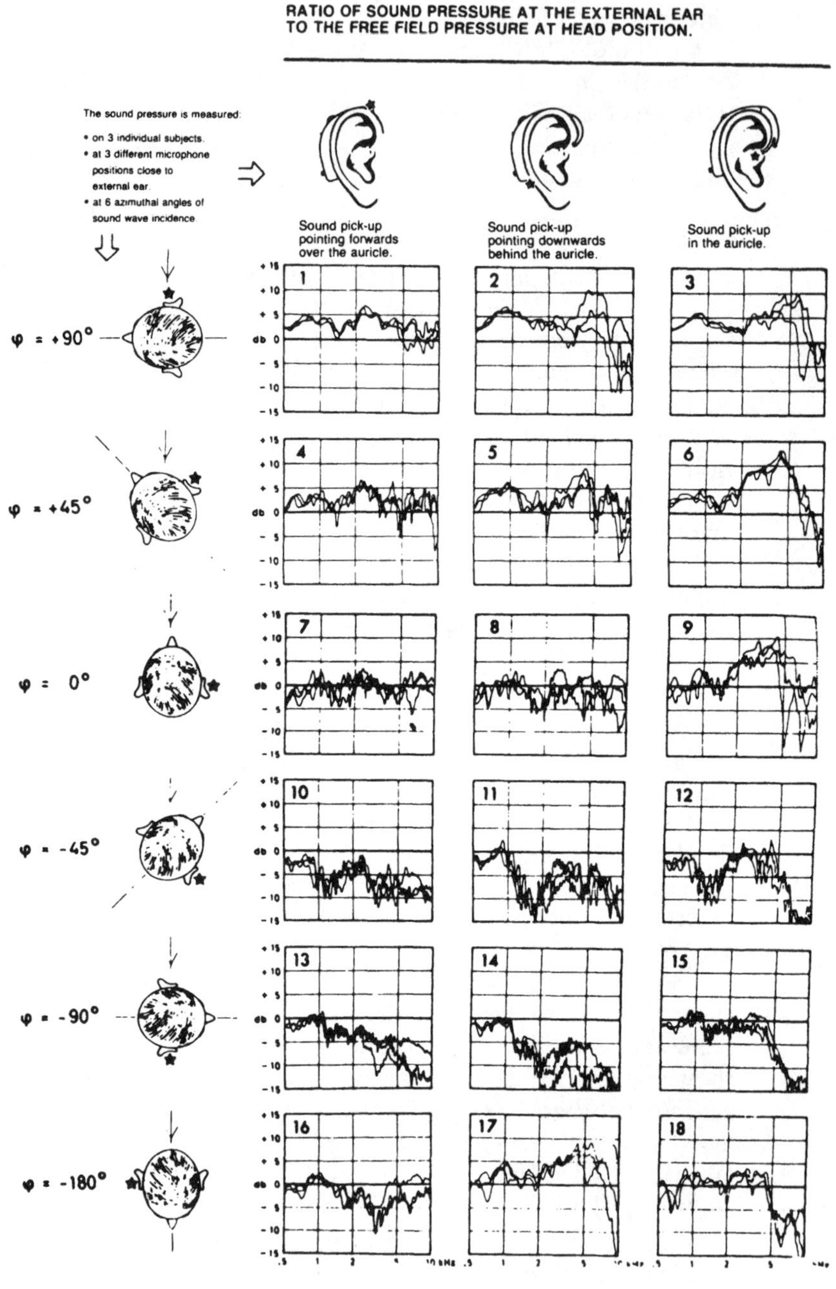

Fig. 9. Ratio of sound pressure at the external ear to the free field sound pressure at head position. (*Berland and Nielson, Sound Pressure Generated in the Human External Ear by a Free Sound Field, Oticon Laboratories, Denmark, 1968.*)

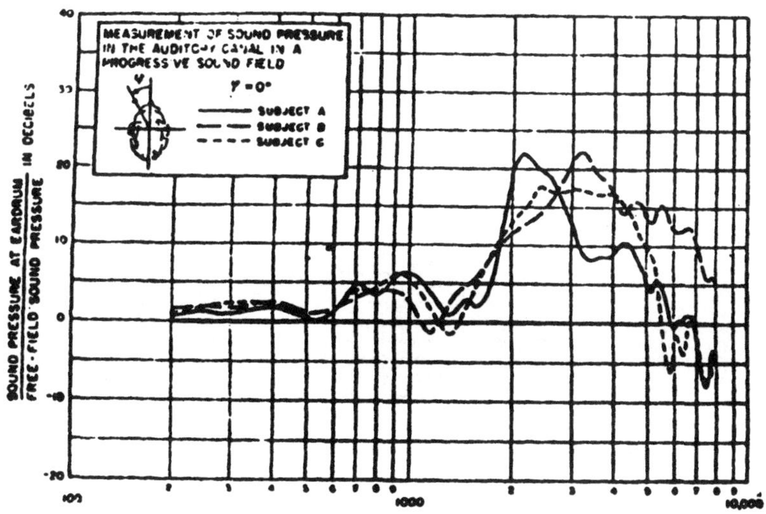

Fig. 10. Changes in ear canal resonance with various sizes and shape ears. (*Weiner, Ross, Journal of Acoustic Society of America, 1946.*)

location, provides its own natural amplification to acoustic signals that arrive. This additional enhancement of the acoustic signal lies in the very range that is most useful for speech reception, namely between 2000Hz and 5000Hz, the region that is most important and critical for speech clarity and intelligibility.

The spectral content of input signals that impinge on the hearing aid microphone in different styles of hearing aids, is affected by the head and body of a hearing aid wearer. For example, a sound striking the microphone of a pocket worn (body) hearing aid will be modified so as to produce more low frequency energy due to reflection off the body surfaces than if it had struck the microphone of an in-the-ear hearing aid. One can view the effect the pinna has on the speech signal by considering what occurs when the position of the hearing aid microphone is changed as the hearing aid is moved to various parts of the head. Although the changes in microphone position are quite small, Figure 11 shows that discernible differences occur as the microphone is shifted from a location below and behind the pinna to just above the top of the pinna and then to the concha plane. The pinna effect is clearly demonstrated when one compares the curves showing the frequency response of the microphone in the behind-the-ear bottom position to that in the in-the-ear (concha plane) position. Although the differences are not dramatic in amount of change,

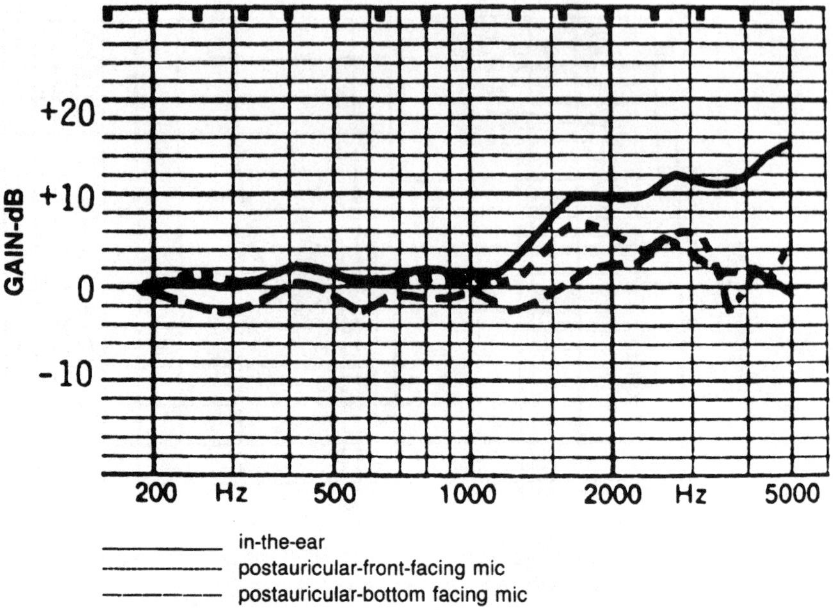

Fig. 11. Effect of hearing and microphone position on diffraction.

their influence on the reception and transmission of important mid and high frequency speech components must not be discounted. Awareness of the natural high frequency amplification provided by the pinna and ear canal resonance may be helpful in selecting the most optimal hearing aid type (behind the ear, in the ear, in the canal, etc.) for a client.

When a hearing aid is coupled to the ear so as to cause an occlusion (blockage or closing) of the ear canal, the natural resonating property of the ear canal is lost; i.e., insertion of a non-vented earmold or in-the-ear ear shell into the canal prevents the ear from having its natural resonance. Substantial loss of ear canal resonance occurs even with earmolds or ear shells with medium diameter vents (see Figure 12). Consequently, the net amplification provided by the hearing aid system is reduced by the amount of the resonance that is lost. This is called insertion loss.

The Pinnae are important for sound localization, i.e., the ability to detect from which direction sound is coming. If a sound is directed to the right side of a person, it will strike the right pinna first, and then the left. This very small difference in the time of arrival of the acoustic signal between the two ears provides the first nec-

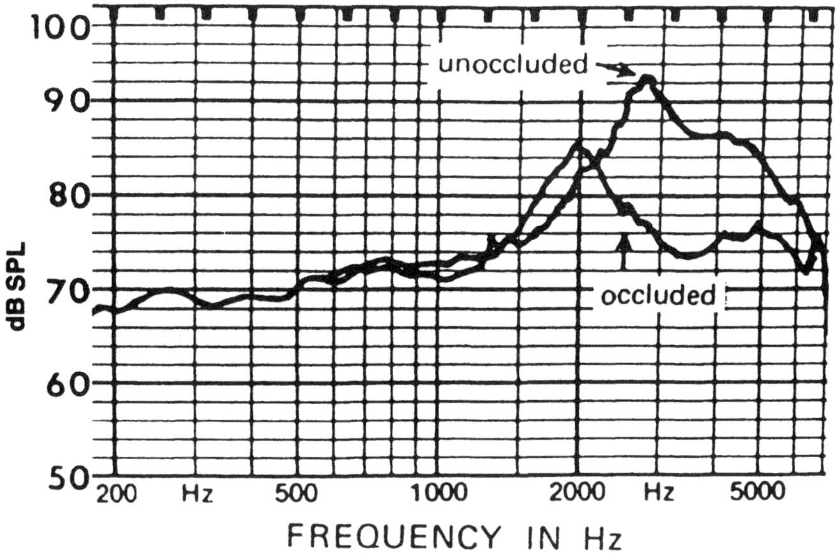

Fig. 12. Insertion loss caused by occluding KEMAR ear with an earmold having a 1/8 inch vent diameter.

essary piece of information which allows the brain to decide the direction of the sound. As a signal passes between the two ears, it also loses a small amount of its energy, especially in the high frequencies. This difference in intensity becomes the second clue necessary for determining where the signal is coming from. Together, the differences in time and intensity of sounds at the two ears provide a series of clues about the direction of sound which is interpreted at the higher auditory centers in the brain. However, without the presence of the pinnae, which are especially sensitive to the high frequencies, the information available to the brain would be incomplete, making the decision task quite a bit more difficult. In addition, the pinnae are especially helpful in distinguishing sounds which come from the back of the head as well as those which arrive from the front. Several futuristic hearing aid noise reduction algorithms are attempting to take advantage of the differences in magnitude and time of arrival of signals at the two ears (e.g., Gao et al., 1994; Kollmeier et al., 1993; and Bodden, 1993).

Recent empirical evidence supports a "duplex" theory of sound localization in an anechoic environment (first advocated by Lord Raleigh in 1907): i.e., the source (direction from which sounds come) of low frequency pure tones is determined by interaural (between the ears) temporal differences, whereas sources of high frequency pure tones are localized by internal intensity differences. An interaural temporal difference refers to the arrival of a sound at two different times at a listener's ears because of the differences in path length traveled between the sound source and each ear. If the sound source is at 90 degrees—or directly opposite one ear, this difference in arrival time at the two ears is about 0.66 milliseconds (660 millionths of a second) for most frequencies (Feddersen et al., 1957). The auditory system is remarkably sensitive to minute differences in time of arrival of the same sound at the two ears. For example, an interaural temporal difference of only 0.02 milliseconds (20 millionths of a second) can be detected by a normal auditory system at 500Hz. At 4000Hz, a difference of about 0.2 milliseconds (200 millionths of a second) can usually be detected (Yost, Wightman and Green, 1971).

Interaural intensity differences are the result of diffraction (bending of a sound wave around an obstacle) produced by the listener's head on arriving sounds. The amount of interaural intensity difference changes according to the frequency content of the sounds. Above about 2000Hz, the average human head is large compared to the wavelength of sound and so considerable interaural intensity differences may be expected. That is, the wavelength of sounds in the high frequency region is much shorter than the distance between the two ears. For example, at 6000Hz, the wavelength of sound is about 2 inches and the interaural intensity difference can be expected to be as great as 20dB for sounds arriving from certain angles. The sounds in this high frequency range bounce off the side of the head rather than travel around the head to the other ear. The result is a loss of intensity in the signal for the high frequencies that reach the other ear. (The purpose of a CROS hearing aid for a person with a unilateral hearing loss is to circumvent this loss of intensity for sounds originating from the unaided ear side). At low frequencies, however, the size of the human head is small compared to the wavelength of sounds. As a result, hardly any interaural intensity differences are expected, for example at 200Hz, for which the wavelength is about 5-1/2 feet. Low frequency signals travel from one ear to the other without much loss of intensity. All of the aforementioned should be tempered by the realization that these effects are true only for sound sources which vary in location in the horizontal plane. Localization of sounds in the vertical plane is accomplished by the pinna and concha altering the spectrum of arriving sounds for frequencies of 8000Hz and higher. Important to good sound localization in either the horizontal or vertical planes is the

Lesson 3 21-27

ability of the listener's head to move. In fact, excellent localization has been observed for some monaural listeners as long as they are allowed to move their heads.

However, in everyday listening situations, sounds to be localized are rarely pure tones but are more complex and transient signals such as those found in speech. These stimuli often have many frequencies present simultaneously and have sharp onsets and offsets in the time domain. In addition, listeners are rarely called on to localize sounds in an anechoic (perfectly non-reverberant) environment, but are frequently confronted first with the original sound and then reflections or echoes arriving at a later time resulting from the sound hitting walls, ceiling and floor of a room. This reflection or reverberation phenomenon makes sound localization more difficult, although the echoes are usually almost totally suppressed within normal auditory systems. One of the most difficult challenges in designing more effective hearing aids is suppressing the undesirable sound reflections in reverberant listening environments. Hearing aids with conventional directional microphones have much less directivity in heavily reverberant real world listening environments than in anechoic chambers. Hearing aids with multiple microphones arranged in arrays show promise in the future of being more effective for suppressing reflections due to reverberation.

At the end of the external ear canal is the eardrum, a semitransparent, conically shaped membrane (Figure 13) which separates the external ear canal from the middle ear. It can be divided into two parts, the pars flaccid at the top, and the pars tensa below. The latter section of the eardrum consists of three separate layers of tissue. A layer of thin skin which is identical to that found in the external ear canal forms the outermost layer, a tough fibrous layer is in the middle, and a lining of mucus membrane forms the innermost layer.

THE MIDDLE EAR

Attached to the inside of the eardrum is the first of three ossicles, a tiny bone called the malleus (hammer). The long arm of the malleus, the manubrium, terminates in the center of the cone and is referred to as the umbo. (See Figure 14.)

Earlier we described the movement of particles of air as they were set into motion by vibration, and emphasized that the motion was a faithful reproduction of the vibratory source. The movement

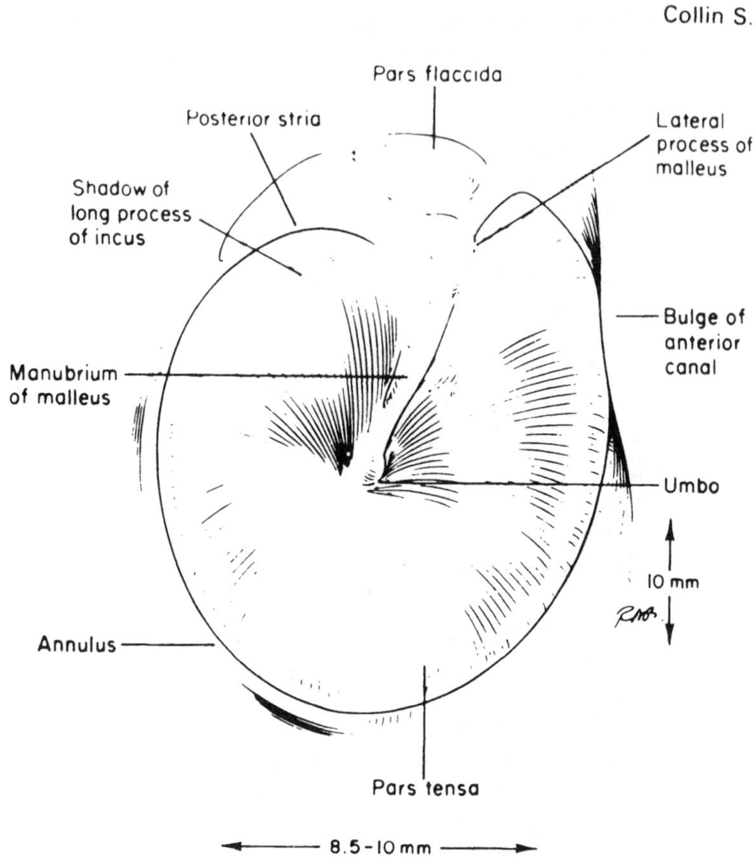

Fig. 13. Schematic drawing of right tympanic membrane. (*Bradford and Hardy, Hearing and Hearing Impairment, Grune and Stratton, 1979.*)

of air particles sets the tympanic membrane (eardrum) into vibration, so that its motion is like the characteristic movements of the particles, which in turn can be traced back to the movement of the vibratory source. The rocking, to and fro movement of the eardrum, causes the malleus, and consequently the other two conected bones, the incus (anvil) and the stapes (stirrup), to move at the same time. The termination of the stapes, that is, its foot plate, is loosely embedded in the oval window in the wall of the inner ear (cochlea). The ossicular chain is suspended in the middle ear space by a network of ligaments and two muscles.

Perforations (holes) in the tympanic membrane, when present, are obviously important to the dispenser, and care must be exer-

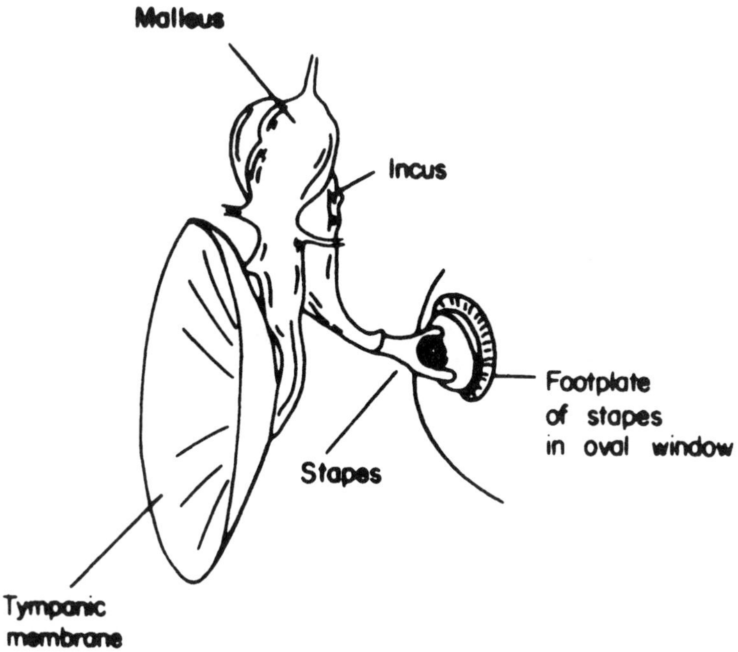

Fig. 14. The three ossicles and tympanic membrane. (*By permission, Pickles, Dr. James O., An Introduction to the Physiology of Hearing, Academic Press, 1982.*)

cised during impression taking to prevent the material from going into the middle ear space. Sometimes it is extremely difficult to close perforations even with the best medical care. Perforations of the tympanic membrane can present problems of hygiene in the event amplification is considered medically desirable. The hearing aid specialist must be acutely aware of the seriousness of the possibility of the introduction or reintroduction of infection into the middle ear when a perforation is present. Care must be taken to aerate the ear canal adequately, usually with some type of large venting, to prevent infection. Interestingly, the amount of hearing loss which occurs specifically as a result of the perforation itself is rarely related to the size of the perforation. Similarly, the frequencies which will be affected in an individual instance are hard to predict, because the eardrum vibrates segmentally; i.e., certain areas of the eardrum vibrate in response to sound energy presented at some frequencies and intensities more easily than others. A conductive hearing loss of up to approximately 30dB across the entire frequency spectrum is commonly found in the presence of large perforations of the tympanic membrane.

Most of the acoustic energy which strikes the eardrum is utilized to move it back and forth. However, some of the sound energy is reflected back off of the eardrum, and "flows" back out of the external ear with a somewhat diminished amplitude. As a result, there is not a perfect transmission of energy into the middle ear and thence into the cochlea. It can be said that the eardrum forms a boundary at the entrance of the middle ear and impedes passage of some of the acoustic energy which is present in the signal striking it.

The eardrum should not be regarded as a free standing anatomical structure unconnected to any other part. Rather, the ossicular chain is connected to the eardrum at one end and to the oval window of the inner ear at the other. Therefore, the eardrum can be viewed as being "loaded" by the ossicles, and also by the fluids and the other structures of the inner ear. Consequently, the entire chain of eardrum, ossicles and inner ear fluids, and not just the eardrum itself, is being moved by the acoustic energy which reaches the eardrum.

The middle ear system as a whole has its own characteristic mass, or inertia, and its own characteristic stiffness, depending on such factors as the size and the elasticity of the tympanic membrane, the muscles and ligaments, and the pressure which is exerted by the fluids within the inner ear. Depending upon how elastic the system is, and how much mass it incorporates in its overall structure, sound energy at different frequencies will be more or less easily transmitted to the cochlea.

Disruptions in the function of the tympanic membrane, or other middle ear structures, will result in changes of normal middle ear operation. It has been suggested that an increase in elastic stiffness (caused, e.g., by fusing and fixation of ossicular joints, decrease in middle ear pressure, etc.) will diminish the capacity to transmit sound vibrations to the cochlea in the lower frequency regions (below 2000Hz). Similarly, any occurrence which tends to increase mass (e.g., fluidic pressure on the tympanic membrane, etc.) will impair high frequency transmission to the cochlea at frequencies above 2000Hz (Johansen, 1948). A disarticulation (disruption or disconnection) of the ossicular chain will cause a decrease in the passage of both high and low frequencies approximately equally, because a major portion of the acoustic signal is used by moving the loose tympanic membrane, or is reflected by it.

Usually, changes in both stiffness and mass occur when the normal middle ear function is altered by disease or trauma. As a result, there often may be an increase in reflection of sound from the tympanic membrane. This condition may make some hearing aid fittings more difficult, especially when a semioccluded (partially vented) or a totally unoccluded (open) earmold is used. The difficulty occurs because as amplification is increased to overcome the impairment, the reflection of sound back out of the external auditory canal increases (by leaking through or around the circumference of the mold), which in turn produces acoustic feedback. Obviously, little can be done to alter the physiology of the middle ear, but by being aware of the heightened potential for acoustic feedback in a given situation, the hearing aid specialist can prepare for the problems which may follow.

As the middle ear system is set into motion, sound energy changes from its original state as an acoustic stimulus, into a form of mechanical energy (i.e., the movement of the tympanic membrane and the middle ear ossicles), and thence to hydraulic energy (the movement of fluids within the inner ear). The middle ear, therefore, transduces* energy; i.e., it causes energy to be changed from one form to another (acoustic to mechanical to hydraulic). In fact, the conversion of sound energy to one form or another can be traced as it travels through the several transducers in the auditory pathway. We have seen that the origin of sound begins with a mechanical vibration acting upon air molecules which, in turn, produces acoustic energy. As this acoustic energy comes into contact with the external auditory meatus, it is converted or transduced to mechanical energy by the movement of the tympanic membrane and the ossicles; this mechanical energy in the middle ear is then changed to hydraulic energy (movement of the cochlear fluids caused by the stapes rocking to and fro), which in turn causes mechanical energy again from the resulting hair cell movement. This hair cell movement is converted to electrical energy as the nerve fibers fire along the eighth nerve. As these pulses travel along the eighth nerve, they are converted to chemical energy by the emission of a chemical transmitter at the auditory synapse, the juncture between successive nerve cells. Thus it can be seen that the original energy resulting from the movement of the vibratory source is changed to other forms of energy on its way through the auditory system.

The inner ear (cochlea), as mentioned previously, is filled with fluid and imbedded in the temporal bone. The fluid is put into motion by the movement of the stapes, and the reciprocal movement of the round window allows the footplate of the stapes to rock back and forth in the oval window. If the tympanic membrane and the

*A transducer is a device which converts energy from one form to another. Hearing aid microphones and receivers are transducers, for they convert acoustical energy to electrical energy (microphone), and electrical energy to acoustical energy (receiver).

ossicular chain were absent, an excessive amount of sound energy (99.9%) would be reflected back into the external ear, because the sound pressure itself would not be great enough to move the cochlear fluids. That is, greater pressure is required to move the fluids in the cochlea than is required to produce particle movement in the air contained in the middle ear space.

For this reason, the middle ear system is commonly called an "impedance matching transformer". Impedance*, in this case, is a term that is used to describe the complex set of events which occur as sound waves reach any barrier, and the reflection and transmission of energy respectively, from and through the barrier interface. In the process described earlier, the lack of a middle ear system (no eardrum or ossicular chain) would make energy transfer from the ear canal to the cochlea quite difficult. This situation is called a "mismatch in impedance". If the inner ear is to be able to take advantage of all of the sound energy being transmitted through the air into the ear canal, some method or device must be available to permit efficient energy transfer to the cochlea, with only a minimal amount of reflection of sound back into the ear canal. The tympanic membrane and the ossicular chain are the intermediary devices which make the cochlear fluid system "look" or act acoustically more like air, and they overcome the mismatch in impedance by their structure and operation.

The transformer effect of the middle ear causes an increase in sound pressure to occur because the operating area of the tympanic membrane is approximately seventeen times larger than the area of the oval window. This difference in area allows the sound pressure that collects at the tympanic membrane to be transferred efficiently to the footplate of the stapes (Figures 15a & b). A pressure amplification occurs because the sound energy has been "funnelled" into the footplate, which moves the oval window membrane to and fro. In addition, because of the construction of the ossicular chain, it acts as a lever, thereby also increasing pressure by a factor of 1.3 times. Since 17 times 1.3 equals 22, the theoretical increase in sound pressure provided by the middle ear structures is about 27dB ($20\log_{10} 22$).

The middle ear space is aerated by the eustachian tube function in order to maintain middle ear pressure equivalent to that of the surrounding environment. If normal aeration is disrupted, a de-

*An Impedance Test is a series of audiological measurements designed to measure the impedance properties of a middle ear. By measuring the reflection of the sound off of the eardrum, as the pressure on the eardrum is increased and decreased, a judgement can be made regarding the condition and functioning of the middle ear.

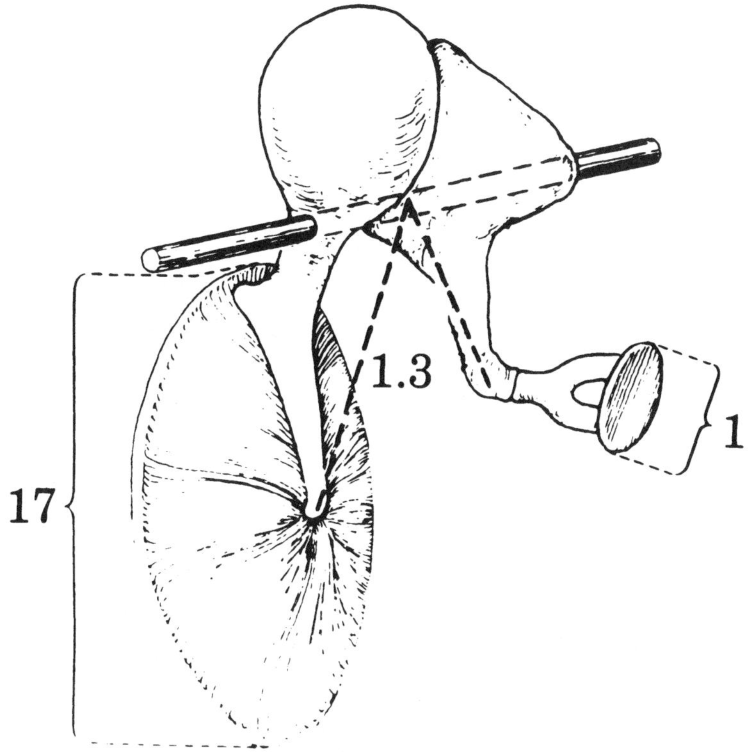

Fig. 15a. Area ratio of eardrum to stapes (oval window). (*Paparella and Shumrick after Otolaryngology, V. 1, 1973 - W.B. Saunders Company.*)

crease in middle ear pressure occurs, which, if prolonged, leads to the absorption of the air molecules in the middle ear by the mucous membrane lining and blood vessels of the middle ear. Eventually a partial vacuum occurs, and fluid is drawn into the middle ear space. A properly functioning eustachian tube is fundamental to maintaining normal middle ear operation because any significant decrease in pressure and fluid build-up impairs the middle ear impedance matching and transformer functions. Children often experience chronic changes in middle ear pressure which lead to mild and moderate fluctuating hearing loss. In some instances, mild gain hearing aids are recommended to overcome the loss, for it is felt that the loss of sensitivity can interfere with the normal development of speech and language processes.

The two muscles of the middle ear, the stapedius (the smallest muscle in the body which is connected to the stapes) and the tensor tympani (attached to the malleus) contract when subjected

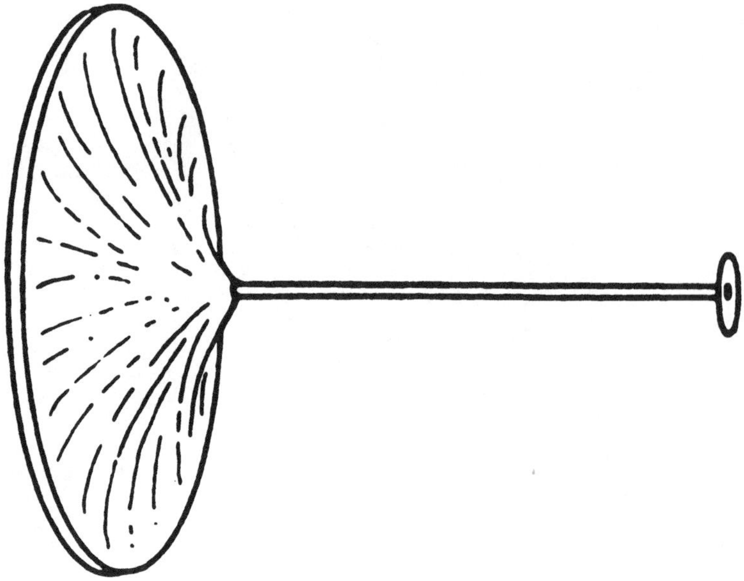

Fig. 15b. Mechanical lever advantage provided by eardrum to stapes area ratio. (*Schubert, Hearing: Its Function and Dysfunction, Springer-Verlag, New York, Inc., 1980.*)

to loud auditory stimuli (80dB SPL or greater for the normal ear). Although the exact function of the middle ear muscles is not well known, the effect of their contraction is to stiffen the ossicular chain. Universal agreement has not been found regarding the degree to which the middle ear muscles protect the inner ear from excessively loud impulsive sounds. However, a 5 to 10dB reduction of low frequency energy transmission occurs when the middle ear muscles contract (Moller, 1965).

Although considerable controversy exists, there is some evidence that the acoustic reflex occurs at a sound pressure level just below the uncomfortable listening level and just above most comfortable listening level for many impaired hearing persons. It has been suggested that one might consider specifying the SSPL90 of a hearing aid from the average of the acoustic reflex levels at 500, 1000 and 2000Hz (Horning, 1975; Rainville, 1976). In other studies, researchers found that the acoustic reflex is more closely related to MCL and may help to set the gain control of a hearing aid (Keith, 1976; Rappaport and Tait, 1976). Thus, the acoustic reflex may be used as another measure of MCL or UCL. Since it is an involuntary response, it may well be a more objective assessment of these parameters.

THE INNER EAR

THE COCHLEA AS A PERIPHERAL PROCESSOR

Whereas many of the functions of the outer and middle ear are comparatively well understood by auditory physiologists and psychoacousticians, the complexities of the inner ear have only been partially explained thus far.

The coiled, snail-like human cochlea is about 1 cm (2/5 inch) wide and is 5mm (1/5 inch) along the length from base to apex. The base of the cochlea begins at the oval window and its apex is at the inner tip. The cochlea houses the basilar membrane which, when uncoiled, is about 35mm (1-2/5 inch) long. A cross-sectional view of the cochlea reveals that three main fluid-filled ducts are present: scala vestibuli, scala media and scala tympani. The oval window interfaces with the perilymph fluid in the scala vestibuli. The round window interfaces with the perilymph fluid in the scala tympani. These outer two ducts are joined only at the apex by the helicotrema. An inner compartment, the scala media, contains the more positively charged endolymph fluid. The basilar membrane separates the scala media from the scala tympani and supports the organ of Corti. Reissner's membrane lies between the scala vestibuli and scala media. A delicate and gelatinous membrane in the scala media, the tectorial membrane, is suspended over the rows of hair cells, which arise from the reticular lamina on the upper surface of the organ of Corti. (See Figure 16).

The organ of Corti is the "transducer" of the inner ear in which the fluid motion (induced by the movement of the stapes) is translated into neuronal (electro-chemical energy) impulses. Because the operation of the inner ear is hard to visualize, there is a certain amount of controversy surrounding its exact behavior when the fluids are set into motion. George Von Bekesy was the first to furnish a documented, reliable description and was awarded the Nobel prize as a result. Although subsequent investigators have offered slightly different details, his work forms a basis for our present understanding.

The basilar membrane is narrow and stiff at its beginning (the base of the cochlea at the oval window), and broader and more compliant at its end (the apex, the helicotrema). Figures 17a, b & c, show cross sections of the cochlea and organ of Corti. Four rows of hair cells are evident, one inner row, and three outer rows, which run from the base to the apex. In total, it is believed that there are about 12,000 outer hair cells and about 4000 inner hair cells, The exact roles played by the inner and outer hair cells recently are becoming better understood (See later section on

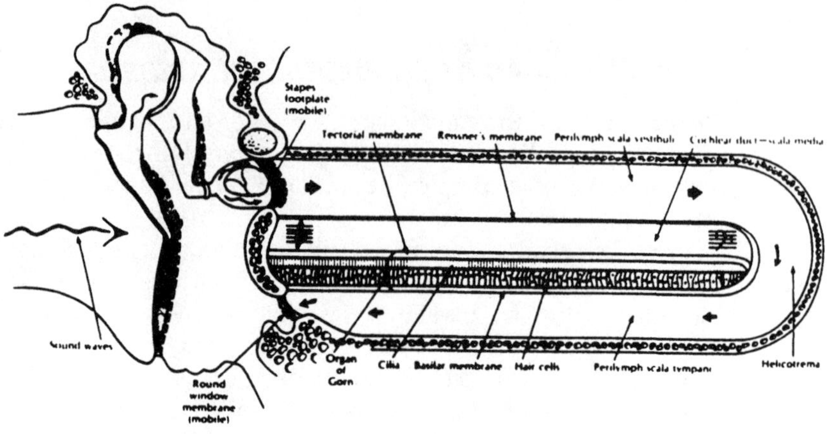

Fig. 16. Schematic diagram of the major components of the cochlea. (*Goodhill, Victor M.D., Ear Diseases, Deafness, and Dizziness, Harper and Rowe, 1979.*)

otoacoustic emissions for a further discussion about outer hair cells). It is believed that the outer hair cells are easily damaged by loud noises and ototoxic drugs. Nerve endings are located near the base of each inner hair cell that are responsible for the afferent or inward-going transmission paths from the cochlea to the brain stem of the auditory system. In total, there are about 30,000 neural fibers or neurons in the human auditory nerve. About 95% of the afferent fibers are connected to inner hair cells and only about 5% to outer hair cells. The outer hair cells make direct contact with the tectorial membrane, but not the inner hair cells.

Figure 18a shows the relationship between the tectorial membrane, into which the tips of the outer hair cells are lightly imbedded, and the basilar membrane, upon which the organ of Corti rests. Since the tectorial membrane is hinged at one end, whenever the basilar membrane is displaced, the tectorial membrane pivots. The pivoting action causes the hair cells to bend. This is referred to as "shearing displacement", and it, in turn, causes an activation of the neural response discussed in a later section of this chapter.

An inward movement of the stapes causes a displacement wave in the fluid, which travels along the basilar membrane from base to apex. When the oval window is displaced inward, at the same time, the round window is displaced outward. The fluidic wave motion sets up a travelling wave pattern (see, for example, Fig. 19b) on the basilar membrane. The traveling wave has a sharply-tuned peak at different locations along the basilar membrane, depending on the frequency of the sound wave. The sharp peak of the

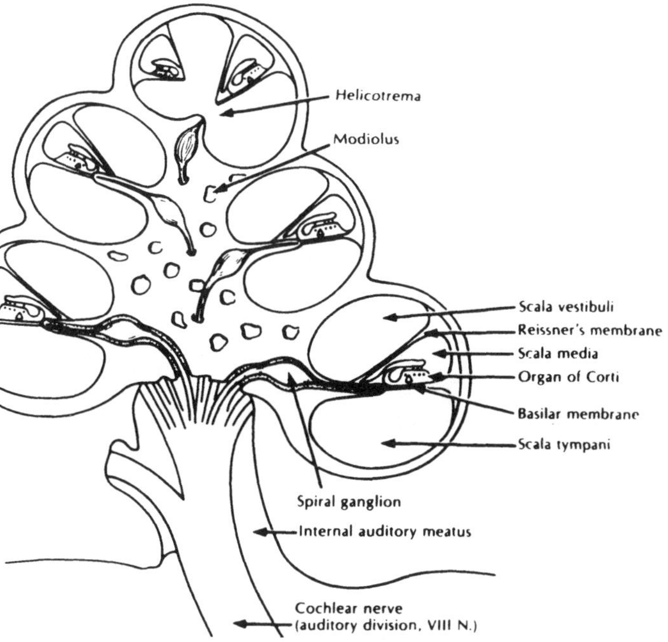

Fig. 17a. Schematic diagram of the midmodular section of the cochlea.

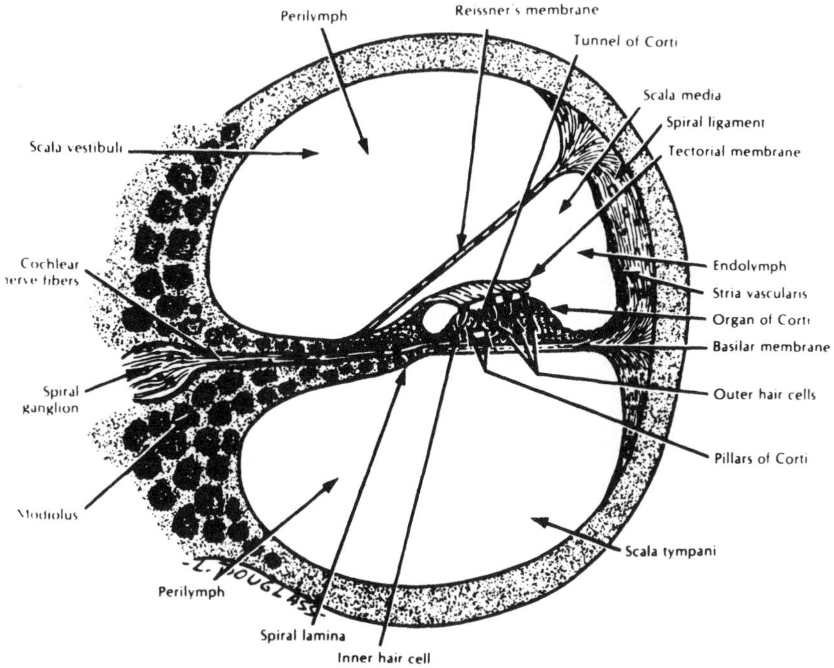

Fig. 17b. The three cochlear compartments.

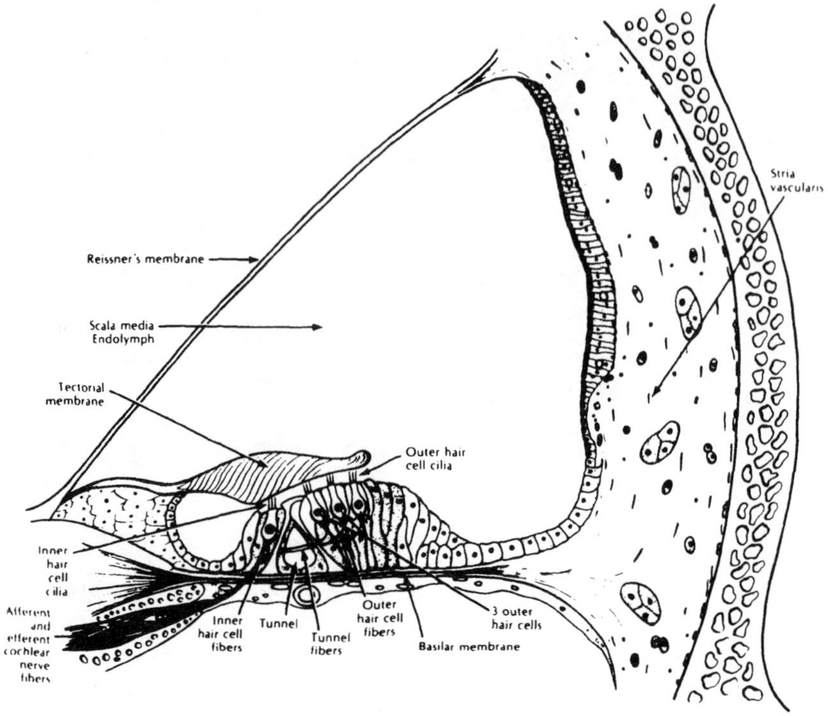

Fig. 17c. Adult organ of Corti within scala media. (*Goodhill, Victor, M.D., Ear diseases, Deafness and Dizziness, Harper and Rowe, 1979.*)

travelling wave cannot be explained solely by the passive mechanical vibration of the basilar membrane. It is thought that the OHC's are responsible for an active mechanical process that could achieve such sharp tuning. The moving basilar membrane, in turn, selectively bends some of the attached inner and outer hair cells as a result of the shearing action of the tectorial membrane and the organ of Corti. (See Figure 18b).

The basilar membrane will vibrate along its length in a unique pattern that depends upon the frequency and intensity of stapes movement. For low frequencies, the point of maximum displacement of the basilar membrane (and consequently, the organ of Corti) will be located near the apex; for high frequencies the maximum vibration amplitude will be located near the base. The point of maximum displacement will move up and down the length of the basilar membrane in synchrony with the movement of the stapes. The lower the frequency transmitted, the further along the

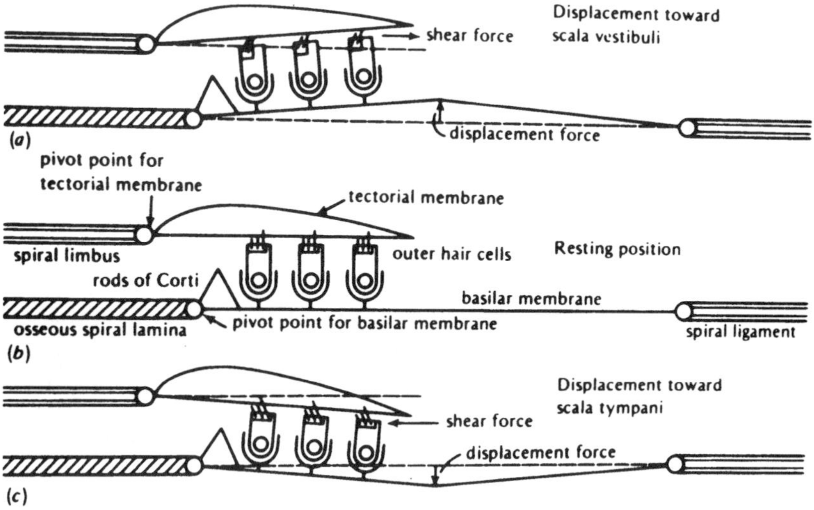

Fig. 18a. Schematic diagrams of shearing forces created between the hair cells and the tectorial membrane as a result of basilar membrane displacement. (a) Shearing force that results from displacement of the basilar membrane toward the scala vestibuli. (b) Relationship between hair cells and tectorial membrane with no stimulation. (c) Shearing forces in the direction opposite to that in (a) for displacement in the opposite direction. The shearing of the cilia is thought to activate the neurons at the base of the hair cells. (*Zemlin, Willard R,. Speech and Hearing Science Anatomy and Physiology, 1960, p. 244, 247. Reprinted by permission of Prentice-Hall, Inc., Englewood Cliffs, N.J.*)

basilar membrane towards the apex the point of maximum displacement occurs. However, all low frequencies cause some movement of the basilar membrane throughout its entire length, but very little of the movement due to low frequencies occurs at the basal (high frequency) end. (See Figure 19a). If more than one frequency is being transmitted at the same time by stapes movements, there will be separate points of maximum displacement or depression on the basilar membrane, each reflecting the separate pure tones or frequencies that are contained within the stimulus. The reader is reminded, however, that a complex of tones rather than pure tones are most often present in typical listening environments. As a result, complex motions are typically produced on the basilar membrane.

Each specific point of maximum depression or displacement on the basilar membrane, therefore, reflects a place where a particular frequency is being analyzed and generated. Thus, the cochlea acts like a bank of filters in performing a spectral analysis of incoming signals. This is why the cochlea has often been viewed as

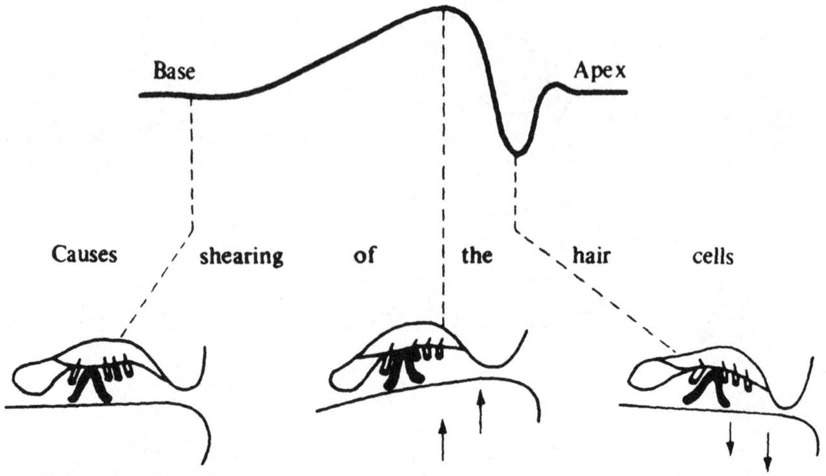

Fig. 18b. Shearing action in the cochlea. When the basilar membrane is displaced due to stimulation, the resulting action on the cilia of the hair cells is a lateral shear. This is due to the interaction of the relative displacements of the tectorial and basilar membranes. (*Minifie, Hixon and Williams, Normal Aspects of Speech, Hearing and Language, 1973, p. 305, 416. Reprinted by permission of Prentice-Hall, Inc., Englewood Cliffs, N.J.*)

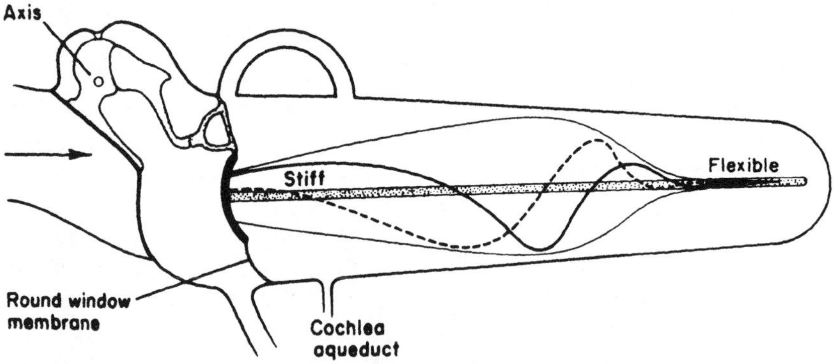

Fig. 19a. Conceptual diagram of the traveling waves. The waves move along the basilar membrane from the base toward the apex. the amplitude of each wave increases gradually, but speed decreases toward the apex. The fine solid line represents the envelope. This increases gradually to a maximal point and then decreases rapidly. The dashed and heavy solid lines represent one-quarter of a cycle out of phase (after Békésy). (*Bradford and Hardy, Hearing and Hearing Impairment, Grune and Stratton, 1979.*)

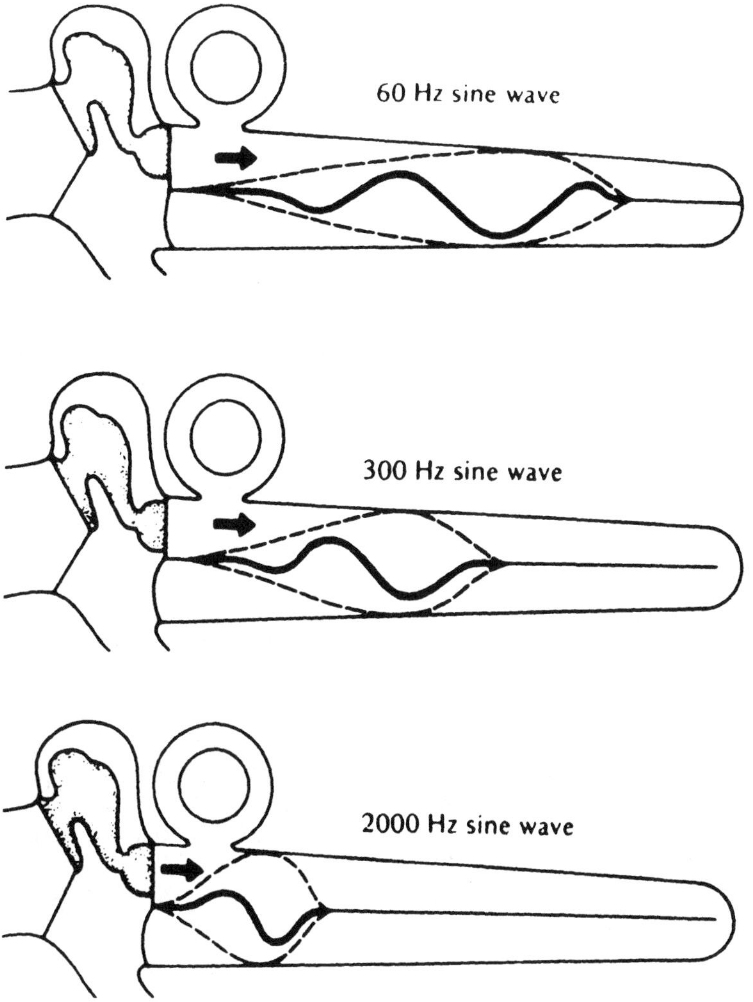

Fig. 19b. Instantaneous waveforms and envelopes of traveling waves of three different frequencies shown on a schematic diagram of the cochlea. Note that the point of maximum displacement, as shown by the high point of the envelope, is near the apex for low frequencies and near the base for higher frequencies. Also, note that low frequencies stimulate the apical end as well as the basal end, but that displacement from higher frequencies is confined to the base. (*Zemlin, Willard R., Speech and Hearing Science Anatomy and Physiology, 1960, p. 244, 247. Reprinted by permission of Prentice-Hall, Inc., Englewood Cliffs, N.J.*)

a kind of Fourier frequency analyzer, having the ability to recognize and break down the constituent parts of a complex signal at any given instant in time. (Figure 19b).

OTOACOUSTIC EMISSIONS

"By all indications, otoacoustic emissions (OAE) will be the test procedure of the 1990s" (Hall, 1992). OAE have helped researchers better understand the innermost workings of the cochlea. With OAE's, the mechanical integrity of the cochlea and the outer hair cells (OHC's) can be studied noninvasively with objective tests. Whereas the presence of normal brain stem evoked response (ABR) requires active neural tramission, OAE's are related to more peripheral cochlear functions (Robinette, 1992). To briefly review, Gold in 1948 hypothesized that the sharp frequency selectivity in the cochlea is due to a feedback system: the cochlea performs a mechanical-to-electrical transduction together with an electrical-to-mechanical transduction in the feedback path. OHC's are a source of mechanical energy that influence basilar membrane motion. Because these structures can oscillate rapidly and actively, the cochlea not only receives sound but also produces sound. Given that OHC's are not innervated by afferent nerve fibers, their role in the stimulus-transduction process appears to be that of feedback. It appears that the OHC's produce OAE's and that they are responsible for the extremely sharp frequency selectivity of the cochlea. There is strong evidence that positive feedback exists between the basilar membrane and the OHC's. It is thought that this positive feedback contributes amplification to basilar membrane movements, resulting in greater displacement for a given sound input than would occur without the OHC's. There is evidence to suggest that OHC's control basilar membrane motion with changes in their length. Researchers believe that it is this length change that results in mechanical movement in the cochlea being transmitted back out through the middle ear and ultimately sensed as OAE's. These faint sounds are sensed in the ear canal and are recorded.

Ototoxic drugs and high level sound stimili that are known to damage the cochlea reduce or eliminate OAE's. It is thought that this is due to OHC's being irreparably damaged. Thus, OAE's may be used for indirectly determining the integrity of the OHC's. In this application, OAE's have been particularly useful for screening newborns, school-age children, or any difficult-to-test population (Nozza and Sabo, 1992).

There are two categories of OAE's - spontaneous and evoked. Spontaneous OAE's (SOAE) are tonal signals that occur without external stimulation. They are present in many but not all persons with normal hearing and also in persons with hearing loss but only at frequencies associated with normal or near-normal hearing. Thus, a physiological relationship exists between the frequency of the SOAE and the cochlear pathology. The usefulness of SOAE's is somewhat limited because they do not occur in all persons.

Evoked OAE's are elicited in all ears at frequencies of normal hearing in response to external test signals presented to the ear canal. There are two categories of evoked OAE's - transient evoked otoacoustic emissions (TEOAE) and pure tone. TEOAE are like echoes in the sense that they are produced in response to clicks or brief tone bursts presented to the ear canal. Giebel and Redemann, 1992 report that no TEOAE's will be found in a patient with cochlear hearing loss exceeding 30 dB HL. Additionally, because TEOAE's can't be measured in the presence of middle ear disorders, they make an excellent hearing screening tool for children (Nozza and Sabo, 1992). Pure tone OAE's are produced in response to externally-presented long-duration pure tone signals and occur at the frequency of the externally-presented pure tone. Distortion product OAE's (DPOAE), a form of pure tone OAE's, are produced by nonlinearities in healthy cochleas and are thought to be generated by OHC's. They are detected in the ear canal by presenting two pure tones (f_1 and f_2, where f_1 is less than f_2) very close in frequency. The dominant component of DPOAE is the difference frequency ($2f_1$ - f_2) usually present at 50-60 dB below the input level of the two test tones (Osterhammel and Rasmussen, 1992). Although this phenomenon shows considerable diagnostic promise for the future, the clinical utility of DPOAE in differentiating between normal and hearing impaired ears has yet to be agreed upon, especially at frequencies below 1000 Hz (Gorga et al, 1993).

NEURAL RESPONSES AND THE EIGHTH NERVE

Neural responses are initiated by the hair cells in the cochlea as follows: when the stereocilia (fine hairs) of the inner hair cells are deflected by the basilar membrane vibrations, ion channels are opened, thus exciting the hair cells and initiating a chemical transmission at the synapses. This chemical transmitter is thought to be glutamate and causes the individual nerve fibers (primary auditory neurons) that are connected to or are adjacent to the inner hair cells to develop a neural potential. The neural potential is the beginning of the nerve impulse which flows to the brain.

The eighth (VIII) cranial nerve (auditory branch) is a series of about 30,000 neurons (individual nerve fibers) which are interconnected one to the other longitudinally. For each separate pathway to the higher auditory centers, a series of four or five individual interconnected neurons leads up to the brain. The termination and beginning of each of these successive nerve fibers occur in the higher auditory centers of the auditory nervous pathway, where bundles of nuclei are formed as the neurons join together. These interconnected nerve fibers form the pathway for neural impulses that are initiated in the cochlea. A "neural potential" is a discharge of electrical energy which occurs in each neuron, which in turn causes its neighbor also to discharge. Thus a neural response can be likened to a series of small firecrackers connected to each other, exploding one after the other in successive order. The action potentials produced in the auditory nerve are sent to the brainstem nuclei and to the auditory cortex in the temporal lobe. Electrical activity caused by this transmission can be recorded by placing electrodes on the skull and is known as the auditory brainstem evoked response or ABR.

To summarize, bending of the hair cells alters their electrical state and produces an electrical potential, which in turn causes current to flow through the hair cells. The result is that individual fibers of the auditory nerve (neurons or nerve cells) that are associated with specific hair cells are caused to discharge or fire. The exact manner in which the neurons are caused to discharge is still a matter of some debate. Basically, however, a chemical transmitter is liberated by a hair cell which causes an electrical voltage change (depolarization) in the primary auditory neuron, the first neuron connected to the hair cell.

PITCH PERCEPTION AND FREQUENCY RESOLUTION

The "place theory" hypothesis of pitch perception is based on the cochlea acting as a frequency analyzer by distributing various acoustic stimuli according to frequency along the basilar membrane. This hypothesis of pitch perception suggests that the individual neurons that are connected to particular hair cells in the organ of Corti are specifically tuned to only those frequencies that are being excited by movement of the basilar membrane. Interestingly, investigators have found that each nerve fiber (neuron) does have a characteristic tuning frequency. That is, each neuron discharges more easily at a particular frequency or at a narrow band of certain frequencies than to other frequencies. A tuning curve is a graph showing the level of the auditory stimulus at each frequency that is required to significantly change the firing rate of a nerve fiber. Tuning curves are named for their sharply pointed tips at which a minimum amount of sound pressure is required to change the fiber firing rate. The tuning curve tip occurs at a particular frequency called the best frequency or the characteristic frequency for that nerve fiber. (See Figure 20).

When the intensity of the stimulus is increased to a certain level, the steeply sloping high frequency tails of the tuning curves also become activated, leading to further eighth nerve activity. Fibers that have high frequency tuning characteristics are located at the base of the cochlea, and those with lower frequency tuning characteristics are located at the apex. Further, by experiments that are used to study the arrangement of fibers in the higher auditory pathways, it appears that there is a "tonotopic" organization of nerve fibers throughout the entire auditory system. That is, the nerve fibers which transmit higher frequencies are always located in certain places at each higher auditory center, and fibers which respond to lower frequencies are characteristically found in other locations. All of these findings form very strong evidence for a place theory of frequency encoding of neural events and consequently, a pitch perception. The place theory is well documented and has rather broad acceptance. However, it does not account for all the phenomena of pitch perception.

The "temporal" theory of pitch perception has been suggested as an alternative to the place theory. The temporal or rate of neural discharge theory suggests that below 1000Hz, the individual neurons fire at rates identical to the stimulus frequencies. With the temporal theory, a 750Hz tone would result in all events within the cochlea being the same as those that would occur with the place theory, except that the nerve fibers at the point of maximal stimulation of the basilar membrane discharge and recover at the rate of 750 times or cycles per second. Since it has been determined that individual nerve fibers cannot physically fire off faster than approximately 1000 times per second, the temporal theory also suggests that for higher frequencies, the nerve fibers discharge in volleys. Figure 21 is an illustration of this principal. For a 3000Hz signal, in the vicinity on the basilar membrane that is maximally displaced for a 3000Hz tone, neurons will take turns firing perhaps every third time. Then, the combined response of three given neurons firing successively will be equivalent to a rate of 3000Hz. Although there is some debate surrounding the applicability of both theories, most investigators agree that some form of both the place and temporal theories can be used to explain how frequency

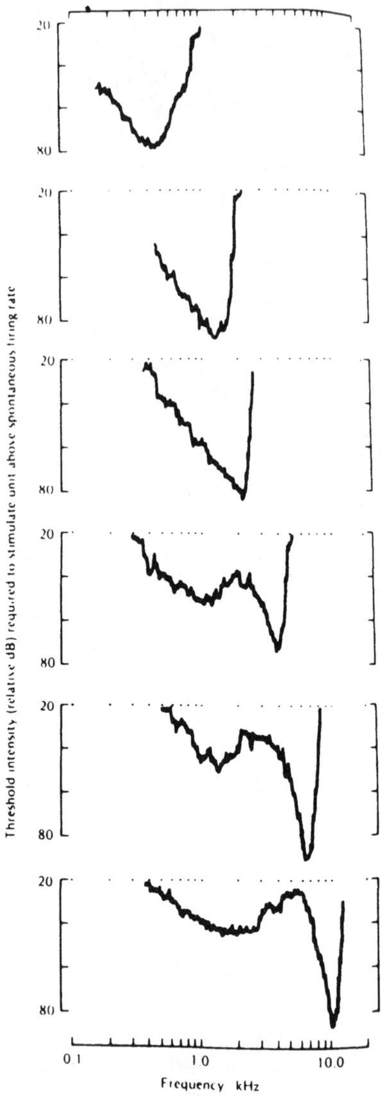

Fig. 20. Tuning curves for six single units with different characteristic frequencies. The stimulus level in relative decibels needed to reach each unit's threshold is plotted as a function of the stimulus frequency. Note the steep slope on the high-frequency side of the curve and the shallow slope on the low-frequency side. The bottom three units have higher characteristic frequencies and show low-frequency "talis" which indicate that they are responsive to a wide range of frequencies of stimulation. (*Kiang and Moxon, Physiological Considerations in Artificial Stimulation of the Inner Ear, Annals of Otology, 81: 714–730, 1972.*)

analysis and pitch perception is accomplished by the auditory system. It is felt that for low frequencies, the temporal theory appears to be more operative, and for the higher frequencies, it is more probable that the place theory is applicable.

The degree of frequency resolution of an auditory system is related to the bandwidth and shape of its auditory filters. (The frequency analyzing capability of the auditory system has been approximated by a bank of filters). The effective bandwidths of the

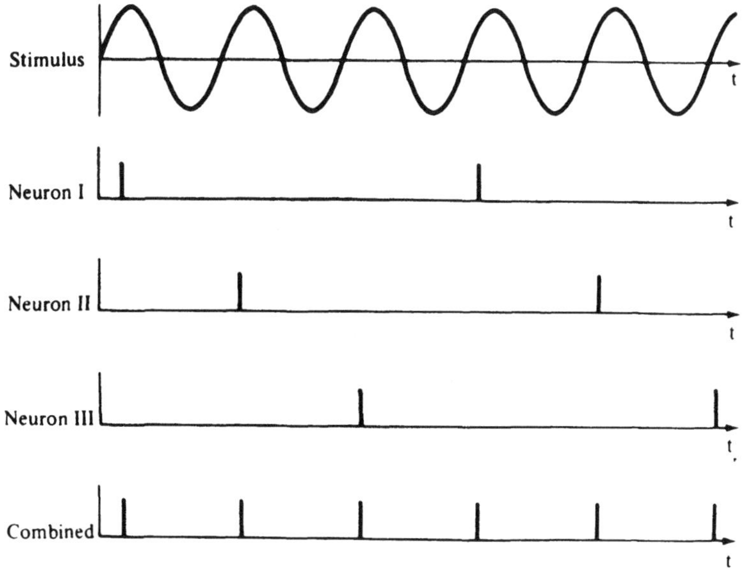

Fig. 21. Volley Principle of neural discharge. (*Minifie, Hixon & Williams, Normal Aspects of Speech, Hearing and Language, 1973, p. 305, 416. Reprinted by permission of Prentice-Hall, Inc., Englewood Cliffs, N.J.*)

auditory filters in normal hearing persons correspond to widely published single number critical bands for auditory filters. However, because the shape of a typical auditory filter has a rounded top and steep skirts, it can not be completely described by a single number (Moore, 1982). The difference limen (DL) of frequency for a just noticable change in pitch varies from less than 1 Hz at low frequencies to about 100 Hz at high frequencies (Moore, 1982).

It appears that normal hearing persons have much better temporal resolution than hearing impaired listeners for signals that have rapid temporal fluctuations or signals that have high frequency amplitude-modulation (Nelson, 1990). The excellent ability of normal hearing persons to follow such rapid temporal envelope fluctuations has been called "listening in the valleys". Persons with cochlear hearing impairment do not listen in the valleys as well as normal hearing persons.

AUDITORY PATHOLOGY AND THRESHOLD OF AUDIBILITY

If there is damage to a specific portion of the cochlea, such as the Organ of Corti and the hair cells, or to the primary auditory neurons and nerve cells in the ascending auditory pathway, the result will be threshold sensitivity loss which will be reflected on the audiogram as some type of sensorineural hearing impairment. For example, violent movement of the cochlear fluids produced by a loud explosion may result in a tearing and destruction of the tissues at the base of the cochlea, and result in a high frequency loss shown on the pure tone audiogram. Or, the growth of a large eighth nerve tumor may interrupt the transmission of some nerve fiber impulses to the brain. Since high frequency auditory neurons are often affected first by the tumor, a high frequency loss may be seen on the audiogram.

However, the audiogram is very limited for diagnostic purposes. For example, reduced blood supply to the basal or high frequency area of the cochlea may produce an audiogram loss similar to that which might be caused by excessive mechanical vibration or high levels of noise. There are any number of causes of neural tissue and structural damage in the auditory nervous system that may appear relatively similar on the pure tone audiogram. Therefore, one can seldom conclude from casual inspection of either the pure tone audiogram or the speech audiogram the exact nature and extent of the underlying pathology. In addition to the loss of sensitivity indicated by threshold shift, other interruptions of normal auditory activity may be present, including distortions in pitch perception and loudness growth, reduced tolerance to intense sounds, reduced ability to localize sound and greater difficulty recognizing speech in noise. All of these abnormal conditions are the result to some degree, of alteration or destruction of various structural tissues, cochlear fluids, and neural tissue in specific portions of the auditory nervous system.

With the considerations in mind, often the hearing aid specialist must rely on the comments of the wearer to know whether or not a specific hearing aid fitting or adjustment is satisfactory. Current auditory tests are not sufficiently advanced at present to consistently reveal the subtle changes in the auditory system produced by adjustment of hearing aid controls.

Traditionally, the term "threshold" has been thought of as a specific value of acoustic stimulus intensity, above which a subject responds and below which the stimulus is not detected by the subject. The threshold level is sometimes difficult to repeat over time due to factors such as the subject's level of attention, external noises in the testing environment and variations in the subject's biological processes such as blood flow that may cause internal physiologic noise to mask the true threshold. Consequently, threshold is really a statistical concept in the sense that it is defined as the point at which the subject responds correctly 50% of the time to a stimulus.

There are two methods of measuring the thresholds for minimum audible sounds: minimum audible pressure (MAP) and minimum audible field (MAF).

Minimum audible pressure is a threshold measurement obtained at a particular frequency using headphones or insert earphones to deliver the stimulus. Minimum audible field is a threshold measurement made in a sound field with a loudspeaker located at a particular direction and distance from the subject being tested. Theoretically, minimum audible pressure may be calculated if minimum audible field is known by subtracting the diffraction effects produced on incident sounds by a human torso and head. However, investigators have determined that 6dB is still unaccounted for after all of the known effects such as diffraction are subtracted out. The difference between the two measurements has been called "the missing 6dB", which appears to be caused primarily by physiological masking effects in the low frequencies that are produced by the pulsing of blood flowing (Killion, 1976).

A plot of minimum audible pressure or minimum audible field versus frequency is usually shown on a graph such as that in Figure 22. The same thresholds, however, can also be converted to hearing level (HL) and be displayed on an audiogram form. The audiogram is used to tabulate hearing threshold levels for a particular subject in dB HL relative to that for normals. The audiometer automatically adds the correct amount of sound pressure required to the setting of the attenuator dial level at each frequency so that, for example, a 0dB HL provides the exact sound pressure level that is required to elicit a response 50% of the time for normal hearing persons. Thus, the actual sound pressure levels produced by an audiometer at one attenuation setting vary as the frequency is changed.

An intensity produced by an audiometer, but referenced to a particular subject's hearing threshold rather than to the average normal hearing threshold, is called dB SL (Sensation Level), and is the number of decibels by which a stimulus is greater than the subject's own hearing threshold level. Whereas dB HL is used to express the audiometer attenuator dial setting, dB SL is often used for describing a stimulus whose intensity is relative to a subject's individual hearing threshold. For example, if a person's threshold is 40dB HL, the presentation of a signal at 70dB HL can also be referred to as 30dB SL. (70dB HL − 40dB HL = 30dB SL).

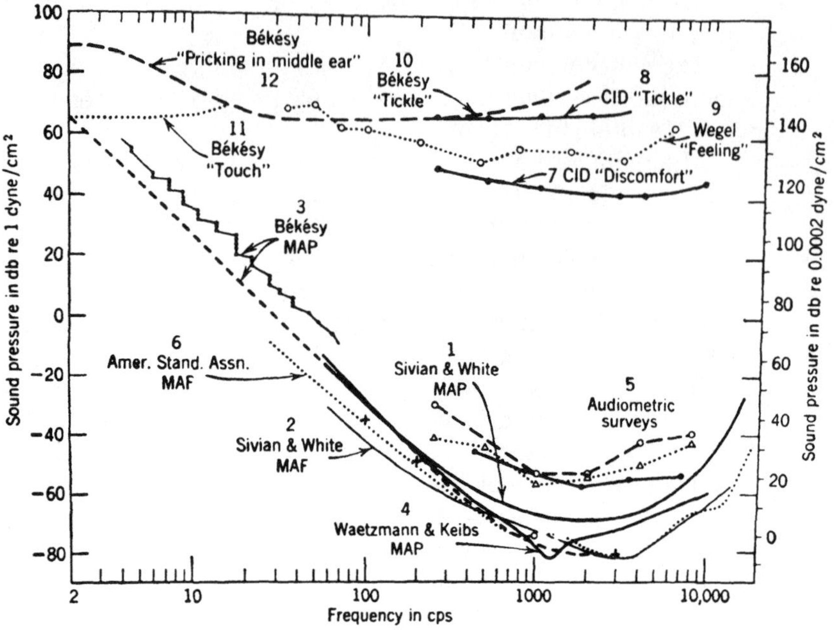

Fig. 22. Minimum Audible Field (MAF), Minimum Audible Pressure (MAP) and Auditory Dynamic Range. (*Licklider in Stevens, Handbook of Experimental Psychology, John Wiley & Sons, 1960.*)

BONE CONDUCTION

Although the usual route of a sound stimulus is by means of the air conduction pathway (through the external and middle ear), stimulation of the inner ear can also occur by conduction of sound via the bones of the skull, which is appropriately called bone conduction. The mechanism for bone conduction bypasses the aid conduction auditory pathway through the middle ear. Bone conduction transmission is believed to initiate the same traveling wave in the cochlea as in air conduction transmission. Skull vibrations create distortional bulges in the cochlea at the oval and round windows that cause traveling waves because of the incompressibility of the cochlear fluids (Tonndorf, 1962).

The ability of a person to hear via bone conduction is readily demonstrated by applying a bone vibrator to the mastoid area of forehead. Since the process of hearing occurs either by air conduction or by bone conduction, a subject's hearing ability can be expressed in dB HL for either air conduction or bone conduction stimuli. Bone conduction audiometry has traditionally been used as a diagnostic tool to determine whether the middle ear of a person is functioning abnormally: if the hearing threshold levels obtained from air and bone conduction audiometry are essentially the same, it is assumed that the pathology that is causing the hearing loss is not occurring in the middle ear, but is either cochlear or retrocochlear in origin.

The pheonomena of air conduction and bone conduction can interact during audiometric testing in some circumstances. Caution is advised if an air conduction signal is presented at a high signal level through an earphone because it may be strong enough to become a bone conduction signal, and thereby stimulate the cochlea. Before an air conduction stimulus can become a bone conduction stimulus, there is about a 35-65dB attenuation through the contact of the audiometric headset and earphone cushions to the test subject's head, depending on frequency and individual subject variations.

The "occlusion effect" gets its name from the sound pressure-build-up in an ear canal that has been occluded with a headphone or an earmold. This increase in SPL for an occluded ear canal relative to the unoccluded condition occurs primarily in the low frequencies. For audiometric headphones used during bone conduction testing, the increase amounts to about 20-28 dB at 250 Hz, 13-20 dB @ 500 Hz, and 6-9 dB @ 1 kHz (Edgerton and Klodd, 1977). The amount of sound buildup is inversely proportional to the degree of earmold venting. For unvented earmolds relative to the unoccluded condition, Wimmer, 1986 and Killion, Wilber and Gudmundsen, 1988 showed comparable increases in low frequency gain to that for audiometric headphones. It is thought that this low frequency energy build-up is related to complaints of hearing aid wearers who report that their own voices sound hollow or too loud.

Relative to hearing aid fittings, Zwislocki, 1953 showed that if an insert earphone ear tip was inserted deeply enough to contact the bony or osseous portion of the ear canal, the occlusion effect could be reduced and even totally eliminated. This phenomenon was confirmed by Khanna, Tonndorf and Queller, 1976 and by Berger and Kerivan, 1983. The deep canal fitting has been utilized for hearing aid fittings to put this knowledge into practical use. The most recent example of reducing the occlusion effect in practice is with a completely in the canal (CIC) hearing aid by extending the canal on the earmold at least 2 mm past the second bend in the patient's ear canal (Killion, Wilber and Gudmundsen, 1988; Staab and Finlay, 1991).

MASKING

In their research into the phenomenon of pitch perception, investigators have also looked closely at related occurrences. The idea of "masking" is closely connected to frequency resolution, because it is well known that the presence of one sound tends to cover up or reduce the presence of another sound under certain conditions. In attempting to distinguish the neural mechanisms and events which account for this phenomenon, scientists have identified two types of masking: simultaneous and nonsimultaneous. The former occurs when two sounds composed of different frequencies and intensities are presented to the cochlea at the same time. By systematically varying frequency and intensity of the two stimuli, using pure tones, white noise, narrow band noise, etc., it has been discovered that low frequency sounds can mask out higher frequency sounds more easily than high frequency sounds are able to mask out low frequency sounds. For example, much less intensity of a low frequency tone is required to suppress the perception of a higher frequency tone than is needed for a low frequency tone to be masked by a high frequency tone. In some instances, it is nearly impossible for certain high frequency stimuli to be made intense enough to cover up or mask low frequency tones.

This masking tendency is thought to be somewhat indirectly related to the behavior of the basilar membrane when it is stimulated at the same time by two tones of different frequencies. Since the traveling wave for low frequency tones is distrubuted along the entire basilar membrane, it will cause some depression of the membrane in the basal turn of the cochlea where high frequency tones are primarily located. As a result, the wave traveling through the basal area may "use up" some of the capacity of the basilar membrane to initiate a neural response for a high frequency tone. The tendency for a low frequency tone to cover up or reduce the perception of a high frequency tone that is presented at the same time, has been called "upward spread of masking". Although the physiological mechanism for upward spread of masking is not entirely clear, the psychological perceptual phenomenon of upward spread of masking is well documented.

The above may help the hearing aid specialist to understand why it is important that low frequencies (below 1000Hz) should not be overamplified in relation to higher frequencies. Too much amplification in the low frequency region may result in a disproportional amount of amplification of background noise, (conversation, street noise, etc.) which usually is made up primarily of low frequency sounds. As a result, the soft, less intense unvoiced speech sounds that are so important for the perception of the speech signal may be covered up or masked even when there is a deliberate attempt to provide primarily high frequency amplification through a hearing aid. Finding the exact level at which low frequencies are being amplified enough so that sound quality is acceptable, but not so much so as to cause masking of the high frequencies, is one of the primary tasks of the hearing aid dispenser. There are few specific, reliable clues to assist in determining the correct balance. Growth of loudness data and testimony by the hearing aid wearer, together with word recognition tests in noise, usually may be relied on to provide some indication as to whether a good compromise between low and high frequency gain has been achieved.

Generally, the higher frequencies in speech are very important for providing intelligibility regardless of the shape (threshold configuration) of the audiogram. Therefore, the masking that occurs is not just a phenomenon that is present in high frequency losses only, but occurs with all types of threshold configurations.

Upward spread of masking is a phenomenon that occurs when two sounds are present simultaneously. Another type of masking, called nonsimultaneous or temporal masking, occurs when sounds follow one another very closely in time. In this case, a preceding loud sound has the ability to mask out or reduce perception of a soft sound that follows it in time, if the time interval between the two sounds is not too great. That is, even though the first sound may have effectively ceased being produced, the listener may still experience some difficulty in detecting a second, less intense sound stimulus that was initiated shortly after cessation of the first. This temporal masking phenomenon is called "forward masking". It may be related to a reduction in sensitivity of recently stimulated cells in the auditory nervous system, or a persistence in the pattern of neural activity produced by the preceding masking sound. Forward masking may be responsible for first formants of speech masking consonants, higher frequency formants and their transitions. For example, in the vowel-consonant pair /at/, the vowel /a/ has a high level of energy in the frequency range of 400Hz to 800Hz. Its presence, especially if overamplified, may cause a loss of perception of the following sound, the soft unvoiced stop consonant, /t/.

A second type of temporal masking is referred to as "backward masking". It occurs when an intense sound follows a less intense sound very closely in time, and because of its intensity and closeness to the preceding sound, reduces the perception of the less intense sound that has preceded it. This phenomenon is more difficult to understand, for it is hard to realize how a stimulus following can have any effect at all on a signal that has not only preceded it in time, but also that has stopped before the stimulus following it has begun. However, the effect does indeed occur, although it is difficult to explain. Temporal masking has special significance for the hearing aid specialist because speech is a sequence of spoken sounds. Some speech sounds have relatively high amplitudes and some have much lower amplitudes (up to 25dB less intense). Consequently, if low frequencies are disproportionately amplified by a hearing aid, it is possible that the speech signal can actually mask itself even when no background noise is present in the environment. That is, if the amplified vowel sounds that precede (or follow) the soft consonant sounds are too intense, they will cause a reduction in the perception of soft speech sounds that are important for speech clarity. Consider the word "thought": the "ou" vowel sound, if made too loud by a hearing aid, actually may have the potential to reduce the wearer's discrimination of the "th" and "t" sounds which follow and precede it. Thus, "thought" may be confused with the words "taught", "fought" or even "talk".

Studies have shown that temporal masking is greater for sounds in the low frequency region than for sounds in the high frequency region. Again, the possibility of low frequency over-amplification exists which will cause, in effect, the low frequency over-amplified voice vowel sounds to mask out the soft, high frequency friction or sibilant sounds, such as /f/ or /s/, which provide much of the intelligibility of speech.

LOUDNESS-SUBJECTIVE CORRELATE OF INTENSITY

Whereas intensity is a physical property of sound, loudness is a psychological attribute associated with an individual's particular auditory system. Although one would expect that if a sound was made twice as intense, it would sound twice as loud, this is not the case with most auditory systems. In fact, loudness for a normal auditory system follows a logarithmic relationship called the power law over much of the range of intensities we encounter: every time the intensity of a sound is increased by 10dB, loudness is doubled. Only a threefold increase in sound pressure is needed to produce a 10dB intensity change and to double the loudness). Thus, as a result of sound pressure increasing repeatedly by the same ratio, e.g., 3 times, the same change in loudness sensation (doubling) is produced repeatedly for normal ears (Fechner, 1860). This phenomenon can be thought of as a logarthmic relationship between sound pressure and loudness sensation. For example, a 1kHz pure tone at 80dB SPL would be twice as loud for a normal ear as a pure tone at 70dB SPL and half as loud as a pure tone at 90dB SPL.

The phon is the unit of measurement used to help compare the loudness level of different tones—the relative loudness of one tone when compared to another at a different frequency. A loudness level scale has been defined on which the loudness level of a 1kHz tone at 40dB SPL is 40 phons. If the loudness level of a 2kHz tone at 49dB SPL is judged to be the same as the loudness level for the 40dB SPL 1kHz tone, the 2kHz tone also has a loudness level of 40 phons. The term sones has been used by Stevens, 1951 for the unit of measure of loudness (not for loudness level for which the unit of measure is phons). On the loudness scale, a 1kHz tone presented at 40dB sensation level (SL)—or 40dB above the hearing threshold of the listener—produces a loudness of 1 sone. A 1kHz tone at 40dB SPL that has a loudness level of 40 phons also has a loudness of 1 sone for a normal ear. At levels greater than 40dB SPL (40 phons or 1 sone), a 10 phon increase in loudness level produces a two-fold increase in loudness (doubles the number of sones) for a normal auditory system.

The hearing aid specialist may be familiar with equal loudness contours (Fletcher and Munson, 1933) the lowest of which occurs at the threshold of audibility. Figure 23a shows that at very high intensity levels of sound, the equal loudness curves are much flatter than they are at the threshold of audibility. This is the rationale behind the "loudness" control found in many high fidelity amplifiers—a switch that adds both high and low frequency boost to the signal for low listening levels to approximate the equal loudness contour found at higher listening levels. Also, the spacing between the equal loudness curves is smaller at lower frequencies than it is at mid frequencies, indicating that less change in sound pressure is required at low frequencies to double the loudness, for example than at mid frequencies. For a recruiting ear, the spacing between the equal loudness contours is often significantly reduced, particularly in the high frequencies. In fact, for some particularly severely recruiting ears, no separation at all is found to exist in the high frequencies between adjacent equal loudness contours (Figure 23b).

Loudness recruitment refers to the abnormal growth of loudness found in clients with cochlear hearing impairment as the intensity of sound stimuli is raised. This phenomenon has important significance for providing a successful hearing aid fitting and should not be confused with an abnormally low uncomfortable level. The top

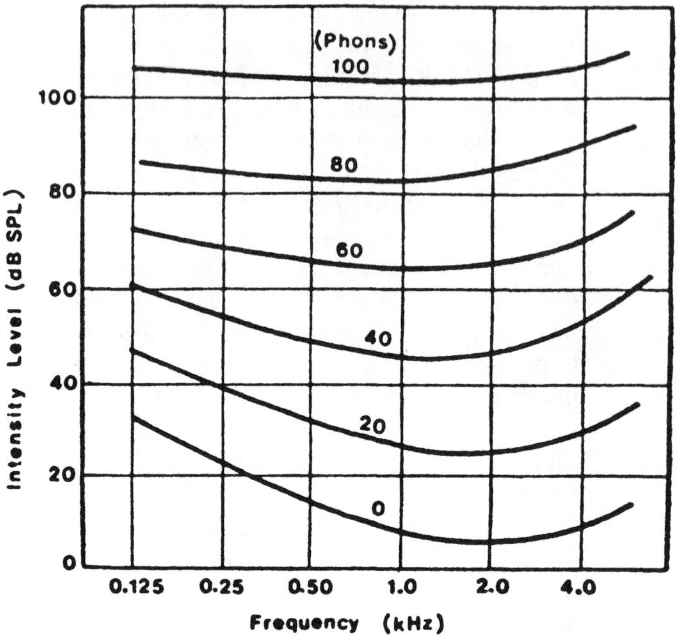

Fig. 23a. Equal loudness contours for normal hearing.

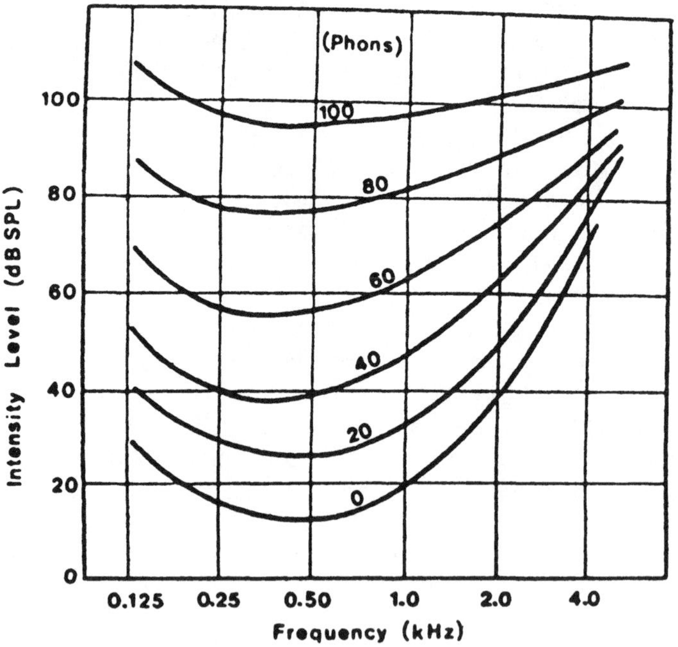

Fig. 23b. Equal loudness contours for a typical sensorineural hearing loss. (*Linear Technology, Inc., 1983.*)

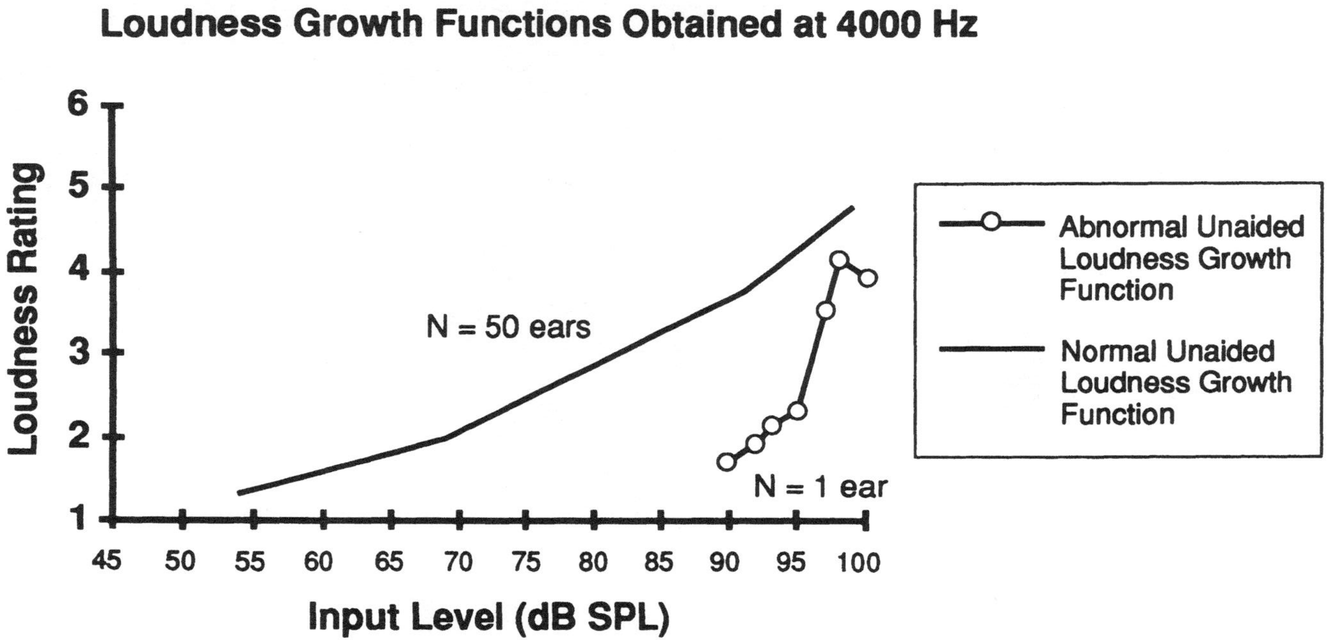

Fig. 23c. Unaided loudness growth at 4 kHz via the LGOB test. Top line - mean for 50 normal ears; Bottom line - for one impaired ear. Reprinted with permission from Fortune, 1992.

line in Figure 23c shows the mean growth of loudness as a function of input level for 50 normal hearing persons for a narrow band of noise one octave wide centered at 4000 Hz using the LGOB protocol advocated by Allen, 1990. The lower line in Figure 23c shows the growth of loudness for one hearing impaired ear using the same test method. The steeper the slope of the lower line, the greater the recruitment. A hearing impaired client may reject a hearing aid if some allowance is not made for compressing the dynamic range of speech and other sounds into the client's restricted dynamic range. Loudness recruitment has a confirmed neurophys-

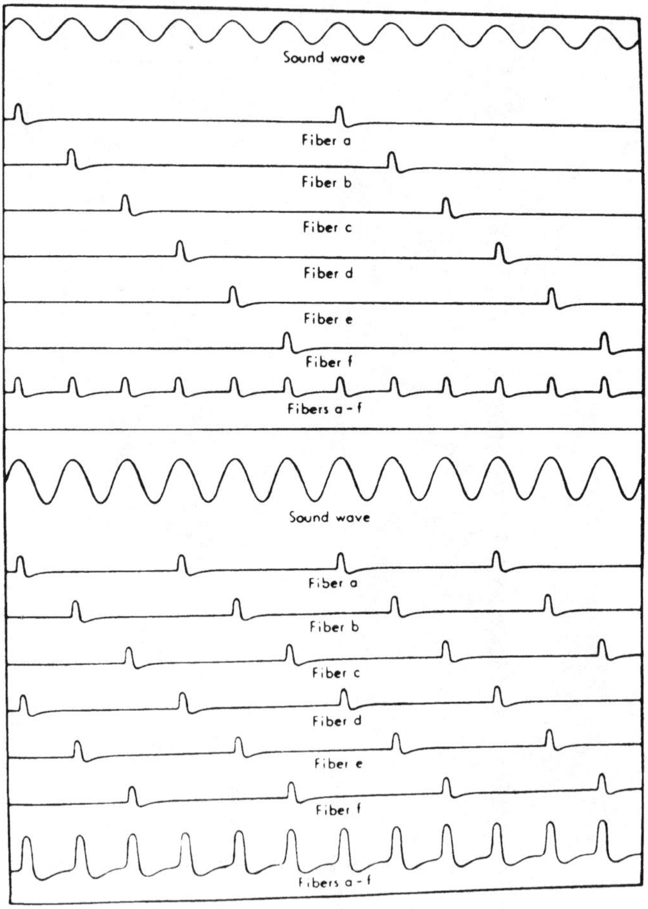

Fig. 24. Schematic of intensity representation in the Volley Principle. (*Zemlin, Willard R., Speech and Hearing Science; Anatomy and Physiology, 1968, p. 429. Reprinted by permission of Prentice-Hall, Inc., Englewood Cliffs, N.J., adapted for Wever, E.G. Theory of Hearing.*)

iological basis and may be a result of damage to the outer hair cells (Moore, 1982), which are particularly vulnerable to ototoxic drugs and to high levels of sound.

How does the auditory system change the intensity of auditory stimuli into a sensation of loudness? Tracing back to what we have learned previously, an increase in sound pressure causes an increase in the amplitude of the to and fro movements of the stapes. That, in turn, produces greater basilar membrane displacement. This increased displacement is accompanied by a certain amount of "spreading" of the area of displacement along the basilar membrane and a greater number of fibers are brought into play. Consequently, it appears that when sound pressure is increased, previously inactive nerve fibers in adjacent areas may begin to discharge. The sensation of loudness appears to be related to the total sum of activity of the auditory nerve fibers. Figure 24 shows how a "volley" of neural discharges could add together on the auditory nerve to provide a greater sensation of loudness.

The just noticeable difference (JND) or difference limen (DL) in loudness is used for the subjective response scale to measure the change in intensity required to produce a particular change in loudness (Fechner, 1860). The JND for intensity has been found to be about equal at all frequencies (Fiesz, 1928). This minimal detectable change in sound pressure level ranges from about 0.4dB to 0.8dB. For example, it is about as easy to tell the differences between a change of 34 to 35dB SPL as it is to distinguish between a change of 95 to 96dB SPL.

OUTER HAIR CELLS, INNER HAIR CELLS AND HEARING AID COMPRESSION PARAMETERS

Kates, 1993 has brought together some interesting facts and assumptions about normal and pathological auditory systems that could form the basis for selecting hearing aid parameters as follows: the OHC's together with the basilar membrane in a normal cochlea provide considerable gain at low input levels (typically 60 dB) and almost no gain at high input levels, making its operation as a system similar to that of a compression circuit (see Figure 25). At a 50 dB SPL input, a normal cochlea would provide about 30 dB of gain so no additional gain is needed from a hearing aid. Consequently, the solid line labelled "0" in Figure 25 has a compression ratio of 1 : 1. According to Kates, the typical compression ratio of a healthy cochlea is about 2.5:1. However, the gain provided in a cochlea with considerable outer hair cell damage is nearly the same (typically 0 dB for severe outer hair cell damage) regardless of input level, making its function similar to that of a linear amplifier. In his model, Kates states that outer hair cell damage therefore causes a reduction in the compression ratio normally provided by the cochlea and a loss of sensitivity evidenced by hearing thresholds as poor as about 60 dB for complete outer hair cell damage.

In order to compensate for recruitment, a hearing aid must fit the dynamic range of speech and other sounds into the abnormally small dynamic range of a hearing impaired person. Compression ratio and gain in such cases may be selected to try to restore the

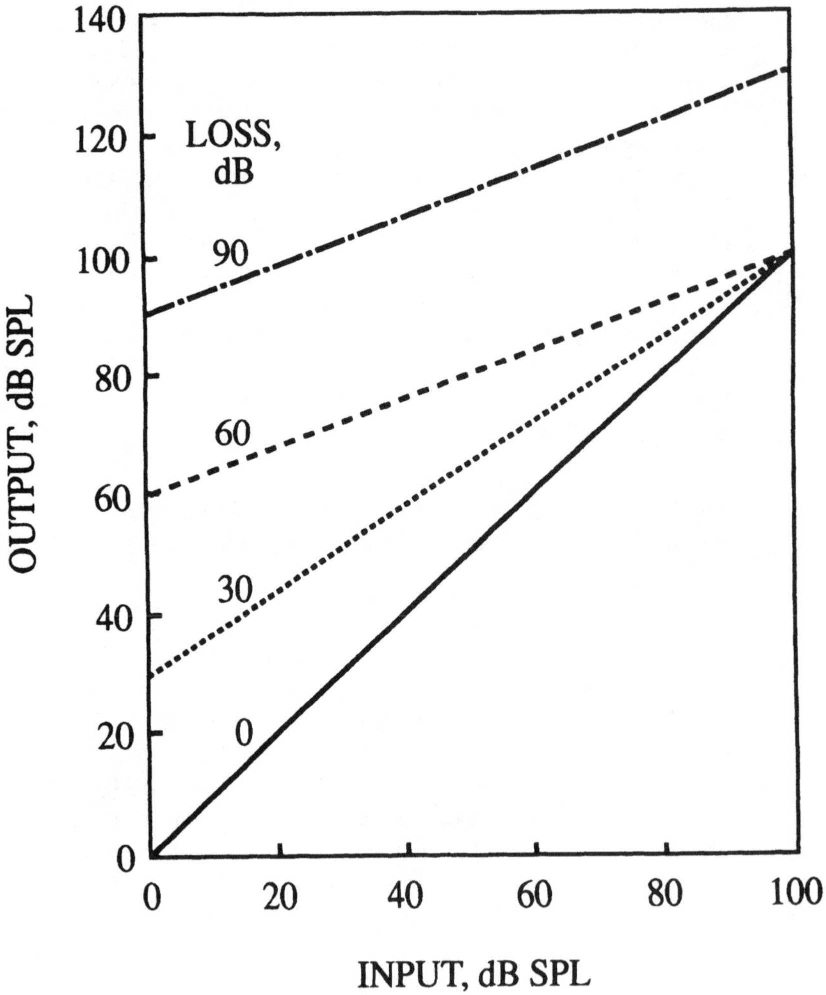

Fig. 25. Compression amplifier input/output curves within an auditory filter band for the model of hearing loss. Reprinted by permission from Kates, 1993.

growth of loudness in the impaired auditory system to near normal. Thus, in accordance with Kates' model, the compression ratio in a hearing aid circuit could be selected by how severe the outer hair cell damage is. Kates states that the popular "half-gain" fitting rule is really an attempt to produce the same gain in a pathological ear as would occur in a normal ear for a given input level. The line labelled "60" in Figure 25 has a compression ratio of 2.5:1 and shows that for a 60 dB loss, about 20 dB additional gain would have to be provided by a hearing aid for sound inputs of 60 dB SPL. The line labelled "30" in Figure 25 suggests that a hearing aid would have a compression ratio less than 2.5:1 for a 30 dB hearing loss because the cochlea itself is healthy enough to still provide some compression. For losses more severe than about 60 dB, inner hair cell damage has also occurred and more gain is needed but still with a 2.5 compression ratio. For example, with a 90 dB loss, the top line in Figure 25 labelled "90" shows that a hearing aid would have to provide about 50 dB of gain for sounds at 60 dB input SPL.

AUDITORY DYNAMIC RANGE

The auditory response area or auditory dynamic range extends from minimum audibility or the threshold curve to the threshold of discomfort as shown in Figure 22. The amount of sound pressure required to elicit either of these thresholds changes as the frequency of the stimulus changes over the range of about 20 to 20,000Hz. At threshold, the maximum sensitivity for hearing is between 2 and 5kHz (Fletcher, 1953) and is, with trained listeners under optimum conditions, about 0dB sound pressure level (SPL) or 0.0002 microPascals. However, for most people, it is quite difficult to hear a sound at 0dB SPL. At lower frequencies, e.g., 250Hz, about 25dB SPL is required to reach the threshold of audibility. The threshold of feeling (sometimes called threshold of tickle) is elicited at about 120 to 130dB SPL and the threshold of pain at about 130 to 140dB SPL, and 20 to 30dB above the levels at which sound becomes uncomfortably loud (UCL) to normal ears.

The physiological basis of the uncomfortable loudness level is cochlear in origin and, as such, is to be differentiated from the tickle or pain sensations that are tactile in nature and may involve nerve endings from the pinna, external auditory canal, eardrum and/or middle ear muscles and bones. For a person with cochlear hearing impairment, the uncomfortable level (UCL), or loudness discomfort level (LDL) as it is sometimes referred to, may occur at a somewhat lower level than that for normal hearing persons (McCandless and Miller, 1972; Schmitz, 1969). The level at which uncomfortable loudness occurs can change depending on such factors as whether the stimulus used is continuous or pulsed; the bandwidth of the signal presented; whether the instructions ask for the level at which the sound is just becoming uncomfortably loud rather than the level at which the sound is so loud it cannot be tolerated and whether the loudness discomfort level is estimated by increasing the level or decreasing the level of the stimulus.

THE BRAIN STEM NUCLEI, ASCENDING PATHWAYS AND AUDITORY CORTEX

Neural impulses from each cochlea lead via the eighth nerve to the ascending auditory pathways of the brain stem. Several way stations exist, namely the cochlear nuclei, superior olivary complex, lateral lemniscus, inferior colliculus and medial geniculate body, as shown in Figure 26. The afferent (ascending or inward going) fibers (primary auditory neurons) from each cochlea lead respectively to each cochlear nucleus. At each of the two main paths above each cochlear nucleus and beginning at each superior olivary complex, bilateral representation of the signal occurs. Therefore, nerve cells in these areas would be expected to respond differentially to the time and intensity differences between sounds which arrive at the two ears. However, it appears that some neurons found in the inferior colliculus and in the superior olivary complex are sensitive only to interaural time differences while others respond only to interaural intensity differences.

The auditory cortex of the brain is located in the temporal lobe following the two medial geniculate bodies. Neurons in this area appear to be particularly responsive to complex sounds and to change in sound stimulus frequency. Thus, these cortical centers appear to be responsible for performing more complex central processing tasks such as localizing sounds or decoding the order of the arrival of competing sounds.

EVOKED POTENTIALS

Evoked response audiometry (ERA) allows one to measure the electrical activity due to auditory stimuli at various locations along the auditory pathway. Auditory evoked responses are measured by placing electrodes on the head of the patient. Middle and late au-

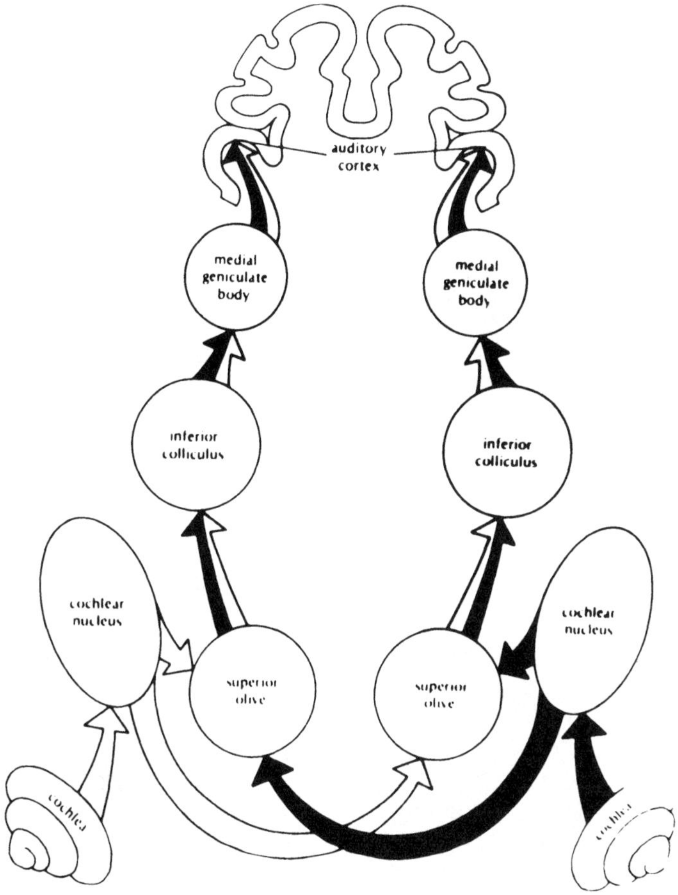

Fig. 26. Schematic diagram of bilateral central auditory system. (*Zemlin, Willard R., Speech and Hearing Science; Anatomy and Physiology, 1960, p. 244, 247. Reprinted by permission of Prentice-Hall, Inc., Englewood Cliffs, N.J.*)

ditory evoked potentials as well as brainstem testing have allowed researchers and clinicians to detect whether lesions are present along the ascending auditory pathways. Such lesions either delay the evoked potential response (increase the latency) or completely eliminate it. Other responses that can be measured include the auditory brainstem response (ABR). The ABR consists of a waveform having 5 peaks (see Figure 27). Considerable research has been done in an effort to determine the physiological origin of each

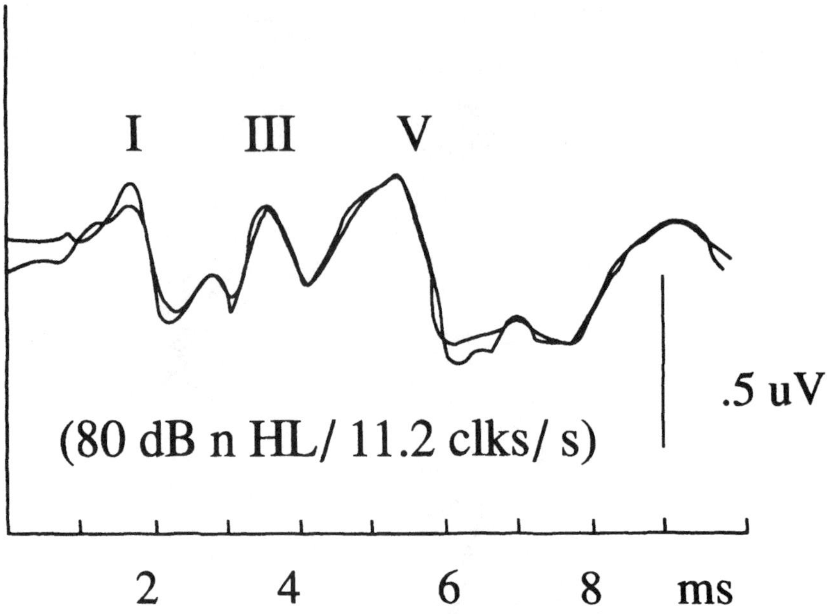

Fig. 27. An example of a normal ABR tracing. Reprinted with permission from Musiek, 1993.

peak. The compound action potential (AP), representing the total activity of the 8th nerve, is generally agreed to be represented by the first peak of the ABR or Wave I. Of interest in the ABR is the amplitude of each peak and its latency or time delay relative to the time of the ABR onset. An increase in latency of Wave V can indicate the presence of a brain tumor (Musiek, 1983). In measuring auditory evoked responses, the electro-encephlagram (EEG) is considered to be noise. Auditory evoked responses have been used for patient monitoring during certain operations. This allows a determination to be made as to whether any neurological injury resulted from procedures used during the operation. In general, however, evoked potentials are not sufficiently developed as clinical tests to assess which portion of the higher order auditory nervous system physiology corresponds to which central function problem, and why individuals with such pathologies often may not utilize hearing aid amplification successfully. Additionally, a current trend is to utilize magnetic resonance imaging (MRI) routinely to determine the site of lesion if an acoustic neuroma is suspected.

Elderly persons often experience greater difficulty understanding speech than younger persons with comparable hearing loss.

Several studies have shown a general age-related decline in the perception of speech in noisy and reverberant environments (e.g., Nabalek and Robinson, 1982; Dubno et al., 1984; Gelfand et al., 1985; Helfer and Wilber, 1990). These increased speech recognition difficulties can not be solely attributed to the amount of hearing loss or even to other auditive factors such as the degradation of frequency resolution and temporal resolution. There appears to be a degradation in speech recognition, as well, from cognitive factors such as reduced memory capacity and mental factors such as the tendency to fatigue easily (van Rooij and Plomp, 1990).

BINAURAL HEARING

When a listener with only one ear (or with only one hearing aid) attempts to function in everyday sound environments, either the good (or aided) ear or the poorer (or unaided ear) will always be favorably or unfavorably positioned with respect to the source of interest at any given moment. One important result of binaural hearing is the elimination of the "far ear" effect (monaural-indirect listening condition) that is caused by a sound source being located at the opposite side of the head from the monaural ear in question. This monaural-indirect listening condition (Olsen and Carhart, 1967) reduces the level of a speech stimulus at the far ear by an average of about 6dB SPL (up to 15dB in the high frequencies), because sound loses intensity as it crosses over the head from one ear to the other.

The binaural "squelch effect" is a phrase coined to document the release from masking or improvement in signal-to-noise ratio that results from binaural listening as compared to monaural listening. Carhart (1965) reported that the binaural squelch effect amounted to about 3dB at threshold. The fact that masking is squelched by 3 or 4dB is extremely significant when considering whether to fit one or two hearing aids for a hearing impaired person because this small amount of improvement can result in up to 20% improvement in speech recognition ability, depending on the speech materials used. For the binaural squelch effect to occur, both ears must have relatively equal sensitivity, and it is absent if the ears are imbalanced.

One theory that has been offered to explain this phenomenon is that of equalization and cancellation (Durlach, 1972). This phenomenon is provided by the higher centers of the auditory system. The output of the two ears is thought to be either subtracted or added in the higher order auditory centers as a result of comparing the inputs processed through the two peripheral systems for differences.

The concept of binaural fusion involves the combination of similar but not exactly identical signals at the two ears into a single sound image. This phenomenon is readily demonstrated with normal auditory systems: when high frequency information is presented to one ear first and low frequency information is presented to the other ear at a later time, they are heard as individual high and low frequency signals, respectively. However, if the same stimuli are present simultaneously to the two ears, the fusion process will render the signals inseparable. It is thought that this process may show promise for hearing aid fitting because masking may be reduced if the low frequency portion of the input is confined to one ear and the high frequency portion to the other ear. This procedure has been called split band or dichotic fitting (Franklin, 1975; Beck,1978).

Binaural summation increases the apparent loudness of an incoming signal if that signal arrives at each ear simultaneously. At supra threshold levels, there may be a 6 to 10dB increase in loudness. Consideration of binaural function can be important in the selection of electroacoustic characteristics for hearing aids. Some researchers have advocated that hearing aids should equalize the signals between the two ears to ensure that the maximum benefit of the binaural system is preserved.

HOW THE AUDITORY SYSTEM RECOGNIZES SPEECH

The purpose of reviewing how the auditory system recognizes speech is to consider how a hearing aid delivers speech and other stimuli to an impaired auditory system.

To review some portions of our previous discussion, we have seen that the relatively weak high frequency components of speech (above 1000Hz) contain the most important energy for recognizing speech sounds. These include second and third formants of vowel sounds (spectral energy peaks produced by resonance of the vocal tract of the speaker), formant transitions (the movement of these energy peaks to other frequency regions at the shape of the speaker's vocal tract changes), and unvoiced friction sounds. Since most hearing impairments almost always affect perception of the mid and higher frequencies, one's ability to hear these critical cues in speech may be greatly affected. As a further complication, the presence of background noise, which usually has most of its energy in the lower frequencies, may mask out the relatively weaker high frequency components of speech. Persons with cochlear hearing impairments generally have more difficulty understanding speech in noisy backgrounds than normal hearing persons (Plomp, 1978). This difference is probably due to a greater susceptibility to masking than for persons with normal hearing (Martin and Pickett, 1970, Nabelek, 1982).

It has been stated that speech recognition within the auditory system depends on how well we use redundant information simultaneously in several psychophysical channels (Barfod, 1979). Hearing impairment lessens the noise rejection ability that is part of a normal auditory system by reducing the number of these channels that are working correctly. Hearing aids that provide frequency-selective amplification may greatly change the speech input to the recognition device via these degraded channels, thus forcing the hearing impaired person to adapt to a new speech input code. Barfod's theory may explain why an adaptation period is sometimes required when first fitting a hearing aid. For some hearing aid wearers, adjusting to the new speech input may never take place. This may help to explain why some hearing aid fittings fail. Understandably, once the hearing impaired person has adapted to the new speech input created by a hearing aid, it is often difficult to improve such a fitting even if the instrument has problems such as high levels of harmonic distortion. Consequently, the common practice of repairing a defective hearing aid so that it meets the original specifications might lead to complaints from the wearer, or even rejection of the aid itself.

One issue which remains unsolved in hearing aid fitting practices involves the speculation that if all speech components are made audible by the hearing aid at a comfortable loudness level, speech recognition will be optimal (Skinner, 1980). That is, if all parts of speech are made audible, because speech is so redundant, hearing impaired persons can usually extract enough information to identify all speech sounds even though their auditory systems have reduced frequency resolution, recruitment and abnormally broad turning curves. Ensuring that the amplification provided by hearing aids makes the less intense high frequency components of speech audible while not making the more intense low frequency speech components uncomfortably loud is not a trivial undertaking. Note in Figure 3 that the spectra of the two sounds /if/ and /ith/ are very similar in the frequency range below 4000 Hz. There are larger differences between the spectra for /ith/ and /if/ only at frequencies above 4000 Hz. Consequently, a hearing aid would have to have sufficient gain at frequencies above 4000 Hz to make these subtle high frequency differences audible for hearing impaired persons.

An opposite view of this appealing but simplistic hypothesis that audibility is all that is needed is as follows: even with all speech components made audible, the distortions created by a severely impaired auditory system are so great that speech recognition can never approach that of a normal ear. Pathological conditions in more severely impaired ears cause certain negative changes, such as reduced frequency resolution. This abnormal condition is detectable using modern psychoacoustic measurement techniques such as the determination of abnormally wide critical bands. In discussing the functions of the auditory system, the critical frequency bands have been likened to band-pass filters. A widened critical band often results in loss of frequency selectivity or a loss of the ability to detect the necessary frequency components of a complex sound (Scharf, 1978). As mentioned earlier, it is thought that the auditory system performs a kind of Fourier spectral (frequency) analysis on acoustic events such as speech and music. It is the passage of sounds through the critical bands which generates this type of analysis. If the bandwidths of these filters become abnormally widened due to hearing impairment, the frequency resolving capability of the auditory system could be significantly reduced.

If this were the case, the formant movements of certain speech sounds, such as those shown in Figure 3 that distinguish /ith/ from /if/, may lie within the bandpass of a single, abnormally widened critical band of an impaired ear rather than in separate critical bands for normal ears. Then, the formant transitions discussed earlier that normally cross the boundaries of adjacent critical band filters may remain within the boundaries of a single abnormally widened critical band filter of an impaired ear, thus making it difficult for the impaired ear to detect these changes.

Another point in considering the mechanism of speech recognition processing within the auditory system is that there is no set of purely acoustic cues that can be used to understand all that is being said by a talker. This is the case because speech recognition depends on syntax and on the context of what is being spoken, all of which can cause significant variability in the acoustic patterns produced by uttering isolated phonemes of speech (Parker, 1977). If the reverse were true, it would be much easier to understand how the auditory system recognizes such features of speech as voicing and place of articulation from the pure acoustic waveforms produced by speech.

To assist the hearing aid specialist to better understand how speech is recognized, it may be helpful to discuss models that attempt to explain the known physiological workings and psychoacoustic phenomena of the auditory system. However, in reviewing models of the peripheral part of the auditory system, one finds that no single model suggested adequately explains all of the phenomena known to occur. However, several early models from the literature of the peripheral part of the auditory system (Siebert, 1970; Duifuis, 1974; de Jonge, 1977; Pfeiffer, 1970) have general agreement as to some of the basic functions (Figure 28). This crude model simulates some but not all of the psychoacoustic behavior of the cochlea and 8th nerve firing.

Relative to the basic model in Figure 28, the normal hearing person understands speech, in part, by being able to detect small changes in frequency (bank of bandpass filters representing the critical bands). For example, the normal ear would have little difficulty in discriminating a 1000Hz tone from a 1030Hz tone; or a 3% change. For the pathologic ear the frequency resolution may be grossly distorted and the hearing impaired person may not be able to tell the difference between a 1000Hz tone and a 1500Hz tone. (The critical band has become too wide to permit detection of small changes in frequency, thereby causing reduced discrimination function.) The process of frequency change detection is mediated in part by the non-linear hair cell transducing mechanism (1/2 wave rectifier in Figure 28). That is, as the hair cell voltage potential changes, it does so in a negative discharge or positive discharge manner. The Poisson process simulates the variable firing rate of the nerve fibers. The addition of noise in each channel of Figure 28 is used to simulate the spontaneous firing rates of the nerve fibers that occurs with no sound input. The resulting nerve

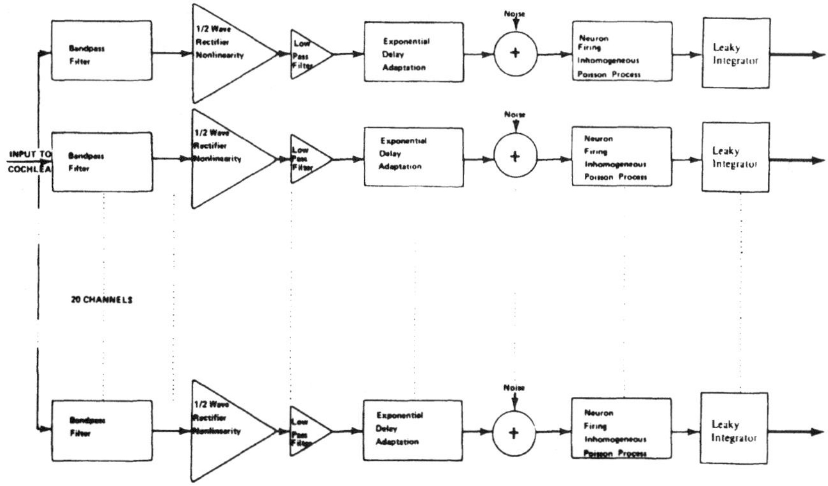

Fig. 28. Block diagram of signal processing portion of auditory system involving cochlea and 8th nerve.

discharges, and the rate of these discharges, are imperfectly summed in a determined order (simulated by the leaky integrator) and the coded bits of neural information are transmitted to the auditory cortex of the brain where they are interpreted as information bearing signals.

FUTURE DIRECTIONS

With the possible harmful effects that auditory pathologies would have on a simplistic model of the peripheral part of the auditory system such as that in Figure 28, it may be doubtful that present day hearing aids could ever hope to be optimum for achieving the best hearing rehabilitation possible. For example, it may be more logical to attempt to correct for the loss of frequency discrimination ability by implanting in the cochlea a set of electrical filters which would narrow or sharpen the response of the damaged critical band filters. Alternatively, cochlear implants may be used to directly stimule the cochlea with electrical signals. To this end, considerable progress has been made in the effectiveness of multi-electrode cochlear implants for severe and profoundly hearing impaired persons. However, in spite of this excellent progress, it still remains to be seen how the anatomy and physiology of the peripheral auditory system should best be coupled physically with such implants. Without a better understanding of the workings of the inner ear and higher brain centers, it is difficult to know how many electrodes to use, where to implant the electrodes and what unique signal processing algorithms to incorporate for each of them. While not of immediate concern for the hearing aid specialist, future dispensers may have to deal with these considerations when selecting appropriate amplification for an impaired ear.

CONCLUSIONS

This overview of the physiology of the human auditory system and its mechanisms reveals the extraordinary capabilities and elegance of the normal hearing process. That our knowledge about the normal operation of the hearing mechanism is inadequate is abundantly clear; the additional effects of auditory pathology on the normal operation even further complicates the picture. Perhaps the hearing aid specialist after reading this chapter, might feel that it is an impossible task to attempt to improve hearing through hearing aid amplification.

However, speech signals are highly redundant, containing more clues than are required for their recognition. The auditory system has exceptional ability to overcome the effects of ear pathology and disease, and the individual can relearn to understand speech again, sometimes under the most unfavorable listening conditions. At times, even a poorly fitted hearing aid is of enormous assistance to a hearing impaired individual. The fact is that the marvelous and complicated function of the auditory system is at the service of the specialist. Our task is to bring to bear on the problem all of the information on how the ear may function, as well as all of the fitting experience we have gained in our practice. Knowledge of the basic hearing processes, therefore, is a fundamental need to improving hearing aid fitting skills.

SUMMARY

Understanding the physical characteristics of sounds includes awareness of a vibratory source which displaces particles within a medium (air), with each particle imparting to adjacent particles a motion coincidental with the vibrating source. Such motion produces a wave form having a compression and rarefaction portion. The resulting sound waves can be said to have frequency and intensity (amplitude) which correlates to subjective sensations of pitch and loudness. The receptor of these sound pressure changes, the human auditory system, is a unique anatomical, neurological and physiological sensory organ. Its description includes the classical division of outer, middle and inner ear structures, as well as the complicated ascending auditory pathways which terminate in the auditory cortex of the brain.

Pathologies of the auditory system can and do interfere with the normal sequences giving rise to the understanding of speech and other acoustic signals.

Hearing aid specialists, as members of the hearing health profession, are encouraged to become acquainted with the contents of this chapter to better understand the complicated sensory apparatus with which they are working.

GLOSSARY

Acoustic Referring to having the physical properties of sound.

Afferent fibers Sensory nerves which carry information inwards for the peripheral sensory organ of Corti to the brain along the ascending pathways of the auditory system.

Air conduction The process by which wound is conducted to the inner ear through the air in the ear canal and via the three bones (ossicles) in the middle ear.

Amplitude The instantaneous value of varying parameters (e.G. sound pressure of a sound wave) at any given time.

Audiogram A graph depicting hearing threshold level at various frequencies.

Audiometer An instrument which measures hearing ability relative to that of normal hearing persons.

Auditory cortex Termination in the temporal lobe of the auditory pathways; the locus where speech recognition, language concepts and meaning are mediated.

Auditory nerve The eighth cranial nerve consisting of fibers which conduct the neural firings from the cochlea to the brain.

Basilar membrane The membrane in the cochlea which vibrates in response to sound, separates the scala media from the scala tympani and supports the organ of Corti.

Bel A unit or level which expresses the logarithm to the base 10 of the ratio of two quantities.

Binaural Pertaining to listening with two ears or two hearing aids.

Binaural fusion The production of one central percept from two independent signals incident at each ear.

Critical band The range of frequencies beyond which noise will not further mask a sinusoid within the same frequency range.

Dichotic Listening with each ear to a different signal.

Difference limen The smallest just-noticeable difference produced by a change in a stimulus. (e.g. intensity of frequency change).

Diffraction The bending of waves around obstacles-e.g. sound waves producing head diffraction.

Equal loudness contour Sound pressure level as a function of frequency required to elicit an acoustic sensation equal to the reference frequency of 1000Hz.

Filter A device that allows energy at some frequencies to pass and discriminates against energy at other frequencies.

Formant Concentration of energy in a sound spectrum produced by resonances in a speaker's vocal tract during speech production.

Fourier analysis Separating a complex waveform into a sum of sinusoids (pure tones).

Frequency The number of complete repetitions of a waveform occurring per unit time (e.g. cycles per second of Hz).

Hair cells Sensory receptors for hearing located within the organ of Corti and attached to neurons.

Impedance The ratio of a force-type quantity to a velocity-type quantity (e.g. force to velocity is acoustic ohms).

Intensity A quantity expressing the amount of sound (e.g. pressure, power, level or amplitude).

Loudness level The perceived loudness of a sound expressed in phons (re: sound pressure level of equal loudness 1kHz pure tone).

Malleus The outermost of the three ossicles in the middle ear.

Masking The process by which the threshold of audibility for one sound is raised by the presence of another sound or sounds.

Middle ear An air filled chamber located within the mastoid process of the temporal bone that contains the three ossicles.

Monaural Pertaining to listening with only one ear or one hearing aid.

Noise Any unwanted sound within a useful frequency band.

Organ of Corti A series of receptor hair cells for hearing and their underlying supporting structures.

Phase The fractional part of a periodic signal through which the waveform has advanced relative to some specified point in time.

Phon Unit of loudness level measurement.

Pitch The subjective auditory sensation correlating to frequency which expresses where on the musical scale (e.g. high or low) a sound is located.

Pressure A measure of force per unit area (e.g. sound pressure).

Pure tone A sound wave whose amplitude versus time course follows a sinusoidal function.

Recruitment Abnormal growth of loudness as sound intensity is increased which results in a restricted dynamic range.

Sensation level The level of a sound in decibels relative to the threshold level for that sound for that listener.

Sensorineural hearing loss Impairment of hearing occurring as a result of damage to the cochlea.

Sinusoidal A waveform whose amplitude versus time variation follows the course of a sinusoid function.

Sone A unit of loudness for a sound relative to a loudness level of 40 phon.

Sound Produced by a variation in pressure, particle displacement or velocity.

Sound pressure level The level of sound in decibels relative to a reference level of 20uPa.

Spectrum level The amplitude of a signal contained in a given unit bandwidth as a function of frequency.

Tuning curve A plot of the lowest sound pressure level at which a single nerve fiber will resound.

REFERENCES

ALLEN, J., HALL, J. and JENG, P. (1990): Loudness growth in 1/2-octave bands (LGOB) - a procedure for the assessment of loudness, Journal of Acoustical Society of America, 88(2): 745–753.

BARFOD, J. (1979): Speech perception process and fitting of hearing aids, Audiology 18:430–441.

BECK, O. (1978): The effect of dichotic amplification on the speech discrimination scores of hearing-impaired subjects, Ph.D. dissertation, University of Maryland, Dept. of Comm. Dis. College Park.

BEKESY, G. V. (1960): Experiments in Hearing, McGraw-Hill, New York.

BERGER, E. and KERRIVAN, J., (1983): Influence of physiological noise and the occlusion effect on the measurements of real ear attenuation at threshold, Journal Acoustical Society of America, 74: 81–94.

BERLAND, O. (1975): No-mold fitting of hearing aids, Scand. Aud., Suppl 5, 177–179.

BODDEN, M. (1993): Modeling human sound-source localization and the cocktail-party-effect, Acta Acustica, 1: 43–55.

CARHART, R. (1965): Monaural and binaural discrimination against competing sentences, International Audiology, 4, 5–10.

DE JONGH, H. (1977): Which stimulus transform controls firing probability of an auditory nerve fibre? In Psychophysics and Physiology of Hearing, ed. EVANS and WILSON.

DUBNO, J., DIRKS, D., and MORGAN, D. (1984): Effects of age and mild hearing loss on speech recognition in noise, J. Acoust. Soc. of Amer., 76: 87–96.

DUIFUIS, H. (1974): A crude quantitative theory of backward masking, in Facts and Models in Hearing, ed ZWICKER and TERHARDT, Springer-Verlag, N.Y., 275–284.

DURLACH, N. (1972): Binaural signal detection: Equalization and cancellation theory, in Foundations of modern auditory theory, V. II, ed. TOBIAS, J., Academic Press, New York.

EDGERTON, B. and KLODD, D. (1977): Occlusion effect in bone conduction tone and speech audiometry, Journal of American Auditory Society: 151–158.

FECHNER, (1860): Elemente der Psychophysik.

FEDDERSEN, W., SANDEL, T., TEAS, D., JEFFRESS, L. (1957): Localization of high-frequency tones. J. Acoust. Soc. Am., 29:988–991.

FLETCHER, H. (1953): Speech and Hearing in Communication, Van Nostrand, New York, 188.

FLETCHER, H. and MUNSON, W. (1933): Loudness: its definition, measurement, and calculation. J. Acoust. Soc. Am. 5:82–108.

FRANKLIN, B. (1975): The effect of combining low and high-frequency passbands on consonant recognition in the hearing impaired.

GABOR, D. (1947): Acoustical quanta and the theory of hearing, Nature, 159, 591–594.

GAO, S., SULLIVAN, J., JAYARAMAN, S., AND SOLI, S. (1994): Method for fitting binaural hearing aids, paper 51PP5 pres. at 127th Acoustical Soc. of Amer. Mtg, Cambridge, MA.

GELFAND, S., PIPER, N., and SLLMAN, S. (1985): Consonant recognition in quiet as a function of aging among normal hearing subjects, J. Acoust. SOc. of Amer.., 78:1198–1206.

GIEBEL, A and EKKEHARD, R. (1992): Screening infants and children by means of TEOAE, Hearing Journal, 45, 11: 25.

GORGA, M., NEELY, S., BERGMAN, B., BEAUCHAINE, K., KAMINSKI, J., PETERS, J., SCHULTE, L., and JESTEADT, W. (1993). A comparison of transient evoked and distortion product otoacoustic emissions in normal-hearing and hearing-impaired subjects, Journal of the Acoustical Society of America, 94: 2639–2648.

HALL, J. (1992): Otoacoustic emissions: the audiologic test procedure of the 1990's, Hearing Journal, 45, 11: 7.

HELFER, K. and WILBER, L. (1990): Hearing loss, aging, and speech perception in reverberation and noise, J. Speech and Hearing Research, 33:149–155.

HORNING, J. (1975): Tympanometry and hearing aid selection, Hearing Aid Journal, 28, 6:8.

JOHANSEN, H. (1948): Relation of audiograms to the impedance formula, Acta Otolaryng, Suppl, 74:65.

KEITH, R, (1976): An acoustic reflex technique of establishing hearing aid settings, Paper presented at Amer. Sp. & Hear. Assoc. Conv, Houston.

KHANNA, S., TONNDORF, J. and QUELLER, J. (1976): Mechanical parameters of hearing by bone conduction, Journal of Acoustical Society of America, 60:139–154.

KILLION, M. (1976): Eardrum pressure at absolute threshold: where is the "missing 6dB?", paper QQ3 and 92nd Mtg of Acoust. Soc. Am., San Diego, CA.

KILLION, M., WILBER, L., and GUDMUNDSEN, G. (1988): Zwislocki was right . . . , Hearing Instruments, 39, 1: 14–18.

KOLLMEIER, B. PEISSIG, J. and HOHMANN, V. (1993): Real-time multiband dynamic compression and noise reduction for binaural hearing aids, Journal of Rehabilitation Research and Development, 30, 1:82–84.

MARTIN, E., and PICKETT, J. (1970): Sensorineural hearing loss and upward spread of masking. J. Sp. Hear. Res, 13: 426–437.

MCCANDLESS, G. and MILLER D. (1972): Loudness discomfort and hearing aids, Hear. Aid J., 25, 8:7.

MOLLER, A. (1965): An experimental study of the acoustic impedance of the middle ear and its transmission properties, Acta Otolar, 60:129–149.

MOORE, B. (1982): An introduction to the Psychology of Hearing, Academic Press, London.

MUSIEK, F. (1983): The evaluation of brainstem disorders using ABR and central auditory tests, *Monographs in Contemporary Audiology.* 4, 2, Instrumentation Associates, Upper Darby, PA, 8–9.

NABELEK, A (1982): Temporal distortions and noise considerations, The Vanderbilt Report, Ed. Studebaker and Bess, Upper Darby, PA, 51–59.

NABALEK, A. and ROBINSON, P. (1982): Monaural and binaural speech perception in reverberation for listeners of various ages, J. Acoust. Soc. of Amer., 71: 1242–1248.

NELSON, D. (1990): Frequency resolution and temporal resolution in hearing impaired listeners, paper pres. at Lake Arrowhead Conference, Lake Arrowhead, CA.

NOZZO, R. and SABO, D. (1992): Transiently evoked OAE for screening schoolage children, Hearing Journal, 45, 11: 29–31.

OLSEN, W. and CARHART, R. (1967): Development of test procedures for evaluation of binaural hearing aids, Bull. Prost. Res., Spring.

OSTERHAMMEL, P. and RASMUSSEN, A. (1992): Distortion product otoacoustic emissions: basic properties and clinical aspects, Hearing Journal, 45, 11:38.

PARKER, F. (1977): Distinctive features and acoustic cues, J. Acoust. Soc. Am, 62, 4:1051–1054.

PFEIFFER, R. (1971): A model for two-tone inhibition of single cochlear-nerve fibers, J. Acoust. Soc. Am., 48:6, 2, 1373–1378.

PICKLES, J. (1982): An Introduction to the Physiology of Hearing, Academic Press, London.

PLOMP, R. (1978): Auditory handicap of hearing impairment and the limited benefit of hearing aids, J. Acoust. Soc. Am., 63:533–549.

RAINVILLE, M. (1976): Impedance measurements in evaluation of hearing aid performance, Hear. Inst., 27, 11–39.

RAPPAPORT, B. and TAIT, C. (1976): Acoustic reflex threshold measurements in hearing aid selection, Arch. Otol., Mar., 102, 129–132.

RIESZ, R. R. (1928): Differential intensity sensitivity of the ear for pure tones. Phys. Rev. 31, 867–875.

ROBINETTE, M. (1992): Otoacoustic emissions in cochlear vs. retrocochlear auditory dysfunction, Hearing Journal, 45, 11:32.

SCHARF, B. (1978): Comparison of normal and impaired hearing II. Frequency analysis, speech perception, in Sensorineural Hearing Impairment and Hearing Aids, eds. LUDVIGSEN and BARFOD, Scan. Audiol. Suppl., 6:90–93.

SCHMITZ, H. (1969): Loudness discomfort level modification J. Acoust. Soc. Am., 12:807–817.

SIEBERT, W. (1970): Frequency discrimination in the auditory system: place or periodicity mechanisms:, Proc. of IEEE, 58,5, May.

SKINNER, M. (1980): Speech intelligibility in noise-induced hearing loss; effects of high frequency compensation, J. Acoust. Soc. Am., 67–306–317.

SMALL, A. (1978): Elements of hearing Science—a programmed text, Wiley & Sons, New York.

STAAB, W. and FINLAY, B. (1991): A fitting rationale for deep fitting canal hearing instruments, Hearing Instruments, 42, 1: 6–10.8.

STEVENS, S. (1951): Mathematics, measurement, and psychophysics, in Handbook of Experimental Psychology, ed. Steens, Wiley & Sons, New York.

TONNDORF, J. (1962): Compressional bone conduction in cochlear models, J. Acoust. Soc. Am., 34:1127–1132.

VAN ROOIJ and PLOMP, R., 1990: Auditive and cognitive factors in speech perception by elderly listeners. II: multivariate analyses, J. Acoust. Soc. Am., 88, 6, 2611–2624.

WIMMER, V. (1986): The occlusion effect from earmolds, Hearing Instruments, 12: 19.

WIENER, F. and ROSS, D. (1946): The pressure distribution in the auditory canal in a progressive sound field. J. Acoust. Soc. Am., 18,2, 401–407.

YOST, W., WICHTMAN, F., GREEN, D. (1971): Lateralization of filtered clicks, J. Acoust. Soc. Am., 50:1526–1531.

ZWISLOCKI, J., (1953): ACOUSTIC ATTENUATION BETWEEN THE EARS, JOURNAL OF THE ACOUSTICAL SOCIETY OF AMERICA, 25: 752–759.

II

AUDIOMETRIC ASSESSMENT AND INTERPRETATION

ROBERT L. MARTIN, Ph.D.

INTRODUCTION

The hearing aid specialist of years past usually limited the hearing test to a puretone, air-conducted threshold measurement done in the client's home. Now, the hearing aid professional has many different tests and many sophisticated instruments. This new diagnostic and prognostic technology helps us make better hearing measurements in less time. The end result is more successful hearing aid fittings. The new diagnostic tools measure ear drum mobility, test hearing with and without hearing aids, analyze the acoustic output of hearing aids, measure battery life, and many other tests. Hearing-aid-testing instruments are changing hearing aid fitting procedures and aiding in the decision-making process.

The improved instrumentation has advanced our understanding of the normal and pathological auditory system. The improved instrumentation can generate a complete information base that the hearing aid specialist can interpret to better serve the client's needs.

CHAPTER OBJECTIVES

The purpose of this chapter is to review the diagnostic, prognostic, and verification tests used to evaluate a client's hearing ability. Basic and advanced tests are discussed. Interpretation and use of the test data are discussed in detail.

The chapter outlines a sequence which a client may go through in being evaluated and fitted with hearing instruments. Hearing tests and data interpretation are discussed.

TOUR OF A HEARING AID OFFICE

The purpose of this tour is to acquaint the reader with the different procedures and types of clinical equipment employed in audiometric assessment and interpretation.

First is the waiting room. Many diplomas and certificates are displayed for the client's inspection. These documents help reassure the client of the hearing aid specialist's professional competence and experience.

Next is the front desk where a receptionist greets the clients and helps them fill out necessary information forms. This area contains patient files, photocopy machine, computer and printer, typewriter, supply of hearing aid batteries, telephones, and work stations. The computer's software includes a data base and word processing software needed for mailings and communication.

Next is the consultation room where one initially talks with the client, obtains pertinent history, and establishes initial rapport. This room contains an otoscope for inspecting ears and a listening tube for checking hearing aids. Hearing aid battery testers and batter drain meters are located here. This area also houses the hearing aid test unit and real-ear system. These instruments are used to evaluate the acoustic output of the hearing aid.

Our next area is the hearing test suite or sound treated room containing the audiometer, impedance screener (also called immittance screener) and associated equipment. The audiometer generates the controls different acoustic signals used to test hearing. Signals from the audiometer are routed to the sound booth where the client is placed during the test. Signals from the audiometer are routed to the sound booth where the client is placed during the test. The audiometer is used to test the client's ability to hear pure-tones and understand selected words. The audiometer generates a calibrated noise called masking. Masking noise is used to preclude one ear from helping the other ear during specific hearing tests.

Next to the audiometer on a rolling cart is the impedance/immittance screener. This unit is used to conduct middle ear tests. These tests are painless and can be done quickly. Basic impedance/immittance tests include ear drum mobility and acoustic reflexes. Other impedance/immittance tests are available, if desired or indicated.

Next is a consultation room where there is a master hearing aid unit and sound field equipment. The master hearing aid unit is a powerful fitting and demonstration tool; it simulates how a person hears with hearing aids. The master hearing aid unit can be adjusted for gain, slope of the frequency response, maximum power output (MPO), and automatic gain control (AGC). The sound field instruments assist in measuring the client's response to sound with and without hearing aid amplification.

Next is the laboratory. This room contains a hearing aid repair facility, and machinery for sanding, cutting, drilling, polishing and modifying ear molds and hearing aids. A work bench is located along one wall. A dental lathe is on the bench. Behind the lathe is a vacuum unit that removes the plastic dust created during the earmold or hearing aid modification process. Use of the vacuum precludes inhaling toxic substances. There is also a cabinet containing batteries, new hearing aids, and a supply of loaner hearing instruments. Spare parts for many models of hearing aids are stocked here.

The last room is the hearing aid specialist's office. Chairs, desk, FAX machine, and telephone allow this room to function as a multipurpose room. The room also houses another computer, printer, and the software needed for word processing and business management.

CLIENT MANAGEMENT SEQUENCES

The following sequence is recommended for effective client management:

1. A telephone appointment is made for the client and a family member.
2. The client and a family member come to an appointed time and complete the intake form.
3. The client and family member are taken to the consultation room where a complete history is obtained.
4. The client's ears are visually examined with a fiber-optic otoscope.

5. Hearing aids, if used by the client, are checked for proper acoustic function.
6. The hearing tests are explained briefly.
7. The client and family member are taken to the hearing testing room. The test sequence is: SRT, aid conduction, MCL, UCL, word recognition, impedance/immittance tests, and bone conduction.
8. The client and family member are returned to the consultation room and function-ability tests are given.
9. If additional client history is needed, it is obtained at this time.
10. The results of the hearing tests are explained.
11. The client is counseled about the benefits of amplification, if hearing aids are indicated.
12. Commitments are obtained from the client. (A) Yes, I have a hearing loss. (B) Yes, the loss is a problem in my life. (C) Yes, I want to hear better.
13. The need for binaural amplification is presented, unless contraindicated by test results.
14. Master hearing aid tests are done to measure use gain, slope, and MPO and to demonstrate the benefits of wearing hearing aids.
15. Ear impressions are taken.
16. The client is referred to a physician specializing in the treatment of the ear-nose-and-throat (ENT) for a medical clearance, unless prior clearance has been obtained or a medical waiver is executed.
17. The next appointment is scheduled and the hearing instruments ordered.
18. The quality of the instruments is checked before the client is called.
19. The instruments are fitted. The client is counseled about batteries, maintenance and care, telephone usage, insertion and removal, use of controls on the instruments, and possible problems.
20. The hearing aid test system is used to set the volume at a comfortable level. The volume setting (use gain) is marked on the aid for the client's future reference.
21. The client's aided hearing is tested to insure adequate gain at appropriate frequencies. This evaluation also shows how

much better the client is hearing with appropriate hearing aid amplification.

22. Clients who have problems hearing in competing noise are evaluated with other hearing aid evaluation protocols.
23. Clients who respond poorly to the initial hearing aid fitting are scheduled for advanced diagnostic and prognostic evaluations.

CLIENT EVALUATION AND CARE CHART

Client's evaluation and hearing aid fitting sequences are outlined in Figure 1. Initially, the hearing aid specialist listens to the client's problems, obtains history, examines the client's ears, and listens to the client's hearing aids through a listening tube.

Next, the hearing aid specialist assesses the problem and decides what is needed to best compensate for the hearing loss. This is called formulating the hypothesis. The tests that are needed come from: (1) basic diagnostic tests, (2) prognostic hearing aid tests, (3) verification tests, or (4) advanced diagnostic and prognostic tests. The selection of the specific test is made based on the client's need.

After the test data are generated, the problem is analyzed again and the hearing aid specialist will decide if amplification is needed. The disposition might include consulting with a technician at the hearing aid factory, or, studying the published hearing aid performance specification sheets.

After the disposition, a plan is developed to resolve the problem as efficiently as possible. This may include making another ear impression, altering the hearing aid response, or instructing the client about the correct use of hearing aid amplification.

The final evaluation is the point at which procedures previously done are rechecked and clinical notes are added to the client's records. The client is then rescheduled, if necessary.

THE HOUSE OF HEARING ANALOGY

INTENSITY, FREQUENCY AND TIME

The auditory system functions within three dimensions: intensity (soft to loud), frequency (bass to treble), and time (instantaneous to delayed). Normal hearing is so sensitive that one can hear the faint sound of a mosquito. The hearing system has such exquisite

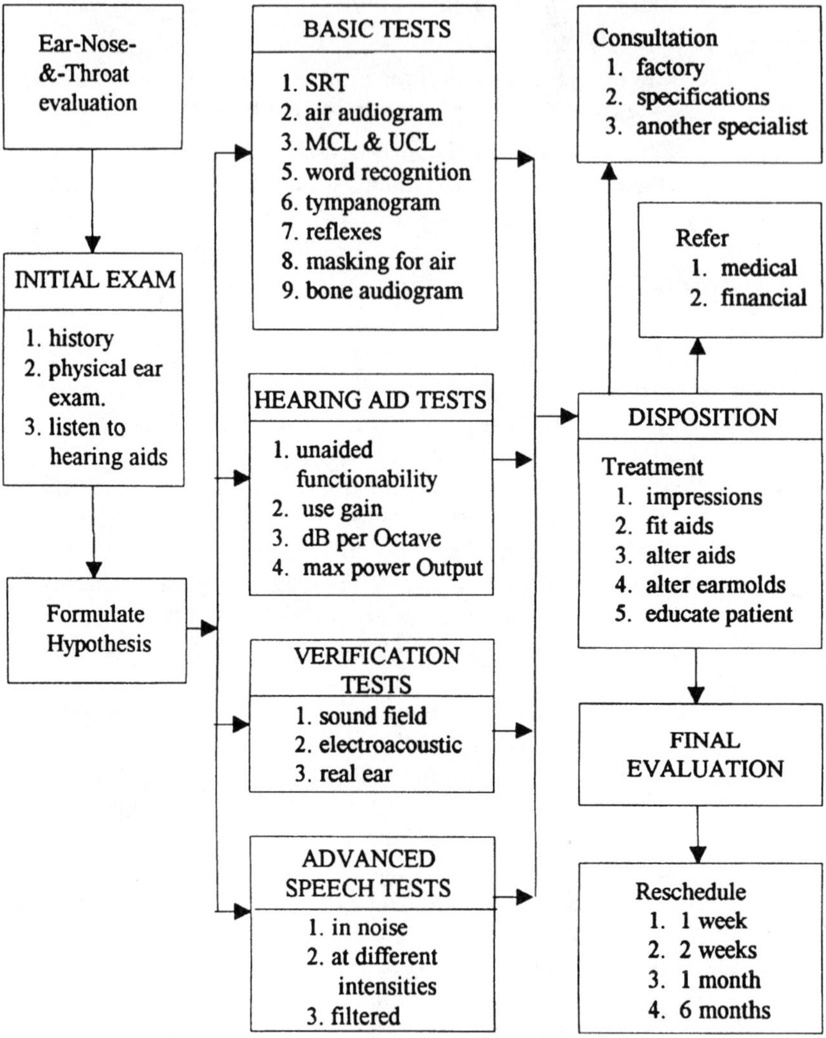

Fig. 1. The patient evaluation, fitting, and follow-up care sequence.

frequency fidelity that one can hear a high frequency squeak occurring ten-thousand times per second and the low frequency rumble of a jet five miles away. Normally, we hear sound in one ear a few thousandths of a second earlier than the same sound in the other ear. This information is used by our brains to locate the sound source.

Hearing loss alters the ears' response to loudness, pitch, and temporal processes. These changes need to be discussed in a straight forward, yet technical manner. The author has developed the following analogy to aid in the understanding of normal and pathological hearing conditions. The analogy is called the House of Hearing. As the name implies, our hearing has all the structures of a standard house.

Terminology such as hearing floor, hearing ceiling, hearing walls, is not intended to replace the conventional terms of threshold sensitivity, uncomfortable listening levels, etc. The analogy is presented here to help one learn the many different aspects of human hearing.

Figure 2 illustrates the three dimensions of hearing; volume or intensity, frequency or pitch, and time or temporality. We can understand these dimensions if we consider the analogous functions of a house.

Figure 3 shows the three variables making up the house. Frequency is shown across the front. Time is displayed along the side. Intensity is indicated between the floor and ceiling.

THE ANALOGY

1. The Foundation

Just as with the foundation of a real house, the foundation of the House of Hearing is the most important, yet most hidden of all the structure. The foundation supports and strengthens the entire struc-

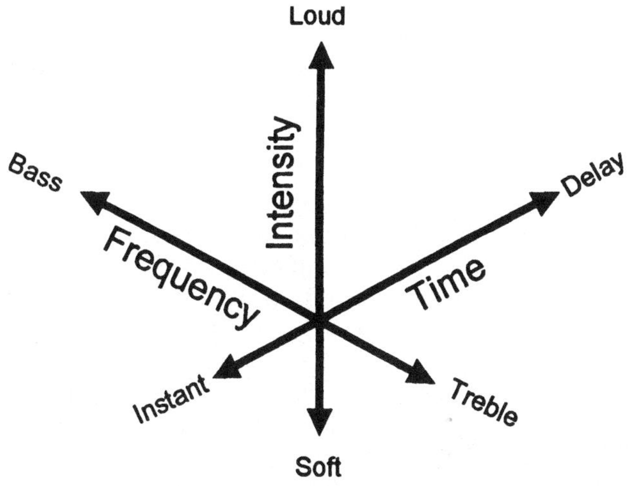

Fig. 2. The three parameters of hearing: frequency, intensity, and time.

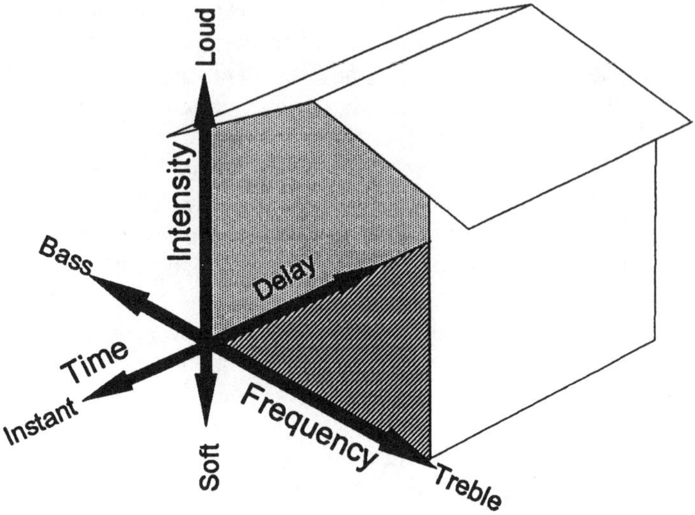

Fig. 3. The three variables of hearing in the House of Hearing analogy.

ture and defines its size, shape, and quality. The foundation is the professional understanding and appreciation of the client's personality, problems, expectations and experiences, especially as these relate to obtaining and using hearing aids. The foundation anchors the house in place, secure against the winds of stress and the tremors of crisis. (See Figure 4).

2. *The Hearing Floor*

The floor is that part of a house with which we have almost continuous contact. We know instinctively where to expect a level floor and where to expect a step up or step down. When an unexpected bunching of a rug or a misplaced piece of furniture gets in our way, we may stumble or fall.

The floor in the House of Hearing is the threshold at which a person just begins to hear sounds and words. The threshold of sensitivity for persons with normal hearing remains level and unchanged. These people do not fumble with misunderstood words. It is the floor that changes the most in many hearing losses.

Hard of hearing people stumble over the unevenness of their floor of hearing because they may hear only part of spoken words. They may fall down emotionally and have great difficulty getting back on their feet. Because they know they can no longer trust their hearing floor, they may suspect the entire structure is decayed and may despair of ever hearing well again.

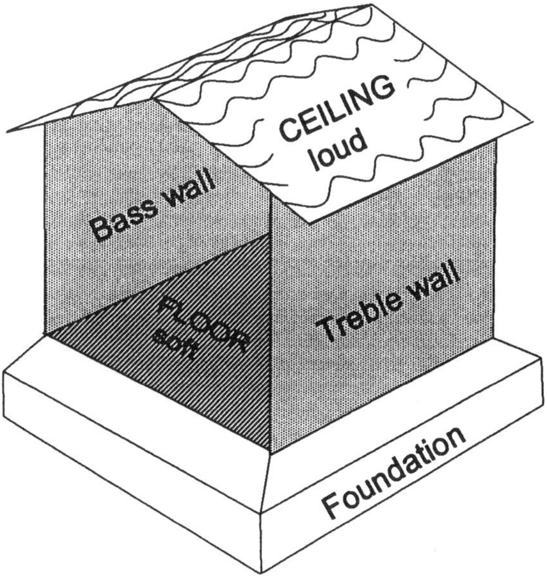

Fig. 4. The House of Hearing analogy. The foundation is client understanding. The floor is the threshold of hearing or soft hearing. The left wall is bass hearing ability. The right wall is treble hearing ability. The ceiling is uncomfortable levels of hearing or loud hearing.

3. The Hearing Ceiling

The ceiling of a house limits the vertical space available for free comfortable movement. Where the vertical space becomes less, the lack of free erect movement makes us uncomfortable and quickly tires us.

The ceiling represents the uncomfortable listening level, or the point of overload of the auditory system. If we get too close to the roof we quickly tire and complain of sounds being too loud. Instead of free movement around the house, we are cramped into a small range of hearing volume that hinders the movement and spaciousness of our hearing ability.

4. The Side Walls

Side walls help determine the amount of space within a house. The greater the distance between the walls, the more space within the room. The closer the walls are placed together, the more restrictive and limiting the available space becomes. Each side wall is independent of the opposite wall; thus, one wall can be short and the other tall.

The side walls represent lower and upper frequency limits. The left wall is the bass or lower frequency limit. The right wall is the treble or upper frequency limit. In normal hearing, side walls are tall and widely spaced. Hearing loss usually produces more deterioration in the treble or upper wall than in the lower or bass wall. The side walls act independently of each other both in normal and abnormal hearing.

Hearing aid amplification can be adjusted in the treble, mid, or bass regions. Adjustments in the amplification of the left side wall—lower frequency or bass—may influence the amount the client hears his own voice. This wall also strongly influences the amount of background noise heard through the hearing aid.

5. The Front and Back Walls

The front of a house is usually the appealing side of the house. The style of the house is most prominently embodied in this wall.

The front and back walls represent time. The front wall is instantaneous time, i.e., zero time delay. The back wall represent the milliseconds of **abnormal** time delay. It takes about 60 milliseconds for the normal ear to conduct sound from the outer ear canal to the brain. In the normal hearing system, no time influencing distortions are present to diminish correct interpretation of the auditory event.

Hearing aids can interfere with the time/intensity function. The electrical activities of some amplifiers change the way sound passes from the ear to the brain. An example of these time (temporal) influences is the action of automatic gain control (AGC) circuits. The attack time of an AGC circuit is that time required for the instrument to sense and reduce (to some desired level) the intensity of an overly loud sound. The release time of an AGC circuit is the time required for the instrument to return to normal posture following the cessation of the loud sound.

Like houses that differ in front and back wall styles, hearing aids differ in their influence on the amount of time needed to process the signal. Linear amplifiers have no AGC function and therefore create no significant change in temporal processing. AGC hearing aids influence temporal processing. Some hearing aid amplifiers allow distortion in time to increase the space available in the intensity domain.

6. The Vertical Space

The distance from the floor to the ceiling defines the headroom within a living space. The smaller this distance, the harder it is to function within the room. Measuring the amount of ver-

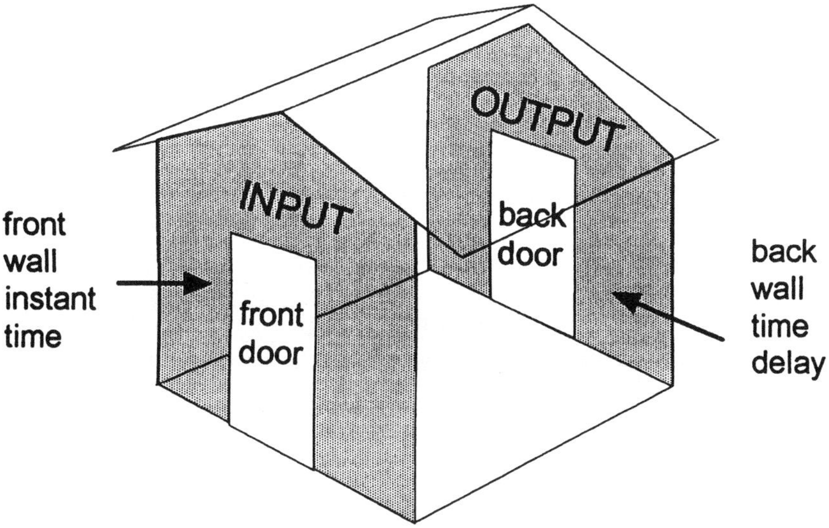

Fig. 5. The House of Hearing analogy. The front wall is instant time. The back wall is time delay. The front door is signal input. The back door is output.

tical space within a room is a prerequisite to planning the efficient use of the space.

The distance between softness (hearing thresholds) and loudness (uncomfortable listening levels, UCLs) is called the dynamic range of hearing, as shown in Figure 6. Figures 6 and 41 contain the same information. In Figure 6 the client's hearing ability for soft sounds (hearing thresholds) is indicated with Xs. The client's uncomfortable listening levels (hearing of loud sounds) are indicated with "ucl" marks. The space between these two lines is the "living space" or the dynamic range of hearing.

It is important to measure the dynamic range of hearing before selecting hearing aids. Many hard-of-hearing people are unable to hear soft sounds, yet they cannot tolerate loud sounds. This adverse reaction to loud sounds suggests a narrow dynamic range. People with this type of hearing problem can be helped. However, it is critically important that accurate clinical measurements are made and appropriate hearing aid amplifiers are selected.

7. The Quality of Space

Most houses have warm cheerful spaces for living. Carefully organized spaces within our homes provide room for comfortable living. Space without light, ventilation, and structural support is nonusable, or greatly limited in use.

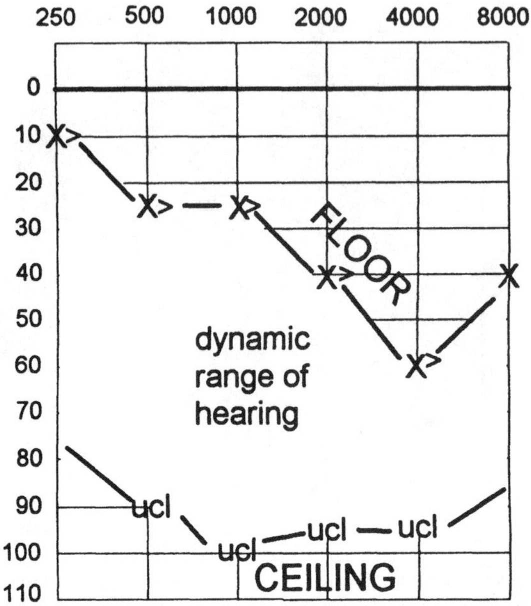

Fig. 6. The space between hearing threshold and uncomfortable listening level, UCL, is the dynamic range of hearing.

The quality of space for the normal ear is excellent and highly functional. Quality is measured by function; "How easily can a mother talk to her children?". "Does the mother have to interrupt the conversation and repeatedly ask the child what was said?"

The quality of space is measured with word recognition tests. Words are presented and the client repeats what was heard. Speech understanding tests can be administered through many different instruments for many different reasons. The ultimate goal of these tests is to find out how well the hearing aid specialist can make an impaired client hear with the use of hearing aid devices. The greater the impairment, the greater the need for diagnostic and rehabilitative procedures. Poor word recognition scores often suggest the need for adjustments in gain, slope, AGC, and distortion. Poor word understanding ability often can be converted into better understanding ability with improvement in the hearing aid performance.

8. The Front and Back Door

People enter a house through the front door. The House of Hearing has the entrance in the front wall. This is at the input stage of the hearing aid (the microphone). The back door is the output stage of the instrument, the receiver or speaker.

Sound control by the hearing aid is sometimes activated at the front door, (input compression), the back door (output compression), or both. In this analogy, an input compressor would squeeze or shorten everyone as they enter the front door, while an output compressor would squeeze or shorten everyone as they exit the back door. The input and output functions are displayed in Figure 5.

The House of Hearing analogy is summarized in appendix A.

HEARING ARCHITECTURE

If our client's hearing is defective, we want to build a highly successful hearing correction framework. As the client's hearing of soft and loud sounds has changed, we need data concerning the floor and ceiling of the amplifiers we will use. To the extent our client's hearing of different tones and frequency bands has changed, we need information about the "walls," that is, we need to adjust acoustic filters that influence hearing aid frequency response (amount of amplification in the bass and treble). The foundation of our entire hearing aid fitting process must be an empathetic understanding of the client's personality, experiences, problems, and expectations. The hearing aid specialist conducts hearing tests to create adequate function in the client's hearing by rebuilding the architecture of hearing.

THE PATHWAY OF HEARING

The pathway of hearing is a teaching technique used to describe the transfer of sound from the outside world, through the ear, to the human brain. Figures 7–9 introduce the normal pathway of hearing through the outer-middle-and-inner ear.

Figure 7 is a basic diagram of the human ear. The outer ear is a tube, open on the outside of the body and closed by the eardrum. The middle ear is normally a closed space that contains the middle-ear bones. The Eustachian tube connects the middle ear to the throat and maintains normal air pressure in the middle ear. The middle ear bones, called ossicles, and Eustachian tube are shown in this figure, but omitted from similar figures in this chapter. The inner ear is illustrated as a coil.

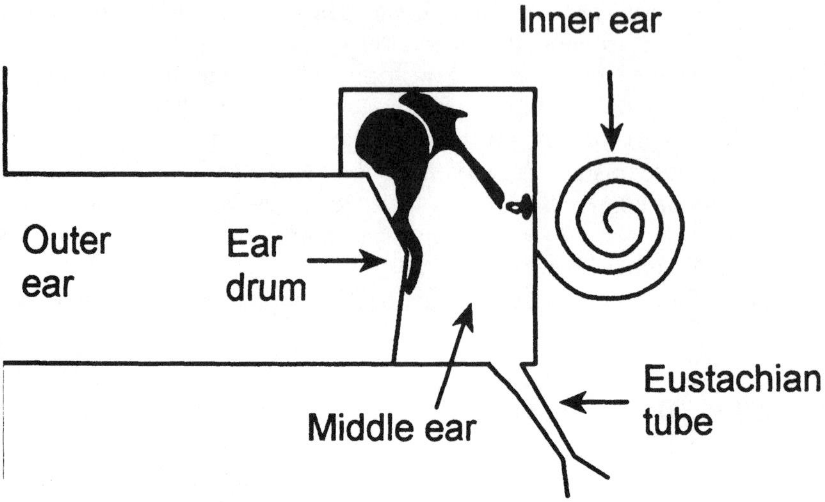

Fig. 7. Schematic of the human ear. Outer ear is shown as an open rectangle. Middle ear is a closed rectangle. Inner ear is a coil.

Figure 8 illustrates a typical hearing testing situation. The earphone emits a test signal that passes through the outer and middle ear, into the inner ear. The sound waves produced by the earphone are shown as a sinusoid. This pathway of hearing is the air-conduction path.

Figure 9 shows an overhead view of both ears during a typical hearing test. The earphone on the left ear is presenting a test signal.

AUDIOMETRIC ASSESSMENT

Figure 11 illustrates audiometric tests that assess different parts of the auditory system. Note that the outer and middle ear can be evaluated by: (1) air and bone conduction; (2) otoscopy; (3) tympanomentry and acoustic reflex tests; and (4) uncomfortable loudness level (UCL) test. This overlap of tests for a single part of the ear greatly improves diagnostic capabilities and test redundancy reduces errors.

An ear that looks normal by casual inspection might have otosclerosis, a hardening of the middle ear bone (stapes) fitting into the oval window. Since the ear drum appears normal, one might incorrectly assume there is a sensorineural hearing loss. A high level UCL might provide a clue suggesting that the ear has a conductive loss component, just as absent reflexes might indicate con-

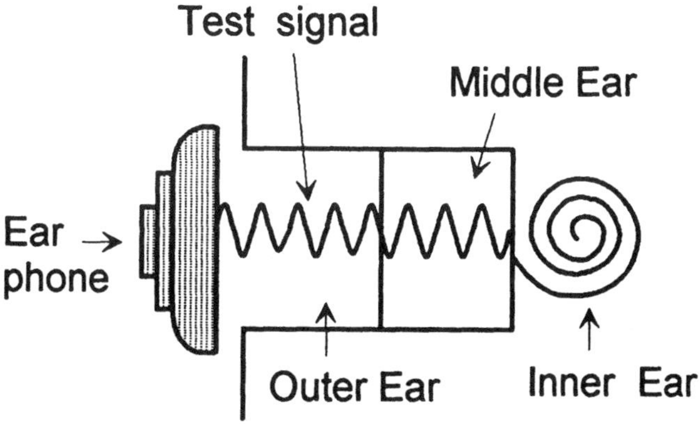

Fig. 8. The test signal goes from the earphone to the outer and middle ear into the inner ear. The test signal is shown as a sinusoid line. This pathway is the air-conduction path.

ductive involvement. An air-bone gap would also direct one's thinking concerning the appropriate circuits to be employed.

The hearing aid specialist must not interpret test data to the client in a way that seems like a medical diagnosis. The physician is the only professional licensed to give a diagnosis. Some tests are easy to learn to do correctly, while others are difficult to do and interpret. Tests such as electronystagmography, brain stem audiom-

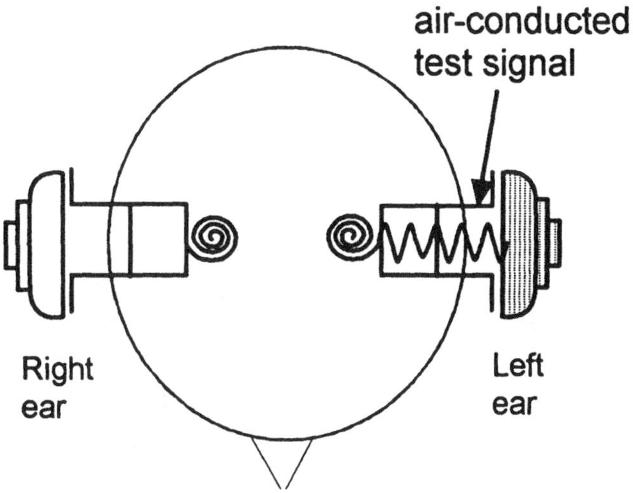

Fig. 9. An overhead view of both ears. The patient is wearing earphones. An air-conducted test signal is presented to the left ear.

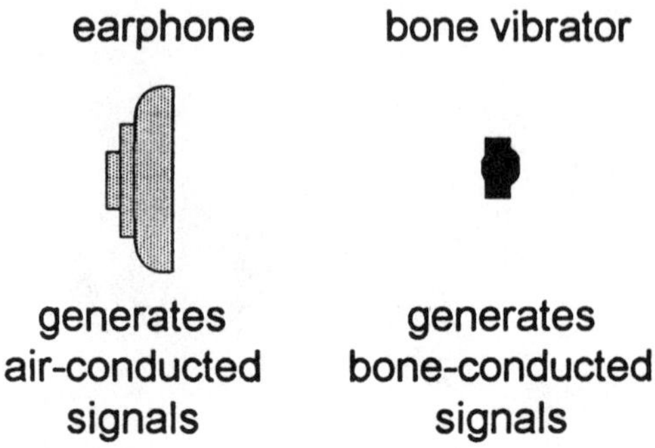

Fig. 10. Test signals are presented via earphones (air conducted signals) and a bone vibrator (bone conducted signals).

etry, and masked bone conduction procedures may require years of study and considerable skill to administer.

There are many hearing tests used as part of a hearing aid fitting. The author recommends the use of those tests that produce the most useful information. The tests selected should be time efficient and include redundancy to guarantee testing correctness. The data produced is used to predict the performance characteristics needed in the hearing aid system. Each test discussed in this chapter was selected for its ability to generate usable information. This information forms the framework of the hearing aid specification which may include power, pitch, and other parameters of the amplifier.

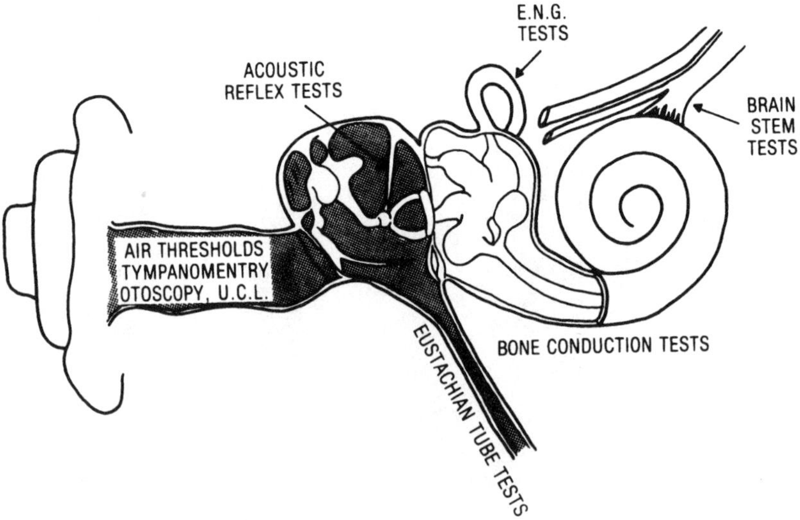

Fig. 11. Numerous tests are used to evaluate each part of the ear.

TEST RELIABILITY AND VALIDITY

Reliability and validity are important in testing. Reliability means repeatability. This is, results obtained at one office can be duplicated at another. Audiometric testing shows good reliability as long as standard tests are conducted using calibrated equipment in suitable test environments.

Validity suggests truth. Tests are valid if they truly represent the client's hearing function. For example, if the client has a total hearing loss in one ear and normal hearing in the other, audiometric tests must be able to prevent the good ear from responding when the bad ear is tested. Invalid measurements might suggest moderate-to-severe hearing loss in the bad ear, where in fact, the ear is dead. Hearing aid specialists must be able to obtain reliable and valid measurements.

THE FOUNDATION: THE HEARING HISTORY

We obtain the client's medical history before the audiometric evaluation to determine which tests are necessary. We need information regarding hearing problems and ear pathology. Pertinent questions often include the topics of tinnitus, vertigo, history of noise exposure, sudden hearing loss, otitis, history of ear surgery, previous hearing aid use, eardrum perforations, history of excessive cerumen, ear pain, etc.

OTOSCOPY

1. PURPOSE

After obtaining the client's hearing history, one examines the client's ears. This procedure is called the otoscopic examination. The otoscopic examination is conducted before the initial hearing test.

The purpose of the exam is to:

1. Evaluate the possibility of ear canal collapse resulting from the pressure of the earphone during hearing testing.
2. Determine the presence of earwax (cerumen) or a build up of dry skin that might interfere with hearing sensitivity.
3. Observe any abrasions, infections, abnormal growths, ear drum perforations, or other obvious disorders.

4. Evaluate the size of the external canal and its ability to accept an earmold or hearing aid.
5. Determine if there are any conductive hearing-related impairments.
6. Look for an enlargement deep in the ear canal that may impede/prevent the extraction of the impression.

2. EQUIPMENT

Test validity is influenced by the quality of the equipment used. Instrumentation used for otoscopy ranges from inexpensive pen light otoscopes to surgical quality binocular dissecting microscopes. Pen light otoscopes and light bars are useful when placing cotton plugs into the ear canal prior to the impression, but are inadequate for viewing the ear canal and ear drum.

Some otoscopes employ the principle of fiber optic light projection. They provide a stronger, focused light source needed for viewing the canal. These otoscopes have the additional benefit of being continuously rechargeable to maintain constant light intensity. Besides an otoscope, one needs an assortment of extra tips (specula) along with containers for sterile and nonsterile tips. Use sterile tips for each client.

The headlights (headlamps) used by physicians are also valuable instruments to view the anatomy of the ear canal. Fiber optic halogen head lights supply an excellent light source and provide a superior three-dimensional view of the ear canal since binocular vision is used. Headlights also have the additional advantage of leaving both hands free while viewing the ear.

3. PROCEDURE

The examination of the outer ear should be done with an otoscopic tip (speculum) slightly larger than the client's ear canal. This maximizes viewing by allowing the most light possible and provides a safety feature, in that the tip will not contact the client's eardrum.

To inspect the outer ear, turn the otoscope on to full power, maximum light. Select an otoscopic tip slightly larger than the client's ear canal and secure it to the otoscope. Project the light on the client's outer ear, studying the cartilage and its hardness. During this part of the procedure, do not look through the otoscope; rather, use the strong light and your natural vision to examine the outer ear. Gently bend the ear forward and look for scars behind the ear. Scars may suggest a history of ear surgery. Next inspect the entrance to the ear canal and the cave of the outer ear (cavum conchae) for active drainage or debris. If there is evidence of an ongoing ear infection, the examination should be stopped and appropriate medical referral made.

Move the pinna forward and backward to see if the ear canal closes easily. Ear canal collapse may invalidate hearing tests. Ear canal collapse produces misleading air-bone gaps, which in turn produce additional problems for the client, the hearing aid specialist, and the physician. Check each ear to see if it has a proclivity to close when slight inward pressure is applied.

Using natural vision under strong light, examine the external canal, pulling the outer ear upward and backward. Now gently insert the otoscope into the outermost part of the ear canal. Look through the otoscope to examine the ear canal and the ear drum. Find the landmarks on the eardrum, especially the umbo and the long process (manubrium) of the hammer.

CATLIN, (1981) stated that:

> "The normal intact tympanic membrane is smooth, translucent, thin, white to gray in color, and tented slightly inward at its center or umbo. A light reflex is usually evident by otoscopy when the surface is smooth. Pneumatic otoscopy reveals that the membrane moves easily to small pressure changes in the external auditory canal. Some of the middle ear structures may be visible when the tympanic membrane is thin and translucent. The malleus, which is attached to the membrane, is usually evident. The long process of the incus, the stapedius muscle tendon, and the chorda tympani nerve may be seen in the posterior-superior quadrant. The pink shadow of the round window niche may be evident in the posterior-inferior quadrant."

Occasionally, hair at the entrance to the ear canal must be trimmed to allow adequate viewing of the ear canal and eardrum. When necessary, explain this to the client and obtain permission. Use dull point scissors to avoid injuring the skin. Note any abnormal changes. Especially notice any surgical altering of the canal size and shape.

When the otoscope examination is completed, some clients will ask, "How is it?" Do not divulge anything that might relate to the health of the ear. The purpose of the otoscopic exam is to give the hearing aid specialist information. Telling the client, "Your ear looks healthy and normal," is practicing medicine without a license. Answer the client's query simply and honestly by saying you are looking to see how much space you have to work with for a hearing aid or earmold. If there is an observable problem, then medical referral is the obvious course to follow.

HEARING TESTING ENVIRONMENT

Human hearing is tested for different reasons. Hearing tests done at the request of a physician are used to determine the medical diagnosis. These tests help locate the pathology and quantify the size of the problem. These tests are the diagnostic battery.

Other tests focus on prognosis. To the hearing aid specialist, these hearing tests show the amount of hearing improvement the client might expect from hearing instrument use. These prognostic tests suggest the amplification needed for optimal hearing.

The hearing professional working in rehabilitation needs both diagnostic and prognostic information. Diagnostic information helps us to understand the hearing abilities of the client before we intervene with amplification. Prognostic information helps us understand how to manage the many ramifications of the hearing aid fitting process. Together, these tests give us a better picture of the client's hearing potential.

The diagnostic battery helps determine the type, degree, and cause of the hearing loss. Most diagnostic tests have been standardized and are conducted under acoustically controlled conditions. The equipment used for these tests is manufactured to perform within permissible limits. The testing environment must be sufficiently quiet to avoid interference during the test. Some argue that since hearing aids are worn in a noisy world, hearing should be tested in a more natural environment. This is not a valid argument. Excessive noise destroys the test quality by elevating pure-tone thresholds and interfering with word recognition results. A quiet environment is essential for diagnostic hearing tests. Usually a quality hearing testing booth or correctly built sound treated room is needed to reduce noise. If the hearing testing booth is not available, as in the case of hearing tests done in the home, the level of the room noise should be monitored with a sound level meter to insure the adequacy of the testing environment. Hearing test results obtained in too noisy an environment are of little value.

The American National Standards Institute (ANSI-1969) has published acceptable norms for hearing testing environments. These norms specify the maximum allowable noise (ambient sound pressure) levels required for no interference (masking) when measuring air and bone conduction thresholds at the zero (0) setting on the audiometer. The values listed below are for the zero hearing threshold level (HTL) setting of the audiometer. If hearing is evaluated at some higher HTL setting (e.g. the 20 dB HTL line) then more ambient noise is allowed.

The acceptable noise levels are different for air-conducted tests and bone-conducted tests. Air conduction tests are done with earphones held in place by standardized earphone cushions, e.g., MX-41-AR. The earphone cushions help reduce unwanted noise. Bone conduction tests do not employ cushions, therefore, the allowable noise levels are more stringent. The ANSI standards set the maximum allowable noise levels for air conducted pure tone tests at: 40 dB @ 250, 500, and 1000 Hz, 47 dB @ 2000 Hz, 57 dB @ 4000 Hz, and 67 dB @ 8000 Hz. The ANSI values for bone conduction pure tone testing are 37 dB @ 250 Hz, 31 dB @ 500 Hz, 25 dB @ 1000 Hz, 23 dB @ 2000 Hz, and 20 dB @ 4000 Hz.

Most ambient noises have energy maximums in the lower frequencies, so the hearing testing problems created by noise are usually confined to lower frequencies. Lower frequency noise is also more difficult to attenuate with standard architectural structures, i.e., walls, doors, and windows.

The hearing aid specialist who evaluates hearing in the client's home can anticipate noise interference, especially in the lower frequencies. These problems can often be circumvented by: (1) selecting a quiet room for the tests, (2) stopping the tests during temporary surges of noise, (3) using earphone cushions designed to attenuate room noise, (4) supplementing the air and bone conduction tests with additional tests that are not degraded by ambient noise, e.g., otoscopy and impedance/immittance testing, and (5) monitoring the ambient noise level with a sound level meter. The reader is referred to Martin (1975) for a more detailed discussion of test environment adequacy.

Prognostic tests are often given under less stringent conditions. Prognostic testing follows the completion of diagnostic testing. Most prognostic tests stress speech clarity; therefore, the frequency region centered at 2000 Hz is considered more important than the frequency region centered about 200 Hz. Most ambient noise has its maximum energy in the lower frequency region. A quiet office room is usually adequate for most prognostic testing.

THE AUDIOMETER

A calibrated audiometer is the instrument of choice to test human hearing. Earlier test methods included whispered speech, watch tick, and tuning fork. These tests served the purpose of checking hearing sensitivity levels. However precision was lacking.

The advancements in electronics have produced many useful hearing testing devices. The most basic of these instruments is the

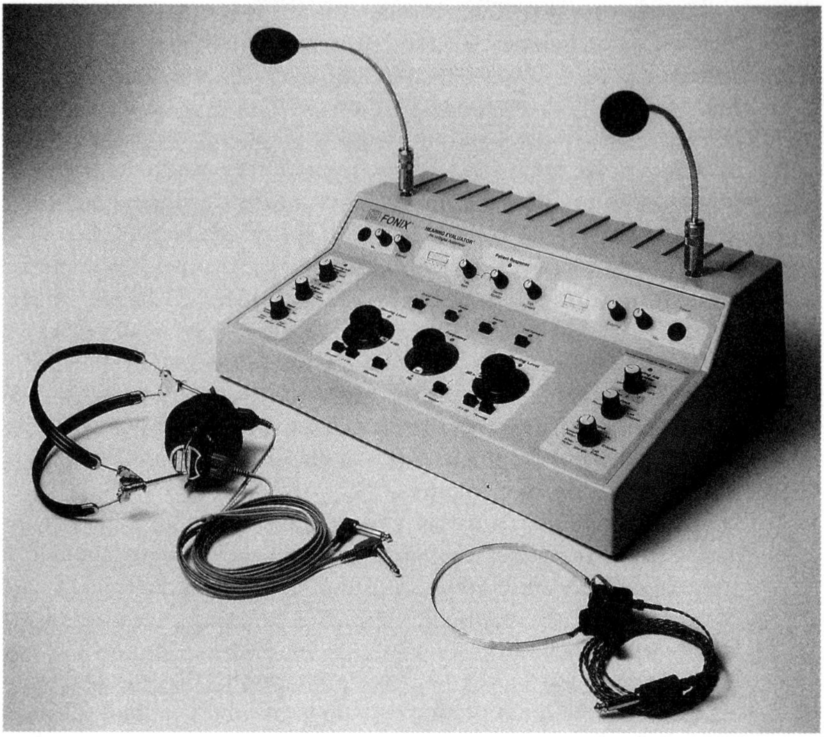

Fig. 12. A modern clinical audiometer. (Photograph used with permission of Frye Electronics).

audiometer, an instrument that produces pure-tones and other acoustic stimuli used to evaluate human hearing ability. A pure-tone is an acoustic signal that has energy at only one frequency. Testing, therefore, with a 1000 Hz tone yields information about the client's hearing at 1000 Hz and no other.

Figures 12, 13, and 14 show a modern audiometer. The intensity, or loudness of the pure-tone is controlled by a dial called the attenuator (marked Hearing Level in Figures 13 and 14). The audiometer is designed so that zero on the attenuator dial represents the level of normal hearing for that frequency. Observe Figures 13 and 14. This audiometer has two attenuators, one for each ear. The attenuators are labeled, "Hearing Level." A close inspection of the attenuator dial in Figure 13 shows that these attenuators operate across a wide range in loudness: from −10 dB, a very soft sound, to +110 dB, a very loud sound.

The test frequencies available on most audiometers are 125, 250, 500, 750, 1000, 1500, 2000, 3000, 4000, 6000, and 8000 Hz.

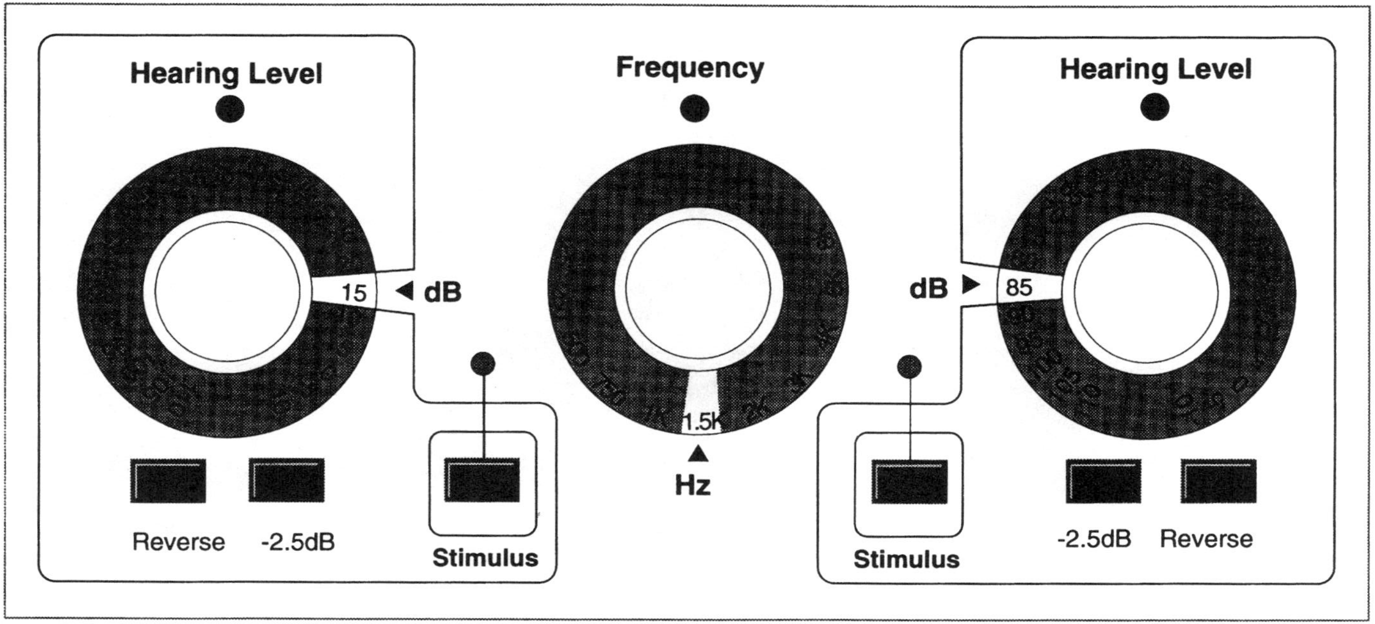

Fig. 13. A simplified drawing of the Fonix FA-10 showing the attenuators, frequency selector, and stimulus presentation buttons. (Photograph used with permission of Frye Electronics).

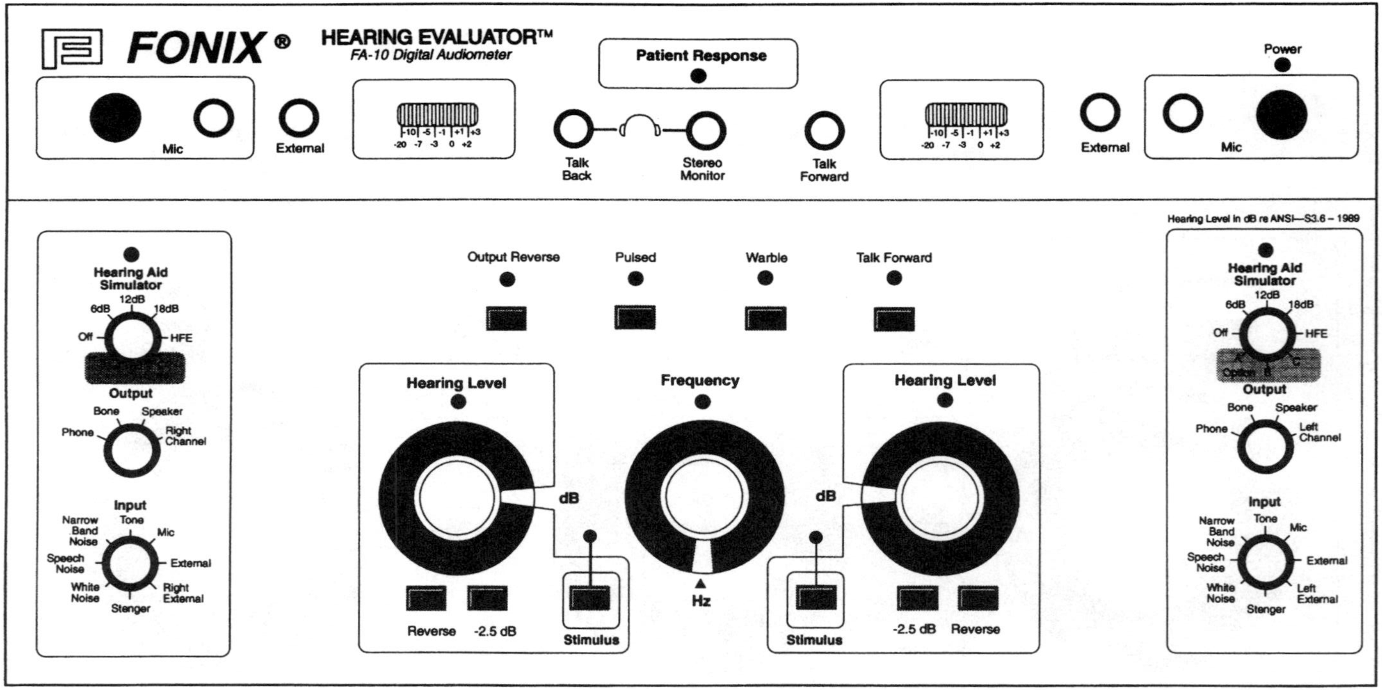

Fig. 14. A schematic of a diagnostic audiometer that includes a master hearing aid unit. (Illustration used with permission of Frye Electronics).

The frequency selector dial in Figure 13 indicates that these same pure-tone signals are available on this unit. Note how the term, "1000 Hz" is sometimes abbreviated 1.0 kHz.

Most audiometers produce signals and noises other than pure-tones to more completely evaluate hearing. Some audiometers control the presentation of speech so the client may be given words at different, controlled intensities. Most audiometers produce a masking noise, which is used for some testing procedures.

THE FLOOR OF HEARING: THE SRT AND THE PURE TONE AUDIOGRAM

Seat the client in a position where you can watch his/her responses to the test signals. Avoid having the client watch you during the tests. Visual signals can elicit artificial responses. You might have the client close his eyes or look to one side of the room.

Before starting the test remove anything (hearing aids, cotton, etc.) from the client's ears that might block the sound from entering the ear canal. Place the earphones carefully on the client, centering them over the ear canals. Be sure the right (red) phone is on the right ear and the left (blue) phone is on the left ear. Check to be sure you are not collapsing the ear canal when the earphone is placed on the ear. If there is a question about ear canal collapse, remove the phone from the headset and have the client or an assistant hold the earphone securely on the ear while lightly pulling the ear backwards to open the canal.

Test the good ear first. This establishes the best hearing of the client early in the test sequence. It helps you learn whether or not you need to use masking when testing the poorer ear.

The hearing tests start with the speech reception threshold (SRT). The client must be placed in a room separated from the tester if live voice stimulus is employed. The client and the tester can be in the same room if recorded speech is used, e.g., when testing in the home. A typical SRT evaluation may go as follows:

By live voice:

"Hello. Are you comfortable?"

"Yes."

"You will hear some words. I want you to repeat them for me. After you hear the words a few times, I will make the words much softer. When you hear the word, just say what you hear. When the words get very soft, guess at the words. OK?"

"OK."

(Switch to recorded speech if environment dictates)

"Say the word, 'baseball'."

"Baseball."

"Say the word 'mushroom'."

The tester gives the client about 10 to 20 two-syllable words taken from the spondaic word test list. (See Appendix B). Initially, the tester presents these words at a comfortable listening level so the client becomes familiar with the words.

After establishing familiarization, the tester reduces the loudness of the words in 5 to 10 dB steps until the client is no longer able to repeat the words. Then loudness is increased until the client responds correctly. Threshold is the softest point at which the client can repeat the words correctly fifty percent of the time.

Two advantages of the SRT bear special emphasis. First, the SRT takes a small amount of time to complete, less than one minute per ear. Second, the SRT provides a substantial amount of useful information. For example, a client with normal hearing will be identified at the outset of the hearing test and can be treated more quickly, thus saving time.

The typical hearing impaired individual has a sloping pure-tone audiogram. Such an audiometric configuration shows better hearing in the bass, and worse hearing in the treble. Take as an example two clients, both having pure-tone hearing as follows: 20 dB @ 250 Hz, 25 dB @ 500 Hz, 35 dB @ 1000 Hz, 55 dB @2000 Hz, 70 dB @ 4000 Hz, and 80 dB @ 8000 Hz. If one of these clients has an SRT of 30 dB, he is proving to us that he can use his residual hearing quite efficiently. His excellent auditory functioning allows him to understand speech when it is presented at what is for him a very soft level. But if the other client with the identical pure-tone audiogram has an SRT of 50 dB, that client needs substantially more power before his brain and ears combine functionally to allow him to hear and understand speech.

The SRT indicates to the hearing aid specialist how the client's hearing loss has affected the ability to hear and understand soft speech. This information is invaluable, as it directly relates to the amount of amplification the client needs.

The SRT can be administered "live" voice or with a tape-recorded voice. Both presentations require an acoustically controlled environment. The live voice SRT should be done in a room where the tester and the listener are acoustically isolated from one another. A diagram of the testing environment for the live voice

SRT is presented in Fig. 15. This equipment routes the tester's voice from the microphone to the audiometer. The tester monitors his voice by watching the VU meter. Voice level is maintained at 0 VU for each part of the two-syllable test word. The tester controls the intensity of the test word presented to the listener by adjusting the attenuator dial to the desired level.

The sound wall between the tester and the listener prevents the tester's voice from reaching the listener's ears. Without this acoustic barrier the client may be able to hear the examiner's voice and the test would be invalid. The acoustic barrier between the tester and the listener can be created in different ways. Most often the client is placed in a sound booth for these word tests.

The SRT can be accomplished also with tape-recorded word lists. A diagram of the testing environment for the recorded word SRT is presented in Figure 16. This procedure is used when the tester is unable to provide the required acoustic barrier between himself and the individual to be evaluated. This test must be done in a quiet room to prevent background noise from interfering with the test results.

The tape-recorded words are presented via earphones and the level of presentation is controlled. Care must be exercised by the tester to avoid needless testing error. The word presentation rate on the tape is fixed. Many elderly people have difficulty with the short time span between words. Remember, the word processing ability of elderly people may be reduced and the speed at which the words are presented may be confusing.

In our analogy of building an architectural framework to help us in rehabilitating the client, the SRT is the floor of hearing. We

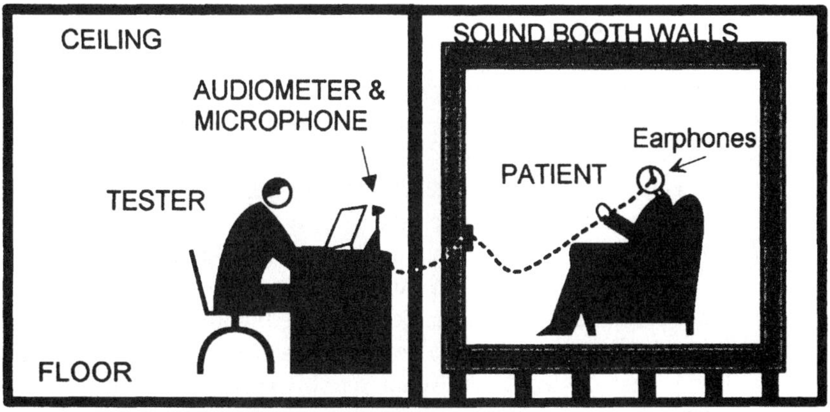

Fig. 15. Instrumentation for the "live" voice SRT.

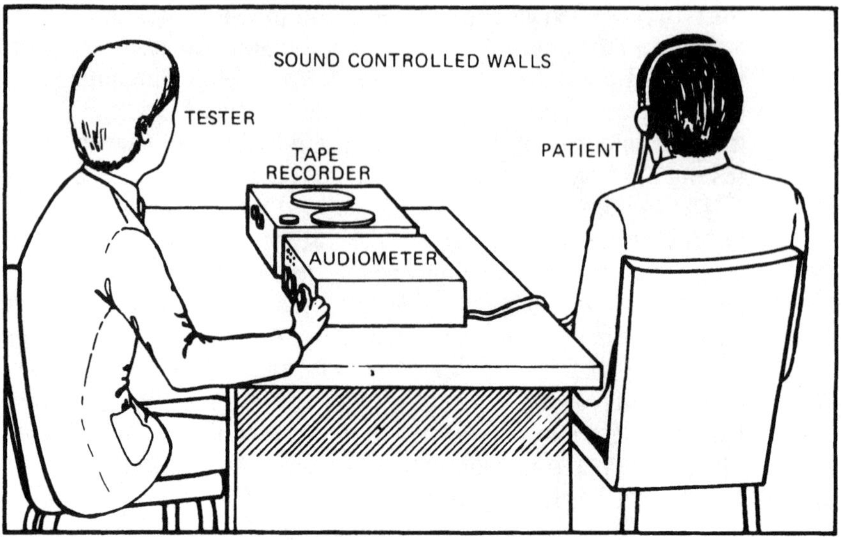

Fig. 16. Instrumentation for the "recorded" voice SRT.

integrate the information we obtain via the SRT with the information we obtain from pure-tone thresholds to better understand the softer limits of our client's hearing.

PURE-TONE THRESHOLD TESTS

The client may indicate his/her response to the pure-tone by voice or hand signal. Instructions for obtaining a voice response may be as follows: "I am going to present some tones. They will become very soft. Each time you hear the tone just say, 'yes'. If you hear something and are not sure if it is a tone, just say, 'I'm not sure.' Do you understand?"

Instructions for a hand response would be: "I'm going to present some tones. The tones will become soft. Each time you hear a sound, quickly raise your hand. Raise your right hand when the tone is in your right ear. Raise your left hand when the tone is in your left ear. Do you understand?"

The essence of a pure-tone hearing testing technique is to start with an easy-to-hear test stimulus and quickly decrease the intensity level to that point where the tone is inaudible. Then in 5 dB steps, slowly increase the level to the point where the client is just able to hear the test tone. Again, quickly reduce the tone to an inaudible level, and then slowly increase the level of the tone until it is heard again to double check the threshold response.

In outline form this procedure is:

1. Refer to the SRT and determine which intensity level will be easy for the client to hear. Present the tone and get a quick, positive response. If the client's response is slow, repeat the instructions and encourage a faster response.
2. Decrease the level of the tone in 10 dB steps. Obtain a response with each presentation level.
3. When the client no longer hears the tone, make a mental note of the last level to which he/she responded. This is the tentative threshold. Increase the level of the tone in 5 dB steps until the client responds to the tone.
4. Increase and decrease the level of the tone several times across the tentative threshold level to be sure the client is responding to the softest, audible level possible about fifty percent of the time.
5. Mark the threshold level on the audiogram. The appropriate symbols are red circles, O, for the right ear, blue X's for the left.

Threshold is the weakest level at which a person can hear the presented tones fifty percent of the time. An individual may make some false "yes" responses. Successively presenting tones above and below threshold will help to determine which tones are audible and which tone are inaudible to the client.

The threshold for 1000 Hz is obtained first. Next the threshold for 500 Hz is obtained and recorded. This is followed by testing at 250 Hz. Before the higher frequency tones of 2000, 3000, 4000, 6000, and 8000 Hz are evaluated, the threshold for 1000 Hz is rechecked to determine test/re-test reliability. The second evaluation of threshold at 1000 Hz should not differ by more the 5 dB from the initial evaluation. If the second threshold obtained at 1000 Hz is greater than 5 dB, a testing error has been committed and all other thresholds obtained at 1000 Hz is greater than 5 dB, a testing error has been committed and all other thresholds obtained may be suspect. If the second threshold obtained at 1000 Hz is within 5 dB of the first, continue testing the higher frequencies in the order recommended.

RECOMMENDED TEST ORDER

Best Ear: 1000, 500, 250, 1000, 2000, 3000, 4000, 6000, 8000 Hz.

Other Ear: 1000, 500, 250, 1000, 2000, 3000, 4000, 6000, 8000 Hz.

The length of the test tone should be held about one second. Sometimes clients confuse the test tones with sounds or noises they have in their heads. In such cases, two or three bursts of the tone, about a half-second long, can be given to help the client differentiate between the test tone and the ongoing tinnitus in his head. Some audiometers have an automatic pulsing tone that, when used, reduces this problem.

Increases and decreases in intensity are controlled with the audiometer attenuator. Most audiometer attenuators adjust the signal in 5 dB steps. The output limit available on the audiometer is normally printed on the frequency dial for each frequency. The output limit for air conducted signals is usually high (about 100 dB HTL) while the output limit for bone conducted signals is much lower (usually about 70 dB HTL).

PURE TONE AIR CONDUCTION TEST

Tone selection is controlled with the frequency dial. Standard test frequencies include: 250, 500, 1000, 2000, 4000, and 8000 Hz. Testing the in-between frequencies helps define more precisely the shape of the hearing loss. These additional frequencies usually include: 750, 1500, 3000, and 6000 Hz.

Sataloff and Sataloff (1980) have developed excellent instructions on obtaining a pure-tone audiogram. It is recommended that the reader refer to this text for additional information.

RECORDING THRESHOLD VALUES ON THE AUDIOGRAM

The audiogram is a graph on which one records pure-tone test results. An audiogram lists frequencies on the horizontal axis. Some individuals have different names for frequency. They may include: tone, pitch, cycles per second (cps), cycles, and musical notes.

The current designation for frequency is Hertz (Hz). A frequency of 1000 cps is called 1000 Hz. Figure 17 shows the frequency axis of an audiogram. Some clinician prefer an audiogram that includes half octave frequencies (750, 1500, 3000, and 6000 Hz). This author prefers the simpler audiogram shown in Figure 18.

Audiograms display hearing levels (intensity) on the vertical axis of the graph. The term intensity or loudness may be referred to in other ways including: sound pressure level, power, quantity, and soft-to-loud. More correctly, the vertical axis of the audiogram is the hearing level (HL) in decibels or hearing threshold level (HTL), calibrated to the appropriate audiometric standard (ANSI 1969).

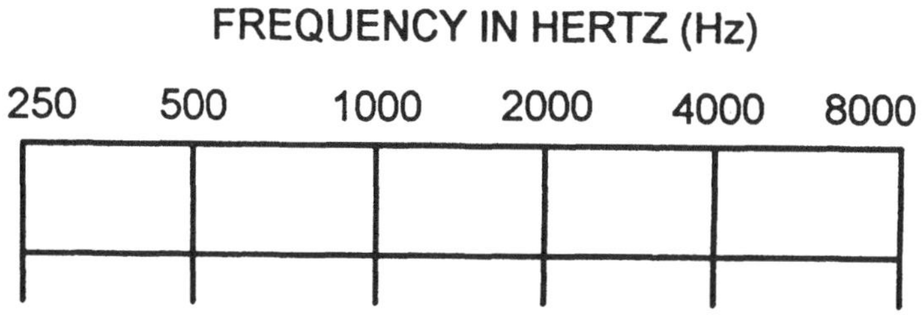

Fig. 17. The upper portion of a puretone audiogram showing the horizontal axis (frequency).

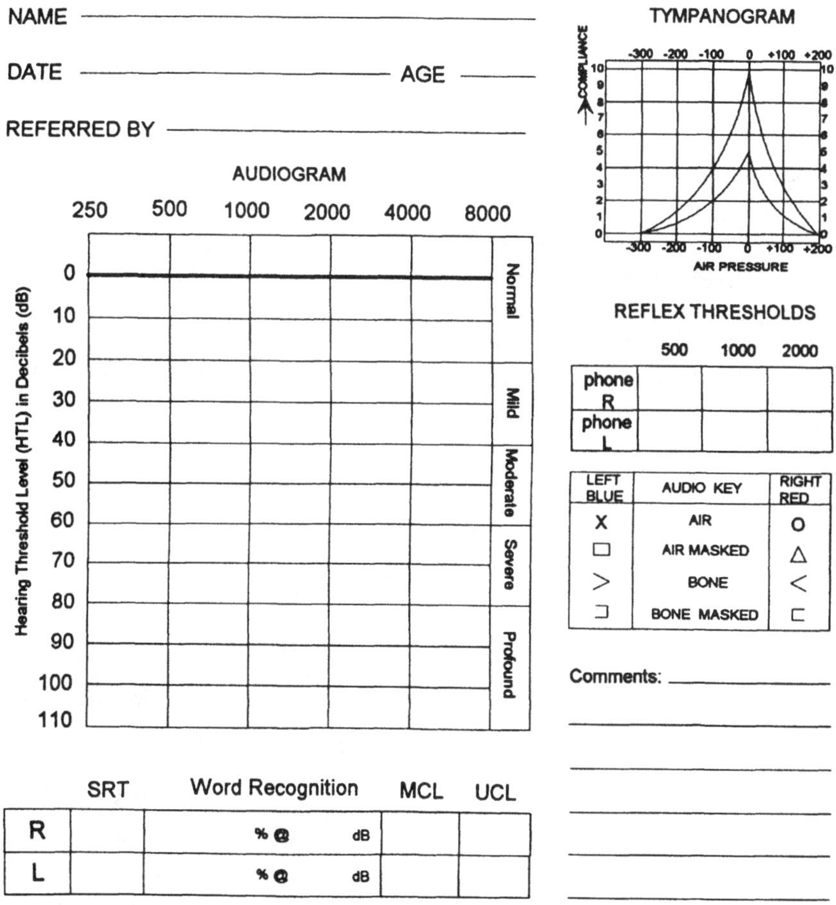

Fig. 18. An audiogram. Note the audio key which specifies the symbols used for the various test stimuli.

Others prefer to organize the vertical scale into hearing loss levels. Lloyd and Kaplan (1978) reviewed these various classifications. Since there is no absolute standard, the author prefers to use the simple system of 0–20 dB as the normal hearing range, 20–40 dB as mild hearing loss, 40–60 dB as moderate hearing loss, 60–80 dB as severe hearing loss, and 80 dB and greater as profound hearing loss. The terms mild and moderate are general terms. These terms should only be used to help the client understand the degree or quantity of his/her hearing loss. A normal human ear can hear all tones presented at 0 dB HTL. See Figures 18 and 19.

Some audiometers and audiograms have minus hearing levels, for example −10 dB HTL. These negative values indicate hearing better than normal. Remember, 0 dB HTL does not indicate absence of sound, instead 0 dB HTL is the level of average, normal threshold of hearing.

THE PURE TONE AVERAGE (PTA)

The pure tone average, PTA, is the arithmetic average of a client's hearing thresholds at 500, 1000, and 2000 Hz. Most practitioners use the PTA as part of the audiological evaluation. Some governmental agencies use the PTA as a criterion to decide who is eligible to receive hearing aids through their agencies. The PTA can be

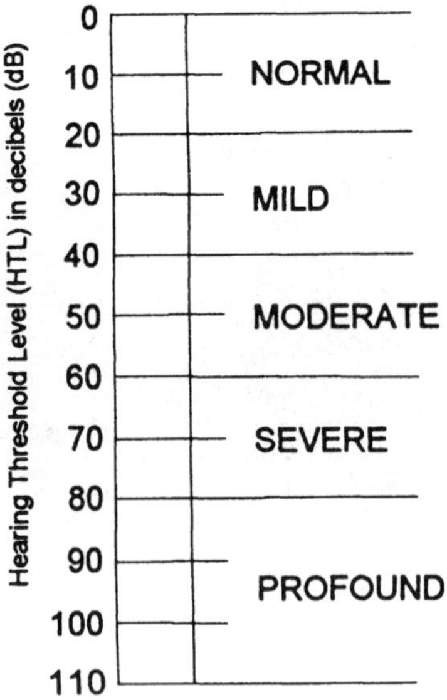

Fig. 19. The left-hand portion of a puretone audiogram and the corresponding hearing loss magnitude.

used as a check of inter-test agreement. The SRT and PTA are both measurements of the floor of hearing and as such they should agree within 5 dB, if the pure-tone values are relatively flat.

Unfortunately, the PTA has become a part of routine audiological calculations. In the author's opinion the PTA has questionable significance in assessing auditory function. The PTA considers the contribution of 500, 1000, and 2000, Hz as equal, when in fact they are not equally important for speech clarity. The PTA omits 4000 Hz, when in fact the octave band of energy centered at 4000 Hz is more important to clarity and speech understanding than is 500 Hz.

The PTA lends itself to simple calculation and is often used as a number that suggests how well or poorly a person hears. The PTA may dramatically underestimate the degree of hearing impairment. It is recommended that the PTA not be considered a criterion measurement used in selecting hearing aid candidates.

MASKING

Masking is illustrated in Figures 20 and 21. Masking is a type of noise applied to the non-test ear to stop that ear from assisting the ear under test. If masking is not used you may present a test signal to one ear and get a response from the other ear. In Figure 20 the earphone makes masking noise which passes through the outer and middle ear into the inner ear. In Figure 21 the test signal is presented to the left ear while masking noise is delivered to the right ear.

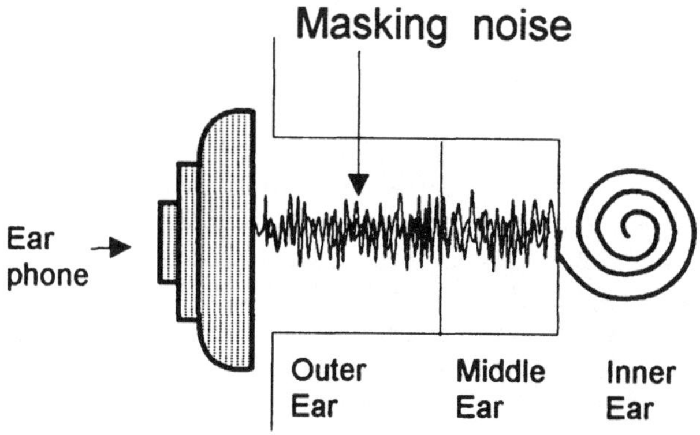

Fig. 20. A masking noise path from the earphone, through the middle ear, to the inner ear.

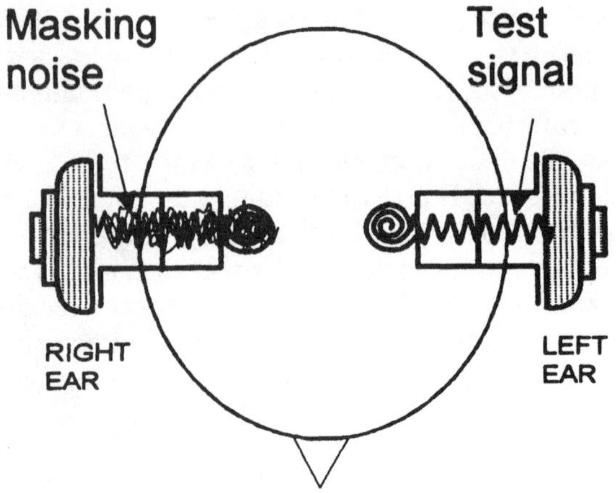

Fig. 21. An air-conducted signal presented to the left ear. Masking noise is routed to the right ear.

If a pure-tone air conducted signal is presented to one ear, it may be heard by the non-test ear, depending upon its intensity. It is, therefore, critical to understand cross-hearing and interaural attenuation. Cross hearing is defined as a condition wherein a sound is presented to one ear and is heard by the other. Interaural attenuation is the loss of acoustic energy in a sound (test tone or the masking noise), as it travels from the receiver, (earphone or bone vibrator) at the test ear across the head to the opposite ear.

Figure 22 shows an example of cross-hearing. The person in this figure has normal hearing in the right ear and no hearing in the left ear. The right pure-tone threshold data are all 0 dB indicating excellent hearing sensitivity. When the pure-tone signals are administered to the **left dead ear** without masking, false responses of 45 dB @ 250 Hz, 55 dB @ 500 and 1000 Hz, and 60 dB @ 2000, 4000, and 8000 Hz are observed. These false thresholds are direct measurements of interaural attenuation. These values show much energy is lost as the signal travels from the left earphone through the skull to the **right normal inner ear.**

Interaural attenuation values vary from person to person. It is less at 250 Hz and greater in higher frequencies. An average value across frequencies might be 50 dB. However, it is recommended that the hearing aid specialist assume a more conservative estimate of 40 dB interaural attenuation.

The air conduction test should incorporate masking whenever there is a 40 dB difference between the air-conducted threshold for the test ear and the bone-conducted thresholds of the non-test ear. Remember in cross-hearing the signal travels through the skull,

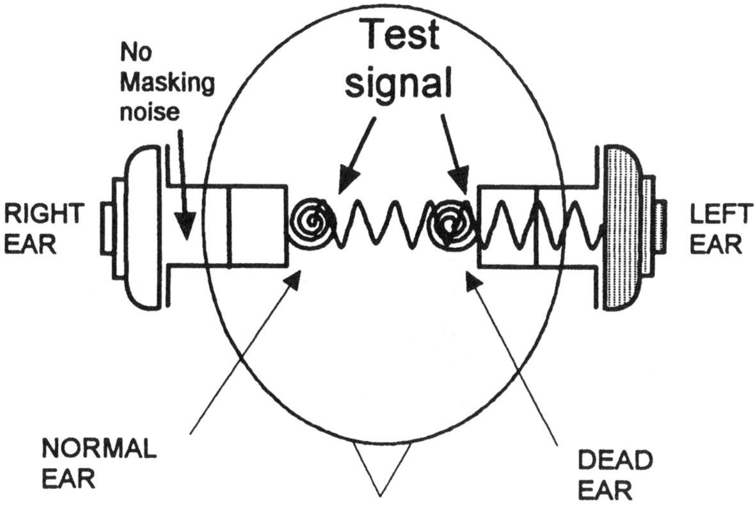

	250	500	1000	2000	4000
right ear	0	0	0	0	0
left ear	45	55	55	60	60

Fig. 22. The right earphone was used to test the right ear and normal hearing sensitivity (0 dB) was observed. In this illustration the left earphone presents a signal to the left "dead" ear. The signal crosses the head and is heard by the right ear.

and the skull is the bone conducted pathway. Therefore, the masking rule refers to the difference between the air conduction threshold on one side and the bone conduction threshold on the other side.

For a more complete discussion of the principles underlying the use of masking, the reader is referred to a later chapter by Donaldson. She presents a definitive chapter on the use of masking.

TYPES OF MASKING NOISE

Audiometers differ markedly concerning the type and calibration of the masking noise utilized. Whenever a new or different audiometer is used, the tester should refer to the operation manual and determine the type and calibration of the masking on that unit.

An appropriate type of masking noise is narrow-band noise calibrated to effective masking levels. The term narrow-band refers to the use of electronic filtering to remove noise energy on either side of the narrow frequency band selected. Narrow-band noise has acoustic energy in the same general frequency region as the test tone. Narrow-band noise is more comfortable to listen to than white or broad-band noise as the overall loudness (power level) is reduced substantially. If the test signal is 2,000 Hz in the test ear, then the narrow-band noise centered at 2,000 Hz would be used as a masking stimulus in the other ear. The actual width of the band may be 1500–2500 Hz.

The term "effective masking" indicated the type of calibration used to adjust the level of the masking noise. Noise has energy at many different frequencies. Pure-tones only have energy in one frequency. For noise to mask, or cover pure-tones, the energy within the noise has to be increased. The term "effective" indicates that the noise level has been adjusted to just barely mask a pure-tone if the two signals were put into the same ear. For example, a 60 dB narrow-band noise calibrated to effective masking will just mask a 60 dB pure-tone if the two are presented to the same ear at the same time.

PURE-TONE LIMITATIONS

Pure-tone threshold testing provides considerable information about the client's hearing sensitivity. However, additional information is needed. Figure 23 illustrates the limitation of the pure-tone threshold test. This figure shows hearing tests for two different individual: Paul, age 35, on the left; and Shirley, age 46, on the right. Both have similar pure-tone thresholds.

Paul has had a hearing loss for about ten years. His hearing loss was caused by Meniere's disease. He has considerable distortion in his hearing. He is unhappy with his hearing aid amplification and has little confidence in his hearing ability, with or without hearing instruments.

Shirley is a manager of a small bank. She wears her hearing aids about fourteen hours a day. She can communicate effectively in person and on the telephone. Her hearing aids are part of her and she depends upon them for everyday functioning. Shirley's aided hearing ability approaches normal hearing sensitivity. Her own evaluation of her hearing ability is, "Without my aids I can just barely hear. Functioning without them would be practically impossible. With them I get along with only minor problems."

Paul and Shirley have similar pure-tone hearing thresholds. In terms of the House of Hearing analogy, they both have the same space between the floor and ceiling. However, it is the quality of the space that is dramatically different. Shirley's space is highly functional. Paul's is not.

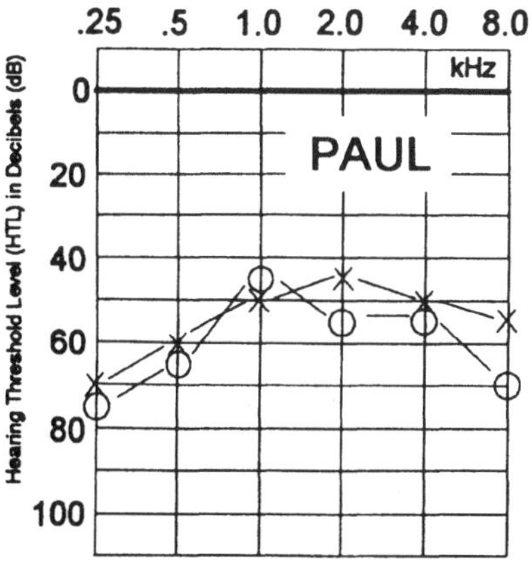

	SRT	Word Recognition	MCL	UCL
R	55	60 % 75 dB	75	90
L	55	62 % 75 dB	75	90

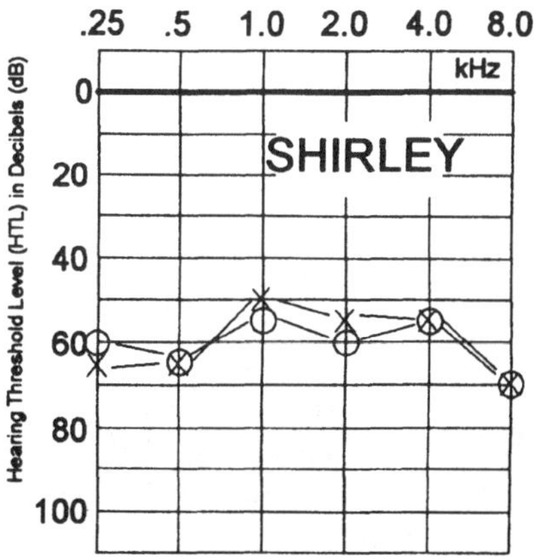

	SRT	Word Recognition	MCL	UCL
R	60	88 % 75 dB	75	90
L	55	90 % 75 dB	75	90

Fig. 23. Hearing tests for Paul and Shirley. The right ear hearing thresholds are indicated with circles, left with Xs. Hearing thresholds are about the same. Word recognition scores are much better for Shirley.

Let us follow the analogy between room space and hearing space. When a contractor evaluates a damaged house, he makes accurate estimates of structural soundness and required repairs so he can correct damages. When hearing aid specialists evaluate a client's hearing, they measure the quantity and quality of remaining hearing. Medically speaking, we need a prognosis. One important hearing evaluation is that of speech clarity. In years past this test was called the "speech discrimination test." We refer to this test now as the "Word Recognition" test. It tells us the degree to which we may help the client hear and understand speech. Paul's best word recognition ability is only about 60% whereas Shirley's word recognition ability is much better, about 90%.

SPEECH TESTS: THE MCL

The Most Comfortable Loudness (MCL) level is achieved by asking the client what loudness or volume he/she prefers. The dialogue might go something like this: "Mr. Jones, you are doing fine. We want to find out what level of sound you like to listen to. If you were listing to me over a radio or TV would this conversation be too loud, just right, or too soft."

After the client's answer, the tester adjusts the attenuator up and down, bracketing the MCL and allowing the client to hear speech at different loudness levels. Frequently one who has not heard very well for years will initially say the louder settings are best. Talk with the client at these settings, but explain that there is a large range from which he/she can choose as the best level. Allow the client to listen to speech levels by experiencing what is too much and too little.

Occasionally a client might show a startle reaction when the intensity is adjusted toward the higher levels. The MCL test may startle or surprise the client. Or, the client may have a damaged inner ear that manifests a phenomenon call recruitment. Hypersensitive reactions to loudness are common responses, if the inner ear has sustained damage. Recruitment may be defined as an abnormal growth in loudness.

The client that displays a hypersensitive reaction to loudness might not have heard loud speech in this manner for a long time. He/she may have recruitment. Some clients are naturally over sensitive and reactive to sound. Regardless of the reason for this overreaction, it is important for the hearing aid specialist to observe and make careful notes about this reaction for future reference.

In contrast to the hypersensitive client, others may absorb energy and tolerate louder intensities rather well. Such a client might respond in this manner because: (1) He/she has a conductive hearing loss and is able to listen to high levels of sound; (2) He/she has a substantial sensorineural hearing loss and wants and needs extra power to hear; or (3) He/she has a tough, macho philosophy and is just underreacting.

THE UNCOMFORTABLE LOUDNESS LEVEL, UCL

THE UCL FOR SPEECH

The Uncomfortable Loudness Level (UCL) is the level at which an individual reports sound to be uncomfortably loud. The author's method for explaining the speech UCL to the client and eliciting responses from him/her involves a sight and sound demonstration similar to the following. This demonstration is for the client who has visual contact with the tester:

"We have tested your hearing for soft and medium sounds. Now we need to test you for loud sounds. Sounds can be soft. Sounds can be medium and comfortable to listen to. Or sounds can be loud.

It is important that we determine how you react to loud sounds. In the category of loud we have three levels."
I now hold up three fingers. "First we have a little loud." I point to one finger. "Next we have loud-loud." I point to another finger, "Last we have terribly-loud." Here I point to a third finger.
"I am not interested in a little loud, nor am I interested in terribly loud. I need to find the level you consider loud-loud. This level is loud enough to bother you, but not loud enough to hurt you."

Having explained the test, adjust the attenuator to 80 dB HL and ask the client if this setting is: 1, 2, or 3; or a little loud, loud-loud, or terribly loud. Depending upon the client's response, adjust the attenuator and find the level the client considers loud-loud (uncomfortable) but bearably loud. Find and record the Speech UCL value for both ears.

THE UCL FOR PURE TONES

Next, measure and record the client's UCLs for the pure tone signals at 500, 1000, 2000, and 4000 Hz. Some clinicians believe it is important to test 3000 Hz. Instruct the client to listen to the pure tone signal, and then point to one of the "Levels of Loudness" (from Hawkins 1987) presented on a large chart show below.

The instructions to the client are, "You are doing fine. Next, I want you to listen to some sounds and indicate how loud they sound to you. I will change the sounds. After you hear each sound, ***quickly*** point to the words on the chart that best describe how loud the sound is to you. If you are not sure, just guess."

LEVELS OF LOUDNESS

- Painfully Loud
- Extremely Uncomfortable
- Uncomfortably Loud
- Loud, but O.K.
- Comfortable, But Slightly Loud
- Comfortable
- Comfortable, But Slightly Soft

A series of pure tones is then presented to the client starting at 75 dB at 1000 Hz. Encourage the client to respond quickly each time the tone is presented. Vary the loudness of the test tone up and down. For this test, the puretone UCL value is the "Uncomfortable Loud" level shown on the *LEVELS OF LOUDNESS* chart, above.

Mark the audiogram with a star. "*", or with the letters "UCL" to indicate the client's response.

Figures 49 and 50, presented later in this chapter, show hearing test results for two clients. The hearing thresholds are identical; however, these people have dissimilar responses to loud tones. The person shown in Figure 49 has a tolerance problem with higher frequency sounds. The person shown in Figure 50 has a tolerance problem with lower frequency sounds.

Pure tone UCL tests are an essential measurement used to localize the zone of greatest intolerance and should be done for all clients. We must know which zone irritates each person so we can select the appropriate hearing aid response, and circuitry. The UCL is represented by the ceiling of the House of Hearing in the analogy.

THE QUALITY OF THE HEARING SPACE: WORD RECOGNITION

Word recognition tests are critical in helping to evaluate potential hearing aid use. Word recognition tests must be obtained to direct the patient's actions and expectations. Low word understanding scores usually indicate a guarded prognosis; the successful use of hearing aids is questionable. High word recognition scores usually indicate excellence in functioning and high hopes for the client when appropriately fitted with hearing aids.

Sometimes it is useful to know how well the client understands speech without hearing aids. Test words given at normal speech levels (about 45 dB HL) indicate how the client is functioning without hearing aids. The 45 dB HL level assumes the talker is one meter from the listener.

The client's **best word recognition score** is determined by testing at varying intensity levels to locate the level which produces the best score. Words used for this test are called PB words; the letter "PB" stand phonetically balanced. The score at this "best" level is called the PB max, indicating maximum word understanding ability. It is important to know the sound level needed to produce a PB max so the appropriate amount of amplification can be selected.

Speech testing provides us with an opportunity to show the client what hearing aid amplification may offer. The clarity obtained during the audiometric word recognition testing approximates the hearing the client may enjoy with hearing aids in a quiet environment. This demonstration can indicate the decided advantage of hearing with both ears.

For a conventional word recognition test, the hearing aid specialist uses a calibrated speech audiometer. Fifty standardized words are presented to the client who is seated in a sound treated room. The more commonly used test words are the CID W-22 words shown in appendix C. The test word is preceded by the instruction, "Say the word ______." This method presents the test word in the context of a sentence rather than in isolation. The last word of the phrase should be presented at O VU. The fifty words are scored 2% per word. The client must repeat the entire word correctly. For example, if the test word is "twins" the client needs to include all parts of the word for credit. Dropping the final "s" results in missing the word.

Non-English speaking clients must be evaluated in their native language. The tester should have good hearing and an excellent, high quality monitoring earphone. Without either of these, the word recognition score becomes a function of the word understanding ability of the tester rather than the word understanding ability of the client.

Some authors suggest the test presentation level be selected at 40 dB above the SRT. Others recommend testing at the MCL. In practice, the level should be the one where the best word understanding score is obtained. When in doubt about which level to use for the word recognition tests, several levels should be evaluated. Also, masking should be used whenever it appears that the opposite ear is helping the test ear to discriminate.

If the speech understanding ability is found to be poor during the audiometric evaluation, speech testing should be done on a master hearing aid unit. The master hearing aid unit incorporates the adjustments of gain, slope, and MPO. Word recognition scores found using an audiometer can sometimes be improved with the help of these extra circuits.

Interpreting the word recognition score is often problematic. Goetzinger (1972) proposed a guide to evaluating the adequacy of word recognition ability:

90–100%	Normal word understanding ability
76–88%	Slight difficulty
62–74%	Moderate difficulty
50–60%	Poor understanding, great difficulty
Below 50%	Very poor understanding ability. Listener is probably unable to understand speech at normal conversation levels.

Using this criteria, one would say that Paul, Figure 23, has moderate (almost poor) difficulty understanding words, while Shirley has normal word understanding ability.

BONE CONDUCTION TESTS

Hearing tests evaluate one of two routes in presenting acoustic stimuli to the inner ear. These routes are the air-conduction path and the bone-conduction path.

Air-conducted tests traverse six different media to bring about inner ear stimulation: (1) earphones; (2) the outer ear canal; (3) the ear drum; (4) the ossicles (middle ear bones); (5) the footplate of the stapes situated in the oval window of the inner ear; and (6) the inner ear structures. The air-conducted path is illustrated in Figures 7 and 8.

Bone-conducted tests only traverse four different media to bring about inner stimulation: (1) the bone vibrator; (2) the skin; (3) the skull; and (4) the inner ear structures. Note that the bone-conducted path excludes the outer ear, eardrum, ossicles, and oval window. The bone-conducted path is illustrated in Figure 24.

The air-conducted path is the path sound traverses in normal hearing. This path starts with earphones as the sound energy transmitter in pure-tone testing. Thus, tests done with earphones give

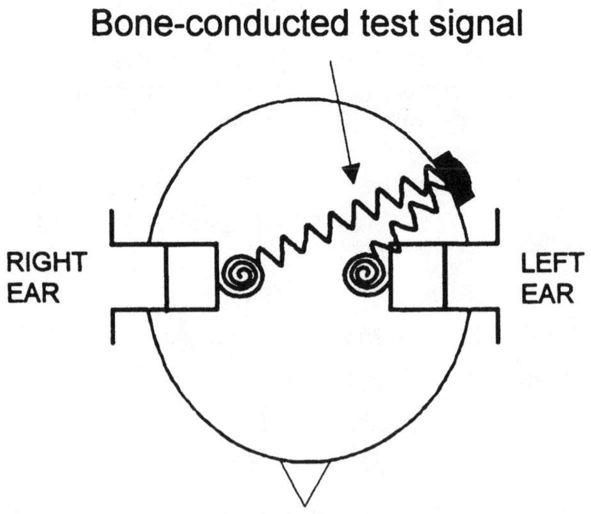

Fig. 24. A schematic indicating that bone conduction vibrations stimulate both ears.

air-conduction hearing thresholds. The bone-conducted path is a much different test. The bone-conduction path begins with a bone vibrator located on the head, not the ears. The vibrator transmits sounds as vibratory energy directly into the skull.

The bone vibrator can be placed at several different locations on the head. The most appropriate location, however, is behind the ear on the mastoid bone. The bone vibrator headband is adjusted comfortably over the head of the client in a manner which holds the bone vibrator tightly against the skull. The metal, spring-loaded band of the bone vibrator applies a steady pressure to secure the vibrator to the head. This pressure is needed to help the vibrator stimulate skull vibrations.

When bone-conducted tests are administered, the energy from the bone vibrator spreads around the skull stimulating both ears, as shown in Figure 24. The energy is only slightly greater in the ear closest to the vibrating source. This two-ear stimulation by the vibrator creates one of the major problems of the bone conduction hearing test, namely, uncertainty as to which ear is really responding to the test signal. Therefore, the hearing aid specialist needs to exercise caution in doing bone conduction testing.

The procedure for obtaining pure-tone, bone-conducted thresholds is initiated by placing the vibrator on the mastoid and asking the client to indicate when the tone is heard. The audiometer has been previously set to produce an audible tone, e.g. 50 dB at 1000 Hz. After the client confirms the tone is heard, the tester moves the vibrator about the mastoid to find the point where the best sound transmission occurs. With each move, the tester asks the client whether the tone is louder or softer. Bone-conduction testing is begun at the site on the mastoid the client identified as having the greatest sensitivity.

Many audiometers produce a warbled, pulsed test tone. This modified pure-tone sound makes it easier for the client to hear the test tone. The warbled, pulsed, pure-tone signal is sometimes easier to hear than a continuous signal.

After determining the location on the mastoid which provides the best transmission, the hearing aid specialist uses bone-conduction testing techniques similar to those used with air conduction testing. The tones presented are at an audible level to insure that the client hears the tone. Next, the tone intensity is decreased in 10 or 15 dB steps until the client no longer hears the tone. The tone intensity is then increased until it again becomes audible. This is usually a stepped increase of 5 dB. Once more the specialist decreases the tone in 10 dB steps until the client is no longer able to hear the sound. The hearing aid specialist makes several passes with the signal from audible to inaudible to obtain the correct threshold. The threshold value obtained is recorded on the audiogram. Figure 18 showed the audio key which specifies the symbols used for the pure-tone thresholds, air and bone conduction, masked and unmasked. The most commonly used bone symbols assume that the patient is facing the tester. This seating position puts the client's right ear to the tester's left. The bone symbol, therefore, for the right ear, faces the same direction as the client's right ear.

Bone-conduction thresholds, like air-conduction thresholds, are defined as the weakest level detected by the client fifty percent of the time. The threshold for 1000 Hz is determined first; then the other frequencies are tested in the usual sequence of 500 and 250 Hz; repeat the assessment at 1000 Hz, then 2000, and 4000 Hz. As each threshold is obtained, the hearing aid specialist records the level on the audiogram.

Following is a sample sequence of a bone-conducted test:

- Locate the point on the mastoid that gives best hearing sensitivity.
- Instruct the client, "Raise your hand each time you hear the tone."
- Set the audiometer at 1000 Hz and present a one-second tone at 50 dB HL.
- When the client responds, nod your head in agreement. This helps reinforce the correct behavior of the client for subsequent tonal presentations.
- Decrease the intensity level to 35 dB and again present a one-second tone.
- When the client raises his/her hand, again smile to reassure him/her the response is correct.
- Decrease the level to 20 dB; give a one-second tone.
- In this example, if the client does not respond, increase the level 5 dB to 25 dB and present the tone.
- If the client does not respond at this level, increase the level another 5 dB to 30 dB and present the tone.
- If the client raises his hand slowly, decrease the level 10 dB to 20 dB and present the tone.
- If no response, increase the level 5 dB to 25 dB and present the tone.
- If no response at this level, increase the level 5 dB to 30 dB and present the tone.

- Now the client indicates he/she hears the tone.
- This point, 30 dB, is the softest level the client is able to hear. Therefore, place a mark on the audiogram at 30 dB for 1000 Hz. The bone conduction symbol is placed beside, not on, the 1000 Hz line. Air conduction symbols are placed directly on the frequency lines.
- Test each of the other frequencies in the same manner and retest 1000 Hz. Remember the test/re-test scores should agree within 5 dB.

Bone-conduction scores have great value when compared with the air-conduction scores. Recall that air conduction is the normal pathway of hearing. Bone conduction is the pathway that bypasses the outer and middle ear. Therefore, air-conducted scores will always be equal to or worse than bone conduction scores. If the outer and middle ear structures are normal, the air scores will equal the bone scores. If the outer or middle ear structures are not functioning correctly, the air-conduction scores will be poorer (farther down on the audiogram) than the bone scores.

Later in this chapter we consider a hypothetical client whose external ear canals are impacted with wax (cerumen). This person's hearing ability—with his ears impacted with cerumen—is shown in Figure 42. The pure tones from the earphones (the air-conducted mode) encounter the wax plug in the ear canal and much of their energy is lost trying to pass through the wax. To compensate for the energy lost, the intensity levels have to be increased and the client's air-conduction thresholds are abnormal by 35 to 40 dB.

When this client is given bone-conduction tests, better thresholds occurred at all test frequencies. Bone conduction hearing values are better than the air conduction values because the conductive impairment did not influence the bone transmission pathway. By drawing one line connecting the air-conduction scores and then drawing another line connecting the bone-conduction scores, the influence of the impacted cerumen is shown as the distance between two lines. This concept is illustrated in Figure 25. This area is the air-bone gap, or the quantity of conductive hearing loss due to impacted cerumen. After the wax plugs are removed, the air-conduction thresholds improve to the level of the bone conduction thresholds.

The function of the outer and middle ear is to conduct sound energy from an external source to the inner ear. An outer or middle ear pathology, which stops or impedes sound from traversing the

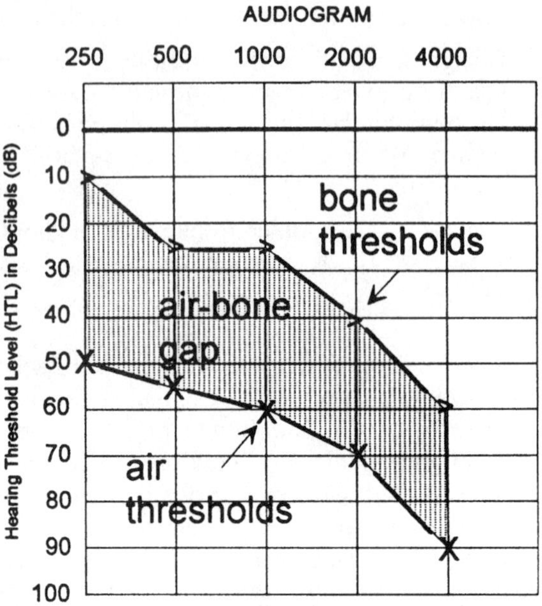

Fig. 25. The air-bone gap is the zone between the bone-conducted thresholds and air-conducted thresholds. Also see Figure 42.

outer and/or middle ear structures, is called a conductive hearing loss, or a loss due to changes in mechanical sound conduction.

The hearing aid specialist often encounters some of the more common outer and middle-ear pathologies, including ear infections, middle-ear fluid, eardrum perforations, and immobile middle-ear ossicles. These pathologies create mechanical interference to sound entering the ear. The result is a conductive hearing impairment.

Hearing aid specialists have two important reasons for doing bone conduction tests: first, to determining if the ear is normal or abnormal, and second, to determine the acoustic power needed to compensate for the loss, if the problem cannot or is not corrected medically or surgically.

Determining whether or not an air-bone gap is present requires the correct administration of air and bone-conduction tests. The major obstacle to correct administration during bone-conduction tests is that the signal from the bone vibrator stimulates the cochlea of each ear. However, the hearing aid specialist must correctly identify which ear is responding to the bone-conducted signal.

Five sources of information exist which help to identify which ear is responding to bone-conduction stimuli. These are: (1) asking the individual, (2) viewing the ear by otoscopy, (3) tympanometry, (4) acoustic reflex testing, and (5) bone-conduction test with masking.

It is tempting to skip over the first four items and discuss the topic of bone-conduction testing with masking. This, however, must not be done. Learning to do correct bone-conduction measurements with masking is like learning to fly an airplane. Though possible for most people to learn to fly, they first must pass several preliminary tests. After so doing, hands-on training begins under the direction an experienced aviator. Mistakes create disasters. Similarly, bone-conduction tests with masking require considerable study and training before the first solo practice. Mistakes in bone-conduction masking can lead to fitting hearing aids on dead, nonfunctioning ears, or over amplifying sensorineural losses. The use of more direct approaches to middle ear assessment are recommended. For example, otoscopy and impedance/immittance testing are very useful testing procedures.

IMMITTANCE (IMPEDANCE) TESTING

For years the term "impedance" was used to describe middle-ear test units. Now the term "immittance" is more clinically popular.

Impedance/immittance tests are valuable tools used to evaluate ear function. Impedance tests can measure eardrum mobility, relative outer ear canal volume, movement ability of the middle-ear bones, stapedius muscle function, eustachian tube function, and other ear functions. Most ear pathologies alter at least one of the impedance functions affecting the normal mechanical function of the ear.

Minimal training is needed to learn to administer immittance tests. The tests are administered quickly. One great value of immittance testing is to give the hearing aid specialist instant feedback to support or place into question the information obtained from the visual inspection of the ear. A hearing aid specialist may be unsure whether or not a small spot on an eardrum is a tympanic perforation or some existing artifact. The impedance test can quickly confirm or reject the visual impression. The hearing aid specialist may be unsure whether or not there is fluid behind the tympanic membrane. Again, impedance testing helps confirm or deny the visual information.

Another valuable application of the immittance tests concerns the evaluation of clients who have hearing losses greater than the output limits of the bone-conducted signals. The typical audiometer has a maximum output of only 70 dB for bone-conducted signals. If the client's bone threshold is at 80 dB, it cannot be measured by bone-conduction testing. The impedance unit, however, can provide excellent outer and middle ear data to substitute for the bone-conduction data.

Immittance testing supplements bone-conduction testing, it should not replace it. Impedance tests provide additional information and insight into the client's hearing function. They help improve the hearing aid fitting and to alert the hearing aid specialist to a needed medical referral.

Many different types of immittance units are currently on the market. Some units have all functions automated. Others require the hearing aid specialist to manipulate the controls.

The ear probe is one main feature of any immittance unit. Figure 26 shows an ear probe, three tubes, and a probe tip. Each tube has its own function. One tube is used to transmit a tone into the ear canal. A portion of this tone's energy is absorbed by the eardrum. The remainder of this tone is reflected back through the second tube and measured. The last tube provides a route for positive and negative changes in air pressure. The probe works like a sonar. It transmits a signal and monitors the reflection of the signal. An easy way to remember the function of the tubes attached to the probe is: (1) tone in; (2) tone out; (3) air pressure change.

Attached to the end of the probe is a rubber plug. Plugs come in different sizes for different ear canals. The probe and rubber plug close the outer ear canal with an airtight seal that holds the sonar-like signal inside the canal. If one plug fails to maintain a seal, a different size plug and/or earmold impression material may be used to achieve the air tight seal. The air tight seal is needed so the unit can conduct a tympanogram.

The tympanogram is the measure of eardrum movement created by changing the air pressure within the ear canal. A rough comparison to the tympanogram is the pneumo-otoscopic test, where a

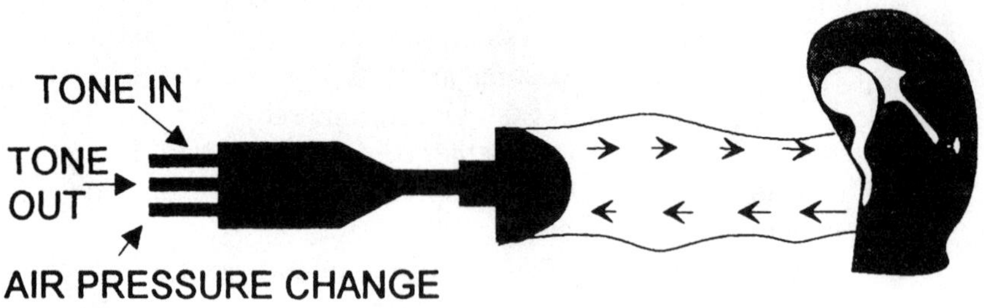

Fig. 26. Impedance unit ear probe.

physician views the eardrum through an otoscope while manually forcing the eardrum to move with air pressure created by a rubber bulb attached to the otoscope.

Many impedance tests have medical diagnostic value. Two tests yield data which aid the hearing aid specialist in understanding the client's ear and aid in determining the amplification needed for the client. The two tests are tympanometry and acoustic reflex threshold measurement.

Automated impedance screening units have been developed which assist the tester in doing impedance tests. A hand held ear probe is inserted into the ear canal and air pressure is changed automatically. After an adequate air pressure seal has been obtained, the machine automatically presents and records the tympanogram and acoustic reflex tests. The self recording and automatic sequencing features of these screeners make them valuable for the busy clinician. See Figure 27 for an example of this type of unit.

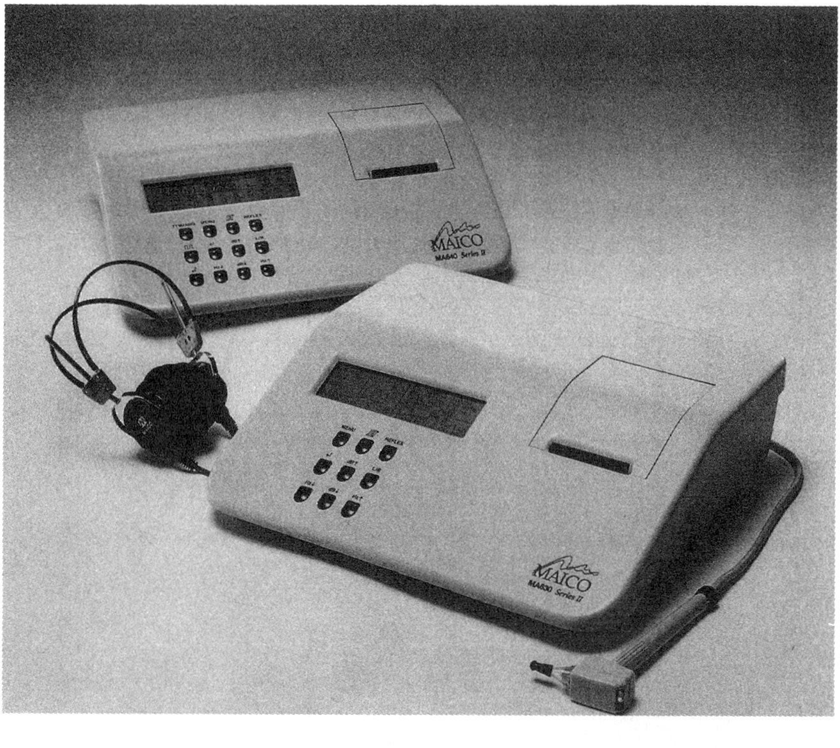

Fig. 27. Impedance screener with automatic Printer. (Courtesy of Maico Hearing Instruments).

TYMPANOGRAMS

Tympanograms are graphs produced by the tympanometric procedure. The graph indicates the change in the mobility of the ear drum (tympanic membrane) and middle ear structures during changes of air pressure within the external ear canal. The graph indicates air pressure along the horizontal axis and ear mobility (also called compliance) along the vertical axis. Figures 28 and 29 show tympanograms. Figure 28 shows the graph used to record tympanograms. The pup-tent shaped area is the area of the normal response.

The procedure to obtain a tympanogram is:

1. Seal the probe tip in the outer ear canal.
2. Adjust the unit and start at a positive 200 mm air pressure, and vary the air pressure from +200 mm air pressure to −400 mm air pressure.
3. Plot the magnitude of eardrum compliance or mobility on the graph. This is done automatically if you have an appropriate recorder. If you do not, chart by hand at each 50 mm increment.

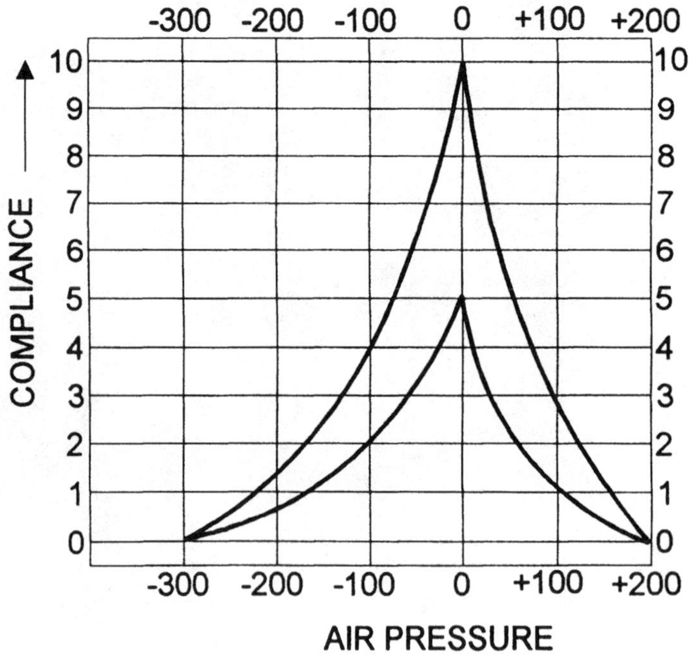

Fig. 28. Tympanogram, the graph is used to record middle-ear mobility.

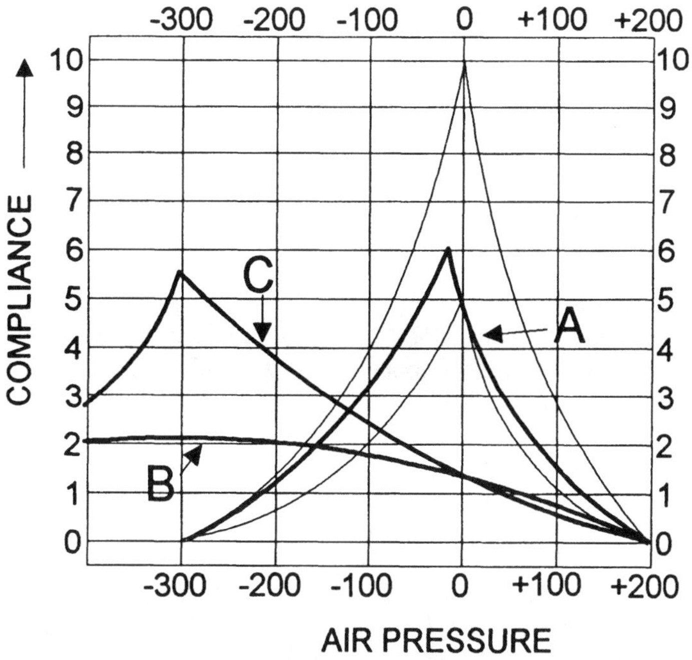

Fig. 29. Examples of A, B, and C type tympanograms.

Tympanograms are classified according to their shape as types A, B, or C as shown in Figure 29. Type A peaks at normal pressure. Type B does not peak at any pressure and is rather flat. Type C peaks at negative pressure.

Type A occurs with the normal conductive mechanism. This type has its point of maximum mobility at or near the zero air pressure line. Type A curves look like the normal curves in Figure 28. One pathological condition, however, which yields a type A tympanogram is stapes fixation and is associated with otosclerosis. A type A graph is obtained because the fixed ossicle does not stop the eardrum from moving during the tympanometric procedure.

Type B tympanograms, also called flat tympanograms, occur when little or no eardrum movement exists. Fluid-filled middle ears, heavily scarred eardrums, and severely retracted tympanic membranes yield this type of tympanometric tracing.

Type C tympanograms indicate negative middle ear pressure. This middle ear condition results from abnormal eustachian tube function. Type C tracing indicates an ear condition which is unstable, i.e., the ear is in the process of getting better or getting worse. If the eustachian tube does not correct itself and allow air to enter the middle ear, the peak of the Type C tympanogram will shift more negatively and the mobility of the eardrum will reduce, producing a flatter tracing.

A more complete discussion of impedance/immittance testing, is presented by Jacobson and Northern 1991.

THE ACOUSTIC REFLEX TEST

The middle ear has several important structures which include the eardrum, three ear bones (ossicles), two muscles (the stapedius and the tensor tympani), and supporting tendons and ligaments. The stapedius muscle plays an important role in the acoustic reflex. This muscle is attached to the stapes on one end and to the middle ear wall on the other end. See Figure 30. The stapedius muscle is enervated (activated) by the facial nerve (VII). Loud sounds cause this muscle to contract. The contracting muscle pulls the ossicles and the eardrum inward.

The acoustic reflex measurement is our second impedance test. An earphone is placed over one ear during this test and the impedance probe is inserted into the other ear. The earphone presents a strong pure-tone signal sufficiently loud to elicit bilateral stapedial contraction. The resulting eardrum movement is observed as a needle deflection on the compliance meter of the impedance unit.

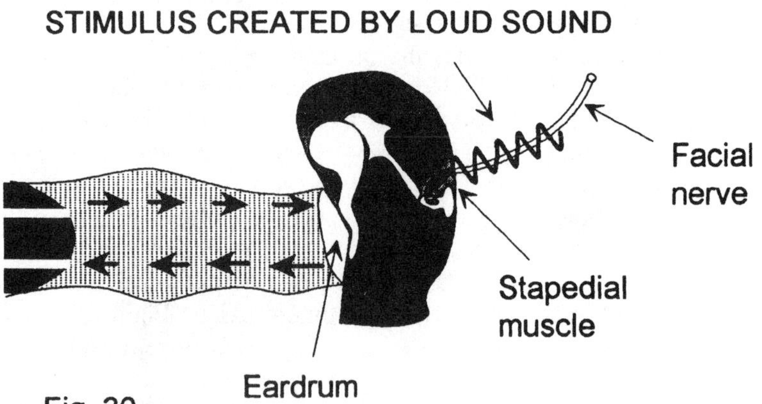

Fig. 30.

Fig. 30. The stapedial muscle in the middle ear contracts when a loud sound is presented. The sonar probe monitors eardrum movement.

The tester observes the needle movement and records the intensity level needed to elicit the reflex. Pure-tone signals of 500, 1000, and 2000 Hz are normally used for the acoustic reflex test.

The acoustic reflex action may be the ear's natural means of protecting itself against the potential damage caused by loud sounds. Intense sound causes the middle-ear muscles to contract. This contraction in turn tightens the eardrum, decreasing hearing sensitivity. If the sound is made even more intense the stapedius muscle increases the pull on the eardrum further reducing hearing sensitivity. Unfortunately this protective mechanism does not adequately protect the ear from very intense sounds.

Figure 31 illustrates the neural pathway of the reflex. Sound passes through the outer-middle-and-inner ear to stimulate the hearing nerve (the VIII Cranial Nerve). The signal is conducted up the hearing nerve to the midbrain in route to the auditory cortex. At the level of the midbrain a small branch of the hearing nerve crosses to the facial nerve. This junction allows auditory signals to activate a branch of the facial nerve which is descending toward the face and ear. This descending nerve enervates the stapedius muscle in the middle ear. The stapedius muscle is attached to the stapes bone and contractions of the muscle pull the middle ear bones and the eardrum inward toward the medial wall of the middle ear. These movements are observable on the compliance meter of the impedance unit.

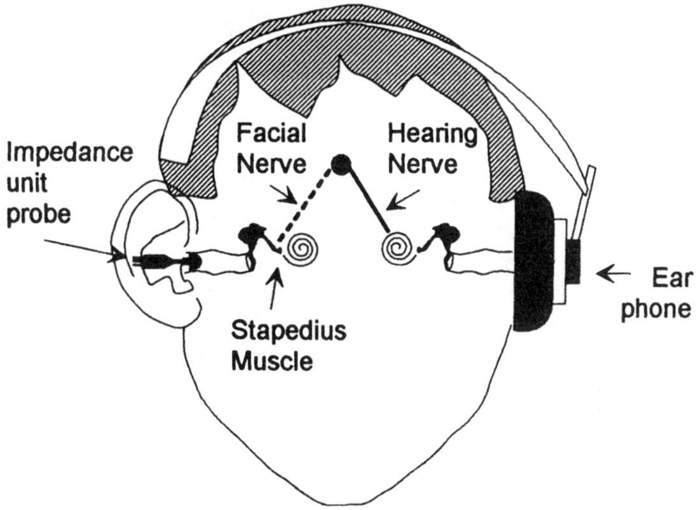

Fig. 31. The stapedial reflex mechanism.

The acoustic reflex test gives us valuable information. Almost all of the conductive hearing pathologies eliminate or reduce the acoustic reflex. Therefore, if the reflex thresholds are observed at their normal levels the function of the middle-ear is probably normal and the probability of a significant air-bone gap is low. The presence of normal reflex thresholds therefore, greatly simplifies and verifies bone conduction tests.

The reflex action is not observed when soft sounds are presented to the ear. Only louder sounds trigger the reflex. Reflex thresholds therefore help define the ceiling of hearing. The level of the reflex may be thought as a physiological reaction or jump response to loud noises. The level of the reflex approximates the overload of the ear and extra sensitive reflexes warn us about a low ceiling, low tolerance to acoustic stimuli.

Reflex thresholds are observed near 90 dB SPL @ 500, 1000, and 2000 Hz in normal ears. Mild and moderate sensorineural hearing losses do not usually change the reflex levels. More severe sensorineural hearing losses may cause the reflex level to be elevated. A sharply-sloping pure-tone audiogram is often correlated with normal reflex level at 500 Hz and elevated reflex levels at 1000 and 2000 Hz.

Acoustic reflexes are not usually seen if the client has a mixed or conductive hearing loss. The reflex action is prevented by the mechanical blockage in the outer or middle-ear due to the conductive component.

Although the frequent recording of an acoustic reflex is that of the contralateral ear, it is also possible and useful to record the acoustic reflex of the same ear for which the tympanogram is to be charted. This reflex measurement is referred to as the ipsilateral acoustic reflex.

RELATIVE PHYSICAL VOLUME TEST

This simple test is the third basic impedance test. It is performed after the tympanogram and acoustic reflex testing. Since all impedance measurements are made using a sonar-like probe sealed in the outer ear canal, the measurement is simply the reading of the cubic centimeters volume (a relative value) of the outer ear canal. This value can be read on the cursor scale of some impedance units.

This test helps evaluate the integrity of the tympanic membrane. A normal ear will usually have a value near or below 2.5 cc. If the tympanic membrane is perforated this value increases dramatically, usually doubling in value. If the tester suspects a perforation in one ear of a client, the relative physical volume measurements from the ear in question and the other normal ear, will provide definitive information.

FUNCTIONABILITY TESTS

Functionability, the client's hearing function without aids, depends not simply on hearing abilities, but also on such factors as intelligence, attention span, and motivation.

Hearing aid specialists may assume too hastily that amplification is the cure-all for every hearing deficiency. One may conclude, without full consideration, that all zones identified as having weak pure-tone hearing levels require amplification. This may or may not be true. The client may be able to function with limited, unaided input by making use of intelligence, auditory closure, and other factors.

The functionability test is a simple procedure. No special equipment is needed. The procedure is: say a word, have the client repeat it, step back, say another word, have the client repeat that one, step back etc.. This procedure is continued until the distance is reached where the client can no longer repeat the given word.

Functionability tests follow the basic hearing tests. Thus, considerable information is already present to help the hearing aid specialist choose the category of words appropriate for this test.

Functionability tests precede the master hearing aid tests and hearing aid demonstrations because we want to know which words at what distances will produce zero word understanding scores. The most impressive demonstration is the black to white example of going from no-hearing to adequate hearing. No-hearing is a condition in which no words are heard correctly or no tones are heard at all. Adequate hearing is being able to correctly repeat all of the test words or hearing the test tone. This demonstration is only possible if the client's functionability has been previously measured.

John Berry, of the Blount Speech and Hearing Center, Maryville, Tennessee, recommends the use of functionability tests as part of all hearing aid evaluations and has helped develop the tonality words listed in appendix D. These words are grouped into five tonal categories of low, low-middle, middle, middle-high, and high pitch.

These words form part of functionability testing by selecting word categories corresponding to frequency zones in which the client's hearing is weak. The tester asks the client to look away from him and then instructs the client to repeat what he/she hears. The tester then presents the words in a normal voice. Each time the client repeats a word correctly, the tester increases the distance between himself and the person. As distance increases, sound energy reaching the client diminishes. Therefore, the tester will find some point at which the client is no longer able to repeat words from that specific category. The tester notes this distance in the record as, e.g., Unable to repeat high tonality words at 12 feet.

MASTER HEARING AID MEASUREMENTS

The master hearing aid unit allows the client to hear and judge the quality of the sound produced by hearing aid circuits before the aids are specified. The hearing aid specialist uses the master hearing aid unit as a testing and demonstration tool. An example unit is shown in Figure 32.

The electronics in master hearing aids approximate the circuitry in hearing aids. The hearing aid specialist utilizes the master hearing aid unit to measure the pitch, power, and protection needs for each ear. The hearing aid specialist controls the gain, slope, and maximum power output (MPO) of the device.

Master hearing aids have complete two channel adjustability to control the sound for both ears. Measurements are first made for

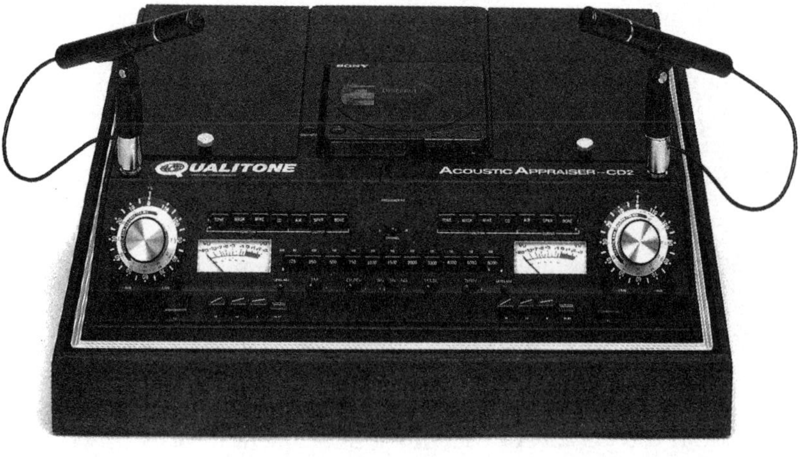

Fig. 32. Acoustic Appraiser desk model C, audiometer and dual master hearing aid. (Courtesy of Qualitone).

each ear independently. Then, the improvement provided by binaural amplification can be demonstrated.

Acoustic gain adjusts the floor of hearing. The gain is increased until the client has sufficient volume or sound. The hearing aid specialist may ask questions like, "Can you hear me?" or "Is this too loud or too soft?" to adjust the gain.

Frequency slope adjustments are made to compensate for the slope of the hearing loss. Slope is also used to equalize aided hearing ability in the bass and treble. The client's unaided hearing thresholds can be easily rechecked with the sound field system, after which slope and gain adjustments are made to produce the desired hearing improvement.

MPO adjustments are made to soften the ceiling of hearing. Tolerance problems are avoided by doing comfort level and uncomfortable level testing with the master hearing aid unit.

Hearing clarity is evaluated and the client is asked to repeat words and sentences. If the settings are adequate, the client will be able to hear and repeat speech stimuli to the best of his/her hearing ability. These word recognition scores should match or be better than those scores obtained during the audiometric word recognition testing. If the speech understanding ability is less than anticipated, adjustments on the master hearing aid unit can be made to improve the fitting.

When the proper adjustment is achieved, this part of the evaluation is often an exciting experience. The client wants to hear, and the quality amplification is demonstrated.

SPEECH IN NOISE TESTS

Some clients report great difficulty hearing in noisy listening environments. Many can be helped by: matching the amplification to a real-ear target, smoothing the frequency response, extending the amplification into higher frequency zones, using directional microphones, reducing distortion, and controlling the MPO. However, sometimes these procedures are of little help. In these cases a more complete hearing aid evaluation is needed.

Jerger and Hayes (1976) reported a hearing aid evaluation procedure which differed from other methods of evaluation. This speech in noise test places the client between two loud speakers. The seating arrangement is shown in Figure 33. The loudspeaker directly in front of the client delivers the primary message which

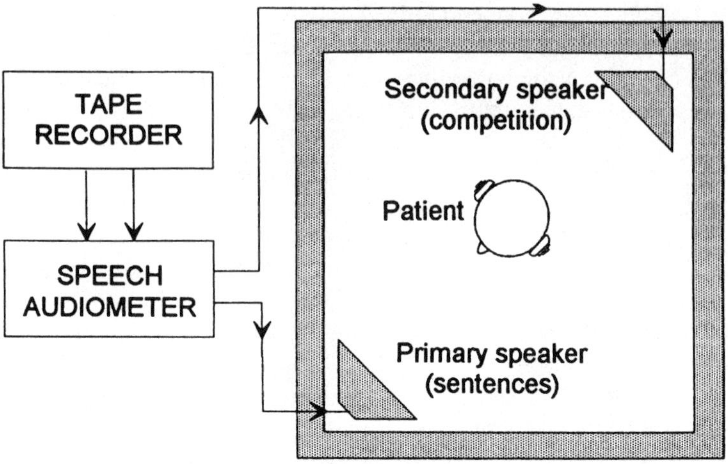

Fig. 33. Seating arrangement for hearing aid evaluations preformed with sentence identification materials. The graphics shown in Figures 33, 34 and 35 are with permission from J. Jerger Ph.D.

is a synthetic sentence. Examples of these sentences are given in Appendix E. The investigators preferred sentences as test stimuli because sentences are most like the speech we normally listen to in everyday life.

An additional speaker is placed behind the client. This speaker presents a competing speech noise. The levels of speech and noise are carefully adjusted to give the client changing speech to noise ratios. Jerger and Hayes refer to the speech signal as the message and the noise as the competition. The signal to noise ratio is called the message to competition ration or MCR. An MCR of +20 dB is called the very easy condition—the speech level is 20 dB louder than the noise level. An MCR of +10 dB is called the easy condition—the speech level is 10 dB louder. At 0 MCR the speech and noise levels are equal. An MCR of −10 dB is called the difficult condition—noise is greater by 10 dB. An MCR of −20 dB is called very difficult.

An example of the Jerger and Hayes hearing aid evaluation is shown in Figure 35. Note that the client's unaided scores are 0% for all conditions of the test. Aided, the client is able to hear 100% for the +20 MCR condition. As the level of the noise is increased the client's ability to correctly identify sentences decreases. When the speech is 10 dB greater than the noise, 80% of the sentences were identified correctly. When the noise level

Lesson 2 pg131-133

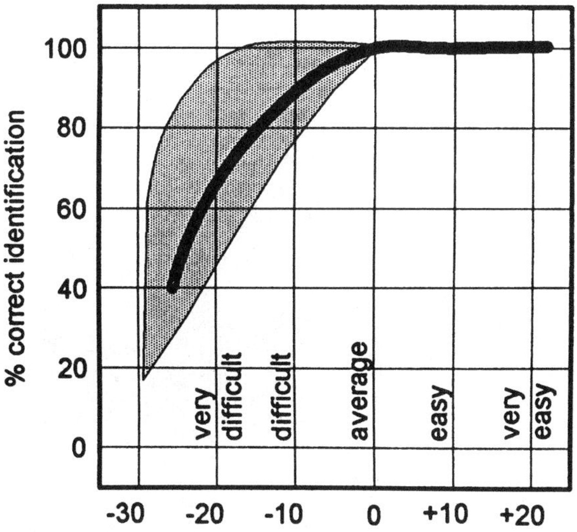

Fig. 34. A hearing aid evaluation summary form used to record the percentage of sentences correctly identified for differing noise levels. The shaded area represents the performance range of normal listeners.

equaled the speech level only about 40% of the sentences were correctly identified.

This procedure has several uses. First, different hearing aid adjustments can be evaluated to determine which adjustment functions best in a noisy environment. Second, the test results provide data helpful in counseling.

Unaided results are shown as the lower black line. The cross hatched area indicates the area of improvement with hearing instruments. The lightly shaded area indicates the residual deficit.

CLASSIFICATION OF HEARING LOSSES

Types of hearing loss share no universally accepted terminology. Lloyd and Kaplan (1978) have reviewed the different classification systems proposed. One system classifies hearing loss according to type (conductive, sensorineural, and mixed), degree (mild, moderate, severe, and profound), and configuration (flat, sloping, sharply sloping, and reverse).

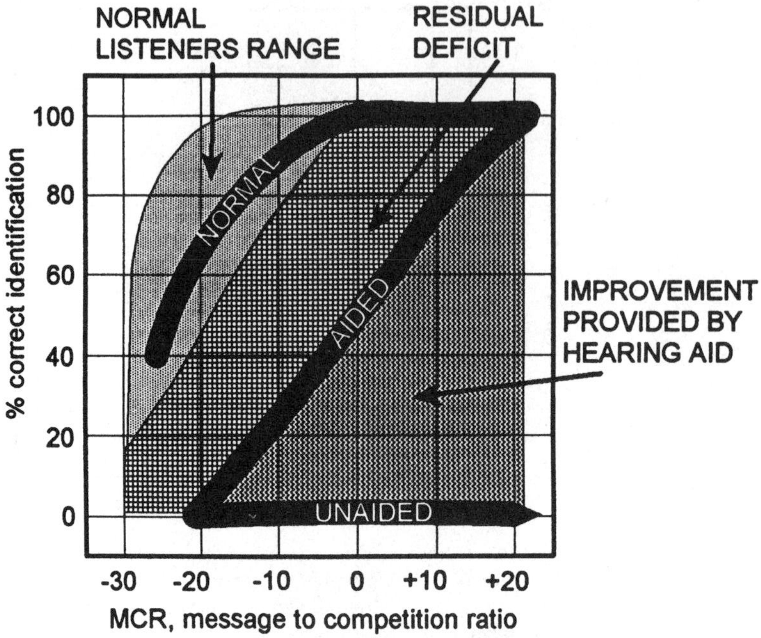

Fig. 35. An example of hearing aid evaluation. Without the hearing aid, the client does not correctly identify sentences. The scores are all 0% as shown by the line marked "unaided." With the hearing aid, the client correctly identifies some sentences, as shown by the line marked "aided."

CONDUCTIVE HEARING LOSS

Conductive hearing impairment is a pathology (blockage or obstruction) in the hearing pathway of the outer and/or middle ear. The term conductive refers to the physical action of sound energy being conducted from the external ear into the inner ear.

Conditions or pathologies which create conductive hearing losses include: impacted cerumen, swimmer's ear, perforation of the eardrum, otosclerosis, fluid in the middle ear, disarticulated (separated) middle ear bones, and cholesteatomas.

Earphones are used to measure air-conducted hearing thresholds. Bone conductors are used to obtain bone-conducted thresholds. Air and bone thresholds are recorded on an audiogram for each pure-tone frequency. When the air conducted threshold differs from the bone conducted threshold an air-bone gap occurs. A client with no conductive hearing loss exhibits no difference between these two thresholds and, hence, has no air-bone gap. If, however, the bone-conducted threshold occurs at a lower dB level than the air-conducted threshold, an air-bone gap exists, that is, bone-conducted hearing is better than air-conducted hearing, and a conductive hearing loss is evident.

Figure 36 illustrates an air-conduction test for a person with a fluid-filled middle ear. The test signal encounters a barrier in the middle ear and loses intensity before passing into the inner ear. Figure 37 expands Figure 36 and shows the bone-conducted test signal passing directly to the inner ear. Normal thresholds are observed for the bone-conducted test because this person has a normal inner ear. The air-conducted thresholds are elevated by 20–30 dB.

Figure 38 shows the hearing test results for a different person with a history of otosclerosis. Data for just the left ear are shown. In this case the third middle-ear bone, called the stapes, is frozen in place, and the air-conducted test signal must be elevated substantially before the patient can hear the test tone. The bone-conducted thresholds show near normal hearing because the inner ear is normal. The SRT is 45 dB indicating the client cannot hear softly spoken words, i.e., until they have an intensity of 45 dB HTL. The MCL and UCL values are also elevated, indicating the patient prefers to listen to loud speech and is not bothered by very loud sounds. The area between the Xs and carat marks is the air-bone gap.

It is technically impossible to have a bone-conducted threshold higher or worse than and air-conducted threshold. Should an audiogram indicate such a situation, either the audiometric equipment malfunctioned or the tester administered the tests incorrectly.

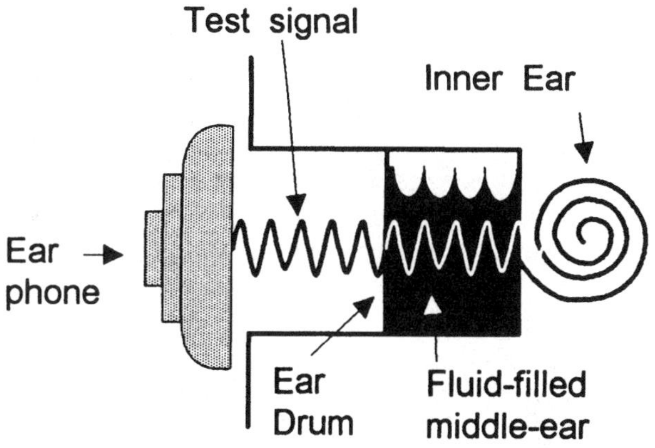

Fig. 36. Schematic drawing indicating loss of energy to the air-conducted signal due to middle ear fluid.

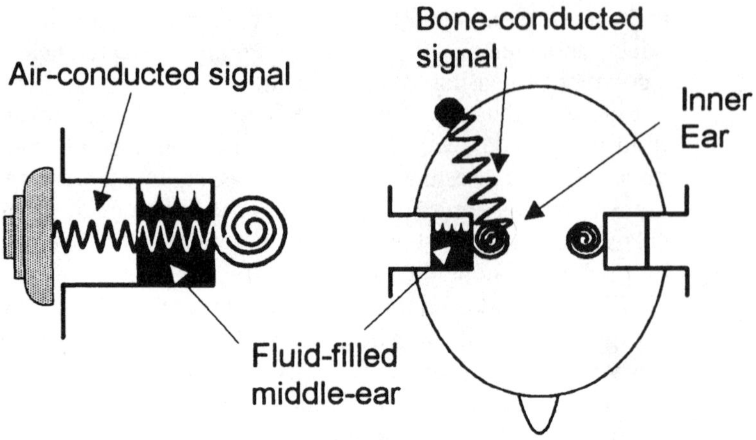

dB \ Hz	250	500	1000	2000	4000
bone	0	0	0	0	0
air	30	25	30	30	20

Fig. 37. A fluid-filled middle ear and normal inner ear. Air-conducted signal must be increased in intensity for the signal to pass through the "barrier" in the middle ear.

SENSORINEURAL HEARING LOSS

Sensorineural hearing impairment involves cochlear (inner ear) or neural dysfunction. Pathologies of the inner ear often damage the sensor cells which electrically stimulate the hearing nerve. Any action which reduces the ear's sensory or neural activity causes a sensorineural hearing deficit.

Figure 39 illustrates a testing situation where the outer and middle ear are normal and the inner ear is impaired. The test signal passes efficiently through the outer and middle ear into the inner ear. Damage in the inner ear is shown by the broken line.

Figure 40 expands figure 39 and shows the bone-conducted test for this person. The air and bone thresholds are the same.

Conditions which generally cause sensorineural hearing loss include excess noise exposure, Meniere's disease, presbycusis, constriction of the blood vessel supplying the inner ear structure, and a host of other possible causes.

To better understand conductive and sensorineural hearing loss, picture them in terms of the House of Hearing analogy. A pure conductive hearing loss causes an elevation of the floor and an equal

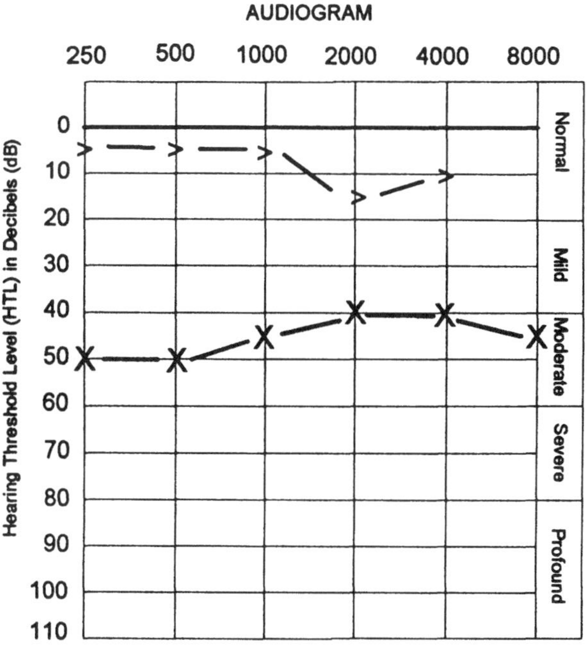

	SRT	Word Recognition	MCL	UCL
R	- - -	- - - - - % @ - - dB	- - -	- - -
L	45	100 %@ 80 dB	80	110+

Fig. 38. A client with a conductive hearing loss and a history of otosclerosis. The air-bone gap is 45 dB at 500 Hz and 25 dB at 2000 Hz. Word recognition is excellent (100%). The MCL and UCL are elevated.

elevation of the ceiling. The usable space retains the same quantity and quality.

For cases of pure conductive hearing loss, a hearing aid specification of increased power (amplification) for the affected ear is the straightforward, presumptive approach. A sensorineural hearing loss, on the other hand, causes an elevation of the floor and frequently a depression of the ceiling. Not only is the usable space of poorer quality, it also has less quantity. In this case, increased amplification will not work by itself, and may, in fact, be counterproductive. Special circuits are needed to protect the client from possible discomfort caused by excessive amplification.

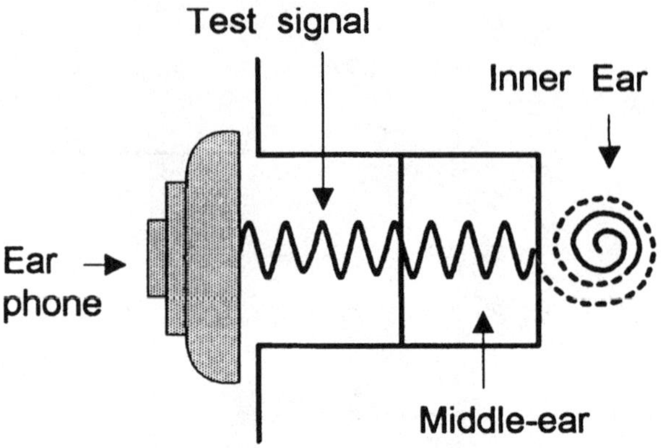

Fig. 39. Air-conducted signals pass through the outer and middle ear to a damaged inner ear. The zone of damage in the inner ear is shown by the broken line.

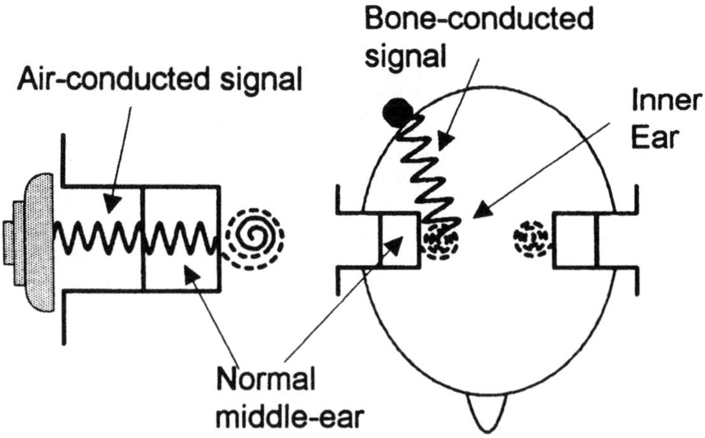

dB \ Hz	250	500	1000	2000	4000
bone	15	35	40	40	50
air	15	35	40	40	50

Fig. 40. Two audiometric tests for a patient having a normal middle ear and a defective inner ear. The air-conducted signal passes unobstructed to the inner ear. The hearing thresholds obtained with the earphone and the bone vibrator are the same.

The client illustrated in Figure 41 has a history of noise exposure and a sloping sensorineural hearing loss. No air-bone gap is observed.

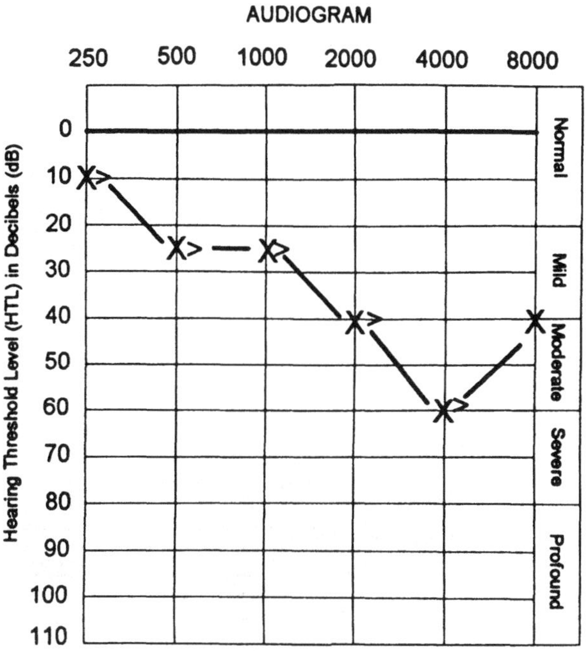

	SRT	Word Recognition	MCL	UCL
R	- - -	- - - - - % @ - - dB	- - -	- - -
L	40	76 % @ 65 dB	65	75

Fig. 41. An example of a client with a history of noise exposure and a sloping sensorineural hearing loss. Air and bone conduction thresholds are equal. The UCL indicates recruitment. The word recognition ability is impaired.

MIXED HEARING LOSS

Mixed hearing impairment is any combination of conductive and sensorineural hearing impairment. A client may have an outer or middle-ear dysfunction as well as an inner-ear dysfunction. The loss of energy due to the conductive problem is added to the hearing loss in the inner ear.

An example of a mixed hearing loss is that of impacted cerumen (conductive blockage) combined with a noise-induced hearing loss. In this example, Figure 42, the client's hearing threshold at 1000 Hz is 25 dB by bone conduction. The air-bone gap (the air threshold minus the bone threshold) is 35 dB. The air-bone gap indicates the degree of conductive hearing loss resulting from the presence of impacted cerumen. The bone threshold of 25 dB, represents the sensorineural hearing loss. This value, 25 dB, will remain after the wax is removed from the client's ear.

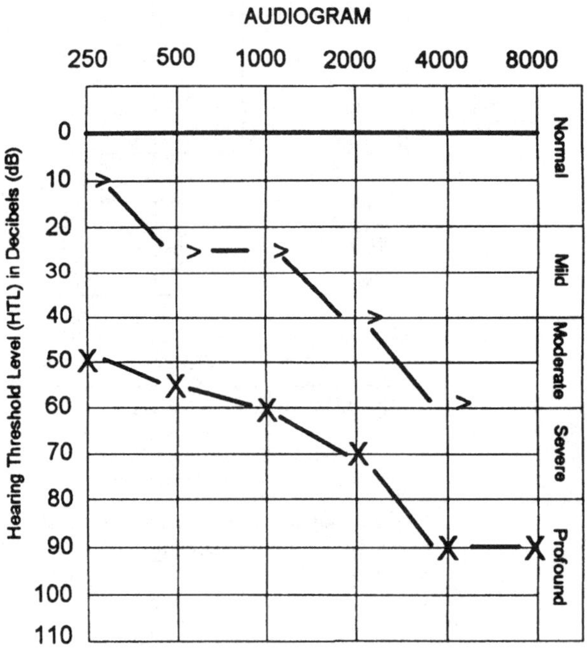

	SRT	Word Recognition	MCL	UCL
R	- - -	- - - - -% @ - - -dB	- - -	- - -
L	70	74 %@ 90 dB	90	110+

Fig. 42. The client has impacted ear wax. After the wax is removed, the hearing levels will return to those values shown in Figure 41.

SUMMARY TABLE ON CLASSIFICATION OF HEARING LOSS

Conductive

Air conduction configuration: flat to gentle rising.

Word recognition ability: excellent.

Air-bone gap: present.

Tympanogram: flat or other abnormal shape.

Recruitment: none.

Acoustic reflexes: absent.

Tinnitus: low pitched, if present.

Sensorineural

Air conduction configuration: sloping.

Word recognition ability: weak to good.

Air-bone gap: none.

Tympanogram: normal (pup-tent shape).

Recruitment: almost always present.

Acoustic reflexes: present if hearing loss is less than 70 dB.

Tinnitus: ringing or hissing, if present.

Mixed

Air conduction configuration: flat to sloping.

Word recognition ability: weak to excellent.

Air bone gap: present, but not equal at all frequencies.

Tympanogram: flat or other abnormal shape.

Recruitment: slight or none, but exceptions are common.

Acoustic reflexes: absent.

Tinnitus: varies.

This is a summary table of general tendencies of the three types of hearing loss. The reader should be aware that there are exceptions to these general tendencies.

DEGREE OF HEARING LOSS

Clients have trouble understanding audiometric thresholds. Therefore, the numeric value of the threshold is often converted to concepts more easily understood. Since there is no standard classification to which all agree, the author uses 0–20 dB as functionally normal hearing; 20–40 dB as mild hearing loss; 40–60 dB, moderate hearing loss; 60–80 dB, severe hearing loss; and 80–110 dB, profound hearing loss. The strength of this system is its simplicity. These values are printed on the audiogram in Figure 18.

CONFIGURATION OF HEARING LOSS

Hearing losses are often described according to the shape of the audiometric pure-tone curve. Normal hearing is seen as a straight horizontal line across the topmost portion of the audiogram.

Hearing loss is observed as a deviation from the normal hearing line with values falling lower on the audiogram chart. The terms flat, sloping, sharply or severely sloping, and reverse draw easily-grasped word pictures of the curve and permit easier use of complex hearing test data.

Flat indicates that the level of hearing is essentially uniform across all the different tones (frequency rate) tested.

Sloping suggests a hearing loss worse in the higher than in the lower frequencies. The audiometric curve slopes downward to the right. Sloping is the most common type of hearing loss. Great variations in the degree of slope are seen.

Sharply or severely sloping hearing loss is indicated by a curve that exceeds some predetermined decibel rate per octave changes. The author prefers to use this term to describe a hearing loss that drops more than 15 dB per octave.

Reverse hearing loss has a curve to the right, rather than falling off to the right. This less common hearing loss suggests poorer hearing in the lower than in the higher frequencies.

The terms selected to describe the hearing loss should represent the complete audiometric results. Where a simple description is inadequate, combined terms are used. For example, "the hearing loss is a mild-to-moderate loss, flat in the lower frequencies and sharply sloping in the higher frequencies."

DISCUSSING THE TEST RESULTS WITH THE CLIENT

After the necessary tests are administered, the hearing aid specialist may follow one of several different approaches. The goals of the discussion are: (1) Help the client understand the type and degree of the hearing loss, (2) Help the client make the commitments: (a) "Yes, I have a hearing loss; (b) Yes, the hearing loss is a problem in my life; and (c) Yes, I want to hear better.", (3) Allow the hearing aid specialist to display his/her professional competence, and (4) Counsel the client about hearing instruments and amplification and how it improves hearing function.

Some hearing aid specialists draw a sketch of the ear for the client. The drawing and associated explanation further educates the client about the physiological basis of hearing while showing the hearing aid specialist's knowledge.

Figure 43 and 44 illustrate the pathway of hearing and the electro-mechanical stimulation of the hearing nerves by the sensory hair cells.

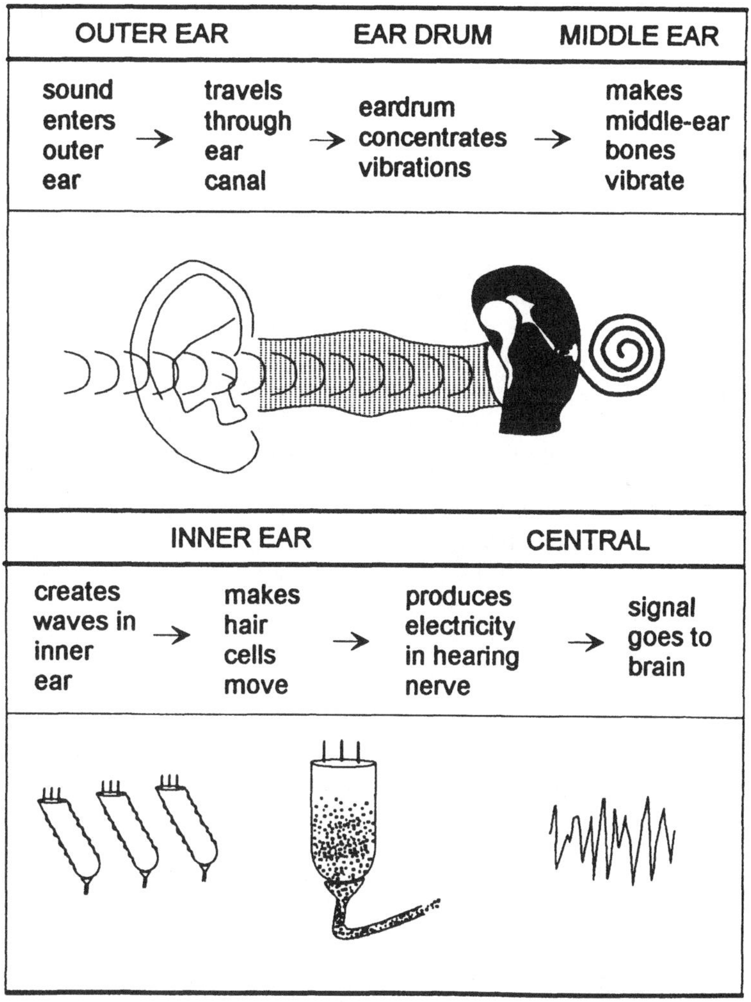

Fig. 43. The Pathway of Hearing.

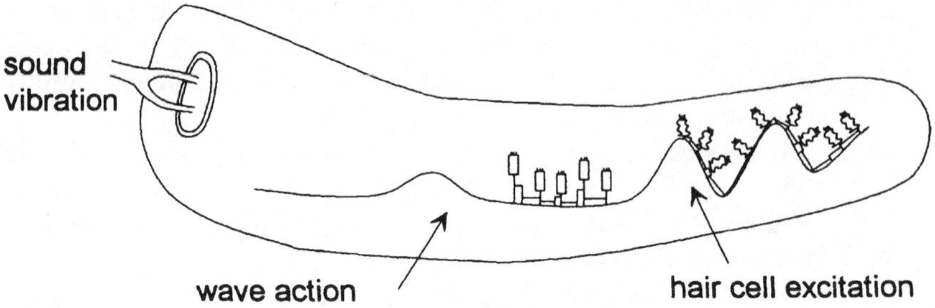

Fig. 44. Sound vibrations from the middle-ear enter the inner-ear where a wave action mechanically stimulates the sensory cells. These sensory cells generate an electrical signal that activates the hearing nerves. The nerves carry the signal to the brain.

These figures can be used to counsel the client. The key point of the discussion is to help the client understand that normal ears produce strong clear electrical impulses for the brain. Ears with sensorineural hearing loss produce weak distorted electrical impulses for the brain. Hearing aid use can increase the strength and clarity of the electrical impulse produced by the inner ear, thereby helping the brain have more easily understood signal.

AUDIOMETRIC INTERPRETATION

AUDIOMETRIC INDICATORS

When we travel by car, road signs guide us through blind curves and around detours. Without them, we may become lost and fail to reach our destination. The hearing rehabilitation process has "road signs" as well. There are audiometric indicators. One must learn to read, integrate, and employ the information from these signs if hearing is to be improved to the maximum level.

1. *Client Attitude*

The client's feelings and attitudes about hearing aid use dominates the prognosis. A positive attitude almost guarantees success. A strongly negative attitude almost assures failure. This information should be part of the case history. If often outweighs all other factors.

2. *Conductive Hearing Loss Indicators*

Conductive pathologies often correlate with air-bone gaps, flat tympanograms, excellent word recognition scores, and absent reflexes. The UCL if often elevated and a wide dynamic range is observed. These pathologies are located in the outer and/or middle ear; therefore, many times they can be observed otoscopically. The client is often aware of the problem and a precise history can usually be obtained.

Sometimes most of the audiometric indicators will point toward a conductive problem, yet one test will disagree. In these cases, it is important to reevaluate the situation. The following recommendations may work as troubleshooting approaches:

If there is an air-bone gap, yet the tympanograms and reflexes are normal, check to be sure the ear canal did not collapse when the air-conduction tests were administered. Normal impedance measures are not consistent with an air-bone gap. It is also possible that the client did not respond to the softest level audible for air conducted signals, so the air thresholds may be artificially depressed. Check to be sure the bone conductor was located appropriately on the mastoid and not against the ear, thereby creating falsely improved thresholds.

If your air-and-bone conduction tests suggest no air-bone gap, yet you observe a flat tympanogram, check to be sure your impedance probe was not against the side of the canal wall or imbedded in ear wax. Also, look at the ear otoscopically. A truly flat tympanogram will most always correlate with an air-bone gap.

If you observe a substantial air-bone gap (e.g., 30 dB), yet your tympanogram is normal, carefully view the eardrum with a fiber-optic otoscope. Sometimes the drum will have one section of highly mobile tissue. This may happen following a perforation when the new tissue forms without the fibrous middle layer. These small highly movable regions can be responsible for the eardrum mobility seen on a normal looking tympanogram even when the larger part of the drum is immobile.

If the ear appears normal otoscopically, yet your audiometric data suggest an air-bone gap, absent reflexes, and a flat tympanogram, recheck the impedance tests. Then, redo and pay particular attention to the UCL. If the impedance values do not change and the UCL is elevated, there is strong evidence sugesting a conductive hearing loss. Otosclerosis can produce anonvisible conductive problem by freezing the ossicles, however, the tympanogram is usually normal. Also, middle-ear fluid can preventhe eardrum from moving, and sometimes middle-ear fluid does not markedly discolor the eardrum and it appears normal to a cursory otoscopic exam.

3. Sensorineural Hearing Loss Indicators

Sensorineural hearing losses often correlate with sloping or sharply sloping high frequency losses, reduced word recognition ability, normal impedance data, high pitched tinnitus, absent air-bone gaps, reduced dynamic range, and recruitment. The pathologies that create sensorineural hearing losses are usually not observable by otoscopy.

The following recommendations may work as troubleshooting approaches related to sensorineural hearing loss.

If the tympanogram is normal, no air-bone gap exists, yet the acoustic reflexes are absent, check to determine the maximum level of signal of the impedance/immittance unit used. Impedance units differ markedly relative to the audio stimulus levels available. Some units only present a single level, other units have maximum levels at 105 dB SPL, while other units extend the upper limit to 125 dB SPL. The absent acoustic reflexes may be explained by noting a low output limitation of the audio stimulus.

If all indicators point to a sensorineural deficit and yet the tympanogram is abnormal, inspect the ear carefully by otoscopy. The impedance tracing is a very sensitive measurement. Sometimes the tympanogram records an abnormal tracing when the problem is not yet great enough to produce an air-bone gap.

If an air-bone gap is observed at 250 and 500 Hz and at no other frequencies, beware of vibro-tactile responses. The bone oscillator is a vibrator. Sometimes the client feels the vibration rather than hears the sound. Vibro-tactile responses are often observed at 250 Hz and 500 Hz. When in doubt ask the client. The client can often tell if they are hearing the test tone or feeling the vibration.

If all audiometric indicators suggest a sensorineural problem, yet the audiometric shape is not sloping, check the known pathologies for abnormally shaped sensorineural losses. Meniere's disease, for example, often yields a flat or reverse loss.

If you are having difficulty obtaining pure tone thresholds, evaluate the SRT, MCL, UCL, and word recognition scores. These tests can be done quickly and are not threatening to the client. An SRT close to 0 dB and excellent word understanding at 40 dB HTL are good, quick indicators of normal hearing.

If all indicators point to a severe or profound sensorineural loss, yet the word recognition ability seems too good, check to be sure the client was not looking at your lips during the word recognition test.

If the hearing loss seems to be a mild or moderate sensorineural hearing loss and yet the word recognition ability seems poor for the degree of loss, check to be sure the word recognition test was not presented at a setting too intense or too weak.

4. Danger Signs

Some types of hearing loss represent potential danger to the client. One type of possibly dangerous hearing problem is retrocochlear impairment. Retrocochlear pathology is located between the inner-ear and the brain. Such pathology is difficult to diagnose and its symptoms vary from person to person. Warning signals for this type of pathology included progressive unilateral hearing loss; poor unilateral word recognition ability and absent reflexes.

Other pathologies of the ear that can be potentially dangerous include cholesteatomas, hemotympanum (blood in the middle ear), infected mastoid, and chronic otitis. Needless to say the symptoms of ear pain, dizziness, and sudden hearing loss all show the need for immediate referral to a physician.

5. Prognostic Signs

The ability to help the hearing impaired client correlates with: the word recognition ability, the degree of slope of the hearing loss, the degree of recruitment, and other non-test factors like the client's manual dexterity and the client's willingness to work with the hearing aid specialist.

The audiometric tests described thus far provide the framework of information from which we develop the hearing aid system specifications. The author has organized the hearing aid system into seven categories. Collectively, they are used to delineate the parameters of hearing aid amplification.

HEARING AID PERFORMANCE PARAMETERS

The results of the hearing tests provide data that help specify the acoustical needs of the client. Seven topics are considered.

1. Power, more appropriately called maximum and use gain.
2. Slope, also called frequency response or pitch. Slope is the dB per octave roll-off of the amplifier.
3. Protection from loud sounds. The use of circuits, like AGC, to control the output so the client is protected from over amplification.
4. Reduction of perceived background noise. The use of filters, multi-memory circuits, and directional microphones to reduce

the amount of amplification in frequency regions perceived by the client to be background noise.

5. Exactness in plastics to enhance performance while maintaining comfort.
6. Optimizing clarity—word recognition. Excellence in clarity means hearing tones clearly and understanding words well. The clarity goal is determined by studying all speech scores, then, ensuring the client can hear an adequate speech spectrum. Lastly, make the amplification accurate as to bandwidth, gain, distortion, overall power, and frequency emphasis.
7. The author believes that all clients need strong, simple proof that they hear much better when the hearing instruments are fitted. This positive reinforcement helps insure the hearing aids are accepted.

POWER

Five items directly influence the amount of acoustic power (use-gain) needed by the client.

1. Personality and history of hearing aid use.
2. Level of hearing loss.
3. Type of hearing loss.
4. Growth of loudness.
5. Overload by power within the ear.

1. Patient Personality and History of Hearing Aid Use

Many new users of hearing instruments overreact to amplification. They are used to a world that has been quiet from their point of view. The return to hearing that comes with their new aids can reintroduce unwelcome crackly newspaper sounds, blaring automobile horns, the raspy-breathed speech of a friend or other ambient noises too long forgotten. Fortunately, the amount of amplification can be easily adjusted thus allowing clients to reeducate their hearing at lower amplification levels and slowly graduate to higher power settings.

2. Level of hearing loss

Hearing loss decreases the ear's ability to hear soft sounds. Consequently, these soft sounds must be amplified to a power level greater than the level of hearing loss. No simple predictive correlation exists between a given hearing loss and the amount of amplification needed. Much research has been done in this area and other sections of this textbook discuss this topic at length.

3. Type of Hearing Loss

A conductive hearing loss usually requires greater acoustic power (use-gain) from the hearing aid than a sensorineural hearing loss. The interruption of the hearing pathway associated with the conductive loss attenuates incoming sound energy before that energy reaches the inner ear. In contrast, damage to the inner ear's sensory hair cells usually makes the affected ear unable to tolerate high acoustic output levels.

A conductive hearing loss weakens sound energy as the signal passes through the point where the pathology exists. Correcting this type of problem requires increasing the amplification (power) to a level great enough to drive amplified sound through the mechanical blockage.

Figure 45 shows a client with a 40 dB air-bone gap. For simplicity, data for only one ear are given. The HTL (Hearing Threshold Level) value is converted to a SPL (Sound Pressure Level) value using the formula: SPL = HTL + 20 dB. In this case, the MCL of 80 dB HTL is equal to 100 dB SPL. If the input to the hearing aid is normal speech, a value close to 60 dB SPL, then this client would need 40 dB gain within the instrument to reach the MCL of 100 dB SPL. Note: 40 dB gain is the same decibel value as that of the air-bone gap.

	pure-tone audiogram					
	250	500	1000	2000	4000	8000
bone	10	10	10	10	10	10
air	50	50	50	50	50	50

speech tests				master hearing aid		
SRT	Wrd Rcgntn	MCL	UCL	gain	dB oct	MPO
50	100 @ 80	80	120	40	6-10	125

Fig. 45. A client with a 40 dB air-bone gap.

A sensorineural hearing loss is an ear condition where damage has occurred to the sensory cells and/or the neural transmitting cells. In some clients the damaged cells are hypersensitive to increases in acoustic power provided by hearing aids.

The pathophysiology of damaged sensory hair cells has been studied by many researchers including Dallos and Martin (1992) and Berlin (1993). The author likes to compare damaged inner ear hair cells to a "scraped" skin bruise. If the skin on the end of a finger is healthy, the finger can be touched without discomfort. If the skin has sustained damaged (scrapped), the tissue is hypersensitive to touch. In a similar manner, most damaged inner ear hair cells over react to loud sounds and the acoustic output must be controlled so it does not irritate the client.

Figure 46 represents a client with a typical sensorineural loss. Note that the air and bone thresholds are equal and that the threshold at 2000 Hz is 50 dB. Note also that the appropriate use gain suggested by the master hearing aid test result is 25 dB. McCandless (1978) stated that clients with sensorineural hearing loss usually set their hearing aids to a level equal to half of their hearing loss.

Compare the SRT, MCL and UCL values in Figures 45 and 46. These values are much greater (higher) in Figure 45 than in Figure 46. People with sensorineural hearing loss tend to reject loud amplified sound, people with conductive hearing loss tend to enjoy it.

In summary, hearing loss type influences the power to be used in the hearing aid. Conductive losses usually require more power.

	pure-tone audiogram					
	250	500	1000	2000	4000	8000
bone	20	30	40	50	60	70
air	20	30	40	50	60	70

speech tests				master hearing aid		
SRT	Wrd Rcgntn	MCL	UCL	gain	dB oct	MPO
30	86 @ 65	65	80	25	12	100

Fig. 46. A typical sensorineural loss.

Sensorineural hearing losses usually require less. Care must be taken in using any estimates, as each hearing aid fitting must be individually determined. Thus, testing is necessary and skilled data interpretation is essential.

4. Loudness Growth

Discussing loudness growth requires making a careful distinction between intensity and loudness. These terms appear synonymous in many usages; both are measured in decibels and both have to do with acoustic power or strength. Intensity is the strength of acoustic energy as it exists in time and space. The sound produced by a jet aircraft is measured in intensity. Loudness is the strength of the sound as perceived by a human listener.

Figures 47 and 48 show the relationship between loudness and intensity. The intensity levels are the horizontal straight lines referenced on the left side. The loudness curves are indicated by the darker curved lines and are referenced on the right side of Figure 47. Loudness curves are called equal-loudness contour lines, since all tones located on a single line would be judged equally loud by a normal hearing listener.

Figure 47 shows only the loudness curves, called phon curves, for 0, 15, 30, 60, 75, 90, and 120 phons. One's judgment of the loudness of a tone changes with age and hearing ability. A young person with normal hearing would judge a sound between the 0 and 15 phon

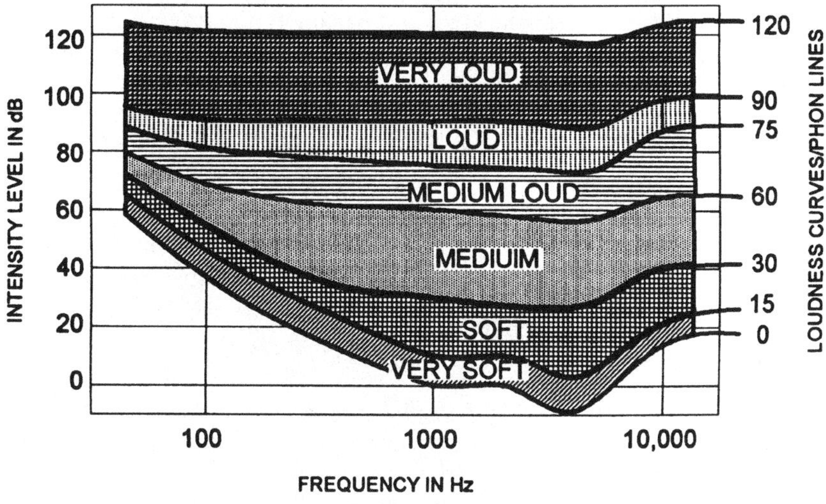

Fig. 47. A drawing showing the relationship between acoustic intensity and the human perception of loudness.

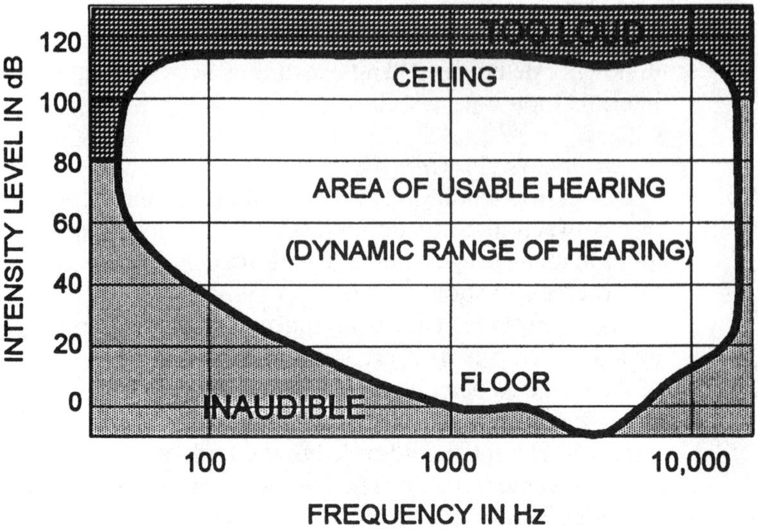

Fig. 48. The usable area of normal hearing.

curves as very soft, 15–30 dB as soft, 30–60 dB as medium, 60–75 dB as medium loud, 75–90 dB as loud, and 90–120 dB as very loud.

Compare human hearing at 100 and 1,000 Hertz. A tone at 100 Hz would have an intensity of about 40 dB to be judged very soft by a normal hearing listener. A tone at 1000 Hz would have an intensity level of only 5 dB to be judged very soft. This example shows that human hearing is more acute in the mid range. It takes much less energy in the mid frequency range for the normal human ear to react to sound.

Figure 48 is essentially the same graphic as Figure 47. It has been redrawn to illustrate the floor, ceiling and usable zone of human hearing for the normal hearing person. The floor of hearing is the zero phon line. The ceiling is the 110 phon line. Sounds with less intensity than the floor line are not audible. Sounds stronger than the ceiling are very irritating to the listener. The space between the floor and the ceiling is the zone of usable hearing, also called the dynamic range of normal hearing.

The 120 phon curve is relatively flat and is closely matched to the 120 dB intensity line. An intensity of 120 dB produces about 120 phons of loudness across most of the frequency range for normal listeners. The 0 and 15 phon curves have steep slopes in their low and high frequency areas. It takes much intensity or signal strength to make very low-pitched sounds equal in loudness to the mid-range sounds. The very high-frequency sounds also require more power than mid-range sounds before they become audible.

Hearing loss alters the ear's response to sound. As discussed earlier, recruitment is an abnormal growth of loudness, i.e., sounds become loud to the listener at softer levels than one might estimate. Some impaired ears recruit at all frequencies. Other impaired ears demonstrate recruitment in specific zones. Figures 49 and 50 illustrate the hearing abilities of two clients with recruitment in different frequency ranges. These cases serve to point out the need of measure Uncomfortable Listening Levels, UCLs, at specific frequency points.

Figures 49 and 50 were developed in a manner similar to Figures 47 and 48, i.e., the "inaudible, too loud, and area of usable hearing" are all labeled. Figures 47 and 48 are drawn like conventional equal-loudness curves, the bottom of the graph shows softer sounds. Figures 49 and 50 are presented as typical audiograms, the "softer zone" is at the top of the graph.

Contrast the area of usable hearing and the ceilings of hearing in Figures 49 and 50. Both clients have equal hearing-sensitivity losses, however, loud sound irritation happens at opposite frequency regions for these two people. The client in Figure 49 can

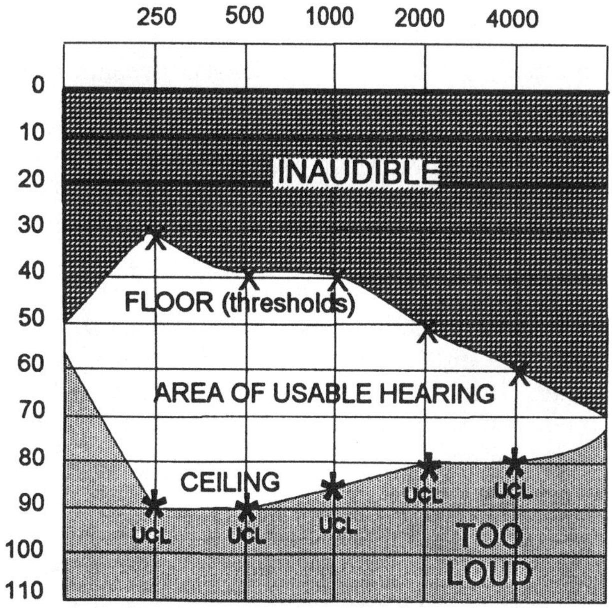

Fig. 49. A moderate loss of hearing sensitivity and a tolerance problem for higher frequency sounds.

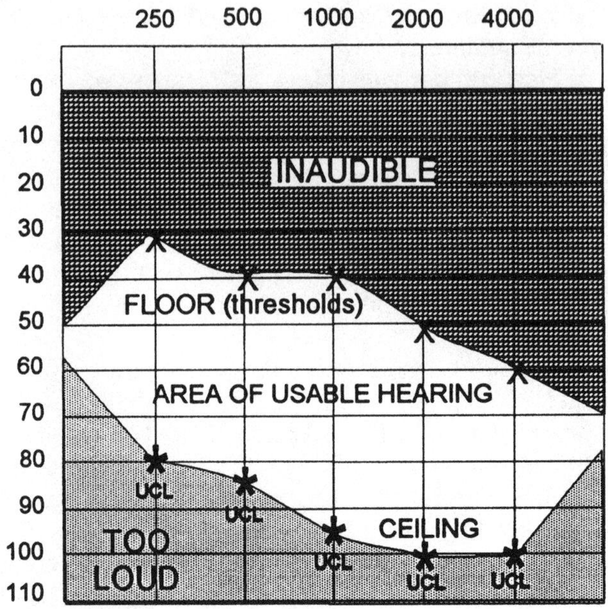

Fig. 50. A moderate loss of hearing sensitivity and a tolerance problem for lower frequency sounds.

tolerate considerable intensity increases in the low frequencies, but not in the higher frequencies. The dynamic range of hearing for this client is greater in the lower frequency range and reduced in the higher frequencies. The client in Figure 50 can tolerate high frequencies at increased intensities.

In the language of the House of Hearing analogy, the ceiling, (uncomfortable listening level) changes across frequency. In Figure 49, the usable space in the higher frequencies is limited, in Figure 50 this space is expansive.

In summary, these cases suggest the need to measure comfortable and uncomfortable levels at selected frequencies for each client. If a flat frequency response were used to measure the uncomfortable listening levels, these frequency differences would not be observed and the client might be misfit with hearing aid amplification.

5. Natural Ear Overload

The last item in the discussion of power is the distortion produced by an ear when subjected to sounds having excessive energy. Some hearing instruments distort sounds at higher amplification levels. However, even with an instrument able to amplify a high intensity sound completely free of distortion, the ear itself may not be able to reproduce the sound without substantial distortion.

Figure 51 is based on the work of Weaver and Lawrence (1954) and shows the inner ear reaction to signals of increasing intensity. Notice the ear responds clearly without distortion to weaker signals. As power increases, signal purity remains until the signal reaches a rollover point. At this high intensity level, the inner ear distorts the signal. This rollover point is the natural upper intensity limit of the ear.

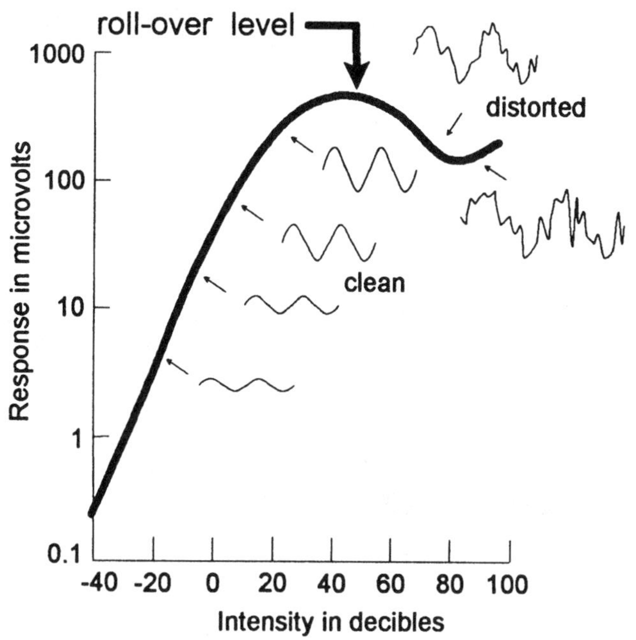

Fig. 51. The ear reproduces sounds undistorted up to a "roll-over" level (dark arrow).

PITCH

The terms pitch, slope, and frequency response are closely related and refer to the selection of the amount of gain within each frequency zone. Pitch assessment in hearing aid selection is of paramount concern. The hearing aid specialist must learn to adjust the basic frequency curve to agree with the general shape of the audiogram. This is not a one-to-one match. Rather, the general shape of the audiogram must guide the selection of the frequency response curve.

The client in Figure 52 illustrates the need to adjust the pitch response of the amplifier in relation to the hearing thresholds. This client has a sloping sensorineural hearing loss that is equal bilaterally. For simplicity the chart presents the data for one ear. The chart shows much better hearing ability in the low frequencies. To avoid low frequency overload, the instrument fitting required an 18 dB rise per octave in the amplifier and earmold vents. This fitting gave the client 25 dB of use gain at 2000 and 4000 Hz and pleased the client. If this client were fitted with a flat-response system, he/she would have difficulty in using such a system, as it would distort (overload) his/her natural hearing in the bass range.

Some people are unable to tolerate the volume of their own voice level when fitted with hearing instruments. Two adjustments help to eliminate this problem: first, reducing bass amplification; and second, increasing earmold vent size. Since the maximum energy in a human voice is in the frequency range of 200 to 500 Hz, a person will hear his own voice as extra loud, if this frequency range is over amplified. Reducing bass may help a client hear her own voice more naturally. Likewise, increasing the size of the vent also reduces bass amplification and makes incoming sounds more natural. Both of these fitting adjustments require skill since acoustic feedback can easily become a problem if earmold venting is excessive.

One of the most important pitch adjustments is that which puts more energy into those frequency regions that are important for

	pure-tone audiogram					
	250	500	1000	2000	4000	8000
bone	15	20	20	50	55	60
air	15	20	20	50	55	60

speech tests				master hearing aid		
SRT	Wrd Rcgntn	MCL	UCL	gain	dB oct	MPO
25	92 @ 65	65	80	20	18	100

Fig. 52. Sloping SN hearing loss.

good speech understanding. Whenever a client reports reduced ability in understanding words, the author first consults Figure 63 along with the client's unaided threshold levels. Real-ear and sound-field tests are administered to ensure adequate amplification within the frequency range labeled important-to-clarity.

Figure 53 is presented to help the reader develop more skill in reading and utilizing audiometric data. The hearing loss is equal bilaterally so only values for one ear are presented. A superficial inspection of the pure-tone values suggests that this person has normal hearing in the lower-frequency zone. The thresholds at 250 and 500 Hz do appear to be good, i.e., 20 dB. However, the 65 dB SRT value suggests the need for substantial power before the client can recognize soft words. Thus, the bass pure-tone thresholds are misleading if viewed in isolation.

Next, observe the severity of the slope. The hearing thresholds drop off rapidly as frequency is increased. Each hearing threshold must be compared with its neighbors. The 85 dB hearing threshold at 2000 Hz must be compared with 4000 Hz that shows no measurable hearing. In cases where hearing levels change rapidly from octave to octave, the hearing aid specialist must be careful in making judgments based on a single point on the audiometric curve. Rather, one must analyze the thresholds above and below the point under consideration.

Figure 53 points out an additional idea. Since the upper frequency range sensitivity is very poor, the hearing aid must accommodate and take advantage of the more functional lower

	pure-tone audiogram					
	250	500	1000	2000	4000	8000
bone	20	20	60	85	NR	NR
air	20	20	60	85	NR	NR

speech tests				master hearing aid		
SRT	Wrd Rcgntn	MCL	UCL	gain	dB oct	MPO
65	48 @ 80	80	95	40	12	120

Fig. 53. Sharply sloping SN hearing loss.

frequency range. While somewhat oversimplified, the concept is that the hearing aid specialist must use the client's existing hearing abilities rather than try correct that what is beyond help.

PROTECTION FROM LOUD SOUNDS

Hearing aid users often experience irritation while listening in noisy environments. Today, there are output-limiting circuits such as automatic gain control (AGC) to protect the user from surges in the noise level.

Output limiting techniques include AGC, peak clipping (PC), signal processing, automatic bandwidth limiting and other circuits. These circuits help control the amplified signal and hold the output to a level within the comfortable range of listening of the hearing impaired person.

Hearing test results contain considerable data that can be used to evaluate the need for output control. It is important to study the audiometric data to find out how much protection (the degree of output limitation) is needed for each person. The following items can serve as warning flags and suggest the need for output adjustment.

1. Low UCL for speech.
2. Narrow dynamic range.
3. Absence of air-bone gap.
4. No history of hearing aid use.
5. Severe loss at 2000 Hz and above.
6. History of stapedectomy.
7. Hypersensitive acoustic reflex thresholds.
8. Low MCL.
9. Low maximum power output indicated by the master hearing aid test.

The hearing test information presented in Figure 54 show a client who is a first time user of hearing instruments. This person is easily irritated by loud sounds. When the speech tests were done (attempted), the client said the speech sounds were, "much too loud." This adverse reaction resulted in MCL and UCL scores at a low intensity level. Because the client could not tolerate loud speech presented through the audiometer the word recognition tests were measured at a too low level. The word recognition score of 48% greatly underestimates the client's actual word recognition potential. The current dynamic range is only 20 dB. The output must be meticulously controlled to protect this client from loud sounds.

Data from the master hearing aid test says that this client prefers a mild-gain low-output hearing aid (20 dB use gain, 6 dB-per-octave roll-off, and an MPO of 110 dB). These numbers differ markedly from numbers one might generate using a hearing aid fitting formula based on the pure-tone audiogram thresholds. Such formula generated numbers might result in 40 dB of use gain, a 12-dB-per-octave roll-off, and a 120 dB MPO. Here, the difference between what the client likes and what the client needs is great. Experience suggests you start with milder gain instruments that contain extra bass amplification (the sound is more mellow). At some time in the future, improve hearing for this client by reducing bass, increasing treble, raising MPO and increasing gain.

Figure 55 shows the hearing test results for a client with a severe-to-profound hearing loss. The question marks in the audiogram show missing information; no bone conduction thresholds were observed at 70 dB, and it was not possible to test bone conduction at higher levels as 70 dB was the maximum limit for this audiometer. Here the MCL and master hearing aid assessment can provide us with the missing information. To illustrate this point, suppose the hearing aid specialist is being forced to choose between two powerful hearing aids. One hearing aid has AGC, lower gain and lower output. The other hearing aid is a linear amplifier

	pure-tone audiogram					
	250	500	1000	2000	4000	8000
bone	40	50	60	70	75	80
air	40	50	60	70	75	80

speech tests				master hearing aid		
SRT	Wrd Rcgntn	MCL	UCL	gain	dB oct	MPO
55	48 @ 70	60	75	20	6	110

Fig. 54. First time hearing aid user.

	pure-tone audiogram					
	250	500	1000	2000	4000	8000
bone	40	60	?	?	?	
air	80	105	105	105	105	NR

speech tests				master hearing aid		
SRT	Wrd Rcgntn	MCL	UCL	gain	dB oct	MPO
100	86 @ 110	110	125	60	12	130

Fig. 55. Severe-to-profound hearing loss.

with higher gain and output levels. Should the hearing aid specialist select the milder or stronger unit?

The answer to this question lies in the correct interpretation of the hearing test data. Two possible types of hearing loss can explain the missing data at 1000 and 2000 Hz: (1) a sensorineural hearing loss at 1000, 2000, and 4000 Hz—no air-bone gaps at these frequencies; or (2) a mixed hearing loss at 1000, 2000, and 4000 Hz—a 35-dB air-bone gap at these same frequencies.

A 35-dB air-bone gap means the energy reaching the inner ear will be 35 dB weaker. Obviously, no air-bone gap means sound energy will reach the inner ear without the 35 dB loss. These two facts translate into major differences in the gain and MPO requirements of the hearing aid fitting.

If we incorrectly believe the client has a sensorineural hearing loss, we would probably fit the AGC instrument and provide approximately 60 dB gain and a 125 dB MPO. Of the 60 dB gain available, 35 dB would be lost before the signal reaches the inner ear. Only 25 dB would be available in the inner ear as actual use gain to improve the client's hearing. This 25 dB assumes the hearing aid is worn at a full-on volume setting.

If we incorrectly assume a mixed hearing loss, we might fit the client with the more powerful linear amplifier. Such an aid may provide 70 dB gain and a peak MPO near 140 dB. We might incorrectly think that 35 dB of the 70 dB gain would be used (lost) to reach the inner ear. In fact no energy would be lost and all of the signal would reach the inner ear. If the client used this fitting unwisely, the excess power could cause additional damage to the ear.

The hearing aid specialist may successfully fit the client illustrated in Figure 55 by using several tests to measure a single aspect of hearing. The client's hearing abilities can be best understood if all hearing tests results are integrated. Tympanometric studies, otoscopy, MCL, and UCL measurements can be used to determine the missing bone conduction values. These tests provide considerable information that can be used to differentiate a mixed loss from a pure sensorineural loss. Observe the MCL value of 110 dB. When this client was asked, "Is this setting: too soft, just right, or too loud?", the client asked for the level to be increased. This strongly suggests the hearing loss is mixed at all frequencies rather than sensorineural in the high frequency zone.

Hearing aid specialists have a number of circuits available to control output—preclude power overload. However, before the client is given the hearing aid system, valid measurements must be made and skilled judgements are needed.

PROTECTION AGAINST BACKGROUND NOISE

The tools available to reduce perceived background noise include: filtering the bass, venting, using directional microphones, employing frequency-dependent AGC, multi-band amplifiers, multi-memory systems, and other hardware.

Most environmental noise has an energy maximum in the lower frequencies. The audiometric thresholds at 250 and 500 Hz can be used to judge the amount of perceived background noise the client will hear with and without hearing instruments. The better the bass hearing thresholds, the more audible the background noise.

Figure 56 illustrates a person with a typical sensorineural hearing loss in both ears. The hearing loss is mild in the lower frequencies and severe in the high frequencies. The data are for only one ear. The typical hearing loss is sloping—in this case 30 dB at 500 Hz, 70 dB at 2000 Hz. This client has worn hearing aids for years and the current hearing aids are five years old. He returned to the office reporting two common problems: poor speech understanding and an inability to understand speech in a crowded noise filled room. Our first goal is to improve speech understanding, especially in the presence of background noise. The data in Figure 56 suggests the following:

1. This person's hearing ability is markedly impaired from 1500-to-6000 Hz. Adequate high-frequency amplification is critical for this person to improve speech understanding.

	pure-tone audiogram					
	250	500	1000	2000	4000	8000
bone	20	30	50	70	70	nr
air	20	30	50	70	70	85

speech tests				master hearing aid		
SRT	Wrd Rcgntn	MCL	UCL	gain	dB oct	MPO
40	72 @ 70	70	80	40	18	125

Fig. 56. Experienced hearing aid user.

2. Hearing sensitivity at 250 and 500 Hz suggest that this person will hear substantial background noises if this zone is amplified too strongly. The existing fitting therefore needs to be checked.
3. The dynamic range of hearing is about 40 dB. The UCL is 80 dB and SRT is 40 dB, so the dynamic range is 40 dB. The master hearing aid tests show 40 dB of use gain and an 125 dB MPO. It appears that this person can use substantial amplification.
4. The audiometric shape is sharply sloping in the mid frequency range, however, hearing sensitivity values are flat between 2000 and 4000 Hz. This suggests the high-frequency hearing ability is stable and usable (can be amplified) rather than becoming worse with increasing frequencies.
5. The history of hearing aid use suggests the client will accept new hearing aids.

The real-ear and sound-field tests for this client's hearing aids showed them to provide substantial amplification in the low-frequency range and little usable amplification in the higher-frequency range.

This client received new hearing aids with a wide frequency response, mild gain in the low frequencies (250 to 500 Hz) and 40 dB of use gain in the high frequencies (2000 to 6000 Hz). Bass amplification was reduced in the new hearing aids to reduce perceived background noise. Treble amplification was increased to improve word recognition ability. AGC circuits allowed the client to increase gain without fear of over amplification.

Many additional electronic devices are available to reduce perceived background noise. These circuits include multi-memory circuits and multi-channel amplifiers. The new digital amplifiers may also be helpful in this regard.

OPTIMIZING WORD RECOGNITION—CLARITY

A major complaint of hard-of-hearing people is that they hear but do not understand what is said. Our primary objective is to resolve the client's main problem. Our quest to improve speech understanding begins by studying the components of speech: (1) speech production, (2) vowel consonant differences, (3) the power curve of speech and (4) the clarity curve of speech.

SPEECH PRODUCTION

Human speech is a composite of articulated sounds and voicing. The articulated sounds are made with our lips, teath, tongue, and other structures in our mouth. The sound /sh/ and whispered speech are examples of articulated sounds.

Voicing is the noise made by the vocal cords. The act of voicing is accomplished by exhaling (gently forcing) the air through the vocal cords. If you want to explain voicing to a client, have him/her lightly touch their voice box while saying /ahahahahahahah/. Vocalization is felt as a vibration.

Figure 57 shows some important anatomical components of the speech production system. Stevens and House (1972) said that the human anatomy of speech can be viewed in three groups: "the structures below the larynx . . . used for breathing; the larynx itself, in which lie the vocal folds, which can be adjusted to vibrate and thus periodically to interrupt the air flow from the lungs; and the structures above the larynx . . . which control the configuration of the vocal tract."

The vocal cords are thin bands of tissue that move into place across the throat tube, called the trachea. We open and close these vocal cords when we talk. When voicing is needed, we close the cords and allow the air from the lungs to push through the closed cords making the voice sound.

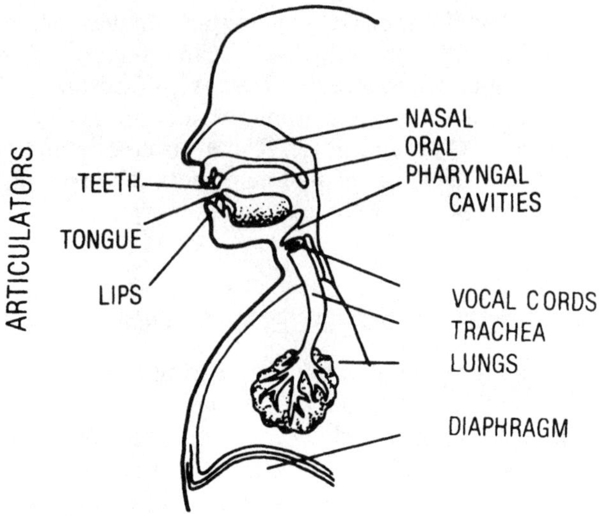

Fig. 57. The anatomy of speech production.

VOWELS AND CONSONANTS

Vowel sounds have more energy than consonants. Vowels are produced by a more open vocal tract configuration and always have the presence of voicing. Vowels are considerably longer in time than consonants. A stressed vowel might be 400 msec (msec = milliseconds) while a short vowel might be 100 msec. Consonants, especially stop consonants (p, t, k, b, d, g) are very short, about 40 msec.

Most of the energy of vowels is located in the bass, whereas consonants have more energy in the higher frequencies. Figure 58 lists many speech sounds by frequency and decibel sensation level. Note that /s/ is a high frequency sound and /j/ is a low frequency sound. The speech sounds shown on the upper part of the chart have more acoustic energy while those on the lower part are softer. Sounds may have more than one frequency component and, therefore, appear on the chart more than once.

Figure 59 shows the energy in the human voice as function of frequency. This graph has considerable utility in hearing aid selection. Frequency is shown horizontally. Relative intensity level in decibels is shown on the vertical axis. Locate 200 and 2000 Hz and notice the approximate 15 dB difference in power between the two frequencies. The graph says the human voice is much stronger in the lower frequencies (vowels) and much weaker in the higher frequencies (consonants).

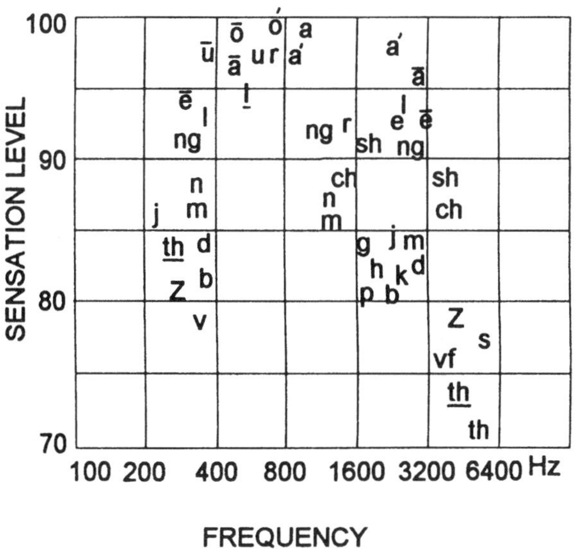

Fig. 58. Frequency and intensity regions of speech sounds. [From Fletcher (1953)].

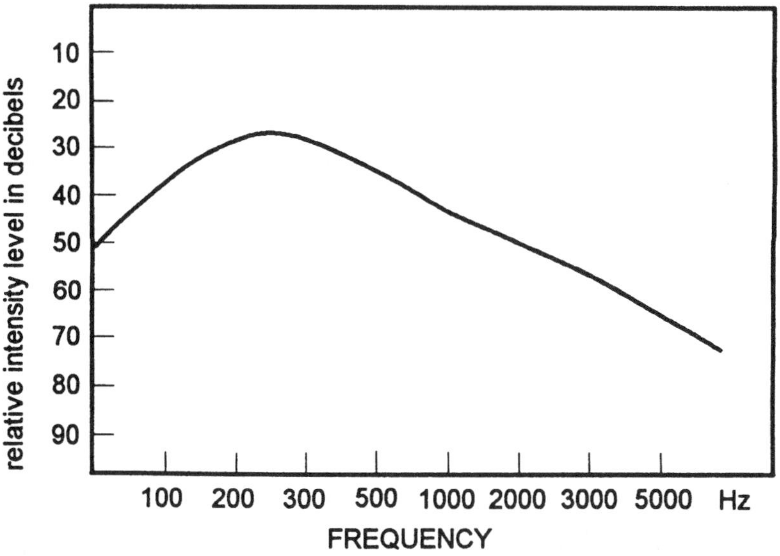

Fig. 59. Average Speech Power Curve.

THE POWER CURVE OF SPEECH

Natural speech is a condition in which we say words at different intensities. When we read aloud, we vary the amount of power in the speech sounds each time we utter them. This natural variation in power is outlined in Figure 60. The upper line shows the upper intensity limit of speech power, while the bottom line shows the lower intensity limit. Between these levels is the average. Sometimes the space between the upper and lower limit is called the speech envelope, meaning that most of the time speech power is within this range.

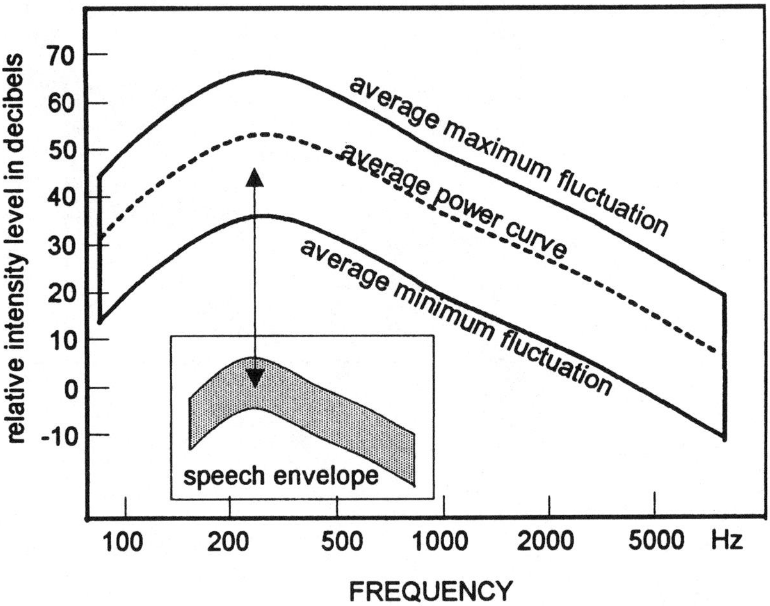

Fig. 60. Long term average of speech.

MAXIMIZING CLARITY IN HEARING AMPLIFICATION

People need to hear and understand for many different reasons. We need to hear cars on the street, music for entertainment, and the singing of the birds. We need to understand what other people are saying to us in order to lead more productive lives.

To create maximum clarity in hearing amplification, one must understand the difference between the power of speech and the frequencies within speech, which are responsible for clarity. The term "power" considers the loudness of speech. The term "clarity" means hearing sounds clearly and understanding words well. The zone of speech that has the most loudness (power) is not the zone most important to word understanding.

French and Steinberg (1947) studied speech clarity. They presented speech through selected filters to normal hearing people. They adjusted the frequency bandwidths of the filters and recorded how these adjustments affected the percentage of words correctly heard. They learned which frequency regions were important for speech clarity.

An outcome of the speech clarity research was the development of the Articulation Index, AI, (ANSI 1969). Using the AI we can measure the intensity of a person's speech, measure the intensity of the interfering noise, then calculate the number of words the listener will understand correctly. The AI has weighting factors that are the numerical values used to show the importance of a given frequency band to speech intelligibility (word understanding).

These numbers (from ANSI 1969) show the relative importance of each frequency zone (octave bands) to word recognition ability. For example, the octave-band centered at 250 Hz contributes 8% to word understanding. The octave-band at 500 Hz contributes 14% to words understanding . . . This information is also shown in Figure 61.

The author prepared Figures 61 and 62 to contrast the clarity curve with the power curve. Notice in Figure 62 that the maximum power region is in the 200–400 Hz region. Observe the region important for speech clarity around 2000 Hz. The information in Figure 62 can be used in counseling clients. One may say, "Please notice, Mrs. Smith, that your hearing loss is in a region important for speech clarity. You are still able to hear louder speech sounds in the bass. Unfortunately, these louder sounds are not the only ones needed to understand words".

Figure 63 illustrates the envelope of speech power and the importance of the higher frequencies to speech understanding. The solid curved lines represent the upper and lower limits of speech power. The dots show the importance of the frequency band for speech and understanding. The greater the number of dots, the more

Table 1. The importance of the standard octave bands to word understanding in percent.

250	500	1000	2000	4000 Hz
8	14	22	33	23%

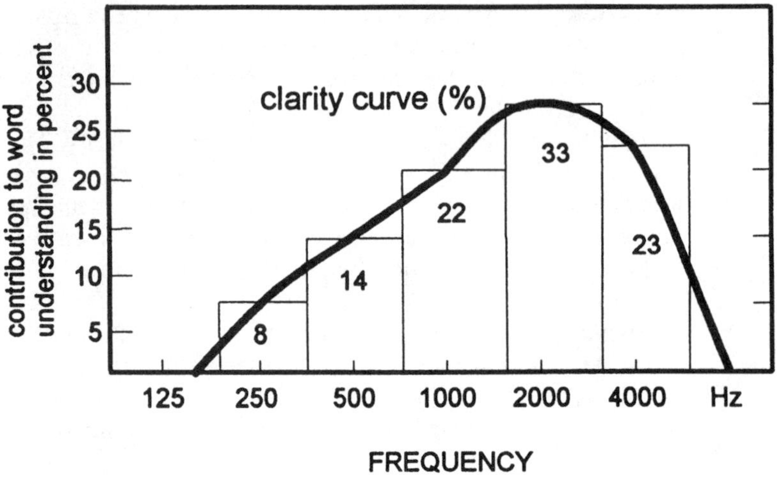

Fig. 61. The Clarity Curve.

important that area is for speech understanding. Each dot represents a 1% contribution to word understanding.

POSITIVE REINFORCEMENT

Clients need positive reinforcement to become successful hearing aid users. Figure 64 illustrates a client who might deny a hearing loss. Successful reinforcement is given to this person by review-

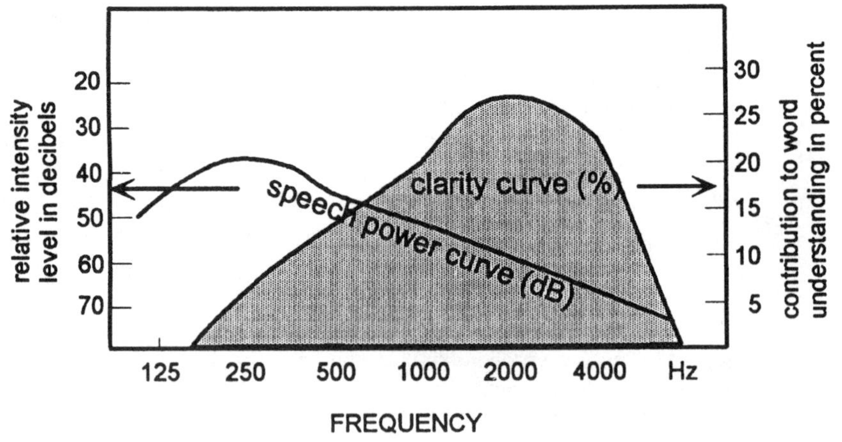

Fig. 62. The speech power curve and the speech clarity curve. Power is referenced in decibels. Clarity is referenced on the right in percentage contribution to word understanding.

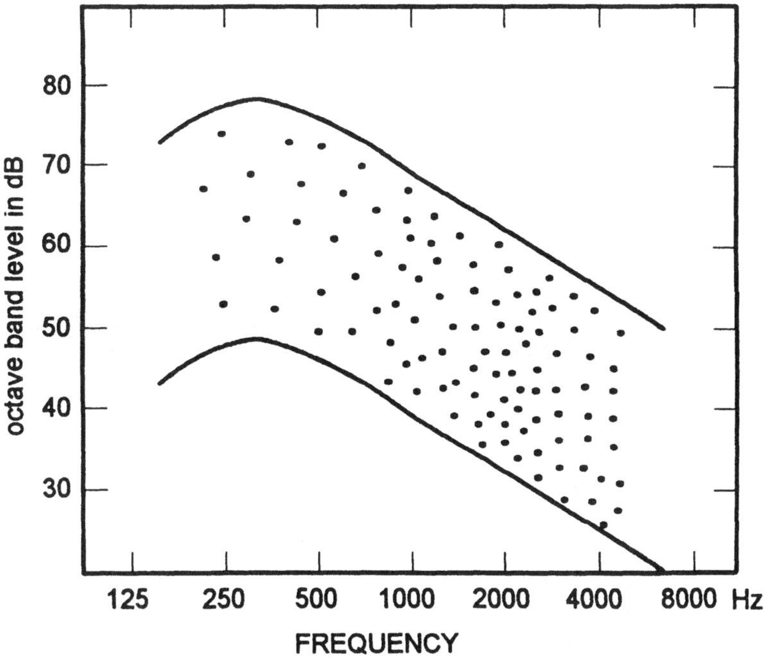

Fig. 63. AI speech region for "conversational level" speech, also called the speech power envelope. The dots show the importance of the frequency band for speech understanding. (With permission by William J. Cavanaugh).

ing the audiogram and locating the zones of "better" and "weaker" hearing. Hearing sensitivity is "better" at 250 and 500 Hz and "weaker" at 2000 Hz and the higher frequencies. The client is seated in a sound field. A 2000 Hz tone is presented at 45 dB and

	pure-tone audiogram					
	250	500	1000	2000	4000	8000
bone	25	25	30	50	70	80
air	25	25	30	50	70	80

speech tests				master hearing aid		
SRT	Wrd Rcgntn	MCL	UCL	gain	dB oct	MPO
30	92 @ 60	60	75	25	18	110

Fig. 64.

the hearing instrument is adjusted to allow the client to easily hear the signal. As the hearing instrument is put on and then removed, the tone is first audible and then inaudible. The client hears the tone clearly and naturally with the hearing instrument, yet does not hear the tone at all without the instrument.

PATHOLOGY

A quote from the International Hearing Society, formerly the National Hearing Aid Society, publication (1979) is representative of the necessity to be aware of the ear pathologies: "Needless to say, the person who fits and sells the hearing aid should not in any way whatsoever, attempt to diagnose or state the cause of a hearing impairment, or attempt any treatment or medical advice. Diagnosis and the medical or surgical treatment of hearing loss is the special task of the physician. The hearing aid consultant should, however, have a basic knowledge of hearing disorders for three reasons: (1) to supplement his knowledge of the workings of the hearing mechanism; (2) to help him understand the medical problems of his customers; and (3) to enable him to refer his client to a physician."

CHOLESTEATOMA

A pouch of skin formed by a retracted ear drum, which fills with sloughed skin cells and invades the middle ear spaces, is called a cholesteatoma. As a cholesteatoma sac fills with epithelial debris, it grows in size and can erode mastoid bone and ossicles.

Perforated eardrums are susceptible to this pathologic condition. Normally a perforated tympanic membrane heals by creating a smooth thin continuous membrane across the area of perforation. Occasionally, the edges of the perforation grow inward into the middle ear space and trapped epithelial skin cells create white "pearls" of epithelium which can form congenitally or after traumatic or surgical perforations. Some cholesteatoma sacs are observable with a good otoscope and appear as white masses.

Cholesteatoma produces conductive hearing loss which increases with time. Clients who exhibit such growths should be referred immediately to a physician specializing in the treatment of the ear.

Audiometric indicators approximate normal test results when the cholesteatoma pocket is small. As the pocket grows, conductive indicators become positive. These include: rounded or flat tympanograms, elevated or absent reflexes, small air-bone gaps and elevated MCL's & UCL's.

GENETIC OR HEREDITARY HEARING LOSS

Congenital deafness occurs during the development stages of the embryo. Congenital hearing loss may be due to medications used by the mother, illness during the pregnancy or a host of other reasons.

Some hearing losses are transmitted from the parents to children because of genetic defects. These hearing losses may occur at any age and may be bilateral or unilateral. Most often, the loss is severe and noticeable shortly after birth.

IMPACTED CERUMEN

Ear wax in the outer ear canal is normal. It serves to lubricate the skin of the ear canal, repelling water and helping to control bacteria. Impacted cerumen, however, has the negative effect of plugging the ear canal and creating a conductive hearing loss.

The production site of cerumen is in the outer part of the external ear canal. When impacted cerumen is observed deep in the canal, it has probably been pushed there by the client. Normally, cerumen migrates out of the ear along with the dead, dry skin.

Since impacted cerumen is a common problem with hearing aid users, it is recommended that the dispenser make arrangements with nearby medical professionals to have this problem efficiently remedied.

> "Under no circumstances should persons with impacted cerumen be fitted with a hearing aid. They should first be referred to a physician for removal of the ceruminous plug, after which audiometric testing may be done and a hearing aid fitted if needed." (National Hearing Aid Society, 1981)

Audiometric indicators include flat tympanograms, an air-bone gap and good word recognition function at MCL.

MENIERE'S DISEASE

Meniere's disease may cause symptoms of ear pressure, hearing loss with tinnitus and imbalance. It is also called endolymphatic hydrops, because it is caused by an excess production of one of the inner ear fluids called endolymph.

Clients with Meniere's disease may have long periods without symptoms. Then, with little warning, the disease may suddenly become active. Individuals sometimes report a "plugged" feeling in their ear during the buildup of endolymph. Any person with a history of hearing loss, vertigo and tinnitus should be monitored by a physician specializing in the treatment of ear. The hearing loss associated with Meniere's disease is cochlear, i.e., sensorineural.

The audiometric indicators include sensorineural hearing loss of varying shapes. Some losses are sloping, while others are flat or slightly reversed. As the disease is altered, the hearing levels change. According to Sataloff et al. (1980), the hearing loss fluctuates, and such fluctuation is more pronounced for the lower frequency range.

NOISE-INDUCED HEARING LOSS

Noise-induced hearing loss can develop slowly from daily exposure to moderately loud noise or suddenly due to a sudden excessive noise. It is estimated that one-third of the industry in this country has a working environment in which noise levels exceed permissible levels. The Occupational Safety and Health Act (OSHA) of 1971 makes mandatory the development of feasible noise controls to reduce the level of noise and the setting up of continuous, effective hearing conservation programs when the noise level cannot be reduced below the permissible exposure level. Permissible noise exposure levels were set at 90 dB-A for an eight-hour duration, a 95 dB-A for a four-hour duration, a 100 dB-A for a two-hour duration, and 105 dB-A for a one hour duration.

There is an abundance of literature relating to noise exposure and subsequent hearing loss, e.g., Sataloff and Michael (1973) and Sataloff et al. (1980).

The audiometric indicators include a sensorineural hearing loss more pronounced in the higher frequencies concomitant with a history of excessive noise exposure. Often the hearing loss is greatest at 4000 or 6000 Hz, with a slight recovery at 8000 Hz.

Early exposure to noise may produce only a temporary threshold shift form which the person recovers after a period away from the noisy environment. However, repeated exposure and frequent temporary threshold shifts will often result in permanent threshold shift.

OTITIS

"Oto" is a word root for ear. "Itis" indicated an inflammation or infection. The terms externa, media and interna define the location of the pathology.

Otitis Externa: An infection of the external ear canal for which there are several causes. The use of hearing aids may aggravate an external otitis. Signs and symptoms of otitis externa include drainage, pain and redness of the ear canal.

The audiometric indicators of otitis externa may be normal testing data except for the otoscopic examination.

Otitis Media: Middle ear problems are more common in children. An otitis media may be caused by bacteria within the middle ear space. Middle ear fluid and pus often collect in the middle ear during an attack of suppurative otitis media. The infected fluid applies an outward pressure on the ear drum, creating severe pain and, possibly, a perforation of the ear drum itself.

The audiometric indicators for otitis media may be flat or rounded tympanograms, absent reflexes, slight air-bone gaps, excellent word recognition ability.

Non-infected (non-suppurative) otitis media is a condition in which the Eustachian tube has failed to allow air into the middle ear and a sterile fluid occurs in the middle ear space. The individual usually does not experience pain, and, if a child, may not be aware of the loss of hearing caused by the middle ear fluids. The problem can be treated medically or surgically.

Otitis Interna: Inflammations or infections of the inner ear are much less common than outer and middle ear problems. The classical symptoms of otitis interna parallel those of Meniere's disease; i.e., tinnitus, vertigo and hearing loss.

The indicators for otitis interna may be varied sensorineural hearing loss, normal impedance data unless the reflexes are absent. As the disease produces varying degrees of hearing loss, the data vary accordingly.

OTOSCLEROSIS (OTOSPONGIOSIS)

Otosclerosis is a disease of the bone tissue which can cause conductive or sensorineural hearing loss. The disease causes the bone to become spongy or vascularized, Sataloff et. al. (1980), after which the bone becomes sclerotic or scarred. The disease sometimes causes the footplate of the stapes to become fixated and immobile in the oval window producing a conductive hearing loss. The process happens gradually with a progressive loss of hearing. The disease is more common in women than men and the disease may be familial. Typical otosclerosis produces a conductive hearing loss with quite good hearing by bone conduction.

POST-OPERATIVE OTOSCLEROSIS

The hearing aid specialist may see cases of otosclerosis years after the client has undergone stapes surgery. These postoperative ears have mixed hearing losses of dramatically differing degrees. The control of hearing aid output and AGC selection is critical. Some postoperative ears are extremely delicate due to the loss of the stapes muscle and the implantation of the artificial stapes. The mixed loss might generally show the need for power. However, the postoperative otosclerotic ear may not be able to tolerate much acoustic power. Each postoperative case must be individually evaluated to determine whether the ear is hyper or hyposensitive to amplification.

Audiometric indicators vary considerably. The hearing aid specialist must be aware of this in reviewing test results of the postoperative otosclerotic ear.

PRESBYCUSIS

Hearing loss that increases with age is termed presbycusis. This is a common type of sensorineural hearing loss. The condition may exist for many years. However, the hearing loss usually does not become a problem until the age of fifty or sixty.

There is much debate about the cause of presbycusis. Some researchers have tested the hearing of populations which are free from noise exposure and modern civilization stress. These tests suggest a much better level of hearing even at extreme old age.

Presbycusis is considered a sensorineural hearing problem. The loss may affect all of the hearing network. It is not uncommon to find a conductive loss present in the presbycusis ear. Equally important are the changes in the auditory cortex. As age increases, the speed of information processing decreases. The presbycusic subject may react slowly to the spoken word. Hearing aids seem to work best when the distortion is kept to a minimum and the speed of the spoken messages is reduced.

Audiometric indicators show sensorineural hearing losses sloping into the higher frequencies and reduced word recognition function.

SUDDEN DEAFNESS

Sudden deafness, as the name implies, is an instantaneous loss of hearing. The degree of loss is usually quite substantial and the type of loss is sensorineural and frequently in one ear only. Sataloff (1980) states that this pathology is commonly observed by ear, nose and throat physicians.

Individuals experiencing sudden deafness may have partial or complete recovery of hearing. The etiology is usually attributed to abnormal constriction of the blood vessels supplying oxygen to the ear.

Sudden deafness can happen with or without other accompanying symptoms, such as tinnitus, vertigo and nausea. Persons may be asymptomatic except for hearing loss.

The hearing aid specialist can help clients reporting a sudden hearing loss by advising them to see a medical doctor as quickly as possible. Sudden deafness is a true medical emergency.

TINNITUS

Subjective tinnitus is an acoustic sensation in the head for which there is no external sound source. Objective tinnitus has known causes which may be eliminated through medical or surgical intervention.

The treatment of subjective tinnitus is of some concern to the hearing aid specialist. Hearing aids or tinnitus maskers are sometimes fitted to the offending ear of the client. A tinnitus masker is a device which produces a narrow band of noise. The intensity of the noise can be controlled by the client. The frequency band of noise produced by the masker is selected in agreement with the frequency region of the client's tinnitus.

Ideally, a client will find the masking noise more acceptable than his/her own head noise. This happens when the masker is adjusted to produce an output which masks the client's ongoing tinnitus. The term "mask" means to cover or hide.

In some instances, the noise produced by the masker will not entirely cover the subjective tinnitus. However, the client may appreciate the partial reduction in his/her tinnitus. Some clients find, after using the masker device over a period of time, that they experience residual inhibition. Residual inhibition is the absence of tinnitus after a period of exposure to noise. This release from tinnitus may last only a few minutes or may extend to several days. Clients who experience residual inhibition are good candidates for masker devices.

The hearing aid specialist should be aware that there are many medical and non-medical treatments for tinnitus. None has proven good enough to find general acceptance among medical practitioners working with the treatment of tinnitus. The hearing aid specialist is cautioned to approach tinnitus management with the awareness that the cause, cure and treatment are not clearly understood. Any claim to the contrary would neither serve the interest of the client nor that of the hearing aid specialist. Without question, if a client is complaining of tinnitus and approaches the hearing aid specialist for assistance through a hearing aid or masker, medical referral is strongly indicated even though the possibility of a causal link between tinnitus and some ongoing disease process may be remote.

TYMPANIC MEMBRANE PERFORATION

Tympanic membrane perforation is best defined as a hole in the eardrum. Hearing loss stemming from a perforation is conductive. The degree of loss depends upon the location and size of the perforation. A small perforation may produce no measurable loss of hearing.

The audiometric indicators include conductive hearing loss. Eardrum perforations dramatically alter the impedance test, especially the relative physical volume measurement. The relative physical volume of the outer ear can be read on some impedance units. Normally, this, value approximates 2–3 cc's. Perforations cause this normal value to increase dramatically, thereby alerting the tester to the probability of a perforated eardrum.

INSTRUMENT MAINTENANCE AND CALIBRATION

Measurement instruments must do what they were designed to do; i.e., produce accurate, repeatable signals in a controlled manner. Instrument calibration is a high priority item. According to Newby (1972), "The accuracy of testing depends upon the proper functioning of the audiometric equipment, as well as upon the skill of the audiometrist and the adequacy of the testing room."

Equipment must be calibrated at a specified interval to insure accurate performance. Some states require this to be done yearly under the licensing regulations. Many manufacturers have local representatives with trained technicians to clean, calibrate, and adjust the instrument in the hearing aid specialist's office. Calibration may include (but is not limited to) the following:

1. Measuring output of each test frequency and adjusting the measured output to comply with the published standards. This must be done for air, bone, and speaker-conducted signals.
2. Measuring the pure-tone frequencies to find any frequency drift.
3. Eliminating any distortion within the system which is not permissible by published standards for that instrument.
4. Checking for crosstalk. Signals in one channel must not cross into other channels.
5. Checking attenuator linearity. The attenuator must correctly control the intensity level of the signal at all settings in the attenuator dial.
6. Insuring that switching is quiet and inaudible to the subject being tested.

Audiometric standards have changed over the years and some equipment still in use was manufactured under an earlier reference, e.g. the ASA or ISO standard. The difference between the ANSI and ASA standard can be of major concern if caution is not exercised. Refer to Newby (1972), David and Silverman (1979), Martin (1975), and Sataloff (1980) for a more comprehensive discussion of audiometric standards.

SUMMARY

A multitude of hearing tests is available. Many of these tests provide information which can be used by the hearing aid specialist. If one chooses to use these tests, they must be administered in a manner which produces valid and reliable information. The specialist must be able to judge the quality of these tests. Correct testing is only possible when the person doing the test controls all of the important variables such as background noise interference, equipment calibration, client instruction and inter-test data correlation.

It is critical for the tester to read, integrate and employ all of the audiometric indicators in the decision-making process. These indicators help determine the type, degree, and class of hearing loss. The indicators provide the information needed to select the acoustical properties needed to achieve maximum hearing aid performance.

The selection and fitting of hearing instruments should be based upon an adequate test battery and the skilled interpretation of the test results. This chapter has stressed appropriate sequences involved in obtaining applicable audiometric data and their interpretation in the decision-making process.

ACKNOWLEDGEMENT

The author wishes to recognize and thank Dr. Dean Echols (ENT) for his assistance with the section on ear pathology.

GLOSSARY

Acoustic reflex Loud sounds presented to the ear cause the muscle attached to the stapes bone to contract. This action is measurable with an impedance testing unit.

Air-bone gap The decibel difference between the air-conducted threshold and the bone-conducted threshold for the same frequency and same ear.

Air-Conduction Sounds routed to the inner-ear through the normal pathway of hearing. The pathway: outer-ear, eardrum, middle-ear-ossicles, oval window, inner ear.

Audiogram The graph used to record pure-tone hearing thresholds. The vertical axis is intensity in decibels of hearing level. The horizontal axis is frequency.

Audiometer The electronic instrument used to test hearing with pure-tones and other stimuli. Audiometers route signals to the client through air or bone conduction. Some audiometers include microphones and audio systems used to test hearing with speech stimuli.

Binaural Hearing with both ears.

Bone-conduction Sounds routed to the inner-ear through the skull. This pathway is: vibrator, skin, skull, inner-ear. Bone conduction measures the hearing integrity of the inner-ear with minimum influence of the outer-ear and middle-ear.

Calibration The measurement and adjustment of the output of an instrument to make the output agree with desired levels. These desired levels are published by the American National Standards Institute (ANSI) for many hearing testing instruments.

Cerumen A wax-like substance produced by the glands in the outer part of the ear canal.

Cholesteatoma A tumor which starts in the tissues of the ear-drum.

Cochlea The inner-ear has two parts; hearing and balance. The cochlea is the organ of hearing.

Conductive hearing loss Hearing loss due to an obstruction in the pathway of sound within the outer or middle-ear.

Cross hearing Stimuli presented to one ear crosses the head and is heard by the other ear.

dB slope A measurement made with the master hearing aid unit indicating the frequency response needed for the hearing aid as measured in decibels (dB) per octave roll-off in the amplifier.

Functional hearing loss An exaggeration in the degree of hearing impairment. Also called nonorganic hearing loss, malingering, and exaggerated hearing loss.

Functionability tests The measurement of the client's ability to hear simple words without hearing instruments. The test uses no equipment.

Genetic hearing loss Hearing loss due to defects in the chromosomes. Also called hereditary hearing loss.

Impedance Impedance means to reduce or retard. Impedance tests measure many physical properties of the ear including ear drum mobility and stapedial reflex levels.

Interaural attenuation The energy loss in a sound as it travels from one ear to the other.

Internal auditory canal The canal within the skull which houses the VIII cranial nerve, the hearing and vestibular nerve.

Masking The use of noise in the non-test ear to preclude that ear from assisting the ear under test.

Mastoidectomy The surgical removal of infected tissue within the mastoid bone behind the ear.

Meniere's disease An inner ear disease which occurs as a result of over production of inner ear fluid called endolymph. The classical symptoms include hearing loss, tinnitus, and vertigo.

Mixed hearing loss Hearing loss produced by both conductive and sensorineural problems in the same ear.

Monaural Hearing with one ear.

Monitored live voice (MLV) Speech hearing tests given with a live voice instead of a recorded voice. The voice level is controlled by monitoring a volume units meter, a VU meter.

Most comfortable level (MCL) The intensity level which the client judges to be the most comfortable; not too loud nor too soft.

Myringotomy A surgical opening in the ear-drum to remove middle-ear fluids.

Noise induced hearing loss (NIHL) Hearing loss that results from exposure to noise which is sufficiently intense to damage the delicate tissues within the cochlea. Also called noise induced permanent threshold shift, NIPTS.

Ossicles The middle-ear bones.

Otitis media An inflammation which affects the middle-ear structures.

Otosclerosis A pathology affecting the bones in the middle-ear. Initially the process is spongy, after which it hardens and fixates the footplate of the stapes in the oval window creating a conductive hearing loss.

Otoscope A light producing unit used to illuminate the outer and middle-ear. Newer otoscopes have a halogen light source which delivers light through fiber optic plastics into detachable ear speculums.

Perforation in tympanic membrane Hole in ear-drum.

Phonetically balanced (pb) words Monosyllable words used to measure the word recognition ability of listeners. Phonetic balancing indicates an equal frequency of occurrence of speech sounds in the test words as in the words used in American speech. For example, an /f/ sound will occur in the test words with the same frequency as /f/ occurs in American speech.

Pure-tone average (PTA) The average of 500, 1000, and 2000 Hz hearing thresholds.

Presbycusis Hearing deterioration as a result of the aging process.

Recruitment The abnormal growth of loudness within an ear due to damage in the cochlear tissues. Hypersensitivity to loud sounds.

Retrocochlear hearing loss Hearing loss as a result of a pathology located medial to (inward from) the cochlea. Retrocochlear indicates the position between the cochlea and the auditory cortex of the brain.

Sensorineural hearing loss (SNHL) Hearing loss within the sensory hearing unit (the hair cells within the cochlea) or within the hearing nerve.

Sound booth A sound treated enclosure which attenuates ambient noise by a fixed amount called the transmission loss. The adequacy of the "quietness" inside the booth must be checked by measuring the noise level in the booth and contrasting this level to the required standards.

Sound field The area close to a loudspeaker from which hearing testing signals are emitted. Sound field tests are conducted a fixed distance from the speaker within a fixed area.

Word recognition score The percentage correct of a word understanding test. PB words are used for the evaluation. Other word lists are used for additional measurements.

Speech Reception Threshold (SRT) The softest level at which spondee words can be heard and repeated correctly 50% of the time.

Spondee words Two syllable words which have equal stress on each syllable.

Stapedectomy The surgical removal and replacement of a non-mobile stapes to improve hearing.

Stapedius muscle The small muscle attached to the stapes bone.

Stapedial reflex arc Sound passes through the outer-middle-and inner ear into the hearing nerve. A small branch of the hearing nerve crosses to the facial nerve within the brain. The facial nerve activates the stapedius muscle in response to loud sounds. The contracting stapedius muscle tightens the ear-drum by moving the middle-ear ossicles.

Sudden deafness The sudden (overnight) loss of hearing. Usually the loss is severe and sensorineural in nature.

Synthetic sentences Speech test stimuli in sentence form but without meaning.

Threshold The softest level a tone or other test stimulus can be heard 50% of the time.

Tinnitus Ear noises not generated by an outside source (head noise).

Tonality words Speech test stimuli. Monosyllable words which are grouped into five tonal categories; low, low-middle, middle, middle-high, and high.

Tympanic membrane The ear drum.

Tympanogram The graph showing eardrum mobility at varying air pressures.

Tympanoplasty The surgical repair of a perforation of the ear-drum.

Uncomfortable loudness level (UCL) Signals presented in increasing intensity until a client responds that the level reached is uncomfortable, a level which they can no longer tolerate.

Use gain The decibels of amplification used by the client at a comfortable listening level.

Vertigo Dizziness resulting from a problem in the balance mechanism of the inner ear. The client usually reports spinning or severe imbalance sensations.

REFERENCES

AMERICAN NATIONAL STANDARDS INSTITUTE: American National Standard Specifications for Audiometers, ANSI S3.6-1969, New York, American National Standards Institute, Inc. (1970).

AMERICAN NATIONAL STANDARDS INSTITUTE: Methods for the Articulation Index, ANSI S3.5-1969. New York, American National Standards Institute, Inc. (1969).

ASP, C. W., "The verbo-tonal method for establishing spoken language and listening skill". In Current Therapy of Communication Disorders Chapter Nine, Edited by W. H. Perkins, Thieme-Stratton Inc., New York, 1984.

BERLIN, C., "When Outer Hair Cells Fail, Use Correct Circuitry to Stimulate Their Function". In The Hearing Journal, Vol 47, No. 4, (April 1994).

BERRY, J., Functionability testing, Blount Speech and Hearing Center, Maryville, Tennessee, Personal communications.

CATLIN, F. I., "Otologic Diagnosis and Treatment of Disorders Affecting Hearing". In Medical Audiology Disorders of Hearing, by F. N. Martin Ed., Englewoods Cliffs, Prentice-Hall, (1981)

DAVIS, H., and SILVERMAN, S. R., Hearing and Deafness. New York, Holt, Rinehart, and Winston, (1970).

DELK, J. H. Comprehensive Dictionary of Audiology, Sioux City, The Hearing Aid Journal, (1975).

DALLOS, P., AND MARTIN, R., "The New Theory of Hearing". In The Hearing Journal, Vol 47, No. 2, (Feb. 1994).

FLETCHER, H., Speech and Hearing in Communication, New York, Robert Krieger Pub. Co. (1972).

FRENCH N. R. and STEINBERG, J. C. "Factors Governing the Intelligibility of Speech Sounds". In The Journal of the Acoustical Society of America, Vol 19 No. 1. (Jan 1947).

GIOLAS, T. C. and RANDOLPH, K., Basic Audiometry including Impedance Measurement, Lincoln, Cliffs Notes, Inc., (1977).

HAWKINS, D. B., "Procedure Designed To Select SSPL 90," Ear & Hearing Journal, Vol 8, pp 162–169, Williams & Wilkins, 1987.

JACOBSON, J. T. and NORTHERN, J., Diagnostic Audiology., Pro-Ed book. 1991.

JERGER, J., and HAYES, M. A., "Hearing Aid Evaluation". In Arch. Otolaryngo. Vol 102, (April 1976).

JERGER, J., and NORTHERN, J. L., editors, Clinical Impedance Audiometery, second ed. C. 1980 by American Electromedics Corp. Acton, Mass.

LIPSCOMB, D. M., "What is the Audiogram Really Telling Us?" Parts I, II, & III, Maico Audiological Library Services (1975).

LIPSCOMB, D. M., "Audiometry in Fluctuant Hearing Loss", Otolaryngologic Clinics of North America., Vol. 8, No. 2, June 1975.

LLOYD, L. L., and KAPLAN, H., Audiometric Interpretation: A Manual of Basic Audiometry, Baltimore, University Park Press, (1978).

MARTIN, F. N. Introduction to Audiology. New Jersey, Prentice-Hall, (1975).

MCCANDLESS, G. A., "Real-ear measures of hearing aid performance". In Yanick, P., Rehabilitation Strategies for Sensoryneural Hearing Loss. New York, Grune & Stratton, (1979).

MINIFIE, F. D., HIXON, T. J., and WILLIAMS, F., Normal Aspects of Speech Hearing and Language, New Jersey, Prentice-Hall, (1973).

NATIONAL HEARING AID SOCIETY, Basic Course for Independent Study, Livonia, Mich. (1981).

NEWBY, H. A., Audiology, Englewood Cliffs, Prentice-Hall, (1972).

POLLACK, M. C., and LIPSCOMB, D. M., "Implications of Hair Cell-Pure Tone Discrepancies For Oto-Audiologic Practice", Audiology and Hearing Education, February-March 1979.

SATALOFF, J. and MICHAEL, P., Hearing Conservation, Springfield, Charles C. Thomas Pub. (1973).

SATALOFF, J., SATALOFF, R. T., VASSALLO, L. A. Hearing Loss, Philadelphia, J. B. Lippincott Co., (1980).

STEVENS, K. N., and HOUSE, A. S., "Speech Perception". In Foundation of Modern Auditory Theory, by Tobias J. V., New York, Academic Press, Vol. II. (1972).

Studebaker, G. A., "Clinical Masking of Air-and Bone-Conducted Stimuli", Journal Speech & Hearing Disorders 29, 1964, 23–35.

Webster, J. C., "The Effects of Noise on the Hearing of Speech". Proceedings of the International Congress on Noise as a Public Health Problem, Dubrovnik, Yugoslavia, (1973). Available from the U.S. Govt. Printing Office, 550/9-73-008, Washington, D.C.

Wever, E. G., and Lawrence, M. L. Physiological Acoustics, Princeton University Press, (1954).

APPENDIX A

HOUSE OF HEARING ANALOGY SUMMARY

Analogy Term	Contemporary Term	Tests
1. Floor	threshold of sensitivity	SRT, pure-tone threshold
2. Ceiling	uncomfortable listening level	UCL
3. Left wall	bass hearing	hearing for 100–300 Hz
4. Right wall	treble hearing	hearing for 3000 Hz & up
5. Front wall	instant time	no test
6. Back wall	natural time delay	storage oscilloscope
7. Front door	input	many inputs are possible
8. Back door	output	many output measurements are possible
9. Ceiling height	dynamic range of hearing	UCL-SRT
10. Room width	bandwidth	obtained from frequency response curve
11. Quality of space	word recognition	word recognition test
12. Rebuild floor	amplify	use-gain in decibels
13. Reduce left wall	reduce bass amplification	measure use-gain in bass

APPENDIX B

MATERIALS FOR SPEECH AUDIOMETRY

WORD LISTS FOR C.I.O. AUDITORY TEST W-1

List A

1. greyhound	10. duckpond	19. baseball	28. oatmeal
2. schoolboy	11. sidewalk	20. stairway	29. toothbrush
3. inkwell	12. hotdog	21. cowboy	30. farewell
4. whitewash	13. padlock	22. iceberg	31. grandson
5. pancake	14. mushroom	23. northwest	32. drawbridge
6. mousetrap	15. hardware	24. railroad	33. doormat
7. eardrum	16. workshop	25. playground	34. hothouse
8. headlight	17. horseshoe	26. airplane	35. daybreak
9. birthday	18. armchair	27. woodwork	36. sunset

List B

1. playground	10. railroad	19. toothbrush	28. eardrum
2. grandson	11. baseball	20. mushroom	29. greyhound
3. daybreak	12. padlock	21. farewell	30. baseball
4. doormat	13. hardware	22. horseshoe	31. hothouse
5. woodwork	14. whitewash	23. pancake	32. iceberg
6. armchair	15. hotdog	24. inkwell	33. schoolboy
7. stairway	16. sunset	25. mousetrap	34. duckpond
8. cowboy	17. headlight	26. airplane	35. workshop
9. oatmeal	18. drawbridge	27. sidewalk	36. northwest

Lists published with permission from Central Institute for The Deaf, Donald Calvert, Ph.D., Director.

APPENDIX C

C.I.O. AUDITORY TEST W-22 (PB WORD LISTS)

List 1A

1. an
2. yard
3. carve
4. us
5. day
6. toe
7. felt
8. stove
9. hunt
10. ran
11. knees
12. not (knot)
13. mew
14. low
15. owl
16. it
17. she
18. high
19. there (their)
20. earn
21. twins
22. could
23. what
24. bathe
25. ace
26. you (ewe)
27. as
28. wet
29. chew
30. see (sea)
31. deaf
32. them
33. give
34. true
35. isle (aisle)
36. or (oar)
37. law
38. me
39. none (nun)
40. jam
41. poor
42. him
43. skin
44. east
45. thing
46. dad
47. up
48. bells
49. wire
50. ache

List 2A

1. yore (your)
2. bin (been)
3. way (weigh)
4. chest
5. then
6. ease
7. smart
8. save
9. pew
10. ice
11. odd
12. knee
13. mood
14. now
15. jaw
16. one (won)
17. hit
18. send
19. else
20. tare (tear)
21. does
22. too (two, to)
23. cap
24. with
25. air (heir)
26. and
27. young
28. cars
29. tree
30. dumb
31. that
32. die (dye)
33. show
34. hurt
35. own
36. key
37. oak
38. new (knew)
39. live (verb)
40. off
41. ill
42. rooms
43. ham
44. star
45. eat
46. thin
47. flat
48. well
49. by (buy)
50. ail (ale)

APPENDIX D

TONALITY TEST WORDS

Low	Low-Mid	Middle	Mid-High	High
bow	blood	hall	tell	itch
pull	book	head	hit	see
pool	up	hot	tie	she
blow	boat	had	lie	ease
blue	pop	met	hide	each
no	numb	toy	hay	ace
wool	bump	joy	light	eyes
noon	ball	void	isle	ice
bone	pump	duck	high	is
broom	mow	jam	it	thigh
prune	gum	rock	ate	teeth
pope	law	cat	tale	this
pole	bum	cot	tear	sheath
bowl	mop	love	tire	seize
room	comb	drum	tide	shy
burn	good	mad	tile	cheese
low	palm	lamb	till	chase
loop	knock	lot	kit	sight
loom	mob	her	at	cease
lop	pup	heart	ledge	say
lope	plow	hurt	ill	sigh
new	mum	add	ear	size
now	paw	have	hate	thick
mood	go	hair	jet	sheet
known	down	hat	sir	sheep
noun	on	talk	edge	shape
own	one	tack	hire	shake
moan	all	dad	tick	cheat
moon	bug	hack	jail	cheap
row	pound	ham	date	cheek
boom	bud	fat	hedge	seat
bloom	done	flock	dare	seek
worn	loud	get	die	sip
warm	wall	rat	dial	sit
rope	hole	red	height	chick
wood	plum	rum	rear	sake
move	plot	far	rare	tea
bough	lawn	fire	rid	east
moo	nut	fad	raid	teach
blown	loan	jar	rail	tease

Common words for younger children

boo	bone	hello	today	see-saw
mama	under	like	knee	tree
apple	banana	lips	keep	catch
bubble	round	play	word	six
baby	bed	give	find	three
open	pony	my	here	show
purple		come		
		night		

List published with permission of Dr. Carl Asp, University of Tennessee-Knoxville.

APPENDIX E

Ten synthetic sentences, from Jerger and Hayes (1976).

1. Small boat with a picture has become.
2. Built the government with the force almost.
3. Go change your car color is red.
4. Forward march said the boy had a.
5. March around without a care in your.
6. That neighbor who said business is better.
7. Battle cry and be better than ever.
8. Down by the time is real enough.
9. Agree with him only to find out.
10. Women view men with green paper should.

III

MASKING: PURPOSE, PRINCIPLES AND PROCEDURES

LINDA L. DONALDSON, M.A. CCC-A, BC-HIS

INTRODUCTION

The task of assessing asymmetrical, unilateral or conductive hearing impairments has long confused and baffled hearing health care professionals. The clinician must have an understanding of masking techniques in order to perform an audiologic evaluation which is without suspicion. This chapter will assist the clinician in the determination of when to mask, how to perform the task of masking and characteristics of the masking process.

The purpose, principles and procedures of masking have been discussed and analyzed since the 1920's. We, as practitioners, have been attempting to understand masking principles and appropriate usage. Not only do we need to have a well founded grasp of its reasoning, but also of its basic rules to enable us to perform the task appropriately. Why is there a need to mask? When is masking necessary for air conduction, bone conduction and/or speech audiometry? Is masking necessary for speciality testing? How much of an air/bone gap must exist before masking is necessary? When does too little (undermasking) or too much (overmasking) masking stimuli create false thresholds?

Masking has been written about and, perhaps, taught as a difficult process to understand. It is not difficult, as long as a few basic rules and variables are considered as in any challenging game. To simplify the procedure of masking, it *is* a part of the evaluation game, titled "Seek and Find the True Hearing Levels". The practitioner must have an understanding of the principles involved. It is also necessary to understand the characteristics of masking to better assess its variables. Goldstein and Newman (1994) view the task of masking "as a continual decision-making process." This is precisely true as it varies at each frequency and for each stimulus.

Many terms have been used to describe the ear presented with test stimuli and the ear being presented with masking noise. For the purpose of these exercises the terminology will be consistent with test ear/stimuli (TE/stimulus) for "the ear being presented the test stimuli" and non-test ear/noise (NTE/noise) for "the ear being presented the masking noise."

CHAPTER OBJECTIVES

A complete description of the following terminology will be discussed in this chapter:

- Interaural Attenuation (IA)
- Overmasking
- Undermasking
- Central Masking
- Occlusion Effect (OE)
- Masking Dilemma

Each of these characteristics must be considered for every individual being evaluated. These characteristics make for a challenging evaluation process and certainly keep the testing procedure from becoming mundane.

PURPOSE OF MASKING

It is understood that an auditory signal is received by the outer ear mechanism (acoustical energy) which then transmits the sound into the middle ear mechanism (mechanical energy). This mechanical energy is transduced into hydraulic energy in the inner ear system and transduced into electrical and electro-chemical energy as energy is delivered to the brain. The breakdown, as it relates to CROSSOVER, occurs within the mechanical energy stage

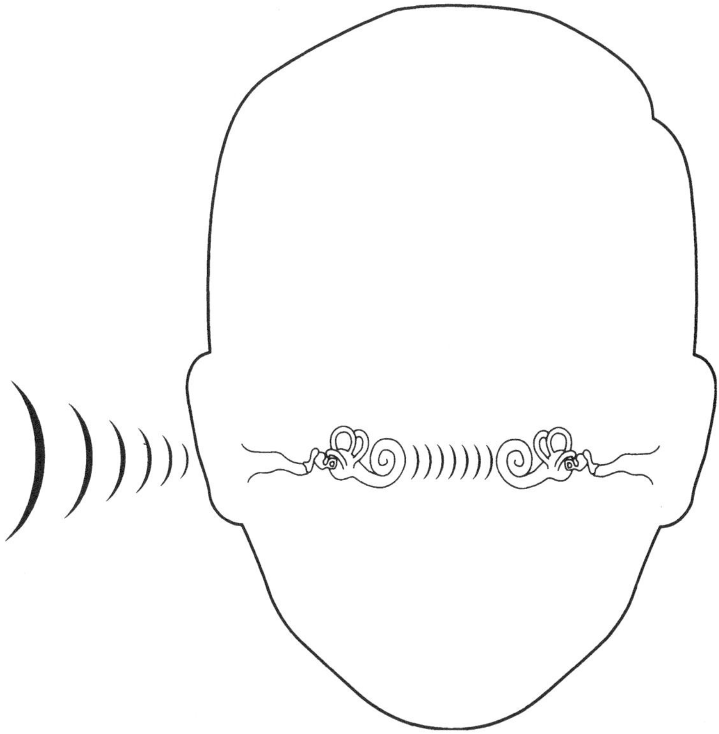

Fig. 1. Crossover (via mechanical transmission).

of the hearing mechanism. (Figure 1) Presenting higher levels of sound energy to one ear will create a cross-over of sound or be audible to the contralateral ear via transcranial pathways (mechanical energy).

To determine degree and type of hearing disorder, it is imperative that the cochlear reserve be ascertained. The cochlear reserve is identified by bone conduction thresholds, or in other words, the patient's cochlear reserve is a determination as to what degree the inner ear is damaged. The answer being sought links the correction of the conductive component with the degree of a sensorineural loss remaining following medical intervention. For an individual client who displays signs of a conductive component (a medically or surgically treatable problem), appropriate masking levels for bone conduction testing may determine the degree of success the patient might expect post-surgically.

Shown in Figure 2 is Hood's plateau method (1960), one of the more popular and widely used masking methods, developed in the 1950's was designed for bone conduction audiometry. Over the

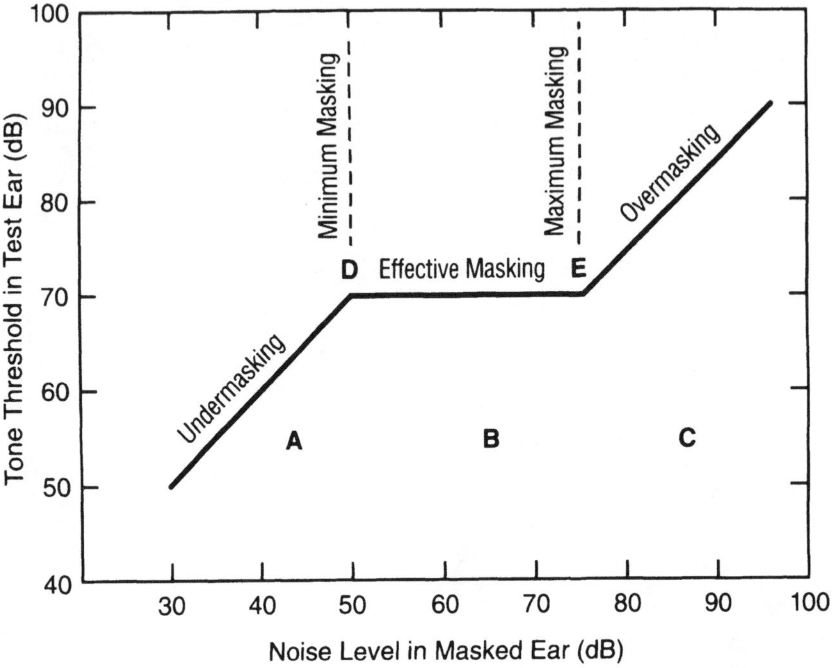

Fig. 2. The plateau method for masking. (A) Undermasking. The tone (by cross-hearing) continues to be heard in the masked ear despite the noise, since the tone level is below the threshold of the test ear. (B) The plateau. The tone has reached the threshold of the test ear. Therefore, raising the masking level in the masked ear does not shift the threshold of the tone. (C) Overmasking. The masking level is so intense that it crosses to the test ear, resulting in continuous shifts in the threshold of the tone with increases in the masking noise. Minimum (D) and maximum (E) masking are found at either side of the plateau. Reprinted with permission from Prentice-Hall, Inc.

years, its principles have also been applied to air conduction and speech audiometry. Three shifts occur with degrees of masking noise indicating insufficient masking or undermasking, the plateau with the appropriate amount of masking noise and finally overmasking with noise levels creating cross-masking.

Masking validates pure tone thresholds and speech audiometry. Without this validation process chances of inaccurate results may occur and misinterpretation of these results arise. An audiological evaluation applying proper masking procedures is one of greater legitimacy.

Before beginning any evaluation procedure, the clinician must have a good understanding of INTERAURAL ATTENUATION (IA). Interaural attenuation describes the amount of energy absorbed when sound crosses from one side of the skull to the opposite or contralateral ear. When a sound is presented to one ear, both cochleas will be stimulated with the sound audible to the contralateral cochlea at a reduced intensity (Martin, 1975). In order to ensure only one ear identifies the test tone, masking of the opposite ear (NTE) is necessary (Fletcher, 1940 and Lusher & Koenig, 1955). When the test stimuli are presented to one ear, how many decibels does it take for the test stimuli to be audible to the opposite ear? Researchers have found that the amount of IA varies dependent upon the frequency under test, intensity of the sound, type of transducer, sensitivity of the contralateral ear, damping effect of the skull and subjectivity of human nature (Hodgson, 1980 and Naunton, 1960). The clinician's primary concern with IA is air conduction audiometry (including speech testing) and bone conduction audiometry.

Procedures of masking need to be routinely implemented for unilateral hearing impairments, conductive hearing impairments or bilateral asymmetrical hearing losses. Often a SHADOW CURVE occurs when no masking procedures or improper masking procedures are used. (See Audiogram 1) A shadow curve is a direct reflection of the better ear responding for the poorer ear due to cross-over. The determination of this "change-over point" is the end goal. For example, as seen in Audiogram 1, without proper masking procedures, the "poorer" ear (the left ear) is displaying a severe mixed loss; whereas, in reality proper masking procedure demonstrates that the left ear may display a profound sensorineural loss (as in Audiogram 2). Without accurate masking procedures, the left ear could show inappropriate responses. Unmasked bone conduction thresholds of the poorer ear may be obtained at the same level as the bone conduction threshold of the better ear due to cross-over and improper effective masking levels (EML). Without proper masking procedures, test reliability is suspect.

Researchers have found IA for air conduction to fall between 40 and 90 dB HL for testing situations under headphones (Liden, Nilsson & Anderson 1959b and Zwislocki 1953). Wegel and Lane (1924) reported that IA is an average difference of 50 dB HL between the air and bone conduction threshold. They describe IA as an "acoustical leakage" between the ears due to bone conduction. Studebaker (1964) suggested an IA of 35 dB in the lower frequencies, 40 dB in the speech frequencies and 50 dB in the higher frequencies. Most researchers since that time feel as Coles and Priede (1975) reported the means and averages shown in Table 1. For example, if the TE/stimulus via air conduction is presented at 60 dB HL, with a 40 dB interaural attenuation, the test stimuli is audible to the opposite ear at 20 dB HL. If the air conduction threshold in

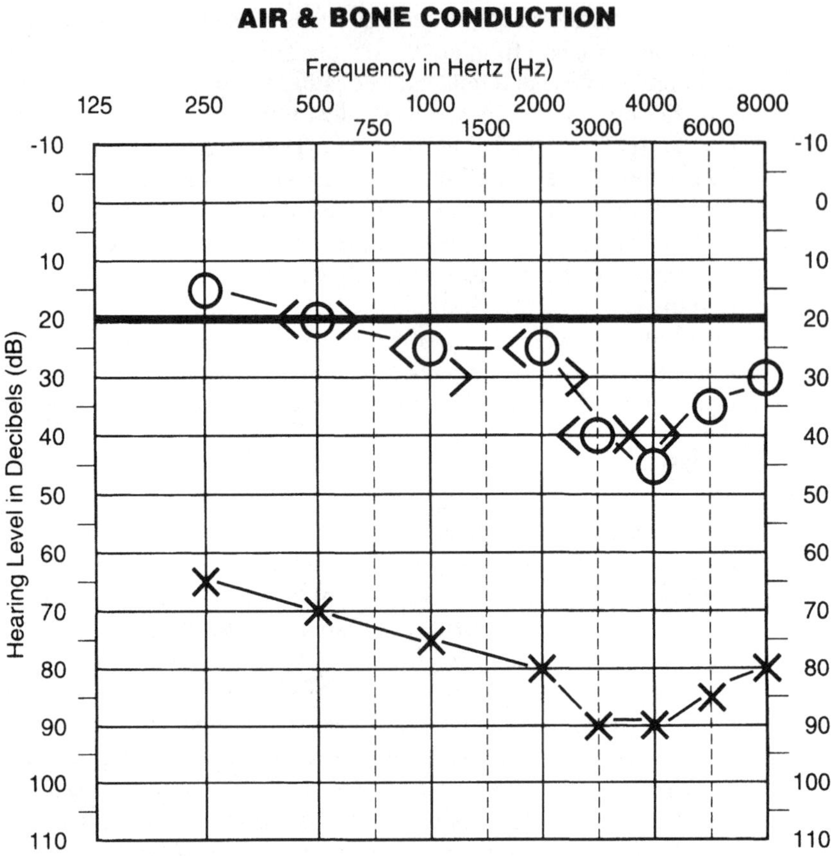

Audiogram 1. Shadow curve. Demonstrates the need to mask with a 40 dB or more difference between the right and left air conduction thresholds.

the NTE is 10 dB, the test stimuli are audible to the NTE. (See Figure 3) Additionally, altering Figure 3 slightly as shown in Figure 4, if air conduction in NTE is 30 dB HL and bone conduction in the NTE is 5 dB HL, the stimulus to the poorer ear is audible to the better cochlea. In this situation, masking to determine bone conduction will be necessary for both ears as the evaluator is not certain which ear is perceiving the bone conducted response.

Chaiklin (1967) cautioned that the lowest IA levels are more useful in an evaluation than average IA due to previously reported variations in subjects, equipment and test modes. In other words, it is best to mask when a question of crossover exists rather than to not use masking techniques when masking may have been indicated. (See Table 1) Therefore, for air conduction, a general guideline is an IA of 40 dB between right and left air conduction

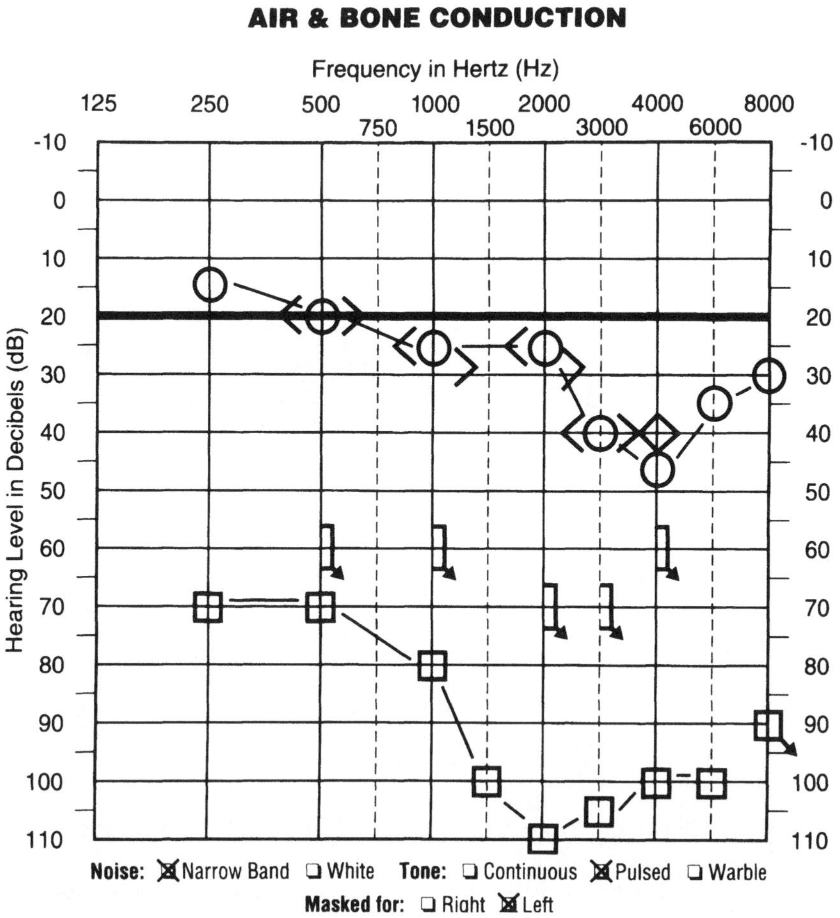

Audiogram 2. Appropriate masking procedures obtain true left ear responses.

thresholds (Rule 1A) or TE/stimuli and obtained bone conduction thresholds (Rule 1B). The three primary rules, Rules 1, 2, and 3 (See Figure 14) will be discussed further in this chapter.

IA for bone conduction occurs as low as 0 dB. This indicates that for bone conduction audiometry the test signal may cross over to the opposite ear as low as 0 dB as both cochleas may be stimulated equally. In order to truly determine which ear is being stimulated, even with a symmetrical sensorineural hearing impairment, one must apply masking noise to the NTE while evaluating the ear under test (Studebaker, 1962). Due to an IA level of 0 dB, theoretically and sometimes more practically, masking should be performed for bone conduction at all test frequencies for each ear.

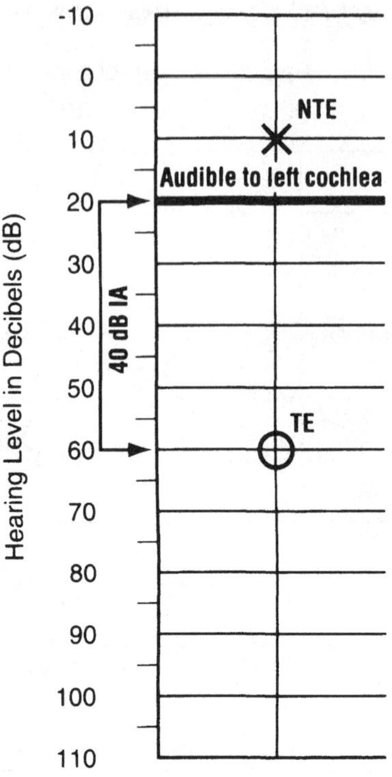

Fig. 3. Shadow curve due to crossover effect.

Many practitioners mask for bone conduction in all cases routinely. Studebaker (1964) disagreed with this conservative plan and followed a more timely and effective approach. This approach to bone conduction audiometry, although interaural attenuation is indicated at 0 dB, employs masking whenever a 15 dB or more difference occurs between the air conduction threshold of the test ear and the obtained bone conduction threshold of the NTE (Rule 2). Especially in the lower frequencies, the test signal may be perceived by the contralateral ear as louder than the ipsilateral (same)

Table 1. Mean and average range of interaural attenuation. Reprinted with permission from *The Journal of Laryngology and Otology.*

Frequency (Hz)	250	500	1000	2000	4000	Average
IA Mean (dB)	61	63	63	63	68	63
Range (dB)	50 - 80	45 - 80	40 - 80	45 - 75	50 - 85	51 - 70

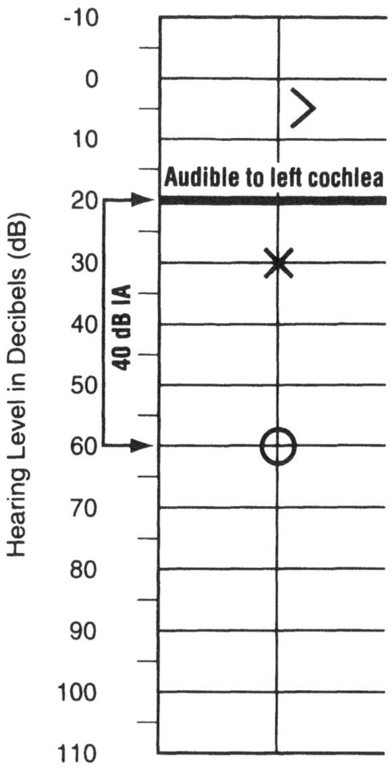

Fig. 4. Crossover relative to a mixed hearing impairment.

ear. When evaluating for bone conduction audiometry, if improper masking levels are used, bone conduction thresholds under test may exhibit the same thresholds as the best ear (Studebaker, 1964). (See Audiogram 1 and 2.)

MASKING CHARACTERISTICS

Masking characteristics must be considered in each phase of evaluating for air conduction, bone conduction and speech audiometry. Without consideration of these variables, inappropriate results may be generated. All of these merely make for a more interesting game to be played. The process of working with hearing diversity is much more challenging than if we were dealt the same poker hand each time.

CENTRAL MASKING

Central masking was noted by Wegel and Lane (1924) when small shifts in thresholds at intensities too low to effect peripheral masking were found. The clinician understands that bone conduction thresholds which fall 5-10 dB below the air conduction thresholds are theoretically not possible and that their occurrence may be quite distressing. The clinician must consider central masking as a potential factor. It is believed that central masking is mediated due to the different pathways in the central nervous system and will potentially shift a threshold 5-10 dB but rarely more than 10 dB (Liden, Milsson & Anderson, 1959b and Zwislocki, 1971). It is felt that central masking may be reduced by the use of a pulsed test stimuli with a continuous masking noise in the opposite or NTE/noise (Dirks & Malmquist, 1965, Dirks and Norris, 1966 and Luscher & Koenig, 1955). As with other testing situations, additional factors such as client fatigue can not be ruled out. A patient who tires easily may have more difficulty following the tasks needed for an appropriate response.

Zwislocki (1971) found central masking to reduce at low and high frequencies (when using a 1000 Hz tone as masking noise) and found central masking to be frequency selective. Central masking is optimal at the onset of the masking noise. Dirks and Norris (1966) concluded that the amount of threshold shift is dependent upon the pulsed or continual temporal presentation of the test stimulus. They observed threshold shifts that increased with frequency when the test stimulus and noise were simultaneously pulsed or continuous. For clients who have difficulty following the task with continuous masking noise and a continuous tone presentation, it may be advantageous to use a pulsed tone presentation with a continuous masking noise. This stimulus presentation mode may be easier to discriminate. Coles and Priede (1975) reported on research work of Spencer and Priede (1974) who found that the central masking effect will decrease speech discrimination approximately one percent for each three decibels of sensation level (SL) using normal hearing subjects and a wide-band contralateral noise.

OCCLUSION EFFECT (OE)

The occlusion effect (OE) occurs any time the pinna and ear canal are tested in a "covered" position as with supraaural earphones. Occlusion results in an improved shift of bone conduction threshold whenever the earphone is placed over the pinna and external ear canal of the contralateral ear (Studebacker, 1979). According to Feldman (1961) when evaluating bone conduction audiometry, the bone oscillator is placed on the side under test (TE/stimuli)

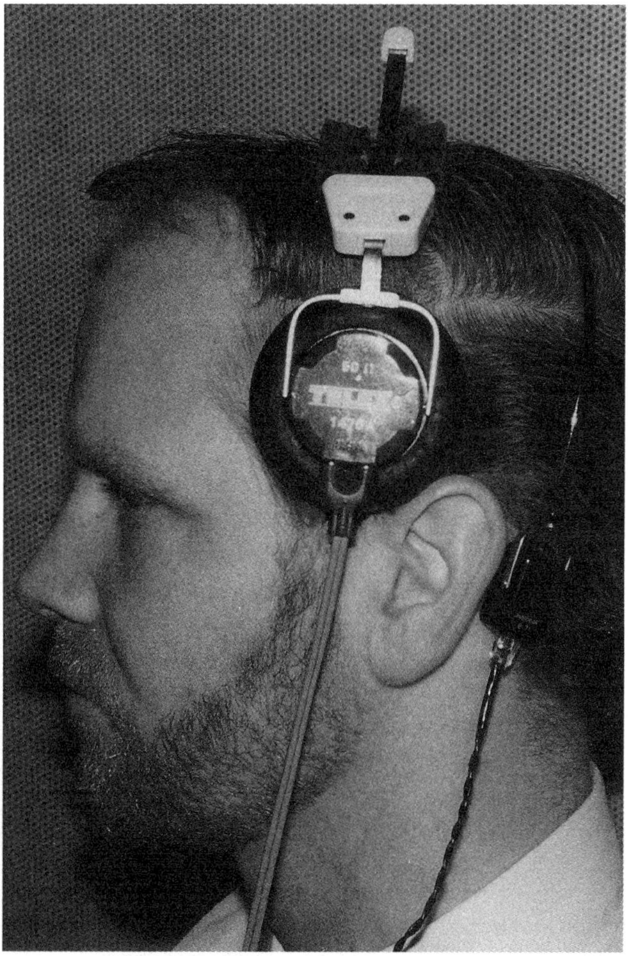

Fig. 5. Earphone and oscillator placement for bone conduction masking.

with the earphone covering only the contralateral ear. The earphone which would be normally placed over the TE pinna and ear canal is seated on the side of the skull off the pinna (See Figure 5). The bone conduction threshold in the occluded NTE ear improves with the placement of the earphone over the pinna (Studebaker, 1962). The occlusion effect occurs in normal and sensori-neural ears, whereas conductive losses have a natural occlusion due to the blockage in the hearing mechanism. A difficulty may arise when only one ear exhibits a conductive component which will increase the danger of overmasking (Studebaker, 1979). The occlusion effect value is factored into the minimum masking level, and will be discussed further in this chapter (See Table 2).

Occlusion Effect (OE) occurs due to the external auditory canal being covered by the earphone which creates additional mechanical energy presented to the cochlea. Conductive components are not affected by OE as energy is sent via mechanical means (Sanders, 1972). The OE values are not added into the effective masking level calculations when evaluating a conductive loss (Studebaker, 1979). Dirks and Swindeman (1967) felt a 30 dB occlusion effect factor may be a necessary addition to the minimum effective level at lower frequencies from 125 Hz to as much as 1000 Hz unless a conductive component is exhibited. The higher frequencies generally do not exhibit any difficulty with occlusion (Goldstein & Hayes, 1965). Elpern and Naunton (1963) stated "since the unoccluded Interaural Attenuation (IA) for a bone conduction stimulus is essentially zero, occluding the untested ear may reduce this value to less than zero. In other words, the threshold in the untested ear may be lowered by an amount equal to the occlusion effect."

OVERMASKING

As seen in Figure 2, overmasking presents above the plateau. Overmasking occurs when a false threshold shift occurs due to too

Table 2. Average occlusion effect values of four studies and recommended values of four studies and recommended values for clinical uses. Reprinted from *Audiology and Hearing Education.*

Study	**Frequency (Hz)**			
	250	**500**	**1000**	**2000**
		(decibel levels)		
Huizing (1960)	13.0	15.0	8.0	1.0
Elpern & Naunton (1963)	28.0	20.0	9.0	0.0 (TDH 39 with firm rubber cushion)
Goldstein & Hayes (1965)	19.4	12.6	5.7	1.1
Dirks & Swindeman (1967)	22.9	20.2	8.8	0.5 (MX 41/AR cushion)
Recommended	15.0	15.0	10.0	0.0

much noise presented to the hearing system. The noise actually covers up the TRUE threshold creating poorer thresholds. The higher the masking noise level, the greater risk of cross-masking or overmasking (Coles & Priede, 1975).

Overmasking occurs more commonly in bone conduction audiometry. This happens when the masking levels exceed the IA level threshold. The clinician must be acutely aware of IA levels. Figure 6 shows the need for masking since a 15 dB or more difference occurs between the bone conduction threshold and the air conduction threshold (Rule 2). Noise is presented to the left ear at 70 dB while the stimuli or pure tone is presented to the right ear through bone conduction at 25 dB. Due to the apparent conductive nature of this loss, no occlusion effect values are included in the effective masking level. The test stimuli presented at 70 dB is 45 dB greater than 25 dB. Therefore, overmasking has occurred which could potentially create a false shift in bone conduction threshold to 30 dB as the masking noise is "covering up" the true threshold. "Overmasking" must be noted on the Audiogram.

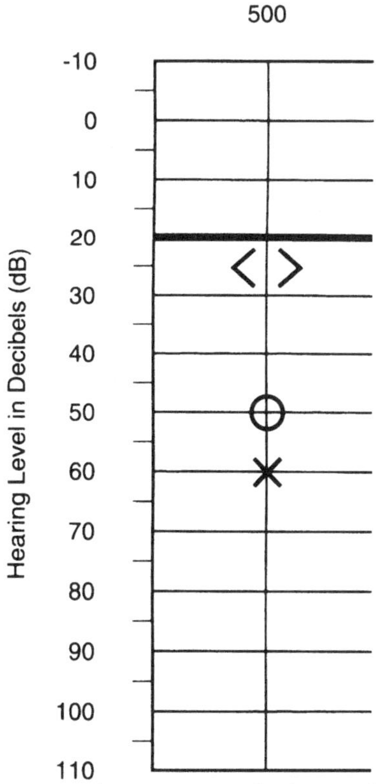

Fig. 6. Overmasking occurs from an excess of noise creating false thresholds.

UNDERMASKING

Undermasking occurs when an insufficient amount of masking noise is presented to the NTE so that the test stimuli presented to the TE are yet crossing over to the NTE. This better ear, not the ear under test, is still responding to the test stimuli.

Undermasking occurs more commonly when performing air conduction audiometry. As in overmasking, the clinician must always be questioning procedures based on the IA. Undermasking occurs when masking levels fall below the recommended IA. (See Figure 7) A rule of thumb adds 10 dB of padding to the obtained better ear threshold for a point of entry on the amount of masking noise necessary. As shown in Figure 7, the right ear threshold is 10 dB with the 10 dB padding figure, therefore, noise should be introduced at 20 dB. The obtained left ear threshold is 70 dB. The difference between 70 dB minus 20 dB is 50 dB. This amount exceeds the recommended 40 dB IA indicating the right

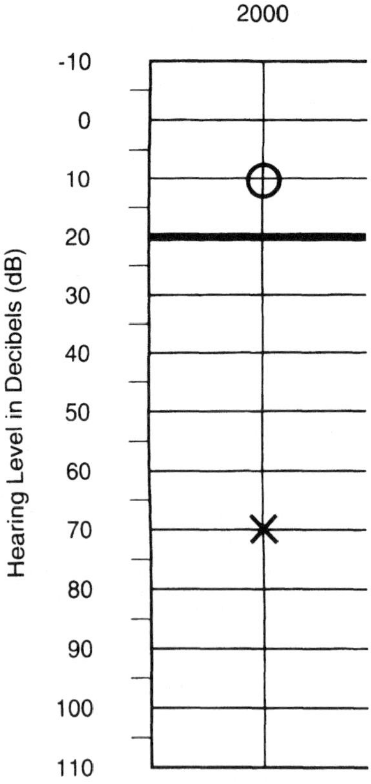

Fig. 7. Undermasking occurs with insufficient amount of noise allows response from the non-test ear.

ear could yet be perceiving the left ear signal. A minimum of 35 dB of masking noise is necessary to negate the response occurring from the right ear.

MASKING DILEMMA

A masking dilemma occurs with a bilateral conductive loss such as is found with bilateral otosclerosis (Naunton, 1960). (See Audiogram 3) This scenario requires excessive masking noise creating overmasking for both ears. Bone conduction thresholds for one ear are at the obtained threshold level but to introduce masking noise for the right or left ear will create an overmasking situation on either ear. Therefore, a masking dilemma occurs and should be so noted on the audiogram. Such notation clearly alters any indi-

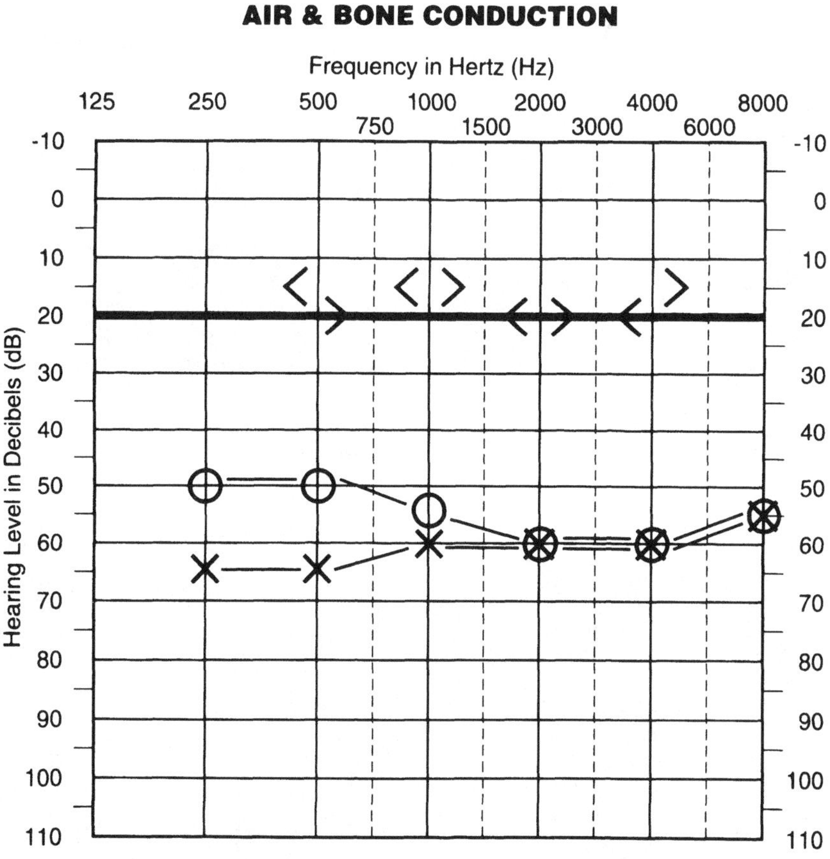

Audiogram 3. Bilateral conductive component creates a masking dilemma.

vidual reading the audiogram at a future date that masking procedures were indicated but could not be completed due to the excessive amount of noise needed which could potentially create false positive thresholds (See Figure 8). At this point other evaluation measures such a tuning forks, otoscopic or microscopic inspection or otoimmitance audiometry should be implemented.

RECRUITMENT

In a practical application of masking procedures, one must keep in mind those individuals who exhibit recruitment. Recruitment is defined as a state when a small increase in intensity results in a large increase in loudness to the patient. Masking noise levels can become quite intense and, to the person with recruitment, these levels may be quite disarming. If such levels are required, it is only

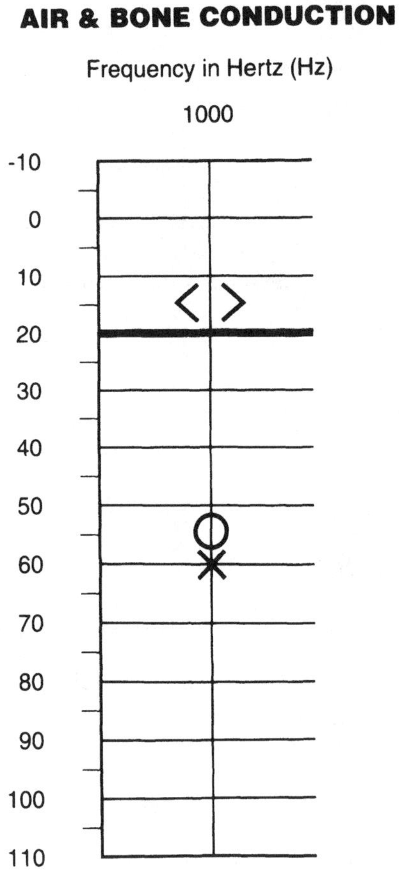

Fig.8. In this example, the effective masking level is equal to 65–70 dB. An overmasking situation is created as this is more than 40 dB over the suspected cochlear reserve, which is 15 dB. For this individual, it is unknown if the cochlear reserve is correct for one ear with crossover to the contralateral ear or if both ears exhibit a conductive component.

courteous for the masking process to be performed as expediently as possible. Excessive noise levels affect clients differently. On a very practical level, the clinician does not want to make a patient angry. Some may become angry enough to stop the testing procedure and lose any rapport the clinician has established with the patient. A patient may make a statement about the noise being "annoying" or may even remove the headphones. These are proof that the signal is at the patient's uncomfortable loudness level (UCL, LDL or TD).

FOREHEAD OR MASTOID PLACEMENT

Early literature regarding masking procedures describe the bone conduction oscillators placement on the forehead or frontal bone of the skull. At this writing, mastoid placement is the placement of choice. Placing the oscillator on the mastoid does appear to be perceived louder with normal hearing individuals and the close proximity to the ear under test assists in the ease of interpretation (Martin, 1975).

Note that forehead placement versus mastoid placement requires different calibration techniques and values. If the forehead placement is used, masking procedures must be employed 100% of the time in testing for bone conduction audiometry.

EARPHONES

Three types of earphones have been reviewed for standardization used with audiometric evaluations. The configuration of a supraaural earphone displays a cushion against the pinna. A second style of earphones is a circumaural earphone whose cushion encompasses the entire pinna. And lastly, insert earphones which are placed into the ear canal itself, much like an in-the-canal hearing instrument. Although supraaural earphones have been recommended for continued usage for standard evaluations, each type has its positive and negative characteristics (American National Standards Institute, 1989b, Killion & Villchur, 1989 and Killion, Wilber & Gundmunsen, 1985). For the purpose of masking, we need primarily to look at the interaural attenuation characteristics of each.

Insert receivers maximize the level of interaural attenuation (IA) as much as 90 dB. IA levels previously discussed were obtained with supraaural earphones. Research by Zwislocki (1953 and 1971) on insert receivers placed into the external auditory canal indicates that a higher IA is due to the stimulation of a smaller area. This high

IA level enables more accurate evaluation of the individual with a large conductive component where a masking dilemma may be present (Hodgson, 1994, Larson-Donaldson, 1988 and Zwislocki, 1953). Killion et al. (1985) reported an IA at 500 Hz of 75 dB with shallow insertion and up to 100 dB with deep insertion of insert receivers (See Figure 9). In addition to the IA advantage, additional advantages are seen in reduction of vibrotactile response such as those found in low frequency corner audiograms; better extraneous noise reduction when evaluating individuals who are not able to be seated in a sound proof booth or room such as in a nursing facility, home or hospital; and the reduction of false responses due

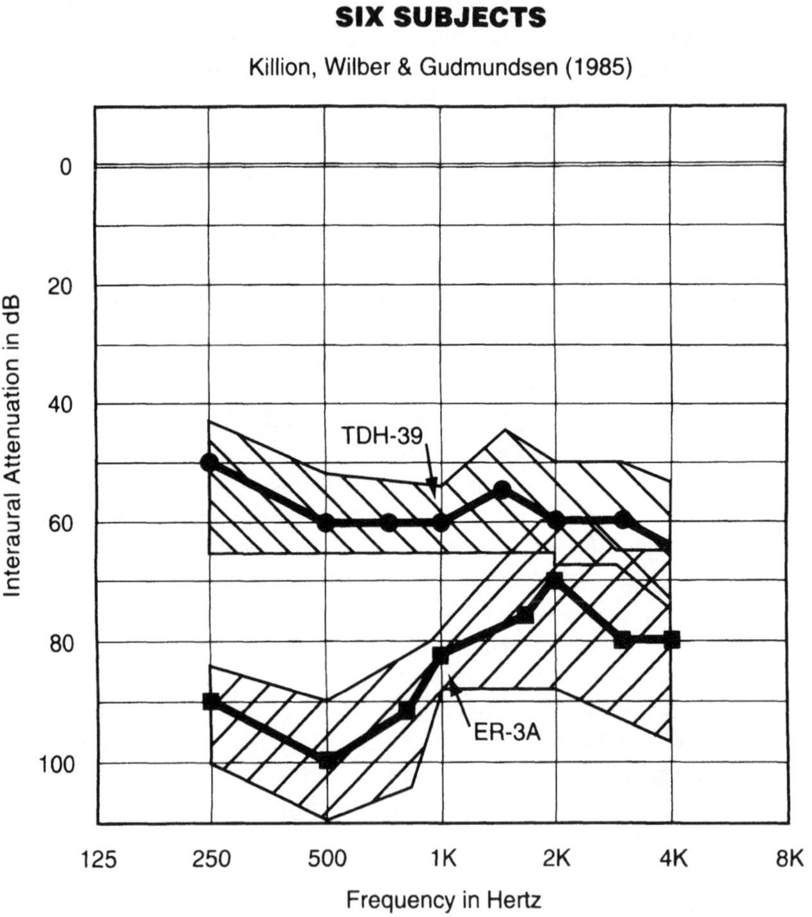

Fig. 9. Average and range of interaural attenuation obtained on six subjects with two earphones: TDH-39 (o) and ER-3 with deeply inserted plugs (+). Reprinted with permission of *Hearing Instruments.*

to a collapsed canal (Hodgson, 1994, Killion & Villchur, 1989 and Killion, Wilber & Gunmundsen, 1985).

Usage of insert receivers instead of standard earphones has been increasing. Insert receivers will assist the validity of masked thresholds to be used in conjunction with otoscopic or microscopic inspection and otoimmitance audiometry assisting in a well rounded evaluation (Naunton, 1960 and Zwislocki 1953).

MASKING NOISE

Various types of masking noises have been used for masking procedures. Masking noise selected should be one of maximum efficiency and minimum intensity. Pure tones as a masking agent were found to be difficult to discriminate between the TE and the NTE/masking.

All masking noise available is a variation of white noise. White noise (also called broadband, wideband or thermal) is found on most audiometers. Until recently, it was standard for portable audiometers. Currently, more portable audiometers are available with white noise, narrow band noise and/or speech noise. White noise is linear noise which researchers feel is most practical for higher frequencies (See Figure 10). White noise is representative

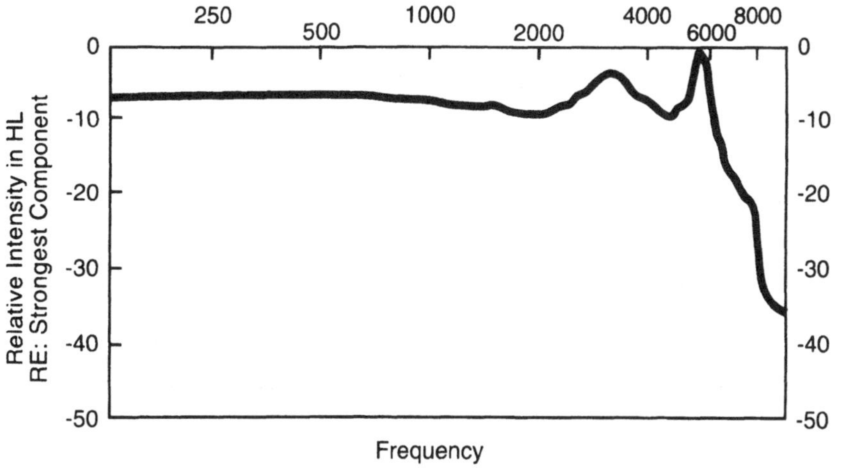

Fig. 10. Acoustic spectrum of a broad band white noise through a TDH-39 earphone. Reprinted with permission of the *Archives of Otolaryngology.*

of all frequencies equally. TDH-39 headphones limit white noise's bandwidth with an extension to 6000 Hz, sharply dropping in the frequencies following 6000 Hz. Since white noise contributes to all frequencies, when one individual frequency is evaluated, the high intensity of the noise may be quite annoying. Therefore, expediency and efficiency when testing with white noise are paramount. Guidelines for masking generators are available from the American National Standard Institute (ANSI) Standards Secretariat, Acoustical Society of America, 335 E. Street, New York, NY 10017-3483 (American National Standards Institute, 1989b).

Speech noise is also a variation on white noise. The frequency response for speech noise is achieved with a "two pole" low pass active filter filtered to a low and middle frequency spectrum (Sanders, 1972). This is shown in Figure 11. Speech noise uses only a small portion of the white noise spectrum providing more emphasis for the speech frequency range than when testing for pure tone audiometry (Feldman, 1961).

Narrow-band noise (a variation on white noise) is produced by selective narrow-band electronic filtering. Each test frequency establishes its own band of frequencies with the test frequency at its center. This critical bandwidth is no more than three decibels below the test frequency. For example, as seen in Figure 12, at 1000 Hz the bandwidth of white noise extends 190 cycles per second en-

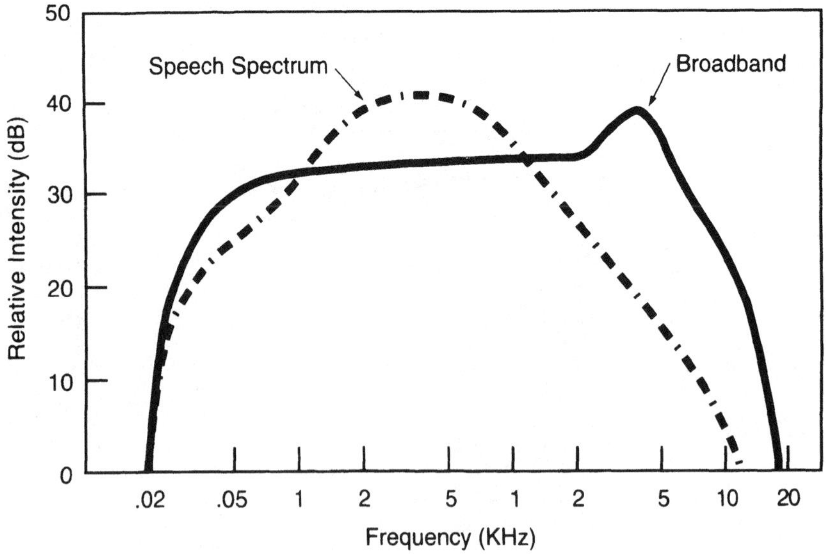

Fig.11. Acoustic spectra for speech and broad band noise through a TDH-39 earphone. Reprinted from University Park Press.

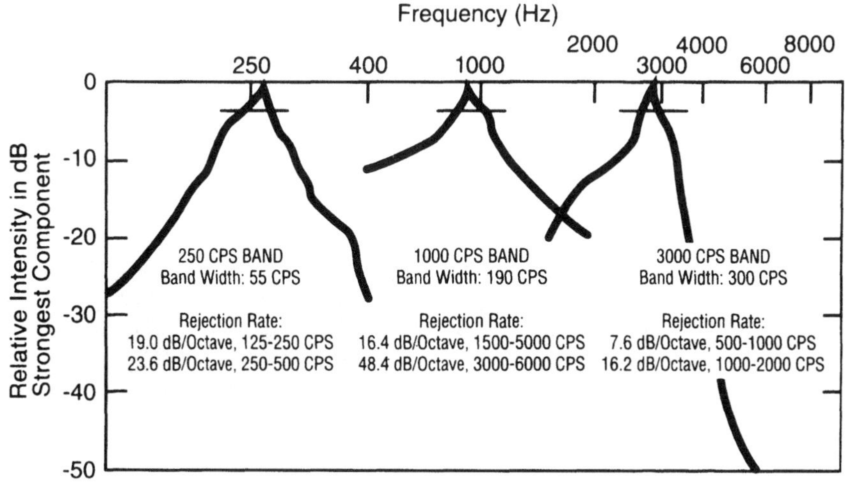

Fig. 12. Acoustic spectra of three narrowbands of noise through a hearing aid type receiver. Reprinted with permission of the *Archives of Otolaryngology.*

compassing the 1000 Hz tone. Narrow band noise makes use of its energy more efficiently than white noise with a smaller amount waste of energy outside of its bandwidth. Sanders and Rintelmann (1964) reported narrow-band noise as more effective in masking lower frequencies than white noise.

Not only is narrow-band noise more efficient in regards to energy usage but it provides more practical applications. Narrow-band noise is more comfortable and less fatiguing for the client as well as more effective for the examiner. Even though narrow-band noise and the test frequency may duplicate the same frequencies, differences between the narrow-band noise and pure tones are enough to be easily discernible to the listener.

Narrow-band noise is the noise of choice when masking for pure tone air and bone conduction audiometry and should be chosen over white noise if the option of either noise stimulus is available.

EQUIPMENT CALIBRATION

Maintenance and calibration of audiometers is too often overlooked. Townsend and Schwartz (1976) caution that many portable audiometers exhibit non-linearity, as the noise spectrum is not always as flat as it should be and that the noise level may not be consistent to 6000 Hz. These factors contribute to improper masking levels. The non-linearity may be a result of the transducer, improper audiometer handling or maintenance, and the "heavy" usage of portable audiometers. Audiometers (portable or clinical) should be biologically checked daily and monthly, and calibrated at least annually.

Masking noise is calibrated by placing an earphone on an "artificial" ear or coupler comprised of a condenser microphone and a 6 cc coupler.39. A 500 g weight is placed on top of the earphone while the output is read in voltage and changed to dB reference 0.0002 dynes/cm2 (29). White noise requires the output to be evaluated at all test frequencies with a linear setting or no filter (39).

Goldstein and Newman (1994) and Wilbur (1994) state the American National Standard Institute (ANSI) 1989 (American National Standard Institute, 1989b) specifies a linear attenuator within .3 dB of the interval stop or one decibel but no higher than one dB. The intensity dial should display 5 dB increments of masking noise. It must attenuate between 3.5-6.5 dB with a resulting intensity of 3 dB or less between the indicated intensity value and actual intensity. A maximum of a 4 dB error is allowable at frequencies from 250-4000 Hz and 5 dB at frequencies below 250 Hz or above 4000 Hz.

The 1989 standards set by ANSI provides definitions for white noise as well as weighted random noise for pure tones, speech and narrow-band noise. One-third octave minimums and one-half octave maximums are recommended for narrow band noise. To calibrate narrow-band noise, it is necessary to employ a frequency analyzer and graphic recorder to determine conformity specifications. Wilbur (1994) cautions the clinician that it is best to use a spectrum analyzer with storage capabilities due to variations and random responses of noise. For narrow-band noise, the SPL value should be within +3 dB of the test frequency (American National Standard Institute, 1989b).

Older audiometers were calibrated in one-half octaves while newer equipment calibrates with one-third octaves. Audiometers are currently calibrated to a 0 dB effective masking level re: hearing level (HL). It is advisable to consult with the users manual for specification and calibration information on audiometers used in the scope of practice.

CALIBRATION OF EFFECTIVE MASKING LEVELS (EML)

Either a biological method or formula method should be used to routinely determine calibration of effective masking levels. Effective masking levels may be calibrated in either hearing level (HL) or sound pressure level (SPL) depending upon the audiometer manufacturer. Check the audiometer equipment manual to determine if calibration is in HL or SPL. Equipment should be calibrated to 0 dB EML equal to 0 dB HL.

Internal calibration is not feasible for effective masking levels using white noise. Calibration of effective masking level for white noise must be performed by either a biological or formula method. These correction factors should be posted on or by the audiometer. The effective masking level varies by frequency and by equipment. Therefore, each frequency must be individually calibrated. To yield the effective masking level, the tone and masking noise must be presented to the same earphone simultaneously, such as on a dual channel audiometer (Wilbur, 1994). Townsend and Schwartz (1976) feel that the spectrum of the noise from portable audiometer is not flat and may offer a miscalculation of effective masking levels due to this non-linearity if the bandwidth is assumed to be flat to 6000Hz.

Two methods exist to determine effective masking levels relative to the functioning of each audiometer. The first method is based on the biological or behavioral responses. The second method is based on the critical band concept of Fletcher (1940) and on the critical ratio data of Hawkins and Stevens (1950). Fletcher's critical band concept indicates a bandwidth of noise not too broad nor too narrow which will exhibit a maximum masking effect with a minimum intensity level. Additional energy above or below this critical ban contributes only to its perceived loudness and not to masking of test stimuli.

Studebaker's biological calibration of effective masking level is executed with six to ten normal hearing subjects. This method may also be used for speech effective masking levels (Lusher & Koenig, 1955 and Studebaker, 1967). A pure tone threshold is established at each frequency with a pre-set amount of masking noise (50 dB, 70 dB and 90 dB intensity levels) presented to the same ear (Sanders and Rintelmann, 1964). Either a two channel audiometer with noise and test stimuli being presented to the same ear simultaneously or some type of mixing system is required. At each frequency a mean threshold value is determined which represents the effective level for normal listeners. This derived value represents the amount a tone will be shifted by noise at each individual frequency. An effective masking level table is then placed on or near the specified audiometer. Biological calibration has been found impractical due to its time-consuming nature (Studebaker, 1964 and Studebaker, 1967).

Coles and Priede (1975) reported a 0 dB EML for speech audiometry to be determined when a 95% or greater speech discrimination score in quiet is reduced to 10% or less by introducing masking noise in normal hearing individuals. Calculating EML for a masked SRT should be the same as that of the PTA (Coles & Priede, 1975, O'Neill & Oyer, 1970, Sanders & Rintelmann, 1964 and Studebaker, 1979).

Veniar's (1965) behavioral approach evaluated the effective masking level with hearing impaired ears, as she felt pathologically affected ears behave differently from normal ears. As with Studebaker's method, test stimulus and noise are presented to the same earphone. The noise level is increased in 10 dB steps until the signal is eliminated. The level of noise required to mask the test stimulus is derived to be 0 dB EML.

Difficulties presented by biological or behavioral methods are several. These difficulties include the requirement to present noise and test stimulus to the same earphone with complete masked audiograms for each subject, a daily calibration, the low number of subjects increases the chances of flawed results, and it is quite time-consuming. On the positive side, this method is less costly monetarily than formula or electroacoustic analysis methods.

Formula methods such as that described by Sanders and Rintelmann (1964) for broadband or narrow-band noise result in less variability due to a higher number of subjects, greater expediency, standardization with good reliability, and calibration performed by a special instrument company. Formula methods are more difficult than biological methods to understand and more sophisticated equipment is necessary (Sanders, 1972, Sanders & Rintelmann, 1964 and Townsend & Schwartz, 1976). Procedures described by Sanders and Rintelmann (1964) determine EMLs based on the critical ratio data of Hawkins and Stevens (1950). This process is used for both one-third octave analysis and one octave filter analysis for which only the bandwidth will be different (see Table 3) (Hawkins & Stevens, 1950 and Sanders & Rintelmann, 1964).

Three formulas:

1. LPC = OA SPL − 10 log BW in Hz

2. E in CB = LPC + 10 log CBW (10 log CBW in Hz = CBW in dB)
3. Z (EM) = E in CB − threshold in quiet (SPL)

Formula one introduces the Level per Cycle (LPC) equal to the overall sound pressure level minus 10 times the log of the bandwidth in Hertz. The bandwidth is based on a frequency component of white or narrow band noise and is modified by the earphone frequency response (Goldstein, 1979, Sanders, 1972 and Townsend & Schwartz, 1976).

Formula two is based on work by Fletcher (1940) who developed the masking effect relative to a band of frequencies of critical width. This critical band hypothesis determines that effective masking level is dependent upon energy in a restricted band of requencies (31). Energy of the critical bandwidth is equal to the level per cycle plus 10 times the log of the critical bandwidth.

The final formula tabulates effective masking of "z" based upon energy in the critical bandwidth minus the normal threshold in quiet measured in sound pressure level (SPL). These formulae predict accuracy and efficiency of masking noise better with one-third octave measurements than behavioral measurements. This concept (or level per cycle) considers overall intensity divided by the width of the noise band. The masking of a pure tone is dependent upon the restricted frequency band width. If this width is narrowed to be less than the critical width with no added energy, a decrease in masking effect occurs.

In widening the bandwidth, efficiency of the masking is also decreased. A narrower bandwidth presents with more intensity centered around primary frequencies. White noise displays a wider bandwidth, therefore intensity is spread over a wider range producing less energy (Sanders & Rintelmann, 1964). White noise displays inefficiency as the majority of its energy falls outside of the critical bandwidth. Narrow-band noise is the most efficient noise due to its range within the critical width for each frequency.

MINIMUM AND MAXIMUM EFFECTIVE MASKING LEVELS FOR PURE TONE AUDIOMETRY

To obtain an effective masking level for each patient the following criteria must be met. First, the masking noise employed must have an intensity level to effectively cover the test stimuli. Second, the masking noise employed must not be so intense as to cover the test stimuli elevating the true "test ear" response. And lastly, the stimuli must not exceed the client's Uncomfortable Loudness Level (UCL) as each person's level of tolerance for noise varies (Larson-Donaldson, 1988).

The minimum effective masking level is defined as the lowest amount of masking noise in the NTE that will effectively cover the test stimuli in the TE without the NTE participating for the TE. The maximum effective masking level is defined as the greatest amount of masking noise in the NTE that will not decrease falsely the TE threshold. These two levels assist the testing situation so that neither undermasking nor overmasking occur. Minimum and maximum effective masking levels have been calculated with a number of different formulas. Do not confuse EML's with previously discussed calibration methods.

Effective masking levels may be calculated by formula or psychoacoustic method. Formula methods determine if masking is necessary, provided the amount of masking noise needed to prevent crossover, and calculate for undermasking or overmasking levels. These methods are not always practical unless all information to be used in the formula is available (Hodgson, 1980). In a

Table 3. Critical band widths* for eleven test frequencies. Reprinted with permission from *The Journal of the Acoustical Society of America.*

Critical Band Widths* for Eleven Test Frequencies

Center Frequency	Critical Band Width	
	In Hz	10 log CBW
125	70.8	18.5
250	50	17
500	50	17
750	56.2	17.5
1000	64	18
1500	79.4	19
2000	100	20
3000	158	22
4000	200	23
6000	376	25.75
8000	501	27

practical sense, formula methods slow down the evaluation process as they are quite time-consuming compared to psychoacoustic methods.

The psychoacoustic methods such as those developed by Hood (1960) and Studebaker (1964 and 1967) search for a "plateau" or "shadowing". Hood's method was developed by 1960 to be used for bone conduction audiometry. It has been adapted for air conduction audiometry as well.

To implement Hood's plateau method, obtain the unmasked threshold for both ears evaluating the better ear first. Determine the need to mask based on the Interaural Attenuation (IA) levels. To the

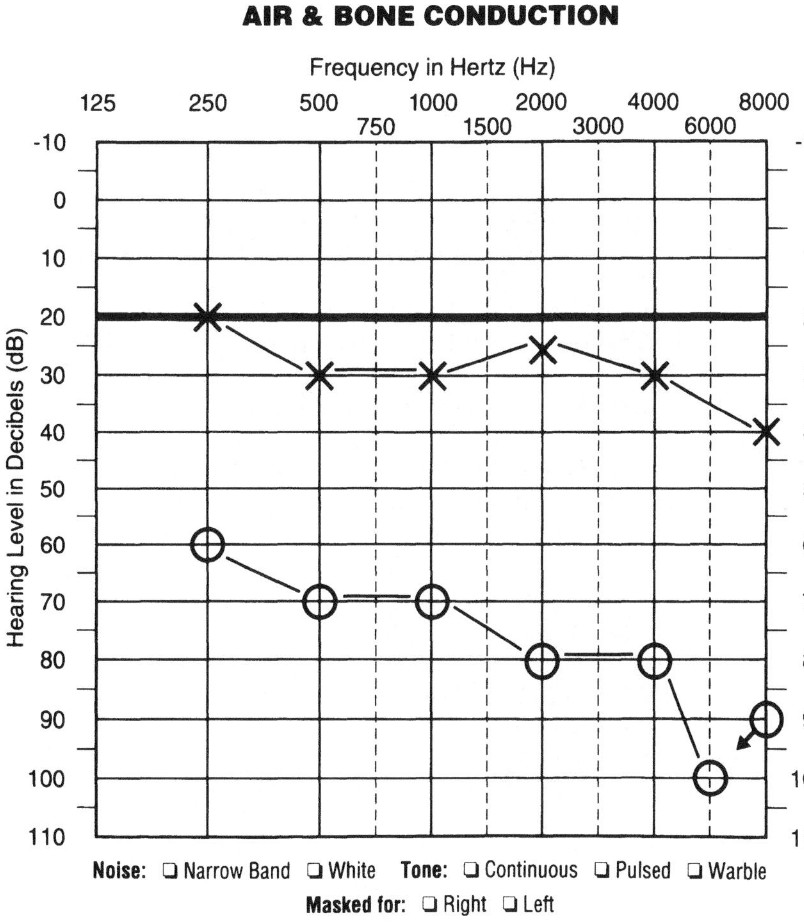

Audiogram 4. Hood's psychoacoustic method.

better ear (NTE) add a padding of 10 dB on to the threshold of the NTE so that at this level, masking noise will be audible to the NTE. (See Audiogram 4) Add 10 dB to the RE obtained threshold of 0 dB. Begin the TE/tone at the obtained unmasked threshold. If a response occurs with 10 dB of masking noise, increase the masking noise in 5 dB steps until an increase of 15 to 20 dB in the NTE results in no change in response from the TE. Thus, the "plateau" has been achieved with no undermasking or overmasking occurring. A more detailed example of this method may be found further in this chapter under "Masking Procedures for Air Conduction, Bone Conduction and Speech Audiometry" (Hood, 1960).

Veniar (1965) and Naunton (1957) have felt that Hood's method and other formula methods do not take into account that more than one plateau may be found with some individuals. Plateaus often were not proceeded or followed by a rise. This aspect might indicate that insufficient masking develops in some people even with extreme noise levels. It is often difficult to compare a normal ear to a hearing impaired ear due to subjectivity of the test process and subjectivity of human nature.

Veniar determined a minimum and a maximum effective masking level at each frequency for each individual. Her process introduced the masking stimulus into the same ear as the air conduction signal at the threshold of that particular frequency. Noise stimulus was increased until the test tone threshold is no longer audible. This level is then recorded as the minimal effective masking level (MEML). With MEML of masking noise presented to the NTE, if the unmasked bone conduction threshold is audible with this level of noise, the decibel level is determined to be a true threshold. If the bone conduction threshold is not audible with this level of noise, it is determined that this is not a true threshold and bone conduction presentation level is increased until a response is obtained. Once a response is obtained, increase the noise level 10 dB to the NTE/masking. If no response is obtained, continue to increase the bone conduction presentation level until a response is obtained. Continue to raise the masking noise in the NTE until two increases of noise (in 10 db steps) does not change the threshold. This is determined the true threshold. Venier describes the primary advantage to this method as the MEML ascertaining enough masking noise so not to undermask or overmask. The methodology determine the limit of noise which is sufficient to mask the NTE (Naunton, 1957 and Veniar, 1965).

White noise variations were better controlled with this method. However this method is applicable to all noise types. Finally, this method allows the client to take an active role and minimizes adjustment to "central noise".

A one-level masking rule of either 50 or 70 dB has been suggested by several educators and researchers to simplify masking. Martin (26) describes this rule as the "Hit or Myth" method. Too often the clinician uses this rule in all situations. This method is an elementary masking procedure and inappropriate in more complex evaluations. This method works in situations with no variables. However, caution with this method must be taken. As with any method, the basic rules and principles must be adhered to (Martin, 1975 and Martin, 1985).

Lucsher and Koenig (1955) calculate a bone conduction minimum effective masking as follows: (See Audiogram 5)

Minimum Effective Masking = MB + BT + (AM − BM)

MB = minimum masking for normal ears
BT = bone conduction threshold in TE
AM = Air conduction threshold in masked ear
BM = Bone conduction loss in same ear

Liden et al (1959a) suggested the following formulas for minimum and maximum effective masking for air and bone conduction audiometry. (See Audiogram 5).

Air conduction formula:

Mmin = At − 40 + (Am − Bm)
Mmax = Bt + 40, provided Mmax is less than D

Bt = bone conduction threshold in TE
Am = air conduction threshold in NTE
Bm = bone conduction threshold in NTE

Actual air conduction threshold of the ear under test is "At". "Am" represents the air conduction threshold of the NTE which is 20 dB. "Bm" is the bone conduction threshold of the NTE.

Mmin = At − 40 + (Am − Bm)
Mmin = 60 − 40 + (20 − 10)
Mmin = 60 − 40 + 10
Mmin = 60 − 50
Mmin = 10 dB

Mmax = Bt + 40, provided Mmax is less than the threshold of discomfort (D)
Mmax = 10 + 40
Mmax = 50 dB

Bone conduction formula:

Mmin = Bt + (Am − Bm)

Mmax = Bt + 40, provided Mmax is less than D
40 represents IA and D represents discomfort

Bt = bone conduction threshold in TE
Am = air conduction threshold in NTE
Bm = bone conduction threshold in NTE

$$\text{Mmin} = \text{Bt} + (\text{Am} - \text{Bm})$$
$$\text{Mmin} = 10 + (20 - 10)$$
$$\text{Mmin} = 10 + 10$$
$$\text{Mmin} = 20 \text{ dB}$$
$$\text{Mmax} = \text{Bt} + 40, \text{ provided Mmax is less than D}$$
$$\text{Mmax} = 10 + 40$$
$$\text{Mmax} = 50 \text{ dB}$$

Formula methods are time consuming and more suitable for research as four different formulas are required to interpret EML for each air and bone test frequency. In addition, formula methods assume that the masking level has been calibrated to appropriate effective masking levels.

Studebaker (1962) suggested a mid-masking level (Mo) formula to reduce formulas for maximum and minimum levels. This formula also eliminates undermasking and overmasking as a potential hazard.

$$\text{Mo} = \frac{(\text{Mmax} - \text{Mmin})}{2} \qquad \text{Mo} = \text{Mon} + \text{Bt} + \frac{(\text{ABm})}{2}$$

Mo = Mid masking level
Mon = Mid masking level for normal hearing
Bt = Bone conduction loss in the Ear under test
ABm/2 = one-half the air/bone gap in the masked ear

This formula is quite workable until a masking dilemma arises wherein ABm approaches minimum and maximum masking levels. Overmasking and undermasking are then kept to a minmum.

$$\text{Mo} = \text{Mon} + \text{Bt} + \text{ABm}/2$$

EFFECTIVE MASKING LEVELS FOR SPEECH AUDIOMETRY

Masking is necessary for speech audiometry especially for tests such as speech discrimination, when the presentation level is much higher than the pure tone average (PTA) or speech reception threshold (SRT) of the better ear. Phonetically balanced (PB) words used for speech discrimination testing are presented at threshold levels well above the pure tone average or speech reception threshold of either ear. Masking for speech audiometry must be employed whenever a 40 dB or more difference occurs between the presentation level of the poorer ear and the PTA or SRT of the better ear (Rule 3). This rule and procedure is often overlooked.

To effectively mask for speech audiometry, speech noise is the most appropriate choice. White noise would be the next option if speech noise is not available. Hawkins and Stevens (1950) found with normal listeners good agreement between masked speech reception thresholds and masked pure tone averages.

Spencer and Priede as reported by Townsend and Schwartz (1976) commented that the higher the level used for speech masking, the greater the chance of the intensity level being close to the uncomfortable listening level of the client. In addition, as mentioned previously, the higher the intensity of the masking signal, the greater the chance of cross-making.

Coles and Priede (1975) calculated the following formula for speech masking levels in the NTE:

Ds − Cs − BBCnt − 30 = masking noise level for speech audiometry

Ds being the presentation of speech stimuli

Cs being the calibration of equipment and speech material which is procured with a group of normal hearing subjects (for purpose of their study and their equipment, a 4 dB level was achieved)

BBCnt is the best bone conduction threshold in the NTE found at 250 to 4000 Hz

Using data from Audiogram 1 the computation is as follows:

Ds − Cs − BBCnt − 30 = masking noise level for speech audiometry

80 − 4 − 15 − 30 = masking noise level for speech audiometry

31 = masking noise level for speech audiometry

Martin (1972) utilizes the following formula for speech masking:

EM for Speech Audiometry = PL − 40 (IA)

It has been the experience of this author that the above formula does not allow for enough "padding" of noise and may result in undermasking. The following formula is suggested:

EM for speech audiometry = PL − 40 (IA) + 20 (Padding)
EM for speech audiometry = PL − 20

Example 1:	Right		Left
	23	PTA	75
	20	SRT	70

The need to mask exists in this example based on the PTA and SRT results. If the SRT results are not available, masking is required here judging from the PTA alone. A 52 dB difference exists between the right and left PTAs which is greater than 40 dB of IA for air conduction testing.

Example 2:	Right		Left
	25	PTA	43
	20	SRT	45
	55	MCL	70

The clinician needs to be acutely aware that there is no need to mask for speech audiometry based upon the PTA or SRT, even though a 40 dB difference does occur between the PL of the left MCL and the right PTA and SRT. A 45 dB difference exists between the MCL of the left ear and PTA of the right ear with a 50 dB difference between the MCL of the left ear and the SRT of the right ear. A need to mask for MCL and speech discrimination exists and proper procedures must be followed.

Using Example 2, the PL may be based upon the SRT plus 30 or PTA plus 30. Either formula may be used in your scope of practice to determine the presentation level of the MCL and speech discrimination. For this exercise the formula of SRT plus 30 will be used which is 45 dB plus 30 or 75 dB for the presentation level. The masking formula which will be employed is:

EM for speech audiometry = PL − 20
EM for speech audiometry = 75 − 20
EM for speech audiometry = 55 dB of speech noise to the better ear

In cases where recruitment or low tolerance to the noise is suspected, the formula may be adjusted to:

EM for speech audiometry, D = PL − 30 (D = discomfort)
EM for speech audiometry, D = 75 − 30
EM for speech audiometry, D = 45 dB of speech noise to the better ear when discomfort is suspect

INSTRUCTING THE PATIENT

When utilizing masking techniques with children, effective instructions depend upon the child's language levels. When evaluating a young child who is pre-lingual or a child with poor language skills, no instructions may be necessary. If the child's language level allows, simplified instructions may be given (Hodgson, 1994). The initial presentation of noise may induce a false response. It may be best to leave the noise in a continual "on" state to decrease any confusion caused by noise in obtaining appropriate test results. Keeping the NTE/noise in a continual "on" state also works well with patients who are confused by masking noise.

Instructions to the patient of any age must be simple and concise. Lengthy instructions only confuse the patient. It has been this author's practice to keep instructions to a descriptive minimum and to keep instructions positive. To say "this is a difficult procedure for clients to respond to" or "you may have some difficulty separating the noise from the tone" only creates confusion. Keep the instructions to a minimum such as "You will be hearing noise in your ____ ear. Ignore the noise and listen only for the tone in your ____ ear." Negative "loading" instruction procedures result in negative outcomes.

To test for air conduction, earphones are placed over the pinna as described in previous chapters of this text. The patient should be instructed, "Raise your hand only whenever you hear the tone, ignoring the noise in the opposite ear." A pulsed tone may be used as it is sometimes easier for the client to discriminate a pulsed tone rather than a continuous tone. Remember to mark on the audiogram which test presentation method is utilized.

Instructions for bone conduction audiometry are much the same. It is important to let the patient know that earphones will not be placed over both pinnas. Example instructions are: "Raise your hand only when you hear the tone. Ignore the noise in the opposite ear. The earphones are not placed as they had been when both ears were covered. Should you hear the tone in the ear with the noise, please let me know."

If masking procedures were used for pure tone audiometry, the individual is an experienced listener for evaluation of speech audiometry. Simple instructions for speech audiometry may be, "You will be hearing noise in the right/left ear, please ignore that noise. Listen to the words in the opposite ear."

Masked test results should be suspect, such as when the masking noise is not sufficient to adequately mask the signal. This may occur if the loss is great and the limits of the masking stimuli on the audiometer had been reached. This should be noted on the audiogram as "insufficient masking noise." A shadow curve might be noted in this situation. For some individuals, the masking signal becomes extremely confusing and distracting (Carhart, 1960). Should the masking noise result in inappropriate responses due to a client's distraction or inability to separate noise from the tone, this should be so noted on the audiogram.

The patient's threshold of discomfort and/or the noise intensity of the audiometry may affect masking procedures (Coles & Priede, 1975). The client's threshold of discomfort must be heeded when employing masking stimulus. Common consideration of the patient's tolerance to the uncomfortable loudness level and to reduce the masking noise stimulus must be employed. Remember, by this point during an evaluation a patient has been toiling to respond to a multitude of stimuli (Larson-Donaldson, 1988 and Liden, Nilsson & Anderson, 1959b).

As previously stated, masking is a decision making process, a challenging game (Goldstein & Newman, 1994 and Larson-Donaldson, 1988). Figure 13 illustrates the complexities of masking where clinicians must choose from the following strategies.

1. Based upon Rule 1A, no masking procedure is necessary due to lack of a 40 dB or more difference between the right and left ears by air conduction.
2. A masking procedure may be initiated since one may assume bone conduction could potentially be 35 dB or better which would result in a 40 dB or more difference between the better

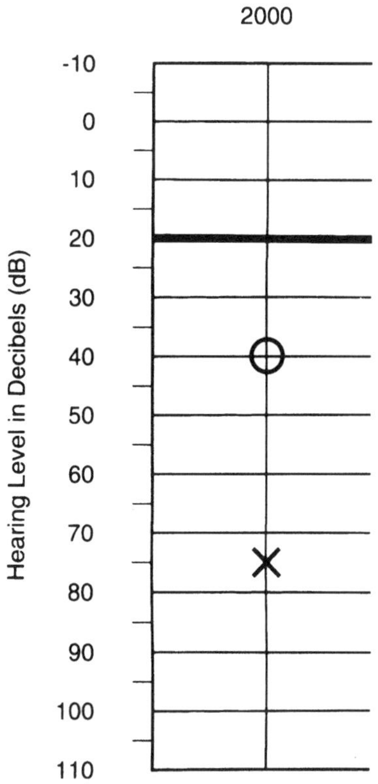

Fig. 13. Complexities of masking techniques.

ear bone conduction and the poorer ear air conduction. This procedure would allow a more even flow in testing.

3. If a need is found to mask for the left ear air conduction, using the test order of unmasked air conduction, then bone conduction; the air conduction testing will need to be repeated, using masking techniques if the bone conduction thresholds fall between 0 & 35 dB.

The second option is more conservative, heeding the advice that it is better to mask when it is not necessary than to not mask when it is necessary. The final scenario may be time consuming due to the repetition of the air conduction testing. This is all part of the strategy for determining the true threshold for each individual frequency.

For the beginning clinician, or even a seasoned clinician, it is advisable to post on or near the audiometer notes on masking procedures. These notes should be neatly written or typed. (See Figures 14 and 15) It is also helpful to use a worksheet such as found in the appendix for organization with the procedures of masking.

RULES FOR MASKING

Rule 1A

Mask for air conduction audiometry whenever a difference at an individual frequency of 40 dB or more exists between air conduction threshold of the better ear and air conduction threshold of the poorer ear.

Rule 1B

Mask for air conduction audiometry whenever there is a 40 dB or more difference between air conduction threshold of the poorer ear and bone conduction threshold of the better ear at any test frequency.

Rule 2

Mask for bone conduction testing whenever there is a 15 dB or more difference between the air conduction threshold of the poorer ear and bone conduction threshold of the better ear.

RULES FOR MASKING

1A: When a 40 dB or more difference between right and left air conduction exists.
1B: When a 40 dB or more difference between poorer ear air conduction and better ear bone conduction exists.
2: When a 15 dB or more difference between better ear bone conduction and poorer ear air conduction exists.
3: When a 40 dB or more difference occurs between PL of speech audiometry and the PTA or SRT of the better ear.

Fig. 14. Rules for Masking.

MASKING PROCEDURES
Starting Points

AIR	
Better ear/Noise	Threshold + 10 dB (padding)
Poorer ear/Tone	Obtained unmasked air threshold
BONE	
Better ear/Noise	Threshold + 10 dB (padding)
Poorer ear/Tone	Obtained better ear bone threshold
SPEECH	
Better ear/Noise	PL of poorer ear − 20 dB
	PL of poorer ear − 30 dB should discomfort exist

Fig. 15. Masking procedures.

Rule 3

Mask for speech audiometry any time there is a 40 dB difference between the presentation level of the poorer ear and the pure tone average or speech reception threshold of the better ear.

PRACTICAL APPLICATION OF MASKING PROCEDURES

Using supraaural earphones, both right and left earphones should be placed against the pinnas. Instruct the client by stating "You will hear noise in your ____ ear (better ear). Please ignore this noise and listen only for pulsed tones in your ____ ear (poorer ear)." Present the masking noise at 10 dB above the obtained threshold to provide a "padding" of sound to make the masking noise audible to the better ear. In the poorer ear begin at the obtained poorer ear air conduction threshold.

To put into use the practical application of this chapter observe Audiogram 4. The right ear displays a moderate to severe loss of hearing while the left ear air conduction thresholds indicate a mild hearing loss. No determination may be made as to the type of loss without bone conduction thresholds or impedance audiometry results. A need to mask exists for right ear air conduction thresholds at all frequencies due to Rule 1A which states "Mask for air conduction audiometry whenever a difference at an individual frequency of 40 dB or more exists between the air conduction threshold of the better ear and air conduction (AC) threshold of the poorer ear." The masking noise of choice is narrow-band noise. If narrow-band noise is not available, white noise is the second choice.

Appropriate symbols should be employed as specified on the Audiogram Key. An example of an Audiogram Key may be found in Figure 16.

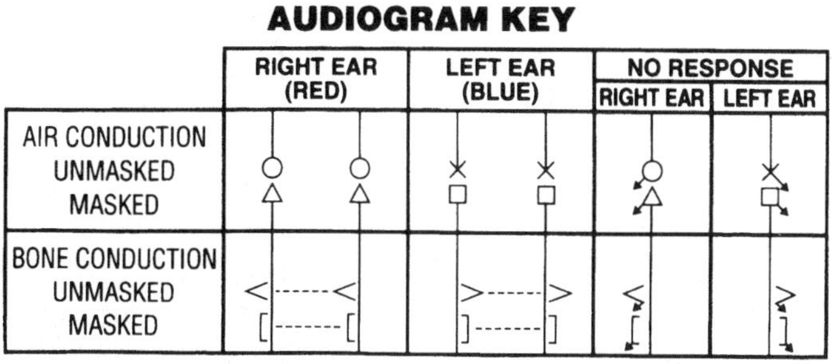

Fig. 16. Audiogram key.

To employ Hood's Plateau method with thresholds obtained at 1000 Hz, the basic rules of starting points in the poorer ear and the amount of masking noise to the better ear will be applied in Audiogram 4.

1000 Hz

Right Ear/Tone	Left Ear/Noise
Begin at the obtained unmasked AC threshold	Begin at the obtained air conduction threshold + 10 dB
70 dB	30 + 10 (padding) = 40 dB

Present tone-Response

With a response to the test tone in the right ear, raise the masking noise 5 dB.

70 dB	45 dB

Present tone-Response

A "rule of thumb" suggests that if a response occurs to the TE/tone, raise the NTE/masking noise. Should no response occur, raise the TE/tone.

70 dB	50 dB

Present tone-Response

A 15 to 20 dB increase in the NTE/masking noise must occur in order to accept the TE/tone as a true threshold. At this point only a 10 dB increase presents itself.

70 dB	55 dB

Present tone-Response

ACCEPT 70 dB HL AS THE TRUE TE/tone RESPONSE. Mark the appropriate symbol on the audiogram. In this case place a red triangle at 70 dB HL on the audiogram.

250 Hz

Right Ear/tone	Left Ear/Noise
Begin at the obtained unmasked AC threshold	Begin at the obtained air conduction threshold + 10 dB
60 dB	20 + 10 (padding) = 30 dB

Present tone-No response

With no response to the test tone in the right ear, raise the TE/tone by 5 dB.

65 dB 30 dB
Present tone-No Response

Again, a "rule of thumb" suggests that if a response is given to the TE/tone, raise the NTE/masking noise. Should no response occur, raise the TE/tone.

70 dB 30 dB

A problem with undermasking is occurring at this point. The TE/tone is 40 dB greater than the NTE/noise level. With the difference being 40 dB HL this creates a situation where, due to Interaural Attenuation (IA), the better ear may be perceiving the TE signal therefore undermasking exists. Raise the NTE/noise by 20 dB to be well within a level where undermasking will no longer create false thresholds.

70 dB $30 + 20 = 50$ dB
Present tone-Response

With a response to the test tone in the right ear, raise the masking noise 5 dB.

70 dB 55 dB
Present tone-Response

Again, with a response to the test tone in the right ear, raise the masking noise 5 dB.

70 dB 60 dB
Present tone-Response

As in the example of 1000 Hz, a 15 to 20 dB increase in the NTE/masking noise must occur in order to accept the TE/tone as a true threshold. At this point only a 10 dB increase presents itself.

70 dB 65 dB
Present tone-Response

ACCEPT 70 dB HL AS THE TRUE TE/tone RESPONSE. Mark the appropriate symbol on the audiogram.

Audiogram 5 shows the masked left ear indicating threshold shifts up to 10 dB. These shifts may have been due to the right ear responding, or due to a phenomenon of central masking. Regardless of the reason for shifts, they occurred and true thresholds were

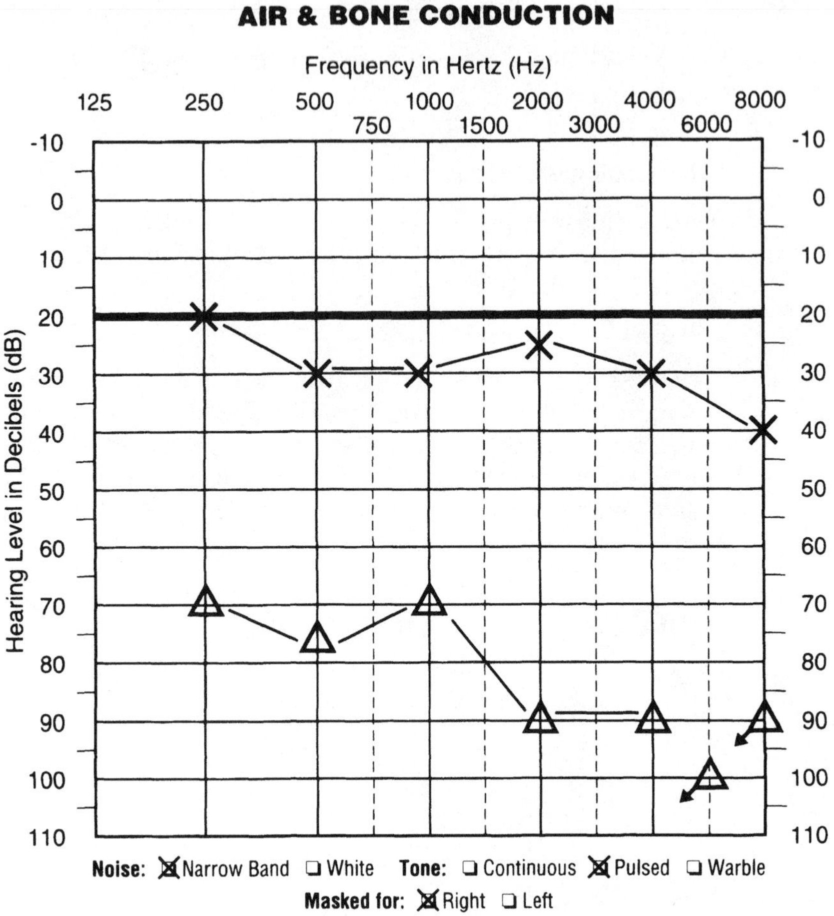

Audiogram 5. Masked left ear threshold shifts.

obtained. Make certain the audiogram is marked with type of noise (white or narrow band) used as well as presentation style of the tone (pulsed or continuous).

The next step is to evaluate for bone conduction audiometry. A rule of thumb is to begin with the better ear or the ear to which the tuning fork lateralizes. In Audiogram 6, the better ear is chosen with unmasked left bone conduction results. Now the need to mask for bone conduction for the right ear is present based on Rule 2. Rule 2 states "masking methods must be put into place when a 15 dB or more difference between the better ear bone conduction and the poorer ear air conduction exists".

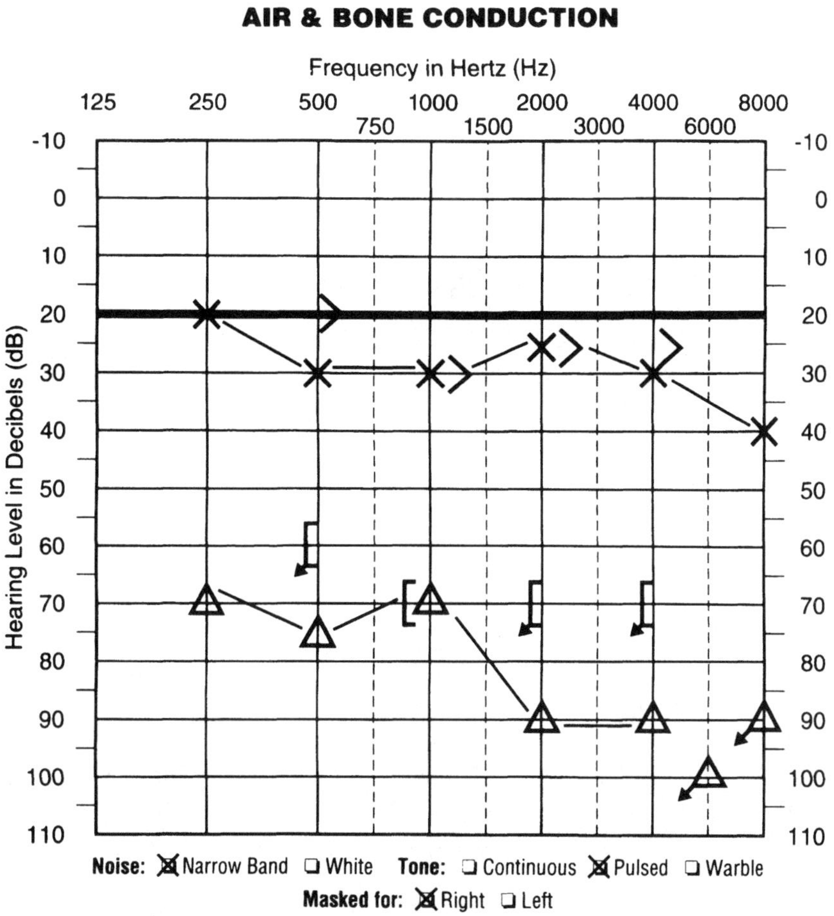

Audiogram 6. Masked results for left bone conduction thresholds.

The air conduction earphone is covering the better ear. As shown in Audiogram 6, it is the left ear. Therefore, masking noise must be audible to the left ear. The same rule applies to bone conduction as to air conduction testing: "Obtained air conduction threshold plus a 'padding' of 10 dB." The TE/tone (in this case the right ear) begins at the obtained bone conduction threshold. The variable for testing bone conduction audiometry is to begin the ear under test at the obtained better ear bone conduction threshold.

The clinician knows that the bone conduction threshold will be no better than the obtained better ear bone conduction score and no poorer than obtained poorer ear air conduction threshold. The challenge begins in determining where exactly that threshold does

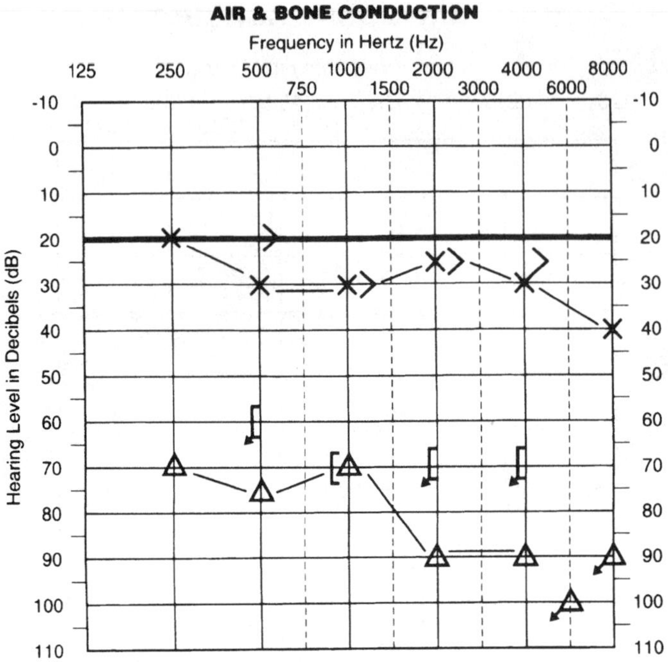

Noise: ☒ Narrow Band ☐ White Tone: ☐ Continuous ☒ Pulsed ☐ Warble
Masked for: ☒ Right ☐ Left

PTA = R - 78
L - 28

SPEECH AUDIOMETRY

	SRT	MCL	UCL	DISCRIMINATION • QUIET		DISCRIMINATION • NOISE	
RIGHT EAR (HL)	dB	dB	dB	%	Presented at: dB HL	%	Presented at dB HL ____ dB S/N
MHA (SPL)				%		dB	
LEFT EAR (HL)	20 dB	55 dB	80 dB	100%	Presented at: 55 dB HL	%	Presented at dB HL ____ dB S/N
MHA (SPL)				%		dB	
BINAURAL (HL) R / L	dB / dB	dB / dB	dB / dB	%	Presented at: R ____ dB HL L ____ dB HL	%	Presented at: R__ L__dB HL ____ dB S/N
MHA (SPL) R / L				%		dB	

Noise: ☒ Speech ☐ White Masked for: ☒ Right ☐ Left ☒ Live Voice ☐ Recorded Voice

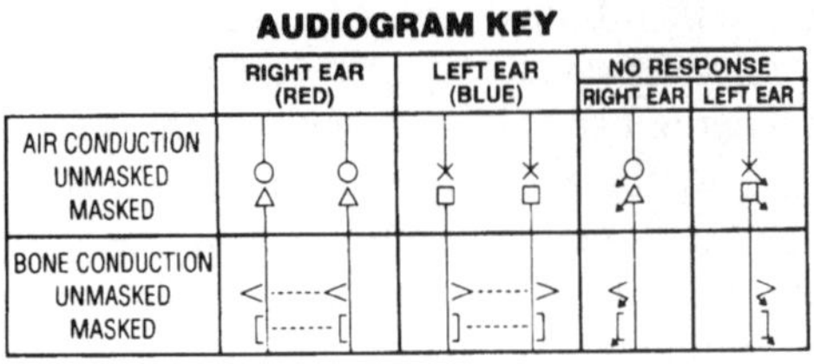

Audiogram 7. Masked right and unmasked left air & bone conduction thresholds.

fall and what type of hearing impairment is created based upon that result.

As an example, let us use 1000 Hz (see Audiogram 6) to perform steps necessary to mask for the right ear bone conduction. Using Hood's plateau method (Hood, 1960), as with the air conduction process, the clinician must determine where to start in the poorer ear and how much masking noise to use in the better ear.

1000 Hz

Right Ear/tone	Left Ear/Noise
Begin at the obtained better ear BC threshold	Begin at the obtained air conduction threshold + 10 dB
30 dB	30 + 10 (padding) = 40 dB

Present tone-No Response

With no response to the test tone in the right ear, raise the tone 5 dB and represent the test tone.

35 dB	45 dB

Present tone-No Response

Again, A "rule of thumb" suggests that if a response occurs to the TE/tone, raise the NTE/masking noise. Should no response occur, raise the TE/tone.

70 dB	50 dB

Present tone-Response

A 15 to 20 dB increase in the NTE/masking noise must occur in order to accept the TE/tone as a true threshold. At this point only a 10 dB increase presents itself.

70 dB	55 dB

Present tone-Response

ACCEPT 70 dB HL AS THE TRUE TE/tone RESPONSE. Mark the appropriate symbol on the audiogram. In this case place a red triangle at 70 dB HL on the audiogram.

Based upon masked air and bone conduction thresholds obtained in Audiogram 7, the right ear displays a severe to profound sensor-neural loss of hearing sensitivity while the left ear presents with a mild sensorineural loss.

Speech audiometry should be performed for the left ear. Rule 3 states "Mask for speech audiometry any time there is a 40 dB difference between the presentation level of the poorer ear and pure tone average or speech reception threshold of the better ear." To mask for speech audiometry one must determine the presentation

AIR & BONE CONDUCTION

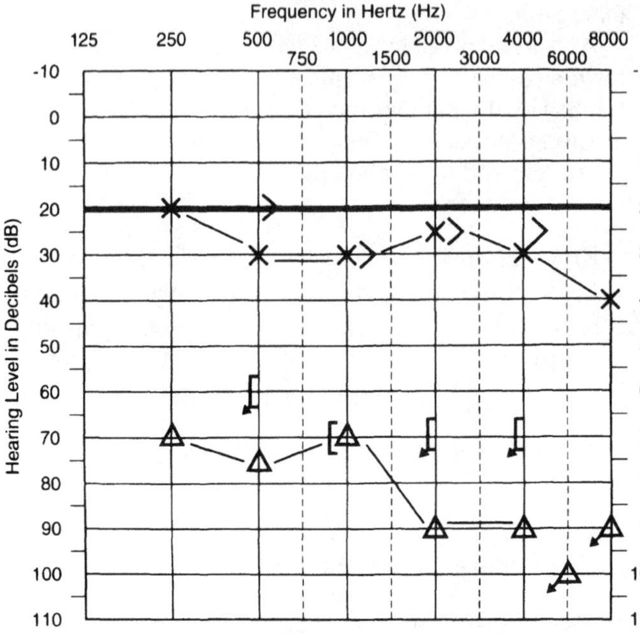

Noise: ☒ Narrow Band ❑ White **Tone:** ❑ Continuous ☒ Pulsed ❑ Warble
Masked for: ☒ Right ❑ Left

SPEECH AUDIOMETRY

	SRT	MCL	UCL	DISCRIMINATION • QUIET		DISCRIMINATION • NOISE	
RIGHT EAR (HL)	80 dB	95 dB	110 dB	68 %	Presented at: 95 dB HL	%	Presented at dB HL ___ dB S/N
MHA (SPL)				%		dB	
LEFT EAR (HL)	20 dB	55 dB	80 dB	100 %	Presented at: 55 dB HL	%	Presented at dB HL ___ dB S/N
MHA (SPL)				%		dB	
BINAURAL (HL) R / L	dB / dB	dB / dB	dB / dB	%	Presented at: R ___ dB HL L ___ dB HL	%	Presented at: R___ L___dB HL ___ dB S/N
MHA (SPL) R / L				%		dB	

Noise: ☒ Speech ❑ White **Masked for:** ☒ Right ❑ Left ☒ Live Voice ❑ Recorded Voice

AUDIOGRAM KEY

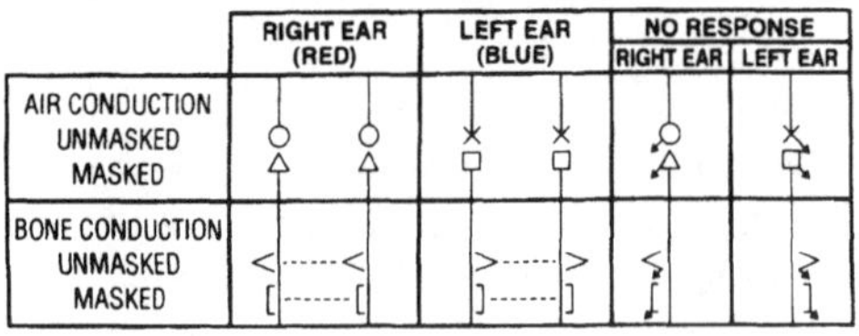

Audiogram 8. Masked results for air & bone conduction thresholds and speech audiometry.

level (PL) of the ear under test and compare this level to the PTA or SRT of the NTE. If this PL is 40 dB or greater than the PTA or SRT of the NTE. masking for speech audiometry is essential. Based on the presentation level in the TE of approximately 108 dB HL (PTA plus 30) in comparison to the NTE PTA of 28 dB HL, due to interaural attenuation differences of 40 dB or more, masking is necessary when evaluating the poorer (right) ear.

A presentation level of 108 dB HL may be beyond limits of output speech on some audiometers as well as being close to a patient's UCL. If either is the case, use as much intensity as the patient may be able to tolerate comfortably. For the sake of this example, let us assume that 100 dB HL is a level that is tolerated comfortably. With a previously discussed formula of PL minus 20 dB equaling the amount of masking noise in the contralateral ear, the presentation level of noise in the left ear will be 80 dB HL of speech noise. Again, if speech noise is not available, the next noise of choice is white noise. Never is narrow band noise used for the purpose of masking with speech audiometry. Make certain to note on the audiogram the type of masking noise used and if the presentation of speech stimuli was recorded or live voice. With the masking noise at a level of 80 dB HL in the left ear, present all speech audiometry tests to the right ear. Remember, should a client have recruitment or a discomfort for the masking noise, use the formula of PL minus 30 dB.

Audiogram 8 is a complete masked audiogram to review. Appropriate masking levels and noise type were recorded. This is a valid evaluation without suspect of error.

SUMMARY

Masking procedures have been discussed and debated for decades. The clinician must use masking techniques which are most comfortable for the scope of practice to which they are exposed. The clinician in an otology practice will find the need to mask more frequently than the clinician in a dispensing practice. However, knowledge of when to mask and how to proceed are the same for either individual. Masking is a challenging test procedure, but one that is easily mastered with time, patience and a knowledge of psychoacoustic variables and auditory behavior.

GLOSSARY

Central Masking Central nervous system phenomenon which creates a 5 dB to 10 dB decrease in threshold in the TE due to noise presented to the NTE even at levels barely audible to the TE.

Cross-Over Also known as cross hearing. A tone, if the intensity is high enough, will be audible to the opposite ear by transmission through the skull.

Interaural Attenuation (IA) Amount of energy taken to allow sound to cross from one ear to the contralateral ear via bone conduction. Air conduction IA levels occur as low as 35 dB whereas bone conduction IA occurs at 0 dB.

Masking Dilemma Commonly occurs in the presence of bilateral conductive components. To properly mask with enough intensity for masking noise to be audible in the poorer ear(s), false thresholds are created, as masking noise "covers up" the true threshold.

Effective Masking Level (Minimum and Maximum) Effective masking levels (EML) describes amount of masking to just cover up the NTE without the possibility to undermask (minimum). Amount of masking noise necessary to cover the NTE without the possibility to create a false shift in threshold.

Narrow-Band Noise Energy of narrow-band noise is centered around the test frequency and is the noise of choice in masking for air and bone conduction audiometry.

Non Test Ear (NTE) : Ear to be presented with masking noise.

Occlusion Effect (OE) Effects the low frequencies to 1000 Hz, due to the pinna covered during the masking process for bone conduction audiometry.

Overmasking Too much masking noise to the NTE which creates false thresholds.

Plateau Method Hood's method creates a level of undermasking (too little masking noise in the NTE) to disallow the NTE to participate in "answering" for the TE. Following this, a level of sufficient masking noise to "cover up" the NTE is obtained known as "plateau". Finally, a rise indicating overmasking is determined with too much masking noise affecting NTE and the TE response.

Shadow Curve Thresholds of the poorer ear assimilate the same pattern as the better ear with at least a 40 dB difference between ears. Opportunity through masking allows the clinician to determine if the better ear is actually "answering" for the poorer ear, or if obtained thresholds are actual.

Speech Noise Noise of choice for speech audiometry. It is a white noise weighted in the primary speech frequencies.

Test Ear (TE) Ear to which test stimuli (pure tones or speech stimuli) are presented. For masking purposes, it is the poorer ear.

Undermasking Occurrence of too little masking noise to sufficiently "cover up" or create the better ear from "answering" for the poorer ear.

White Noise White noise is secondary noise of choice for both pure tones and speech audiometry. It is commonplace on portable audiometers. It has a fairly flat spectrum to 6000 Hz.

REFERENCES

AMERICAN NATIONAL STANDARDS INSTITUTE. Specifications for Audiometers. ANSI S3.6–1989. New York, American National Standards Institute, 1989b.

CARHART, R. Assessment of sensorineural response in otosclerosis. Arch. Otolaryng. 71:141, 1960.

CHAIKLIN, J. Interaural attenuation and cross-hearing in air conduction audiometry. J. Aud. Res. 7:413, 1967.

COLES R. and PRIEDE, V. Masking of the non-test ear in speech audiometry. J. Laryngol. Oto. 89:217, 1975.

DIRKS, D. and MALMQUIST, C. Shifts in air conduction thresholds produced by pulsed and continuous contralateral masking. J. Acoust. Soc. Amer. 37:631, 1965.

DIRKS, D. and NORRIS, J. Shifts in auditory thresholds produced by ipsilateral and contralateral maskers at low intensity levels. J. Acous. Soc. Am., 40:11, 1966.

DIRKS, D. and SWINDEMAN, J. The variability of occluded and unoccluded bone-conduction thresholds. J. Speech Hear. Res. 10:232, 1967.

ELPERN, B. and NAUNTON, R. The stability of the occlusion effect. Arch. Otolaryng., 77:376, 1963.

FELDMAN, A. Problems in the measurement of bone conduction. J. Speech Hear. Disor. 26:39, 1961.

FLETCHER, H. Auditory Patterns. Rev. Mod. Physics, 12:47, 1940.

GOLDSTEIN, B. To mask, and how to mask: teaching masking to students. Audiol. Hear. Educ. 5–1:5, 5–2:8, 5–3:7, 1979.

GOLDSTEIN, B. and NEWMAN, C. Clinical masking: A decision-making process. pp.109 J. KATZ, ed. *Handbook of Clinical Audiology.* Ed. 4. Williams & Wilkins, Baltimore, 1994.

GOLDSTEIN, D. and HAYES, C. The occlusion effect in bone conduction hearing. J. Speech Hear. Res. 8:137, 1965.

HAWKINS, J. E. and STEVENS, S. S. Masking of pure tones and of speech by white noise, J. Acoust. Soc. Amer. 22, 6–13, 1950.

HODGSON, W. *Basic Audiologic Evaluation.* Williams & Wilkins, Baltimore, 1980.

HODGSON, WILLIAM R. Evaluating Infants and Young Children. pp465 J. KATZ, ed. *Handbook of Clinical Audiology.* Ed. 4. Williams & Wilkins, Baltimore, 1994.

HOOD, J. The principles and practice of bone conduction audiometry. Proc. Roy. Soc. Med. 50:689, 1957. Reprinted in Laryngoscope 70:1211, 1960.

KILLION, M. and VILLCHUR E. Comments on "Earphones in Audiometry" J. Acoust. Soc. Am. 85:1775, 1989.

KILLION M., WILBER, L. and GUDMUNDSEN, G. Insert earphones for more interaural attenuation. Hear. Inst. 36:34, 1985.

LARSON-DONALDSON, L. *Masking: Practical Applications of Masking Principles and Procedures,* National Institute for Hearing Instrument Studies, Livonia, Michigan, 1988.

LIDEN, G., NILSSON, G. and ANDERSON, H. Narrow-band masking with white noise. Acta Otolayng. 50:116, 1959a.

LIDEN, G., NILSSON, G. and ANDERSON, H. Masking in clinical audiometry. Acta Otolayng. 50:125, 1959b.

LUSCHER, E. and KOENIG, E. Die vertaubung des gegenohres bei der audiometrischen bestimung der knochleitung. Arch. Ohr-usw. Heilk. u. Z. Hals-usw. Heilk., Bd., 168–68, 1955.

MARTIN, F. Clinical Audiometry and Masking. pp. 1 in A. Halpern. *Studies in Communicative Disorders*. Bobbs-Merrill Co., Inc. Indianapolis, 1972.

MARTIN, F. *Introduction to Audiology* (Third Edition), Prentice-Hall, Inc.; 1975.

MARTIN, R. Audiometric Assessment and Interpretation pp 63 in R. Sandlin ed. *Hearing Instrument Science and Fitting Practices,* National Institute for Hearing Instruments Studies, Livonia, Michigan, 1985.

NAUNTON, R. Clinical bone-conduction audiometry. Arch. Otolaryng. 116:281, 1957.

NAUNTON, R. A masking dilemma in bilateral conduction deafness. Arch. Otolaryngol. 72:753, 1960.

O'NEIL, J. and OYER, H. *Applied Audiometry.* Dodd, Mead and Co., Inc., New York, 1970.

SANDERS, J. Masking. pp. 111 in J. KATZ, ed. *Handbook of Clinical Audiology,* E. 1 Williams & Wilkins, Baltimore, 1972.

SANDERS, J. and RINTELMANN, W. Masking in Audiometry. Arch. Otolaryng. 80:541, 1964.

STUDEBAKER, G. On masking in bone-conduction testing. J. Speech Hear. Res. 5:215, 1962.

STUDEBAKER, G. Clinical masking air- and bone-conduction stimuli. J. Spech Hear. Res. 29:23, 1964.

STUDEBAKER, G. Clinical masking of the non-test ear. J. Speech Hear. Disord. 32:360, 1967.

STUDEBAKER, G. Clinical masking pp. 51 in W. RINTELMANN, ed. *Hearing Assessment.* University Park Press, Baltimore, 1979.

TOWNSEND, T. and SCHWARTZ, D. Calculation of effective masking using one octave and one-third octave analysis. Audiol. Hear. Educ. 2:27, 1976.

VENIAR, F. Individual masking levels in pure-tone audiometry. Arch. Otolaryng. 82:518, 1965.

WEGEL, R. and LANE, C. The auditory masking of one pure tone by another and its probable relations to the dynamics of the inner ear. Physics Rev. 23:266, 1924.

WILBUR, L. Calibration, puretone, speech and noise signals. pp. 73 in J. KATZ, ed. *Handbook of Clinical Audiology.* Ed. 4. Williams & Wilkins, Baltimore, 1994.

ZWISLOCKI J. Acoustic attenuation between ears. J. Acoust. Soc. Am 25:752, 1953.

ZWISLOCKI, J. Central masking and neural activity in the cochlear nucleus. Audiology 10:48, 1971.

APPENDIX

WORKSHEET

____Air Conduction ____Bone Conduction

___Hz			___Hz			___Hz		
R	Response	L	R	Response	L	R	Response	L
___	___	___	___	___	___	___	___	___
___	___	___	___	___	___	___	___	___
___	___	___	___	___	___	___	___	___
___	___	___	___	___	___	___	___	___
___	___	___	___	___	___	___	___	___
___	___	___	___	___	___	___	___	___
___	___	___	___	___	___	___	___	___
___	___	___	___	___	___	___	___	___
___	___	___	___	___	___	___	___	___
___	___	___	___	___	___	___	___	___

___Hz			___Hz			___Hz		
R	Response	L	R	Response	L	R	Response	L
___	___	___	___	___	___	___	___	___
___	___	___	___	___	___	___	___	___
___	___	___	___	___	___	___	___	___
___	___	___	___	___	___	___	___	___
___	___	___	___	___	___	___	___	___
___	___	___	___	___	___	___	___	___
___	___	___	___	___	___	___	___	___
___	___	___	___	___	___	___	___	___
___	___	___	___	___	___	___	___	___
___	___	___	___	___	___	___	___	___

___Hz			___Hz			___Hz		
R	Response	L	R	Response	L	R	Response	L
___	___	___	___	___	___	___	___	___
___	___	___	___	___	___	___	___	___
___	___	___	___	___	___	___	___	___
___	___	___	___	___	___	___	___	___
___	___	___	___	___	___	___	___	___
___	___	___	___	___	___	___	___	___
___	___	___	___	___	___	___	___	___
___	___	___	___	___	___	___	___	___
___	___	___	___	___	___	___	___	___
___	___	___	___	___	___	___	___	___

IV

HEARING INSTRUMENT SYSTEMS TECHNOLOGY & PERFORMANCE STANDARDS

E. ROBERT LIBBY, BC-HIS

INTRODUCTION

The hearing aid is the single most important tool in the rehabilitation of a hearing impaired individual. A hearing instrument can be described as any instrument or device, designed to bring a signal more effectively to a listener's ear from a cupped hand behind the ear, to an ear trumpet, to an all-in-the-ear canal hearing instrument.

The modern hearing instrument is a marvel of advanced technological development. The basic principles, components and functions of a hearing instrument system will be described in this chapter.

CHAPTER OBJECTIVES

It is the intention of this chapter to review in sufficient detail hearing aid performance with respect to amplifier type and function. Attention to hearing aid type (BTE, ITE, Canal and CIC) and the advantages and limitations of each focuses on what the reader should know to adequately perform dispensing tasks. Special hearing aid systems beyond the basic hearing aid are presented and a defense for their application is offered for analysis by the hearing aid specialist.

CONTEMPORARY HEARING AIDS

The hearing aid market (1994) is dominated by the in-the-ear (ITE) and in-the-canal (ITC) hearing aids. Together they represent about 80% of total hearing aid sales. Body and eyeglass types represent less than 1%. Behind-the-ear (BTE) represent less than 20% of the marketplace.

In the past decade, hearing aid technology has experienced a more rapid revolution than in any other similar time. Developments in component parts, integrated circuit amplifiers, and broad band receivers along with better coupling techniques and improved chassis design have resulted in hearing aids that are more versatile, smaller, and of higher quality than earlier models. Developments in low voltage integrated circuit technology have made it possible for hearing aid designers to incorporate new performance features in analog hearing aids (Preves, 1993).

ANALOG V. DIGITAL

Most currently produced hearing aids use analog circuitry. The challenge of incorporating "true" digital technology in ITE and ITC devices is difficult because of the size and battery limitations. Instead, many hearing aid manufacturers have introduced digitally programmable hearing aids, which perform analog signal processing under digital control. The digital memory and control are normally used in place of a screwdriver-actuated mechanical trimmers to store and modify the programmed digital parameters. Benefits of digital programmability include reduced returns for adjustments, and the ability to access different hearing aid characteristics for different environments. If the analog portions of the circuitry are not substantially different for an all analog hearing aid, the hearing impaired person may not enjoy better hearing, solely as a result of adding digitally programmable capability. Programmable hearing aids cost substantially more than analog hearing aids. The cost-benefit ratio of a programmable hearing aid system must be carefully evaluated for each hearing impaired individual.

Dramatic improvements in hearing aid sound quality continue to be made with important advancements in analog circuitry such as amplifiers with compression. (K-AMP and Manhattan circuitry), adaptive frequency response shaping, Class D amplifiers, wideband transducers, multi-channel hearing instruments, and active

Lesson 19
238-239


```
Recommended basic classification of signal processing
    schemes based on electronic technology.
                 /----------------------\
                 |   Signal Processing  |
                 |         (SP)         |
                 \----------------------/
                            |
      /---------------------|---------------------\
      |                     |                     |
      |                     |                     |
/------------------\ /------------------\ /-----------------\
|  Analog Signal   | | Digital Signal   | | Hybrid Signal   |
|   Processing     | |  Processing      | |  Processing     |
|     (ASP)        | |    (DSP)         | |    (HSP)        |
\------------------/ \------------------/ \-----------------/
```

Fig. 1.

filtering. Digital signal processing offers the promise of superior hearing aids as compared to those with analog electronics. Proven digital algorithms however, that are much more effective than those used in analog hearing aids do not yet exist in miniaturized form to reduce environmental noise without introducing undesirable audible artifacts. In the meantime, the capability of integrated circuitry is just beginning to be used in analog and hybrid analog-digital hearing aids (Preves, 1993). For more detailed information on programmable hearing aids, refer to the chapter by Valente.

Modern signal processing hearing aids can be subdivided into three groups:

1) Analog hearing aids in which conventional analog circuits (filters, amplifiers, limiters) are used to process the audio signal.
2) Digital hearing aids in which the audio signal is processed by digital means.
3) Hybrid Analog-Digital which combines analog and digital techniques. A common form of the hybrid analog-digital hearing aid is that in which analog circuits process the audio signal while the analog circuits are controlled by digital means (Levitt, 1991).

CONTEMPORARY HEARING AID TYPES

Current hearing aids types can be classified as either ear level or body styles, according to their placement on the person.

The behind the ear type (BTE). Also called post auricular and over the ear. Fits behind the ear, with a sound tip attached to a plastic tubing, which transmits the sound through a coupler (earmold) into the ear canal.

The in the ear type (ITE). Is designed so that all the components fit into the concha of the ear. This type can be custom molded into an individual earmold or be of the modular variety.

All in the ear canal type. A relatively new type that fits completely into the ear canal within a custom designed earmold.

Body type. Also called conventional, pocket and on the body type. Typically worn in a harness or garment bag or clipped to the clothing. The receiver is either air or bone conduction which is connected by a cord to the amplifier. Most often recommended for severe or profound hearing losses. Also for geriatrics with limited motor capabilities.

Eyeglass type. All components fit into the temples of eyeglasses. The signal is transmitted through tubing into the ear canal. Well suited for CROS and BICROS hearing aid fittings.

Completely in the canal (CIC) type. A recent development is the completely in-the-canal hearing instrument. It is the smallest and most cosmetically acceptable hearing aid ever created. CIC hearing instruments will be discussed in greater detail later in this chapter.

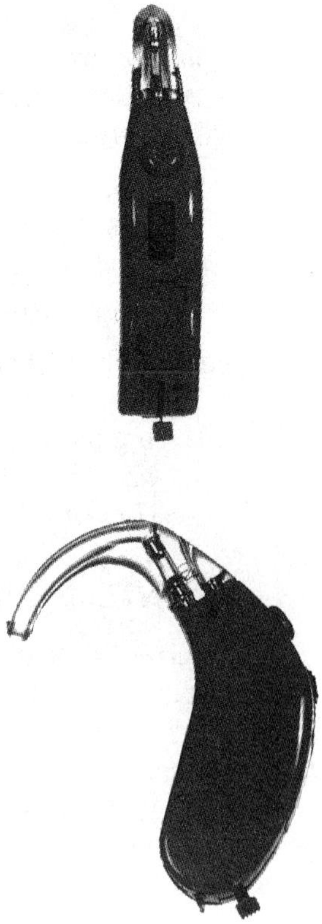

Fig. 2A. Behind the ear hearing aid. BOSCH 33 PPD

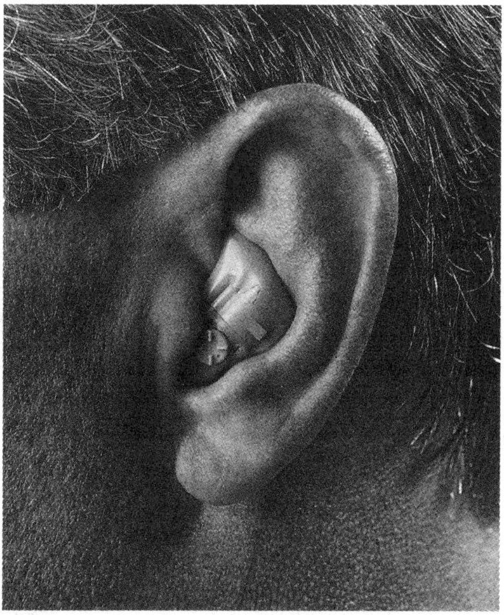

Fig. 2B. In the ear hearing aid. STARKEY CE-9

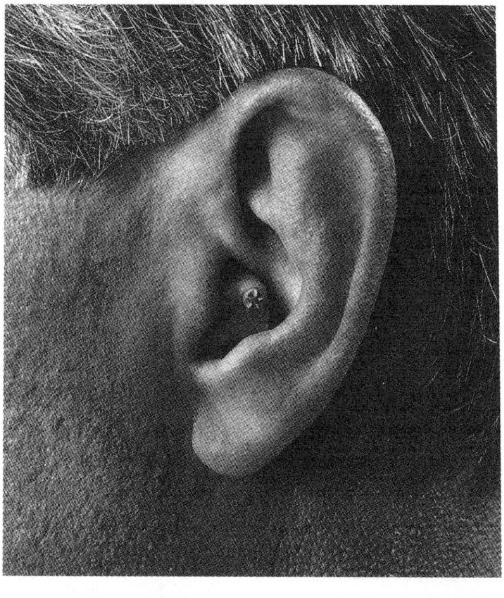

Fig. 3A. All-in-the-ear canal hearing aid—Starkey Canal Hearing aid. STARKEY INTRA V

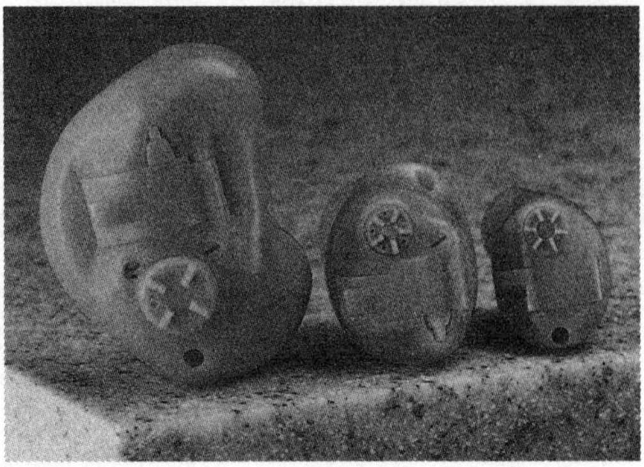

Fig. 3B. Comparison of In-the-ear, Half shell, and Canal hearing aids. (STARKEY)

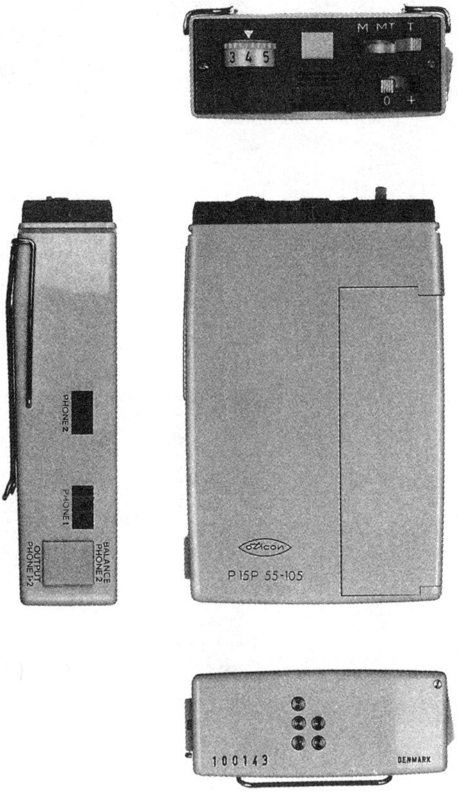

Fig. 4. Body Type Hearing Aid. Oticon body hearing aid.

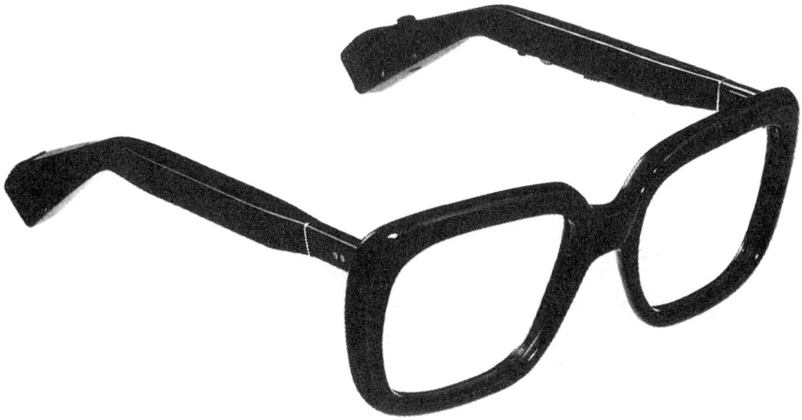

Fig. 5A. Eyeglass Hearing Aid (air conduction). Oticon eyeglass hearing aid.

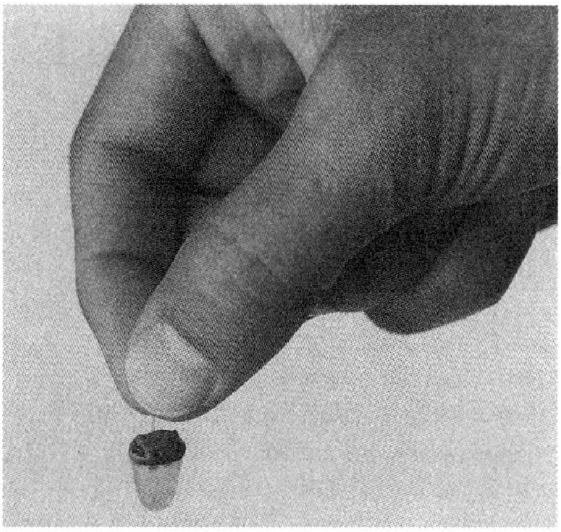

Fig. 5B. Completely in the canal (CIC) type (STARKEY)

THE ANATOMY OF HEARING AID SYSTEMS: THE BUILDING BLOCKS

Motor vehicles may look different, however they are all constructed from the same building blocks—motor, steering system, brakes etc. Hearing aid systems are certainly no different because they are also built from elementary units.

Typical hearing aid system building blocks consist of:

1. a microphone
2. an amplifier
3. a volume control
4. an earphone (receiver)
5. a power source
6. a coupling to the ear (earmold)

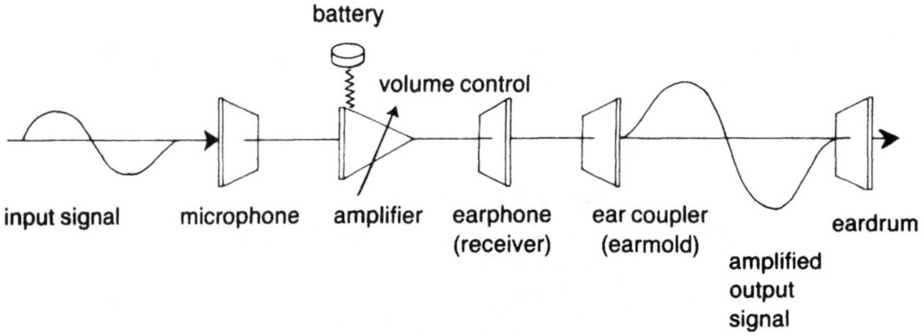

Fig. 6. Basic building blocks of a hearing aid.

Adequate function of each component is critical to the overall performance of the amplification system. The microphone responds to acoustic stimuli and produces the tiny amounts of electricity which contain the speech of music information. The signal is then processed and sent to the amplifier where the information is amplified (strengthened). The gain of the amplifier is monitored by a volume control which can vary according to user needs. The strengthened signals are then routed to the earphone (receiver) where they are converted into acoustic energy (sound). The acoustic energy is further modified by the coupling system and transmitted to the eardrum. It should be emphasized that all hearing aids, no matter how simple or complicated they may appear, contain these basic building blocks.

LAW OF CONSERVATION OF ENERGY

To better understand how these basic building blocks interact with one another we should first turn to a basic and universal physical law. Many different forms of energy exist which are familiar to most of us: nuclear energy, electrical energy, chemical energy (such as that stored in a battery), and acoustic energy (sound waves). The basic law which governs all these energy forms is called the *law of conservation of energy.*

Law of conservation of energy. Energy can neither be created nor destroyed. It can, however, be converted from one form to another. Let us now examine how this law applies to hearing aid systems as acoustic energy is continuously being converted from one form to another.

The acoustic energy from the sound source is converted to mechanical energy which, in turn, is converted to electrical energy by the microphone. The electrical energy is strengthened (amplified) by the amplifier and converted back to acoustic energy by the earphone. The acoustic energy is modified by the coupling system (earmold) and transmitted to the eardrum.

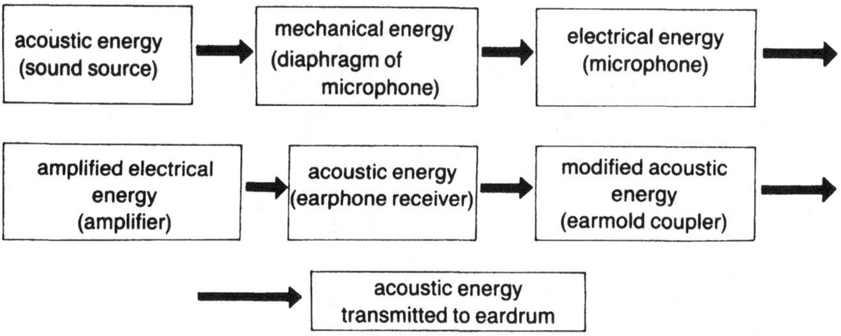

Fig. 7.

PHYSICAL CHARACTERISTICS OF HEARING AIDS

MICROPHONES

Microphones and earphones (receivers) are known as *transducers,* which are devices designed to change electrical energy into acoustical energy and vice versa. Microphones are classified as *input transducers* and earphones (receivers) as *output transducers*.

A microphone is probably best defined as an acoustic mechanoelectric transducer in that it converts acoustic energy to mechanical energy, which in turn is converted to electrical energy. The acoustic-to-mechanical conversion is accomplished by a diaphragm responding to the compressions and rarefactions of the sound waves with corresponding to and from motions (Olsen, 1981). This action of the diaphragm, in turn, activates a dome type of mechanism capable of converting these mechanical vibratory motions into a corresponding flow of electrical energy.

MICROPHONE TYPES

The types of microphones in recent use are:

1. Magnetic
2. Ceramic
3. Electret
4. Directional (Cardioid)

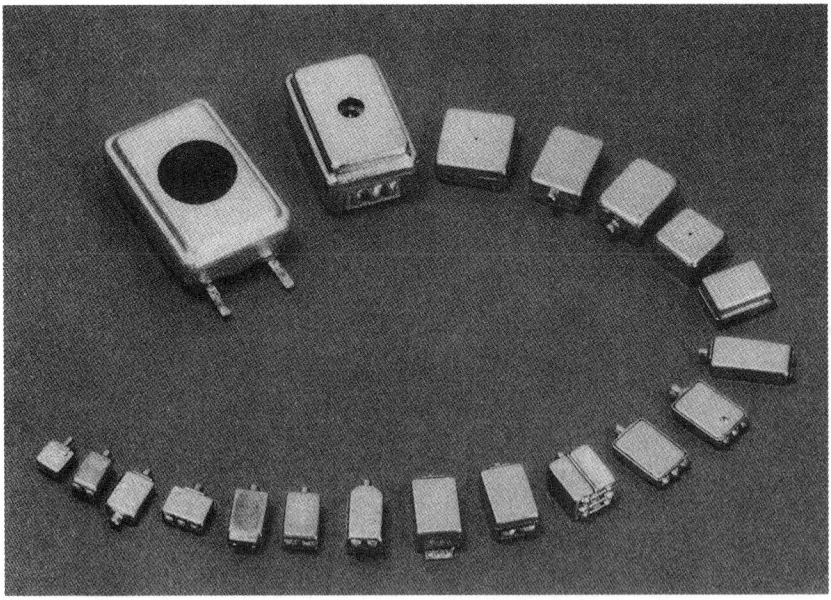

Fig. 8. Knowles transducers—(microphones and earphones).

Magnetic, ceramic and electret microphones are classified by physical design, and directional (cardioid) microphones by polar patterns.

Crystal microphones were used with vacuum tube applications. With the advent of transistor instruments, a microphone of lower impedance was needed. The magnetic microphone became the instrument of choice with transistor hearing aids. The magnetic microphone has a reasonably ideal frequency response over the speech range. Unfortunately very high and very low frequencies needed to be sacrificed when the magnetic microphone was miniaturized (Berger, 1980).

In time, an improved version of the old crystal microphone was developed—the ceramic microphone. Its high impedance problem was solved by employing a field effect transistor (FET). The ceramic microphone permitted extended low frequency amplification of hearing aids, and was virtually free of temperature and humidity problems.

In recent years, a new type of hearing aid microphone has been developed—one based on condenser microphone technology (Staab, 1978). This is the electret condenser microphone more popularly known as the electret microphone.

The electret microphone has an extremely broad and quite flat frequency response and like the ceramic microphone is rugged and sensitive. It is also virtually free of mechanical feedback problems and clothing noise (Berger, 1980). The electret microphones have applications not only in hearing aids, but in virtually all other audio amplification, recording, and communication applications as well.

A wide variety of microphone frequency responses are available today. Figure 10 illustrates some of the responses. When the effect of the various coupling tubes commonly used with these microphones is included, a much wider variety of responses can be obtained (Killion, 1980).

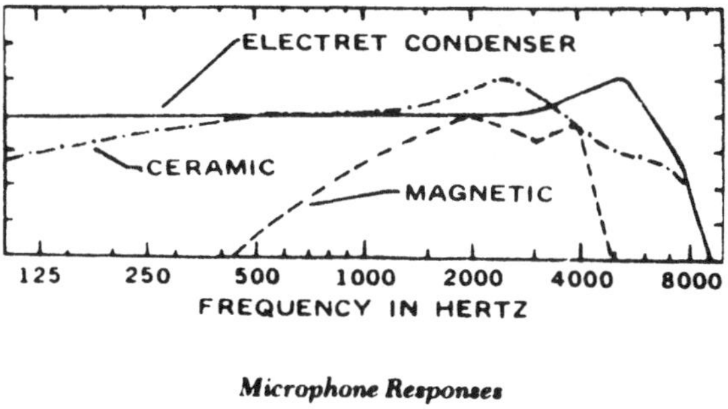

Fig. 9. With permission K. W. Berger, 1984.

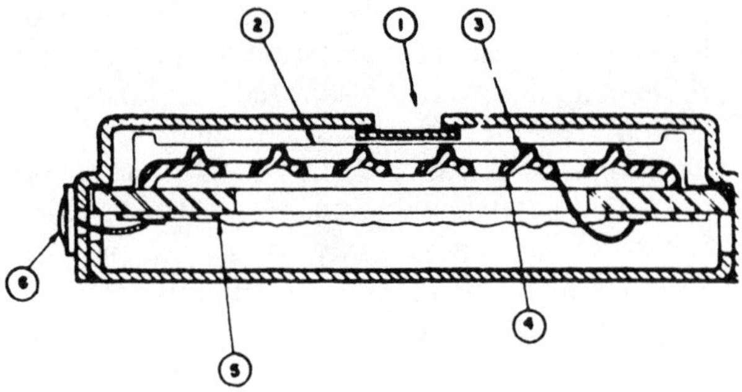

Electret Condenser Microphone

Fig. 10. Cutaway diagram of an electric microphone. Sound enters the microphone. Sound enters the microphone case (1) to act upon the thin film diaphragm (2) the diaphragm presents a conductive surface toward the electret (3) which is mounted on the conducting back plate electrode (4). Both the diaphragm and the back plate are connected to the FET preamplifier (5) that is constructed on the under side of the diaphragm and back plate ceramic substrate. The preamplifier is connected to exterior terminals (6) which lead the signal out of the preamplifier to the amplifier.

Another development in microphones for hearing aids is the *directional microphone*. The directional microphone is more responsive to sound originating from the front of the microphone than from behind it. Such devices have been used for public address systems, etc. for many years. The directional microphone has two acoustic inlets or microphone openings, one on each side of the diaphragm. This results in greater sensitivity to sounds coming from the front (or direction toward which the head is turned). Sounds from the rear are attenuated by various amounts. The motion of the diaphragm is dependent on the pressure difference on the two sides of the diaphragm.

Directional electret microphones are so constructed that the rear facing sound inlet is extended with tubing so that the separation of the front and back sound inlet is approximately ½ inch. An acoustic time delay element is placed at the back sound inlet. The intent is to create a delay in the sound entering the back opening, causing the two sides of the diaphragm to essentially cancel one another. The directional effect covers a range of about 200–2000 Hz, and the microphone is about 15–20 dB more sensitive to

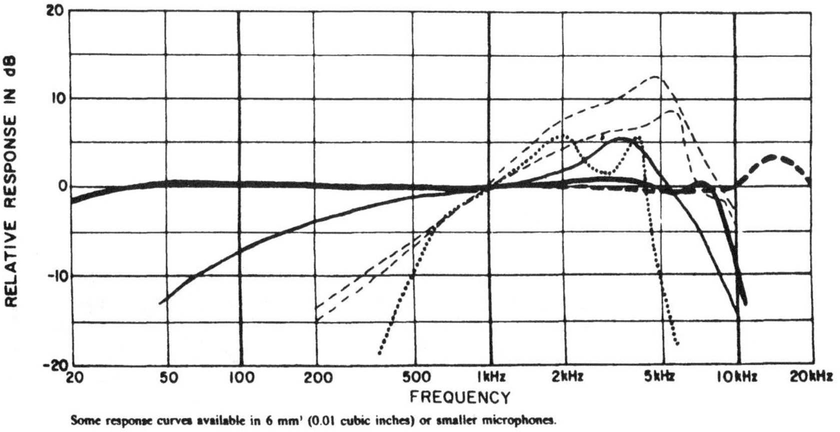

Fig. 11. Some response curves available in 6mm³ (0.01 cubic inches) or smaller microphones. (With permission M. C. Killion, Acoustic Factors Affecting Hearing Aid Performance Studebaker and Hochberg ED. University Park Press 1980).

sounds originating from its front than to sound originating from the back (Olsen, 1981).

Directional microphones and real ear response is discussed in a later section of this chapter.

EARPHONES (RECEIVERS)

Hearing aid earphones are frequently labeled as receivers in the literature. However, with the advent of radio frequency, auditory training units, in which the unit worn by the student is commonly called a "receiver", it is preferable to refer to the electromechanical acoustic transducers of hearing aids as earphones in order to avoid some confusion in terminology (Olsen, 1981).

Earphones are microphones in reverse. Just as *microphones* were labeled *input transducers,* the earphone can be defined as an electromechanical acoustic *output transducer.* The output transducer converts the amplified electric signal of the hearing aid to an acoustical or vibratory output. The earphone is of two types, either *air conduction* or *bone conduction (bone vibrators).*

The most common type is the air conduction earphone which converts the electrical impulses from the amplifier back into acoustical energy. Air conduction earphones are classified as either internal or external. Ear level instruments use the internal type earphone and body-type instruments, in general, use the external type

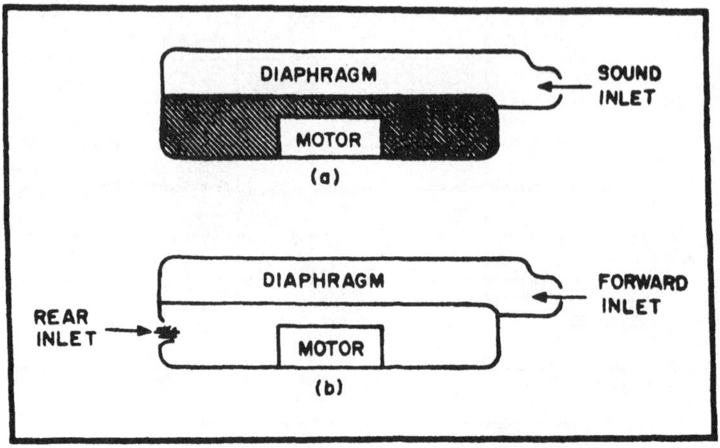

Fig. 12. Comparison of a conventional microphone (a) with a directional microphone (b). The latter shows a delay element (damping material) in the rear inlet opening. (With permission W. J. Staab, the Hearing Aid Handbook, Tab Books 1978.)

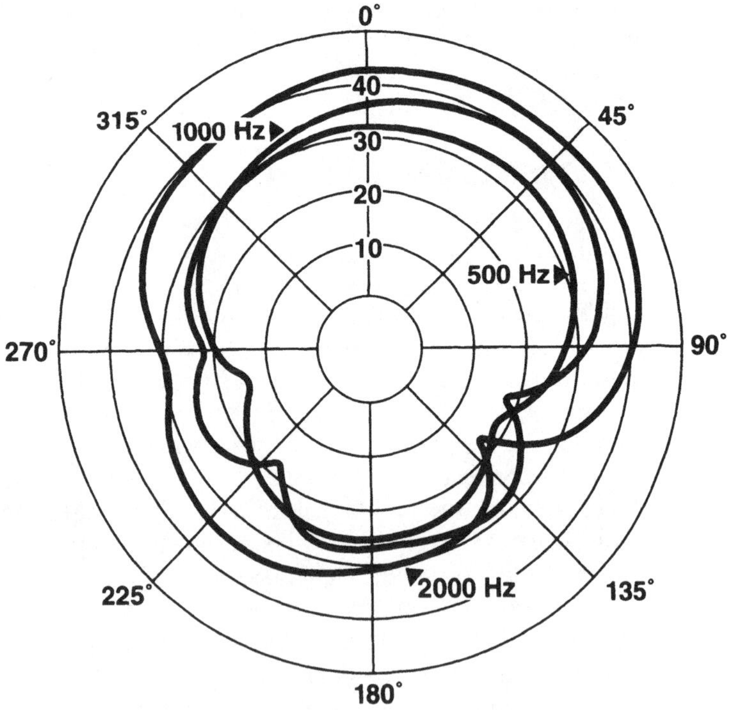

Fig. 13A. Polar response of directional hearing aid obtained on KEMAR (Zwislocki occluded ear simulator) right ear, anechoic chamber, (Maico Series G 117).

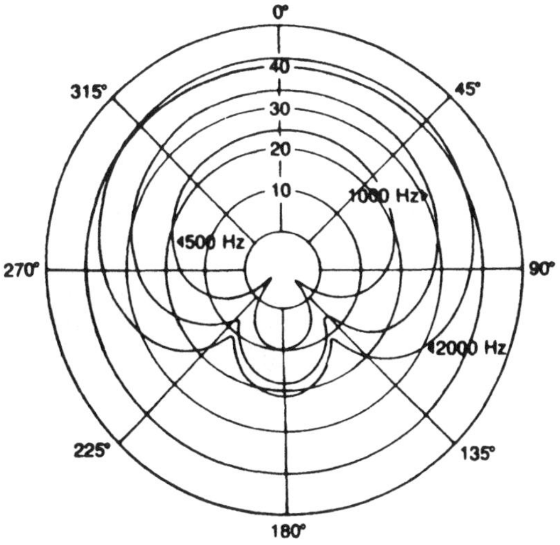

Fig. 13B. Polar response pattern of directional hearing aid measured in a 2 cc coupler, anechoic chamber. (Maico Series G117).

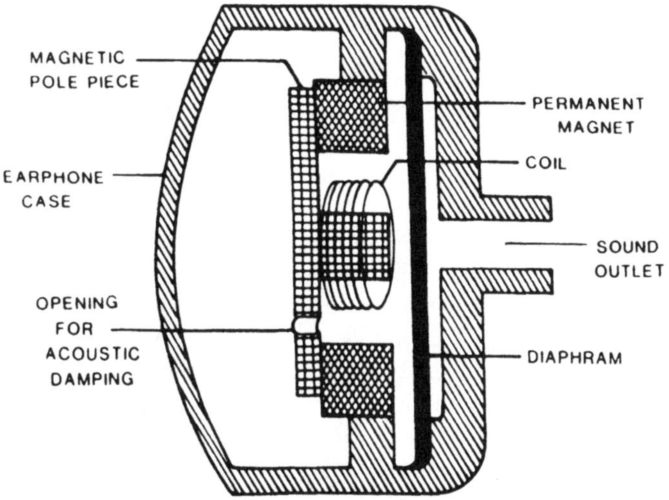

Fig. 14. Cross-section of external type hearing aid earphone. (With permission W. O. Olsen, Hearing Aid Assessment and Use in Audiologic Habilitation, Hodgson and Skinner Ed., Williams and Wilkins, 1981).

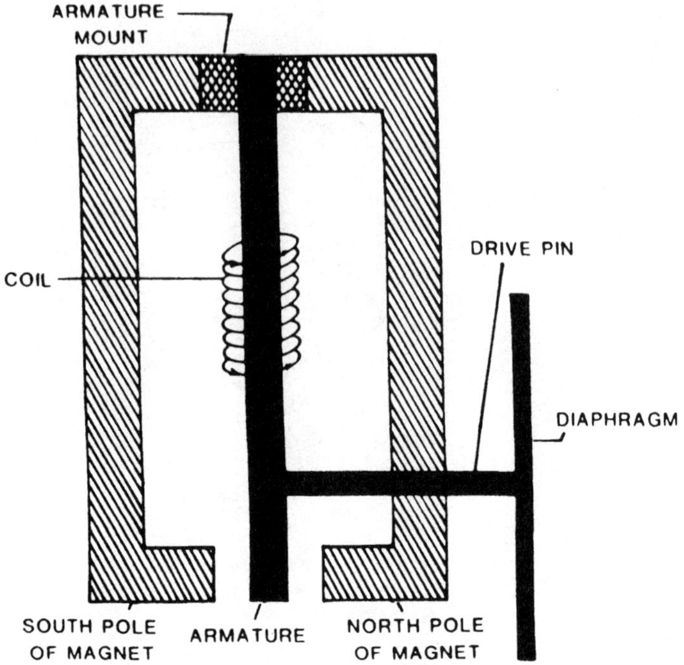

Fig. 15. Cross-section of internal-type hearing aid earphone (earphone housing and connections to coil not shown). (With permission W. O. Olsen, Hearing Aid Assessment and Use in Audiologic Habilitation, Hodgson and Skinner Ed. Williams and Wilkins, 1981).

earphone. Earphones have a resonant frequency, a frequency at which they are most efficient, determined primarily by a combination of the mass and elasticity of their mechanical system. Acoustic damping is used in the earphone assembly to smooth and extend its response.

Both transducer (microphone and earphone) and amplifier technology have reached the point when the hearing aid designer can produce, electro-acoustically, almost anything one might ask for in a hearing aid, including high fidelity (Killion, 1980). Wide band earphones are now a reality. A crucial factor in earphone and hearing aid response is the coupling system. A so-called broad bank hearing aid can be reduced significantly by an incorrect coupling system. Figure 16 illustrates a wide variety of response curves that can be obtained with a single earphone by changing the coupling system (earmold construction).

Bone vibrators are used in those instances when the hearing impaired person cannot benefit from air conducted sounds, such as with atresia of the ear canal. Bone vibrators are not only used in body type instruments, but also in specially constructed eyeglass arrangements, where cosmetic appeal plays a significant role. The bone conduction unit held tightly against the skull sets the bones of the skull into vibration and stimulates the inner ear. The shape of the case conforms to the mastoid bone posterior to the auricle. The bone conduction vibrator frequency response is poor at the high frequencies, and it does not have sufficient output to fit more severe of profound hearing impairments. A significant amount of acoustic energy is lost traveling through the skin and fat surrounding the temporal bone.

POWER SOURCE - BATTERIES

Hearing aid batteries require not only extreme miniaturization, but also complete reliability, with as long a life as possible. Longer life necessitates the development of new types, as well as new designs, for merely to reduce the size of the normally used battery cells by clever design techniques would not give the length of life requires (Berger, 1974).

WHAT IS A BATTERY?

A battery is a common type of "electrical pump", and its strength is rated in volts. The battery achieves its pumping action by separating and holding the positive and negative changes onto two separate terminals. When an external wire is connected between the two terminals, the electrical force of attraction draws the electrons

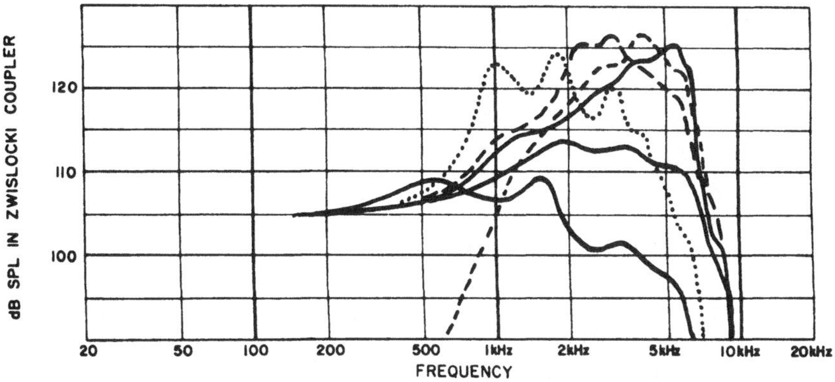

Fig. 16. Wide variety of response curves obtained (with a single earphone) by changing the earmold construction. (With permission M. C. Killion, Acoustic Factors affecting Hearing Aid Performance, Studebaker and Hochberg Ed., University Park Press 1980.)

to the positive terminal, thus creating a current in the wire. The interior of the battery is filled with a chemical substance known as an electrolyte. The electrolyte is crucial because it removes electrons from one terminal, leaving it with a net positive charge, and deposits them on the other. The process of charge separation results in an energy transfer between the electrolyte and electrons. The continuous flow of current implies that the electrolyte must continually expand its reserve chemical energy by separating the electrical charge. However, the law of conservation of energy (energy cannot be created or destroyed) requires that the electrons gain this energy in the form of electrical energy. When the electrons leave the negative terminal, they may, in turn, expend this energy into heat or some other form of energy such as that carried by sound waves.

Technically, a battery consists of two or more cells. The word battery and cell are often used interchangeably in reference to hearing aids.

Carbon and vacuum tube hearing aids employed *zinc oxide* batteries. The zinc cell had a sloping characteristic and therefore needed to be reasonably large to be practical. This means, that with continued use, the battery produced a smaller and smaller voltage. It was necessary to turn up the volume of the hearing aid as voltage was reduced. For ideal use, these batteries needed time for rest and recuperation, and hot weather reduced their life (Berger, 1980).

Dr. Samuel Ruben developed the *mercury cell* during World War II to fill the need of a battery with a high capacity and one which could be stored and used over a wide range of temperatures. The mercury cell admirably filled this need and is still in wide use today. The discharge characteristic is such that the voltage drops significantly only at the end of the cell's useful life.

In addition to *mercury,* there are five main systems for miniature batteries for microelectronics applications—*silver oxide, alkaline-manganese, nickel cadmium, lithium, and zinc-air.*

Silver-oxide—operating at 1.55 V and being relatively stable throughout the discharge cycle, silver oxide cells were the automatic choice for many miniaturized applications including hearing aids. The escalating silver price, however, relegated it to applications where higher operating voltages were essential-older, high gain hearing aids and some watches. Though silver prices have fallen, some manufacturers phased out the production of this type of battery because of the uncertainty of raw materials; in turn this led to hearing aid manufacturers discontinuing models needing silver oxide batteries.

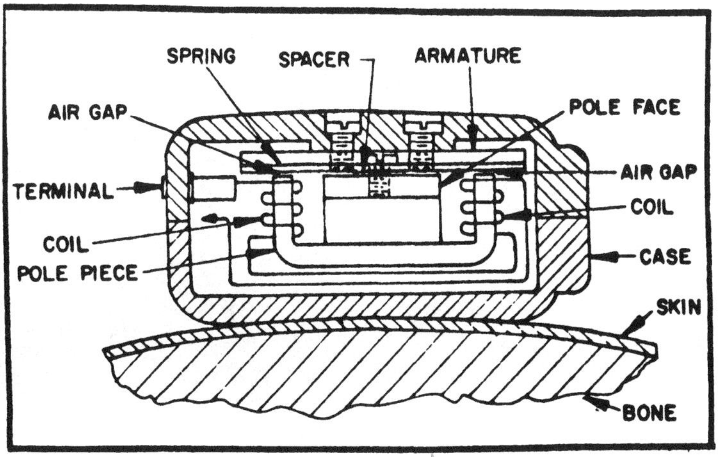

Fig. 17. Schematic of a bone-conduction vibrator. (courtesy Radioear Corp. With permission W. J. Staab, and Tab Books, 1978.)

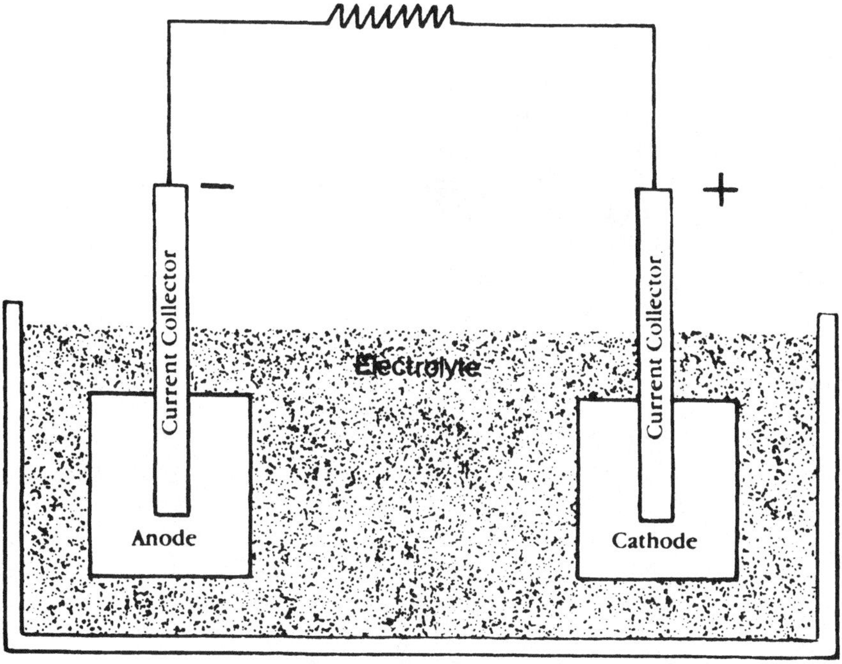

Fig. 18. The Basic Cell. (Duracell International Inc., 1981).

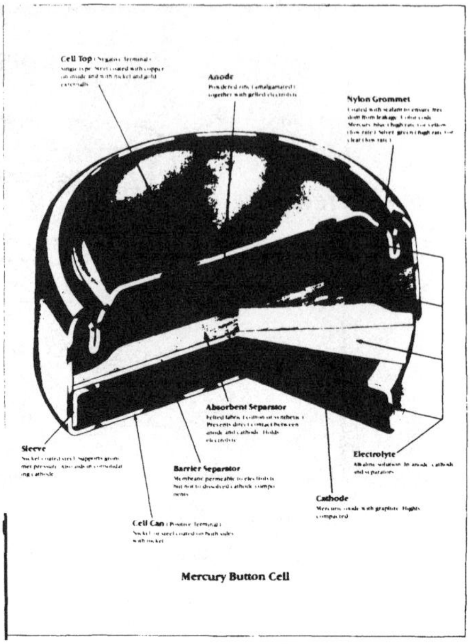

Fig. 19. Mercury Button Cell. (Duracell International Inc., 1981).

Mercuric oxide—was the primary battery system until recently. In 1984 the battery types sold were as follows—mercuric oxide 44.96%, zinc air 52.56%, and silver oxide 2.48%. Oper ating at 1.35 V it is the lowest of any primary miniature battery system. This type falls between manganese and zinc air in energy density. It is losing some of its popularity because of the mercury pollution problem. Mercury cells contain over 30% mercury.

Alkaline Manganese—batteries use the familiar chemistry of the 1.5 V alkaline cell and have recently advanced because of the significant price advantage over silver oxide. However, low energy density, declining voltage output, and poor storage life direct them only to non-critical applications of in areas where low cost is essential.

Nickel cadmium—the familiar "NICAD" technology gives the only rechargeable system available in button configuration. Like mercury cells, however, they suffer from the potential cadmium disposal hazard; but cost less per hour to use than other cells because they can be recharged by the use of a recharger. Recharging usually takes about fourteen hours, and there is risk of damage if they are overcharged. The cell may be recharged five hundred times or more. Typically, the nickel cadmium can be used about twenty hours before recharging is necessary.

Lithium—there is considerable interest at this writing in *lithium* because it is a material which is highly reactive and has inherent energy. Lithium batteries would allow for twice the present energy in the same size package; the cost, however, at the present time, makes the lithium battery considerably more expensive. Their high operating voltage of 3 V is proffered as an advantage, but the cells generally are larger, and even in standard sizes, cannot directly replace the more popular battery systems due to the voltage difference.

Zinc-air—batteries are on outgrowth of research done on fuel cells for the NASA space program. The air cells were rapidly accepted and have become the most popular cell in use in today's micro miniature hearing aids. Zinc-air technology utilizes the oxygen in the air around for one half of its energy. This means that a zinc-air cell can be filled with almost twice as much zinc as mercury zinc or silver zinc cells. Zinc-air cells feature longer life performance (about twice as much as mercury) and more constant voltage needing fewer volume adjustments. No warm up time is necessary. Shelf life is excellent with less than 2% loss per year. Normal office and room conditions are adequate for storage. Air cells are safer than mercury cells containing only a few percent of mercury versus 30% for mercury oxide. The operating voltage varies between 1.45 and 1.35. The battery starts operating when the tab is removed on the top of the cell.

CELL CAPACITY

The amount of electricity which a cell (battery) will hold is known as the *capacity of the battery*. The amount of electricity flowing from a power cell through the circuit at any moment is called the *current*. It is measured in *milliamperes*. (1 milliampere = 1/1000 of an ampere). When a current of 1 milliampere flows through the circuit for one hour, the total amount of electricity that has passed is 1 milliampere hour. Thus, the capacity of any particular power cell can be expressed as the number of milliampere hours of electricity it can produce. Knowing the battery current required of a hearing aid and knowing the capacity of a cell permits one to calculate the hours of service expected of that cell: battery life = battery capacity divided by battery current. If a hearing aid takes a current, for example of 2mA, a battery rated as 250 mmAH should last for about 125 hours.

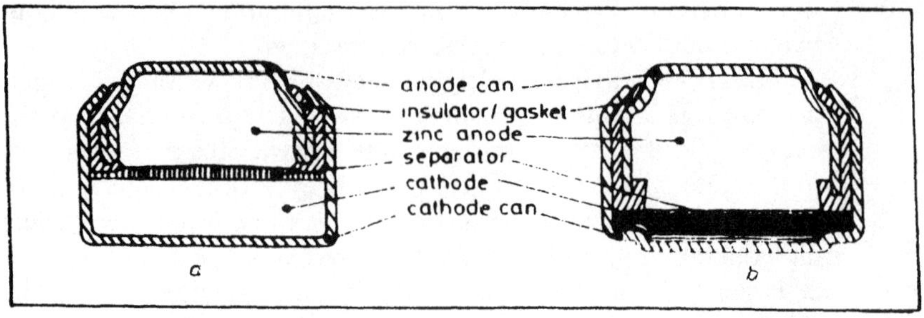

Fig. 20. Cross-section of a zinc-air cell: (a) Conventional (b) Activair, (Gould Electronics).

Battery life = Battery capacity (milliampere hours)

Battery current drain (milliamperes)

The results of this formula is an approximate figure depending on certain variables such as the age of the battery and variations in different units of the same hearing aid model.

As the battery ages over a period of months, the capacity will diminish. The user may notice a reduced battery life and fault the aid. (Zinc-air batteries are an exception and may not lose more than 2% of shelf life a year).

AMPLIFIERS

Another basic building block of a hearing aid is the amplifier. *Amplifiers* play such an important role in sound reproduction that they are found extensively in almost all phases of audio equipment. As it has been mentioned, the main purpose of an amplifier is to amplify. Not only must an amplifier produce an enlarged copy of its input signal, but it must produce a completely accurate and undistorted copy while compensating for the individual hearing loss. The amplifier receives the electrical signal from the microphone and enlarges it and transmits to the output transducer (earphone).

The amplifier consists of transistor, capacitors, resistors, and switches, and comprises the most complex portion of the hearing aid. The amplifier may have a number of stages of amplification and maintains an electric signal at both its input and output stages. Modern hearing aids achieve amplification primarily through the use of the transistor. The transistor is a *semi-conductor* device which has replaced the vacuum tube because of its smaller size and

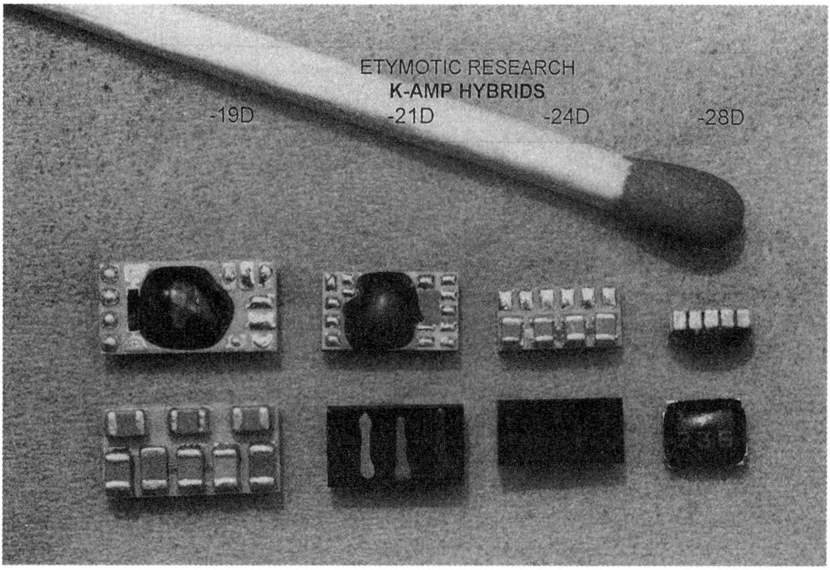

Fig. 21. K-Amp Hybrid Integrated Circuits (Etymotic Research).

weight, low power requirements, good reliability, and longer life expectancy (Staab, 1978).

A transistor is an electronic valve. It is a *solid state device in which the input current controls the amount of current in the output circuit. A transistor is designed such that small changes in the input current lead to large changes in the output current.*

The semi-conductor is so called because it lies between metals and insulators in the ability to conduct electricity. Semiconductor technology is commonly referred to as *solid state*. Refinements in transistor production and solid state electronic circuitry have led to the development of *integrated circuits (IC),* variously referred to as chips, micro modules, microcircuits, or microlithic circuits. Thin films of the desired materials are deposited on a substrate; tiny canals and holes are etched into the film deposit, and other materials in minute quantity are added, all under precise automated control. Provision for making appropriate connections to other components which cannot be built into the integrated circuit are included in the production process. Provisions are made for capacitors, which are too large physically to be incorporated into the integrated circuit, and for the microphone, battery, controls, and earphone (Olsen, 1981). For the production of hearing aids, integrated circuits have the advantages of small power requirements, low electronic noise characteristics, small size, and the need of few connections which might break. Integrated circuits generally include transistors and resistors. The functioning of the transistors is based on some special facets of electrical conduction in semi-conductor materials, particularly germanium and silicon. Silicon has replaced germanium as a semi-conductor because it is less temperature sensitive, requires lower operating currents resulting in increased amplification and lower inherent noise (Staab, 1978). Integrated circuits are also hermetically sealed against outside influences, allowing for uniform manufacturing conditions using mass production techniques.

Nothing has made a greater impact on the electronics industry than the integrated circuit. It is less than two decades old and yet the integrated circuit has found its way into everything from spacecraft to children's toys. It is virtually impossible to find a piece of recent electronic equipment that does not contain at least one integrated circuit (Cole, 1979). The integrated circuit combines dozens, or thousands of transistors along with other components in a single block of silicon interconnected to perform various operations on electrical signals. They must perform the functions required of hearing aid amplifiers while providing long battery life from a single battery housed in a miniature package.

Because of the relatively small volume of the hearing aid industry (approximately one million, one hundred two units in 1984), specialized integrated circuits entail high development and tooling costs, and as a consequence, the integrated circuit is just now starting to exert its influence on the hearing aid industry. High power behind-the-ear hearing aids and mild to moderate power in-the-ear hearing aids are creating a new demand for integrated circuits. The full potential of integrated circuitry in hearing aids has yet to be realized. The integrated circuits used in calculators and watches contain a thousand times more components than those used in hearing aids. Cole noted (1979) that before the hearing aid can reach the level of technological development, great strides must be taken in the understanding of hearing loss. Further, if these future instruments are to be effectively utilized, those involved in distribution and fitting must become more conversant with the fields of acoustics, electronics, and computer science. For these reasons, future hearing aid designs will be constrained by the market place rather than by technological limitations.

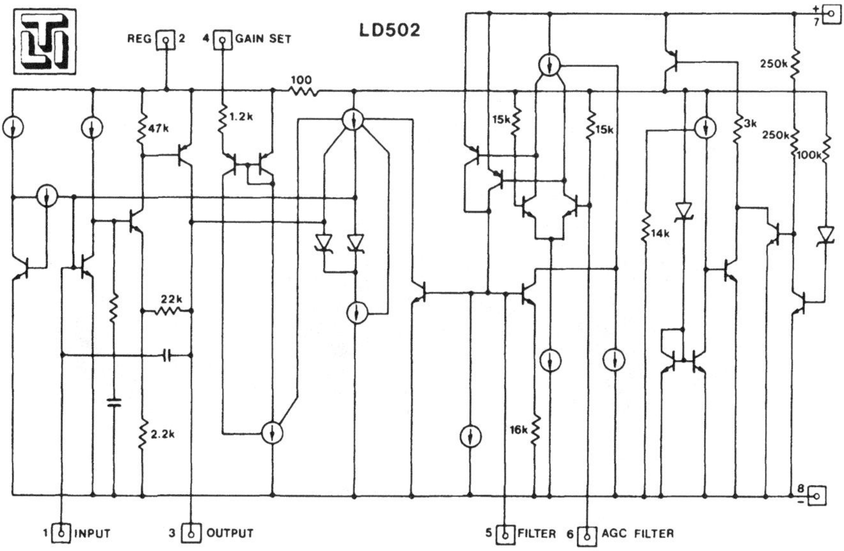

Fig. 22. Circuit schematic of Class A compression amplifier. (Linear Technology, Inc.)

CONTROLS

Most hearing aids employ electronic controls to change the hearing aid frequency response characteristic from that inherently developed by the combined response of the microphone and earphone. The frequency response can also be manipulated significantly by the use of dampers, horns, cavities, etc.

Volume controls and tone controls are the most often used electronic controls in hearing aid technology. They are generally made up of combinations of resistors and capacitors which are switched into or out of the circuitry as desired, or a variable resistor may be used in combination with other resistors and capacitor combinations. Capacitors are often used because of their ability to allow the high frequencies to pass through them more easily than the low frequencies. *The effect is that low frequencies are somewhat attenuated by the action of the capacitor; this "high frequency emphasis" is, in actuality low frequency suppression (Olsen, 1981).*

On some contemporary hearing aids, there are variable controls to choose output limiting options such as peak clipping, output compression and input compression. In fact, at this writing, there is a hearing aid available with six variable controls where the fitter can vary gain, low frequency response, high frequency

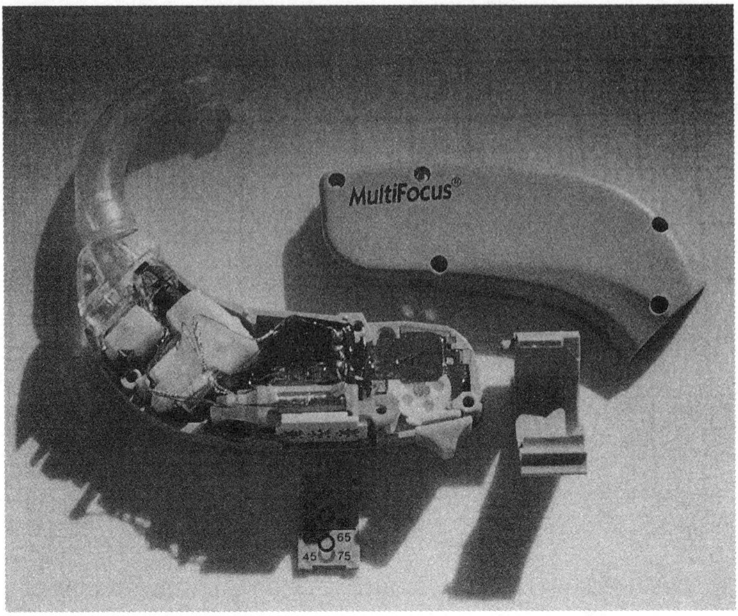

Fig. 23. Components of an Oticon BTE hearing aid.

response, peak clipping option, and output compression or input compression options.

Some controls are designed to be user-adjustable and others fitter adjustable. Fitter adjustable controls are also known as *trimpots, trimmers, or potentiometers.* Some have a continuously adjustable tone control set by a screw driver, others have a fixed response, others are controlled by a receiver; others may have a two position switch (or so). and some are mechanical in nature and are merely restrictions in the microphone or receiver openings (Staab, 1978).

External fitter adjustable controls that control frequency, maximum output gain, type of compression, etc., other than the volume control, extend some freedom in changing the characteristics of the hearing aid, however limited.

CLASS D AMPLIFICATION

One of the recent innovations is the development of the Class D amplifier. Elmer Carlson, Meade Killion, and Knowles Electronics have cooperated to produce the Class D amplifier, which is fast becoming the amplifier of choice for many hearing aid fittings.

The Class A amplifier has dominated the industry in the recent past and has been responsible for a great deal of the early success, of custom in-the-ear hearing aids. Most in-the-ear hearing instruments, however, use a starved Class A amplifier to increase battery life resulting in considerably greater distortion. Class B amplifiers are used when more powerful push-pull amplification is necessary. Class C amplification is used for radio transmitters, and is not suitable for audio classification.

The Class D amplifier appears to have the following advantages, compared to Class A amplification:

1. Decreased battery drain due to increased efficiency
2. Higher output saturation levels and signal head room resulting in lower distortion levels.
3. Increased reliability
4. Improved sound quality

Since Class D amplification is more efficient in terms of energy use, battery life is extended up to 50%. At this time, the Class D amplifier has a 40% penetration in the marketplace and is rapidly increasing.

THE VOLUME CONTROL (GAIN CONTROL)

The volume control is actually a variable resistor. The resistor controls the amount of current transmitted which, in effect, controls the total output of the hearing aid. The volume control is also called a gain control. When the volume control is turned all the way up, the variable resistor introduces very little resistance into the circuit, thus permitting larger currents to flow. Ultimately, these larger currents are translated into louder sounds in the output of the hearing aid. When the volume control is turned down, substantially more resistance is placed into the circuit which causes a corresponding reduction in the current. This produced the quieter sounds when the volume is turned down.

Volume controls on hearing aids do not have linear rotational characteristics. The relationship between volume control rotation and the amount of amplification is referred to as *volume control taper.* Engineers, however, tend to design a hearing aid so that it will function fairly linearly throughout the range of amplification allowed on a particular model hearing aid (Staab, 1978). The end

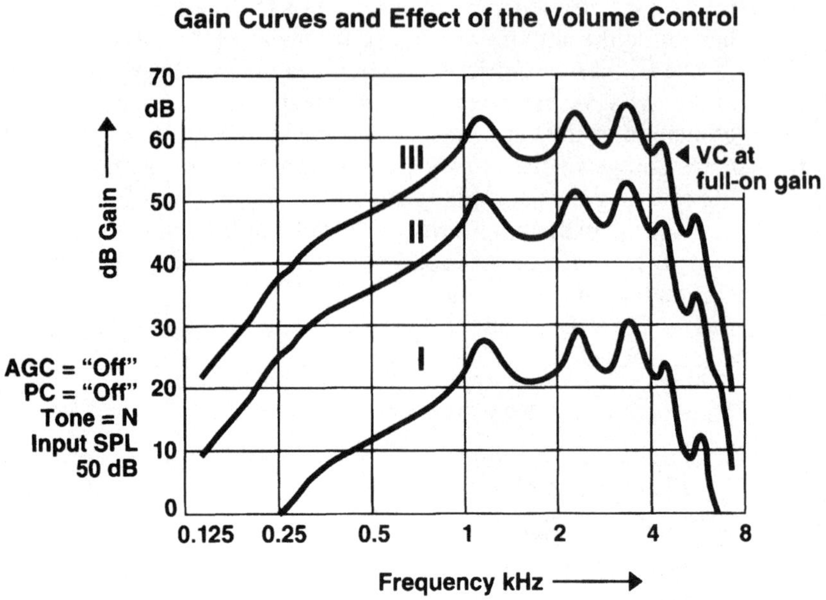

Fig. 24. Notice that the volume control loses its linearity at higher volume settings.

result is a fairly restricted range of amplification in many instruments. It is common to find that the range of amplification in a hearing aid is 30 to 40 dB. This means that a hearing aid with a gain of 60 dB, and a range of amplification of 30 dB, can have a beginning amplification of 30 dB. Volume control taper specifications should therefore be interpreted with caution. The external volume control and tone control can be manipulated by the user. There are internal controls which can be manipulated by the hearing aid specialist to give maximum flexibility in gain, output, or frequency response.

TONE CONTROL (FREQUENCY CONTROL)

Tone controls are used primarily to boost or cut the sound power in selected frequency ranges. In other words, tone controls modify the frequency range of the hearing aid. Tone controls perform a task similar to *bass* and *treble* controls in an audio system. The task is performed by a complicated arrangement of condensers and resistance (filter network) in the circuit. High tone emphasis is obtained by transmitting high frequency efficiently and low frequencies inefficiently. Actually, the low frequencies are attenuated (reduced in strength) more than the high frequencies—hence a high tone emphasis. If the volume control setting of the hearing aid is not changed, a reduced gain will result. If the hearing aid has sufficient gain, however, an advancement of the volume control will enable the listener to hear with sufficient strength.

It is typical of tone controls that only the bass and treble frequencies are changed, and the mid-range frequencies remain unaffected. Many hearing impaired individuals prefer to leave them in the flat position. Others will prefer increased bass for music and high frequency emphasis for speech intelligibility.

TELECOIL (TELEPHONE PICKUP COIL)

The purpose of the telecoil is to allow hearing impaired individuals to utilize their hearing aids to amplify signals transmitted via the telephone. This special circuit utilizes a magnetic induction pickup coil mounted in the hearing case. A switch allows the user to substitute the telecoil for the microphone as the input to the hearing aid. The telecoil is also known as an induction coil.

The telephone earphone is a magnetic receiver which generates a magnetic field through electromagnetic leakage. When the hearing aid is placed close to the telephone earphone, the hearing aid telecoil (induction coil) picks up the magnetic field and changes it to an electrical signal. The signal is amplified and converted into an acoustical signal directly to the ear. In picking up the signal directly from the telephone earphone, the telecoil substitutes for the microphone at the input stage. As a result, no amplified ambient sound is picked up from the environment to interfere with the telephone conversation.

Some hearing aids and auditory trainers used in educational settings have an additional position which allows the microphone and telephone to be used simultaneously. A problem has arisen in some of the newer telephone systems which employ an earphone that radiates little or no usable magnetic field. In this situation, a hearing aid with a telecoil will not function in the telephone position.

A new telecoil and amplifier arrangement which can be built into present day hearing aids has been devised. The device has approximately twice the volume of other telecoils but also incorporates a 28 dB amplifier in it to overcome the difference in the various types of magnetic signals (Goldberg, 1975). Recently, Stoker, et al (1983), completed a comprehensive research study of the use of telephones by the hearing impaired. The results suggest that a large percentage of telephones, now in service throughout the world, are not capable of generating a magnetic field of suitable strength for magnetic coupling of telephones and hearing aids

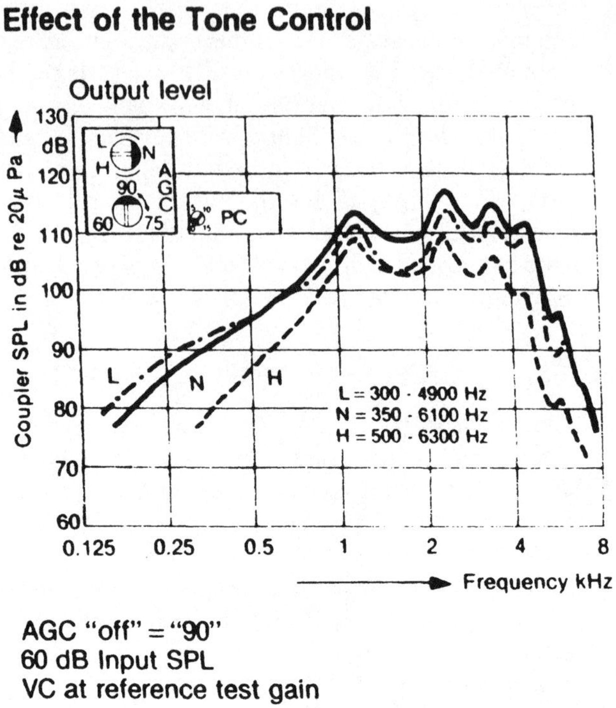

Fig. 25.

via the average hearing aid telecoil circuit. It appears, however, that current technology is capable of producing acoustic coupling of telephones and hearing aids which is superior to the generally accepted capability for such coupling. The difficult problem is the issue of telephone use in noisy environments. There is no indication that acoustic coupling (instead of magnetic) may be improved, at the level of the hearing aid, by providing an alternative frequency response for telephone use for those individuals with precipitous hearing losses. A flat gain response characteristic of the hearing aid diminishes the incidence of feedback and allows for improved word recognition.

HEARING AID OPERATION

The electric signal generated at the microphone is coupled to the amplifier which increases its amplitude or voltage. If all the amplifier needed to do was amplify, one transistor might be designed to provide all that is needed. The more transistors and associated circuitry, the more *stages,* and eventually the greater will be the amount of amplification.

Generally, two types of *amplifier circuits* are used in hearing aid technology. The most common type of circuit is the Class A or single ended amplifier. There is only one output amplifier stage generally using one output transistor. Class A amplifiers are usually used for low and moderate output aids with an average output below 125 dB SPL.

The Class B, or push-pull circuit, is used in high output instruments with an average output greater than 125 dB SPL. Basically, a push-pull output stage consists of two transistors operating, side by side, to develop more current at the earphone. Consequently, a push-pull stage is capable of providing more amplification than a so-called single ended (Class A) output stage.

Recently, a few hearing aid manufacturers have introduced push-pull circuitry for mild and moderate gain hearing aids because of less distortion and more efficient operation. Class D amplifiers, a recent development will be discussed later in this chapter.

AUDIO INPUT

The term audio input describes the electro-mechanical technology for conducting and processing an audio signal through a hearing aid amplifier, usually at the pre-amp stage, without using the hearing aid microphone.

In many listening environments hearing aids may not provide sufficient help. The purpose of an audio-input hearing aid is to improve the signal to noise ratio, thereby enhancing speech discrimination abilities of the hearing impaired person. Because the audio input system utilizes the user's own hearing aid(s), the signals are passing through an already programmed corrective amplification to meet the user's individual hearing needs for intelligible and familiar sound reception (Pimentel, 1984).

Audio input systems for hearing aids were developed originally for hearing impaired school children who used hearing aids but who still needed extra hearing help in certain classroom situations. The audio-input system helps to overcome the adverse signal to noise ration resulting from: (1) distance between teacher and student; (2) classroom noise, shuffling feet, movement of bodies, etc.: (3) reverberation. For adults, audio-input can be directly applied to TV sets, tape recorders, radios, etc. New uses are being found for audio input to help hearing aid users overcome the omnipresent problems of distance, noise, and reverberation (Pimentel, 1974).

ELECTROACOUSTIC CHARACTERISTICS OF HEARING AIDS

INTRODUCTION

A hearing aid is a miniaturized amplification system. What is its main purpose? Its main purpose is to amplify. This statement appears trivial, but there is more to it than meets the eye, or more accurately, the ear. First and foremost, the hearing aid must modify the original signal in order to compensate for the hearing loss of the individual. This process is accomplished by increasing or decreasing the intensity of the signal in certain frequency ranges; for example, boosting the high frequencies in relation to the low frequencies in order to compensate for a downward sloping audiogram. This process of hearing loss compensation should be accomplished by the hearing aid with a minimum of distortion and interference of the original signal.

An understanding of the electroacoustics of a hearing aid is necessary for the more complete explanations of hearing aid performance which follows:

As we have previously discussed, a hearing aid consists basically of a *microphone, electrical amplifier,* and an *earphone*. The energy required for operating the electric amplifier is supplied by a *battery*. The sound pressure impinging on the microphone is called the *input sound pressure level*. Similarly, the sound pressure level which the hearing aid produces at the output is called the *output sound pressure level*. The *gain* indicates how much greater the output sound pressure is than the sound pressure at the input of the hearing aid. For example, if the input sound pressure level is 60 dB, and the output sound pressure level is 100 dB, then the acoustic gain is 40 dB. The output sound pressure level produced by the earphone is usually measured in a standardized 2cc coupler.

Hearing aids usually have a *gain control* by which the output sound pressure level can be varied. This control enables the volume (gain) of the hearing aid to be adjusted. The gain of the hearing aid is dependent on frequency. This dependence on frequency is determined by the transducers: microphone and earphone (receiver). Some hearing aids have a manual tone control with which the transmitted *frequency response* can be adjusted. A hearing aid does not amplify all frequencies equally. A curve which shows the relative gain of a hearing aid, expressed as a function of frequency,

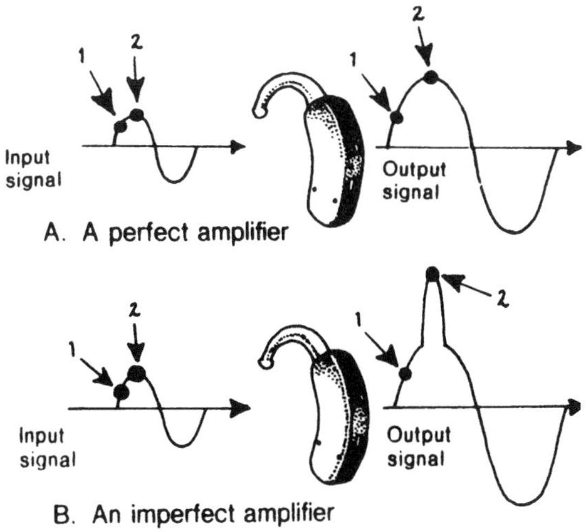

Fig. 26. (A) The perfect amplifier enlarges the signal at points #1 and #2 by the same factor. (B) The imperfect amplifier enlarges the signal at points #1 and #2 by different relative amounts. (Reprinted by permission from Johnson-Walker-Cutnell. The Science of Hi-Fidelity Second Edition-Copyright (c) 1981 by Kendall/Hunt Publishing Company.) (Illustration of hearing aid added to the figure by Libby.)

and a constant sound input is the *frequency response curve.* The frequencies that are of special interest when discussing hearing aids are the frequencies in the range from approximately 100Hz to 8kHz.

The *bandwidth* of the hearing aid must be adequate to transmit the sounds of speech and music with a minimum of *distortion.* The *dynamic range* of the hearing aid is restricted both by the upper and lower limits of the input sound pressure level. The lower limit of the dynamic range of the hearing aid is restricted to the *inherent noise pressure level* of the hearing aid. In hearing aids this level is, in general, relatively small. Moreover, the individual hearing threshold of the hearing impaired person is often so high, with respect to the sound level, that the inherent noise level usually can be ignored (Veit, 1975). Of considerably greater importance, however, is the upper limit of the dynamic range, the *saturation sound pressure level.* This represents the *maximum sound pressure level* the hearing aid can produce with the gain at a given setting and frequency, regardless of the input sound pressure level. A further increase in the input level results in over-driving the hearing aid, and

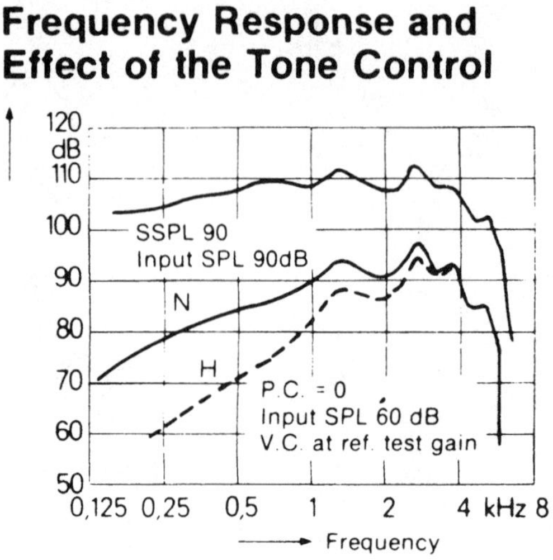

Fig. 27.

non linear distortion occurs. The more the input sound pressure level is increased, the greater the distortion. In the fitting of hearing aids, particular attention must be paid to the output limit. In general, saturation sound pressure levels, with ear level hearing aids, is between 100 and 135 dB; in body worn hearing aids between 130 and 140 dB SPL.

How well a hearing aid will perform its function with a minimum of distortion and interference depends a great deal on the electroacoustic characteristics is often a complicated, frustrating, and confusing task. The many pitfalls that affect the routine measurer of electroacoustic characteristics are disarmingly intricate (Briskey et al, 1966). Artifact appears to abound within the measurement equipment and the hearing aids themselves (Kasten and Franks, 1981). In addition, measures of hearing aid function has less value unless they can be related to listener behavior. Most measures of hearing aid performance are designed to describe hearing aid performance in the absence of a listener with the use of *2cc coupler* or a *manikin* KEMAR©. Another set of measurements can be performed with the hearing aid directly coupled to the listener. Both sets of measurements serve their separate function, and both are necessary to the understanding of hearing aid function. The electroacoustic characteristics of a hearing aid as the signal is transduced from acoustic to electric and back to acoustic are commonly known as electroacoustic characteristics. The Food and Drug Administration (FDA) requires hearing aid manufacturers to

Lesson 30 271 - 281

make available the electroacoustic characteristics of hearing aids. Real ear probe measurements will be discussed in another chapter.

DISTORTION

Hearing aid distortion is the failure of a system to reproduce a signal with accuracy and exactness. It should be stressed, however, that distortion can be built into a hearing system, deliberately, in order to compensate for the hearing loss of the individual.

Distortion occurs when a hearing aid generates additional frequencies of its own which were not present in the original signal. It can result in a change in the perceived quality of the signal and if sufficiently severe, in loss of clarity and quality of the signal. The ability of a hearing aid system to transmit or reproduce a signal with exactness is called the "*fidelity*" of the system. *In other words, a hearing aid with good fidelity and low distortion preserves the loudness relationships of speech and other informational elements entering into the system.* We will discover later in this chapter that certain distortions, such as various forms of compression, may be beneficial, and used in a purposeful way to improve sound comfort and clarity.

If you have ever looked at yourself in a fun house mirror, you immediately grasp the principal of distortion. The image is recognizable but untrue to the original. The wave form of the signal gets twisted out of shape, and while the signal remains recognizable, the sound is no longer true.

The absence of distortion is what truly separates quality hearing aids from its lesser counterparts. A hearing aid may have a wide frequency response, but still it may not be judged "high fidelity" if distortion is present. If the bass notes are boomy and muffled, and the treble (high frequencies) are metallic and harsh, distortion may be present. Now that wide range hearing aids are available, it is essential that the tonal quality be kept as natural and distortion free as possible. What can occur is that marginal distortion, too slight to register consciously, builds up, sublimally, to create a psychological effect known as *listener fatigue*. Fortunately, the detection of distortion has been worked out by physical methods which will be described later.

As we describe the gain of a powerful hearing aid, power by itself means very little in terms of hearing aid fidelity. *What counts is undistorted power.* As a hearing aid approaches its power limit, distortion also rises with output. *Three principal types of distortion——harmonic, intermodulation,* and *transient* - plague hearing aid engineers.

HARMONIC DISTORTION

Harmonic distortion takes its name from the harmonics, or overtones, produced by a signal in addition to its basic frequency. These harmonics are not distortion; they spring from the basic sonic nature of the signal. Harmonic distortion occurs if the hearing aid distorts the waveform and adds overtones of its own, thus altering the proportions of the original signal. These overtones, generated within the hearing aid, are then superimposed on the signal and change the essential natural sound of the signal. Harmonic distortion is a result, primarily, of overloading the hearing aid amplifier or earphone. This distortion results mainly from peak clipping. When output limiting occurs, in its commonest form, the strongest peaks of the signal are clipped, changing the waveform of the signal. No hearing aid is entirely free of this unwelcome tendency to add its own impromptu frequencies to the signal. The object of good hearing aid design is to minimize such additions. Harmonic distortion is the least obtrusive of the three types of distortion. Fortunately for hearing impaired listeners, hearing aid design engineers have succeeded in reducing harmonic distortion (Kasten et al, 1967). It would, therefore, be undesirable to select a hearing aid for an individual that would have to be set at, or near, maximum gain in order to achieve a comfort level (Pollack, 1980).

In order to illustrate harmonic distortion, consider Figure 28 in which a single frequency of 1500 Hz is the input (fundamental frequency). In principle, the output of the hearing aid is supposed to be an exact replica, only enlarged, of the input waveform. This implies that the output must have a frequency of precisely 1500 Hz, with no other frequencies present. Surprisingly, the output waveform is not an exact duplicate of the input, but may have a distorted shape as in Figure 28. The complex output waveform is comprised of the fundamental wave, whose frequency is 1500 Hz, plus all the higher harmonics. Thus we see that it is the presence of the higher harmonics at 3000 Hz, 4500 Hz, etc. which are responsible for the distorted appearance of the output waveform. Since these higher harmonics were not present in the input, they were created by the hearing aid and added to the output signal. *The Total Harmonic Distortion (THD) depends on the amount of power the hearing aid is producing.*

What is considered a good value for Total Harmonic Distortion? In terms of listening, a 2% THD value means that 98% of the amplified output will contain all the frequencies which were present

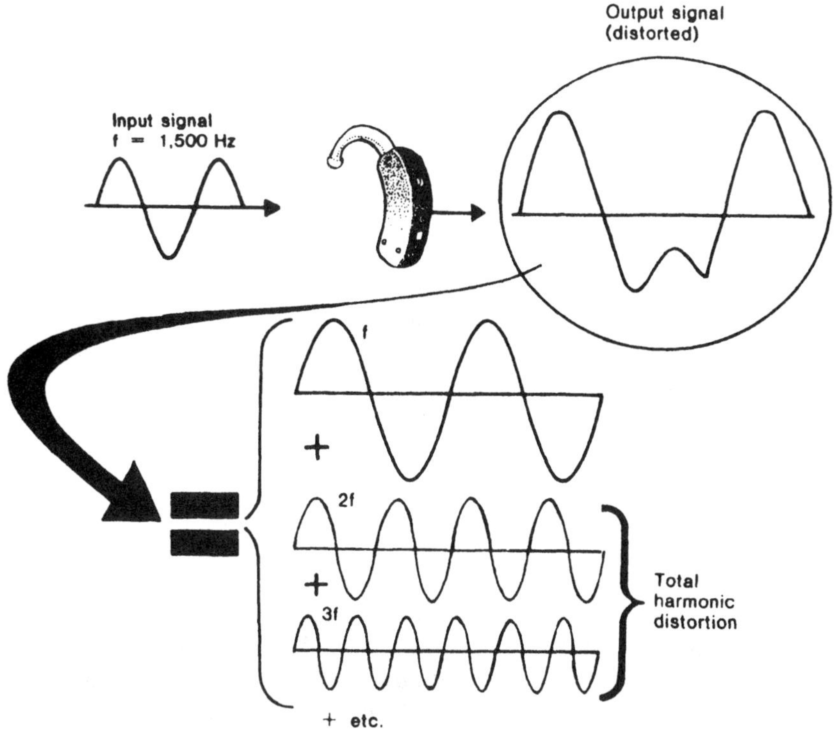

Fig. 28. Total harmonic distortion occurs when an amplifier produces unwanted harmonics of a fundamental frequency. A qualify amplifier keeps THD to an inaudible level. (Reprinted by permission from Johnson-Walker-Cutnell. The Science of Hi-Fidelity Second Edition-Copyright (c) 1981 by Kendall/Hunt Publishing Company.) (Illustration of hearing aid added to the figure by Libby.)

in the original signal; 2% of the output will be the unwanted higher harmonics of the input frequencies.

In a study of the amount of distortion tolerable in a high fidelity system, Olson (1957) found that total harmonic distortion levels of approximately 1% were not considered objectionable in a system with an 8 kHz upper cut off frequency (Killion, 1979).

Distortion levels below 2% are generally inaudible on musical material, and even gross distortion levels (6 to 12%) are sometimes inaudible. In general, the just-audible distortion levels for musical material are at least ten times greater than the just-audible pure tone distortion levels. At low sound pressure levels, the level of harmonic or inter-modulation distortion products may lie below the normal threshold of hearing. At high levels, the increased upward spread of masking, and the distortion of the ear itself, may mask externally generated distortion products. Thus no single number distortion specifications will apply to all listening levels (Killion, 1979).

Difficulties have been encountered in attempting to study the effect of distortion on speech discriminations. Peters and Burkhard (1968) found that the 40% total harmonic distortion produced by one system had negligible effect on speech discrimination, whereas another system whose distortion measured only 20% resulted in a greater loss in speech discrimination scores. ANSI standards dictate that harmonic distortion levels should be measured at one arbitrary input pressure level. It has been this writer's experience that more meaningful harmonic distortion levels are obtained at the user's volume control level. The reference gain level necessary for ANSI often demonstrates distortion levels significantly higher than those obtained at the user's volume level. Before an aid is rejected by the hearing aid specialist for too high distortion levels, this point should be taken into consideration.

In light of available information, a reasonable goal for a high fidelity hearing aid with an 8000 Hz bandwidth would appear to be a maximum THD of 2% for output levels between 50 and 90 eardrum SPL, with a relaxation to 10% at 30 dB and 110 dB SPL. Listening tests should be employed as a final check.

INTER MODULATION DISTORTION (IM)

The most disturbing of the three distortion types is unquestionably inter modulation distortion (IM). The raucous harshness that it adds to speech or music is one of the predominant causes of listener fatigue. And it is present to a certain extent in all audio components, including hearing aids. Unlike THD, however, the unwanted frequencies are not harmonically related to the input frequencies. *IM distortion occurs when two or more waves of different frequencies are simultaneously passing through an amplifier. The output contains the original frequencies plus the sum and difference frequencies created by the IM distortion.*

At this time there are no ANSI standards for maximum allowable IM distortion. In general, a hearing aid with a significant amount of THD will also contain a significant amount of IM distortion. Killion reported that IM distortion becomes objectionable at a value of 3% or 4% when the difference frequency lies in the 400 to 5000 Hz range. IM distortion testing consists of putting two tones through a hearing aid and taking a census of their unwanted byproducts. Because of the greater complexity in testing IM dis-

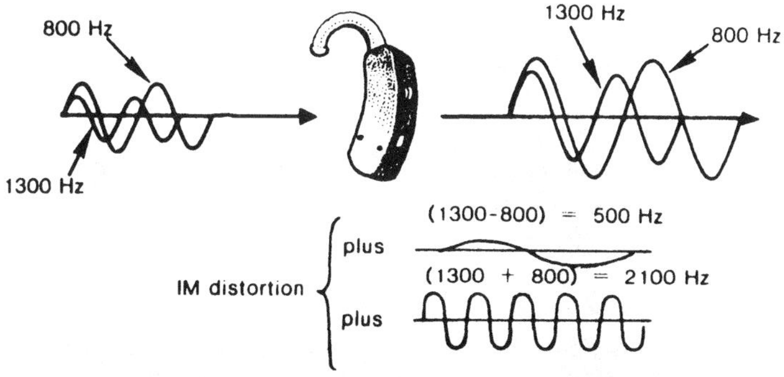

Fig. 29. Inter modulation distortion occurs when two of more waves of different frequencies are simultaneously passing through an amplifier. The output contains the original frequency plus the "sum" and "difference" frequencies created by the intermodulation distortion. (Reprinted by permission from Johnson-Walker-Cutnell. The Science of Hi-Fidelity Second Edition-Copyright (c) 1981 by Kendall/Hunt Publishing Company.) (Illustration of hearing aid added to the figure by Libby.)

tortion, manufacturers' spec. sheets usually print only THD measurements. In high quality audio components, manufacturers strive for IM distortion values of less than one percent. In general, no single number distortion specification will apply to all listening situations. In conclusion, the common complaint regarding hearing aid sound quality may be related more to amplifier THD, and IM distortion due to peak clipping, than to frequency response of the hearing aid per se (Killion, 1979).

TRANSIENT DISTORTION

We will now end the topic of distortion with a "bang". In acoustic parlance, a bang is a transient something that comes and goes quickly. Transients are sounds bursting forth suddenly at relatively high loudness levels and breaking off just as fast. Speech is full of transients—especially consonants. Music is also full of transients, such as the clash of cymbals, or the hard impact of piano hammers against the strings. Transients are difficult for all amplifiers, such as hearing aids, to reproduce. They fall victim to transient distortion, a deplorable process that can turn a sharp, hard click or snap into a fuzzy "thunk". The reason is that electronic circuits are afflicted with *inertia.* They have trouble starting or stopping swiftly enough to reproduce the transient wave shape accurately. When the sudden bang occurs, it causes a fast rising electric pulse, known as a *fast rise time.* This means that the amplifier must replicate the signal's peak with virtually no inertial delay. When the bang is gone, the amplifier must return promptly to neutral. The amplifier's attempt to return to neutral (*known as fall time or decay*), an alteration or lingering of the wave form, often results in what is called "*ringing*". The ear perceives such transient distortion as a pall cast over the whole texture of the sound, clouding the detail of speech or music and resulting in a washed-out quality draining the signal of its tension and excitement (Fantel, 1983).

Unfortunately, there is no altogether satisfactory way of measuring transient distortion. The measure that is often used is the time required for decay at the output when a pure tone input has been abruptly squelched. Like other forms of distortion, transient distortion is frequency dependent and is found in linear as well as nonlinear systems.

These tests, however, provide only presumptive evidence of an amplifier's transient characteristics. The human ear, listening for sharpness of tonal definition and clarity of texture, still remains the most reliable test instrument for transient distortion (Fantel, 1983).

ADDITIONAL DISTORTIONS

Staab and Ely (1978) mention additional types of distortion which can destroy the fidelity rating of a hearing aid; *frequency (linear) distortion, phase distortion, and noise distortion.* We will discuss these types of distortion briefly.

Frequency (linear) distortion occurs when the frequency response curve of the electroacoustic system favors or suppresses some frequencies more than others. This distortion is expressed in the frequency response and is a change in the input spectrum. It should be understood that the shape of the hearing aid response curve can change the harmonic or inter modulation amplitudes.

Phase distortion results when the phase angle between the fundamental frequency and any of its harmonics, or between any two frequencies of a complex wave changes. The effect is a change in the waveform of the original signal in the output. Phase distortion is not easily measured. Ely (1974) stated that amplifying systems tend to shift phase, particularly as they filter out certain frequencies. If this is done in a linear manner, no phase distortion occurs. On the other hand, if the phase shift is not linear with frequency, phase distortion occurs.

Noise distortion can be of two types (Staab, 1978). The first is caused by the amplifier adding noise to an input signal and changing it. The second is an extraneous noise caused by friction against

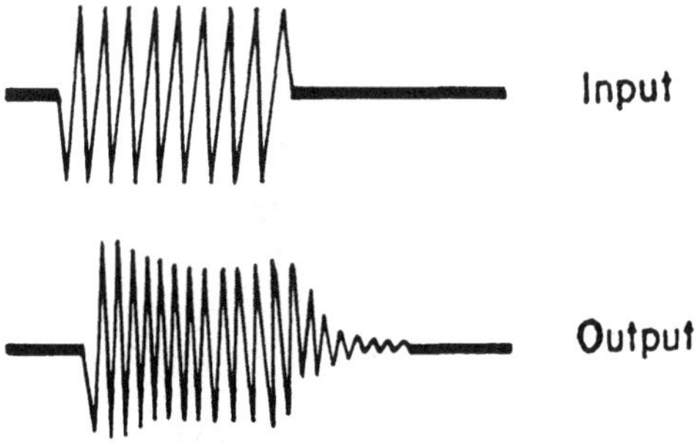

Fig. 30. Response of a hearing aid earphone to a 2000 Hz tone burst. The output builds up gradually and does not terminate immediately or abruptly.

the case of the aid. Both of these types of noise distortion mask the primary signal. Noise distortion is measured as a signal-to-noise ratio with better performance occurring as the difference in levels between the two become greater. This type of distortion, unlike the others, does not involve some form of non linearity of the input signal.

HEARING AID NOISE LEVELS

Unfortunately, all amplifiers, including hearing aids add a certain amount of "noise" to the signal. If you tune in a weak station on the radio, there is the ever present background hiss or static. Hearing aids present the same problem. Hearing aid engineers call this annoying disturbance "noise", and it is created by the electronic components, such as transistors and resistors present in the hearing aid circuit. In designing hearing aids, attempts are made to make them as noise free as possible.

One of the major sources of potential noise is the microphone. Since its noise is amplified by the circuitry, the mass inherent noise level of the microphone is one of the factors which determine the weakest signal the hearing aid can handle effectively. The electret microphone utilized in today's hearing aids offers the best low noise available. (Staab, 1978).

FEEDBACK

One of the most persistent problems plaguing the hearing aid industry has been the control of feedback. Feedback has been variously identified as whistling, squealing, buzzing, howling, or humming. Even with carbon sets dating back 50 years with considerably lower gain than is now common, acoustic feedback was considered a problem. At some time, most of us have experienced a squealing sound from a public address system, tape recorder, or some other type amplification system. Feedback can take many forms, *both desirable and undesirable,* and has been a major engineering consideration in hearing aid design and production (Pollack, 1980). Desirable feedback that is deliberately introduced for a purpose may be categorized as *positive or negative feedback.* Positive feedback is sometimes referred to as *regenerative, or in phase feedback.* Negative feedback is sometimes referred to as *degenerative (or out of phase)* feedback. In the first instance, the feedback serves to add to amplification factor as well as lessening non linear distortion (Berger, 1984).

The farther apart the microphone and the receiver are, the greater the amount of available output before feedback occurs and the less the energy reaching the microphone. With a body aid, the separation may be as much as 18 inches, so higher amplification levels can be used. In the ear *transducers* may be separated by as little as 2.5 mms., and are therefore the most likely to produce feedback at relatively low output levels. Thus, the power of these instruments is severely restricted (Pollack, 1980).

Pollack (1980), Staab (1978) and Lybarger (1982) have presented excellent articles on feedback characteristics.

Four types of feedback are generally identified with hearing aids. Three of these are usually considered to be undesirable - *acoustical, magnetic, and mechanical.* Another type, electrical, is often engineered into the hearing aid.

ACOUSTICAL FEEDBACK

Acoustical feedback occurs when amplified sound escapes via the earmold or ear canal and arrives back at the hearing aid microphone.

There are three possible effects of acoustic feedback:

1. Oscillation can occur, making the hearing aid useless unless the gain is reduced;
2. The frequency response of the aid can be greatly altered, even if oscillation is not occurring;
3. One of the major alterations in response is the creation of sharp peaks as oscillation is reached. These sharp peaks result in very poor transient characteristics or "ringing" when sounds are processed by the hearing aid.

If the response of the hearing aid were perfectly flat, acoustical feedback would be less common because of the absence of resonant peaks. With the trend to smoother responses, feedback has become less of a problem in many hearing transmission systems.

Acoustical feedback may be caused by leakage of sound through or around an earmold or tubing. Another common cause is poor acoustic isolation of either or both of the hearing aid transducers.

The use of heavy wall or double wall tubing can help to reduce the feedback due to tubing effects. A slightly greater output is attainable before feedback occurs. Lybarger (1982) points out that it appears that the "danger area" for open canal fittings lies between 1500 and 4000 Hz although the latter may be related to the high frequency cutoff of the receiver.

Lybarger further points out that some of the most revealing work on acoustic feedback is seen in the Handbook of Hearing Aid Measurements published by the Veterans Administration and reporting tests made for them under the direction of Edwin Burnett of the National Bureau of Standards. Using the *KEMAR* manikin and open earmolds, most hearing aids show a well defined feedback peak between 1700 and 2500 Hz in the majority of cases. The average feedback peak frequency is about 2050 Hz for hearing aids tested. Burnett (1982) reports that where high amplification is used, there is always some possibility that a significant part of the sound put in the user's ear may return to the hearing aid microphone. With sufficient amplification, the instrument will oscillate and produce an objectionable high amplitude sound (howl). At volume control setting short of actual howling, the presence of this feedback will introduce a spurious resonance into the response of the hearing aid. The precise degree of this resonance will depend upon the gain setting. A higher degree of resonance can occur for an actual wearer because of this problem of obtaining a good seal, or in the case of "open earmold" fittings. Thus, a "flat" instrument may be converted into a peak instrument by the presence of incipient feedback.

MECHANICAL FEEDBACK

Increased miniaturization of hearing aids has resulted in an increase in mechanical vibration feedback between the microphone and receiver because they are closer together. The "squeal" is lower pitched than what is heard in acoustical feedback and is caused by low frequency mechanical vibrations (400–500 Hz) from the receiver vibrating the case of the hearing aid. Rubber cushions are used inside the aid to cushion the transducers from the case and from each other. In addition, the transducers are oriented within the case with their sensitivity and direction of

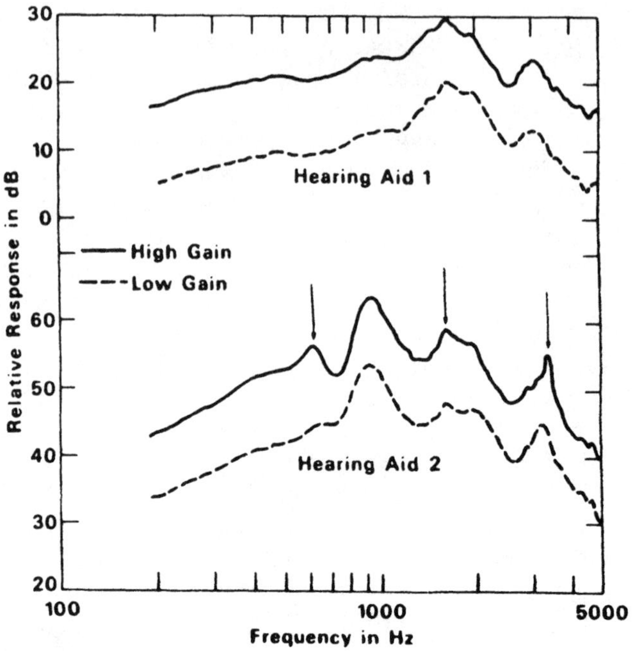

Fig. 31. Examples of the growth of resonance peaks as a function of gain control setting. Hearing aid 1 is a typical mild-to-moderate-gain hearing aid. Hearing aid 2 is a high-grain; its response at the higher gain-control setting shows appearance or growth of resonance peaks (marked by arrows). Such curves are found occasionally for hearing aids, even for the controlled conditions used in measuring the responses shown; closed mold fittings with careful sealing to the manikin. (With permission E. D. Burnett, et al, Vanderbilt Report Monographs in Contemporary Audiology, 1982.)

maximum vibrations output at right angles to each other to take advantage of directional vibration properties and minimize mechanical feedback, as reported by Staab (1978).

MAGNETIC FEEDBACK

Magnetic feedback results from the coupling between the magnetic fields of the receiver and telephone coil or magnetic microphone. The magnetic field of the receiver can be induced to the microphone or telephone coil, resulting in feedback. Today, this is a minor problem.

ELECTRONIC FEEDBACK

Electronic feedback is important, because it is a technique for reducing hearing aid distortion. It involves taking a small portion of this output signal of a hearing aid, turning it around so that it is exactly out of phase with the input signal, and feeding it back to the input. This technique is used in automatic volume control (AVC) situations for beneficial reasons. Other controlled uses of negative feedback include giving some condenser microphones directional response characteristics and sloping amplifier response characteristics (Hillman, 1974).

Pollack (1980) discussed two forms of electronic feedback that can have a detrimental effect on hearing aid performance. The first is *electrostatic feedback* which results from a capacitive coupling from the output to the input stages of the amplifier. The sound that is heard is a very high pitch, hissing sound. Electrical oscillation is caused by inadequate decoupling of the battery and amplifier circuit. As the usable battery voltage decreases, impedance increases and causes oscillation of the amplifier circuit. The sound that is heard is a low frequency "motor boating" which sounds much like saw tooth noise (Staab, 1978).

FEEDBACK CONTROL

Some methods have proved to be beneficial in reducing acoustic feedback for the vented or open mold conditions. Some helpful methods are reduced gain, smoother response by careful application of acoustic damping techniques, reduced high frequency response, notch filters, and reduced earmold opening for open canal molds (Lybarger, 1982). Preves (1982) constructed a number of circuits using adaptive notch and phase shifting techniques which allowed a gain increase of about 10 dB before the onset of feedback. Preves (1982) stated that the circuits could fit into headworn hearing aids and operate from a 1.3 volt battery.

Digital technology lends itself to partially solving this troublesome problem. For example, a promising technique involves canceling the feedback path by placing an adaptive filter in the path of the hearing aid, that is tuned to the inverse frequency response and phase of the acoustic feedback path (Preves, 1994).

This approach is similar to the one used in the Danavox Genius, a true digital feedback rejection post-auricular hearing aid (Drylund, & Bisgaard, 1991). Increased real ear gain before feedback, with an average of 9 dB, can be demonstrated in the Danavox Instrument.

AMPLITUDE COMPRESSION

When a hearing impaired person wears a typical hearing aid at comfort level for normal quiet conversation, a dropped fork or a slamming door entering into the sound environment would also be amplified by the same amount, resulting in discomfort to the user. As a result, the listener reduces the volume of the hearing aid, which in turn would cause him to miss some of the conversation and would further contribute to the user's frustration. In addition, the high sound levels would drive the hearing aid into *saturation or overload* resulting in distortion of the original signal. This scenario has been one of the major reasons for many hearing aid users to relegate their hearing aids to the "dresser drawer".

Another problem is that listeners with sensorineural impairments typically exhibit poorer thresholds, while discomfort levels often remain essentially the same. This results in a smaller dynamic range, thus producing a reduction of usable auditory area and a reduction in channel capacity. Consequently, even if the listener can be aided by amplification, the ability to extract information from the speech signal is reduced.

In addition, the sensorineural listener may exhibit recruitment, an abnormal recovery of hearing sensitivity, as the sound intensity increases above threshold. The person's loudness response becomes progressively closer to normal at higher levels, implying an abnormally fast growth of loudness with intensity and a reduction of the dynamic range of hearing. Complete recruitment, in which sound at some high intensity is heard at normal loudness, is common. (Villchur, 1978), (Killion, 1979). The discomfort levels of those persons with recruitment who do not have an accompanying conductive impairment are likely to be within the range of normal discomfort levels.

In an attempt to solve the problems of decreased dynamic range, tolerance, recruitment, and hearing aid distortion, non linear amplification may be necessary.

LINEAR AMPLIFICATION

All hearing aid circuits which do not compress the input signal exhibit linear amplification. For example, a 20 dB increase in the input SPL would mean a 20 dB increase in the output SPL.

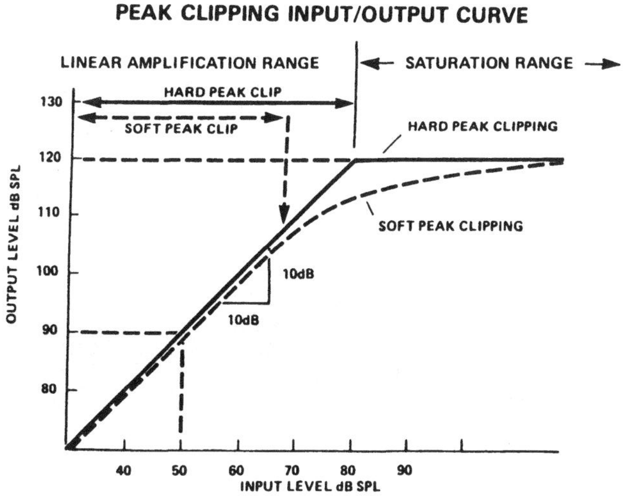

Fig. 32.

This input-output relationship would be maintained up to the level at which further increases in input would no longer result in continued increases in the output. This level is referred to as the saturation output, maximum output, or overload.

When a hearing aid receives more input signal than it can handle, it stops doing its job of amplifying.

Figure 33 Part A shows a hearing aid properly amplifying each part of the input signal. No difficulty arises because even the crests of the wave are not large enough to exceed the amplifying capacity of the hearing aid. This situation occurs while the user is listening to a conversation in quiet. Now, what occurs when a fork drops or a door is slammed? Let us now observe Part B of Figure 33 which shows what happens when the input signal is too large. The most extreme parts of the crests and troughs (compressions and rarefactions) are clipped as if by a pair of scissors. The parts of the wave are simply too big for the amplifier to handle. *Peak clipping* occurs, which distorts the input signal, and can result in discomfort to the user. Under this circumstance, the hearing aid is forced into non linearity in that an increased input does not result in an increase of its output.

Output limiting is therefore necessary to prevent the hearing aid from producing sound beyond a given sound pressure level. It protects the user against high intensity sounds that might otherwise become painfully loud.

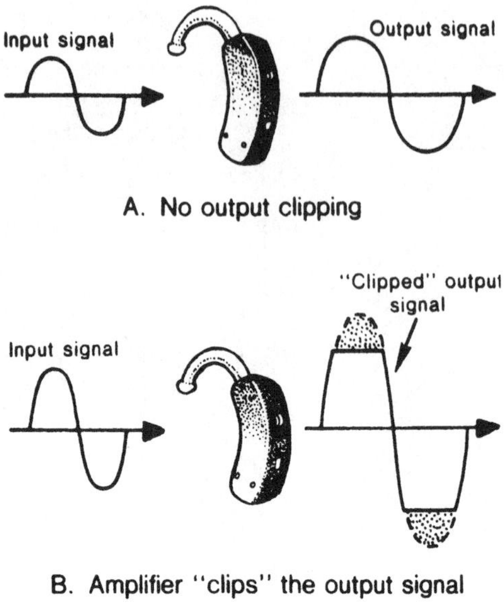

Fig. 33. Part A shows a hearing aid properly amplifying each part of the input signal. Part B shows the clipped output signal when the input signal is too large. (Reprinted by permission from Johnson-Walker-Cutnell. The Science of Hi-Fidelity Second Edition—Copyright (c) 1981 by Kendall/ Hunt Publishing Company.) (Illustration of hearing aid added to the figure by Libby.)

METHODS OF OUTPUT LIMITING

Peak Clipping (Conventional or Hark Peak Clipping)

Most peak clipping hearing aids clip in a *non-symmetrical fashion* by using resistors to vary the clipping or saturation level. This type of circuitry introduces significant amounts of second order harmonic distortion which can result in unpleasant sound reproduction. *Symmetrical peak clippers* also distort but produce third order harmonic distortion which is less objectionable. Some users prefer symmetrical peak clipping which is used in Class B—push pull amplifiers. (Refer to Figure 34).

Some advantages of peak clipping are that construction is simple, needing only a few added components, and very little space to accomplish instantaneous output limiting. Its primary disadvantage is that harmonic distortion occurs above the limiting level. Despite the fact that a strong relationship between harmonic distortion and poor intelligibility has not been proven, significant distortion does occur which can cause discomfort and frustration for many users.

Diode Clipping (Soft Peak Clipping, Peak Rounding, Diode Compression Control)

(Note: Some hearing aid manufacturers use the term "output compression" to define the diode clipping operation even though no AGC circuit is present).

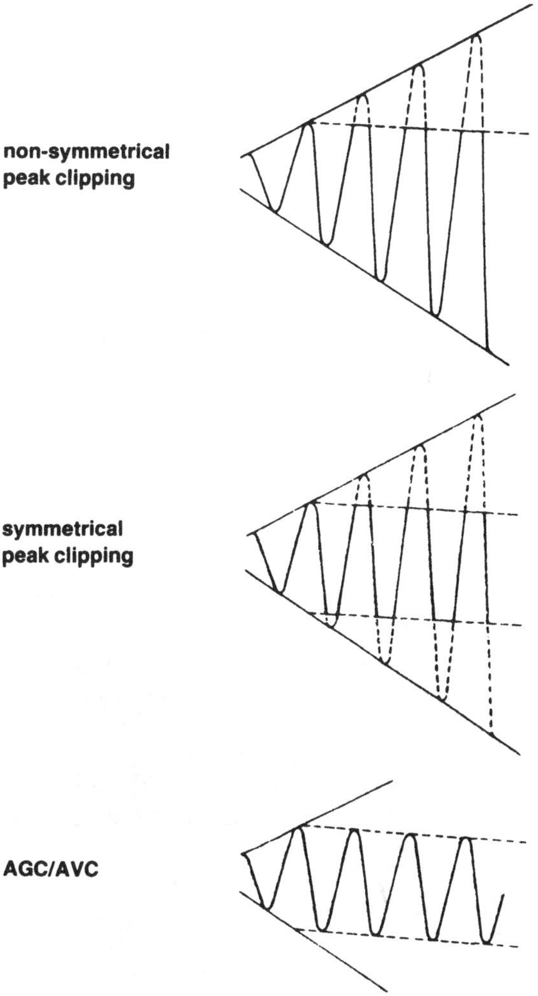

Fig. 34.

Diode clipping is a form of non linear amplification and is evidenced by a gradual, ever diminishing increase in output with each successive increase in input. Characteristically, diode clipping hearing aids have input/output amplifying modes having zero (instantaneous) time constants (attack and recovery times) (Staab, 1978).

Diode clipping methods of limiting are achieved by adding a minimal number of components to hard peak clipping circuitry. Most frequently, they consist of adding two diodes, a capacitor, and sometimes a (variable) resistor. The result of limiting with these systems resemble hard peak clipping in many respects including the creation of harmonic distortion, except that the onset of clipping is more gradual.

The hearing instrument will provide full gain up to the point at which the diodes begin to turn on. The diodes introduce symmetrical peak clipping which provides symmetrical third order distortion, a type generally less objectionable to the listener than second order harmonic distortion produced by standard peak clipping instruments. The advantages of diode clipping are that it is simple in construction, little additional space is necessary, and provides instantaneous output limiting. Its primary disadvantage appears to be that amplification is restricted to comparatively low gain setting to avoid distortion.

COMPRESSION

Compression is a type of automatic gain control which alters the gain of the amplifier in such a way that strong signals are amplified less than weak ones without the undesirable distortion occurring in simpler peak clipper hearing aids.

This type of hearing aid circuit is known widely as automatic gain control (AGC) or automatic volume control (AVC). ANSI hearing aid standards (322–1982) prefers the term AGC. Other terms for compression are Dynamic Range Compression, Linear Dynamic Range, High Level Compression, just to mention a few.

The term compression can be used as a generic term covering the process of compressing an amplified dynamic range into a smaller dynamic range without altering the amplitude relationships of the signal components. Neither peak clipping nor adjustable peak clipping hearing aids should be considered as compression instruments (Berger, 1984). Curran (1973) proposed that the term compression, when applied to hearing aids, should be used as a generic term to denote a particular class of hearing aid. Those hearing aids which qualify as a compression instrument should have some of the following criteria:

- The instrument utilizes a form of feedback around several gain stages in order to achieve compression
- The feedback introduces a *time delay* as the amplifier uses the feedback signal to react and adjust to changes in the input signal
- The signal is reproduced without introducing significant *non linear distortion* (harmonic or intermodulation)

Killion (1979) speculated that in order to avoid constant adjustments of the volume control, an AGC circuit is necessary. In order to introduce the minimum degradation in perceived sound quality, the operation of the compression system must be unobtrusive. Compression amplification has found wide acceptance in the broadcast and recording industries for such purposes.

The prime feature of compression systems is a negative feedback or sensing circuit which reacts to changes in the input or output level. These sensing or feedback circuits lower the gain automatically, similar to a volume control, if excessively loud sounds are fed into the instrument. Early compression designs had noticeable delays or gaps immediately following high level input sounds. This gap was caused by the fact that time was required to generate the control voltage and have the circuits gain turned down. After the loud sound passed, it took time for the gain to come back. This led to a great deal of dissatisfaction with early compression circuitry. Another important contributing factor to lack of acceptance of compression circuits, was that the research used speech intelligibility as the prime measure of compression utility. The careful studies of Barfod (1978) and of Lippmann (1978) have shown no advantage in intelligibility for compression amplification over carefully chosen linear amplification.

Perhaps the major utility of compression amplification involves nothing more than convenience. Compression amplification may alleviate the annoyance of having to readjust the volume control every few minutes. For someone who has trouble manipulating the volume control in the first place, that could well be a major factor (Killion, 1982).

In addition, the reduction of distortion with compression hearing aids will become more significant when wideband amplification gains greater acceptance.

The terms *AGC* and *AVC* are well defined and used in audio engineering. AVC stands for *Automatic Volume Control*, an acoustical term which relates to a change in intensity of a given sound pressure level. AGC or *Automatic Gain Control* is an electrical term which relates to an electrical gain of an electronic amplifier (Cole, 1978). In reality, they are almost inseparable, since one arises from the other. For example, as you turn up the hearing aid volume control, you are changing the electronic gain of the instrument which in turn produces an increase in the volume at the output of the instrument.

As was mentioned before, compression circuits use a sensing mechanism termed *negative feedback* (or watch dog circuit) which is used widely in the audio industry. Negative feedback involves

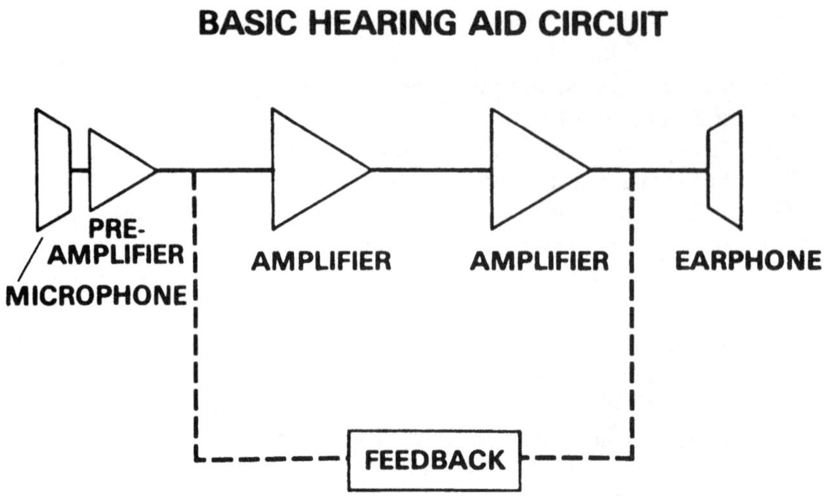

Fig. 35.

taking a small portion of the amplifier signal, turning it around so that it is exactly out of phase, and feeding it back into the input (Figure 35).

Virtually all amplifiers manufactured commercially for the audio industry use some form of negative feedback to keep the audio signals from distorting. This circuit is also known as a *feedback loop*. Since the signal which is fed back into the circuit is subtracted from the original signal, the process is called negative feedback. One obvious consequence of negative feedback is that the combined input signal is somewhat reduced; however, only a relatively small amount of distortion remains in the output. As the feedback circuit adjusts the output, it has an effect on the amplifier which is similar to that obtained by quickly adjusting the volume control except that it occurs much more rapidly and accurately than could be accomplished by manual operation.

It appears likely that any hearing aid which controls the maximum sound pressure output by means other than hard peak clipping or diode clipping could be labeled compression. We must remember that compression hearing aids contain a time factor and peak clipping hearing aids do not. Also, non-compression hearing aids will distort a puretone, and compression hearing aids have sharply reduced distortion factors.

Neither peak clipping nor adjustable peak clipping hearing aids should be considered as compression instruments. Peak clipping

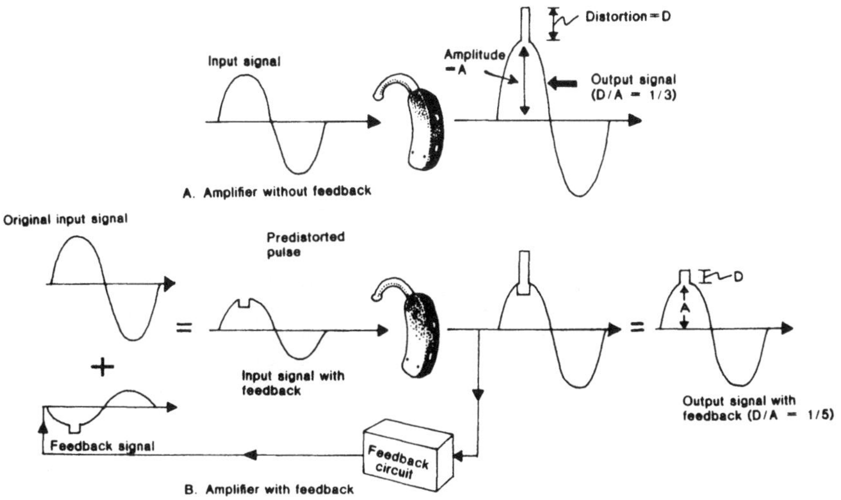

Fig. 36. (A) Amplifier without negative feedback produces a large amount of distortion. (B) Amplifier with negative feedback produces an output which has relatively less distortion. (Reprinted by permission from Johnson-Walker-Cutnell. The Science of Hi-Fidelity Second Edition—Copyright (c) 1981 by Kendall/Hunt Publishing Company.) (Illustration of hearing aid added to the figure by Libby.)

instruments have an instantaneous action without time constants. A compression circuit could be defined as a system which has been employed in efforts to reduce the dynamic range of the amplified signal to that of the individual's dynamic range.

Some compression terms should be defined at this time.

The *compression knee* or *compression threshold* is the point where the hearing aid departs from linearity and goes into compression. For example, if 70 dB is the compression threshold or knee, the instrument behaves as a linear amplifier up to that point, and only at 70 dB goes into compression. Figure 37.

The *compression ratio* (Figure 37) is a term which indicates the amount of compression taking place. The ratio is expressed arithmetically of input level change in decibels to output level change. For example, if compression is first engaged when the output reaches 123 dB SPL, and the ratio is 10:1, a 20 dB increase of gain or of level will increase the output by only 2 dB to 125 dB.

The *range of compression* indicates the limits of compression. Forcing the compression circuit to adjust beyond the limits for which it was designed will distort the sound by exceeding the limiting level. Some compression circuits can only handle 20 to 30 dB (Berger, 1984).

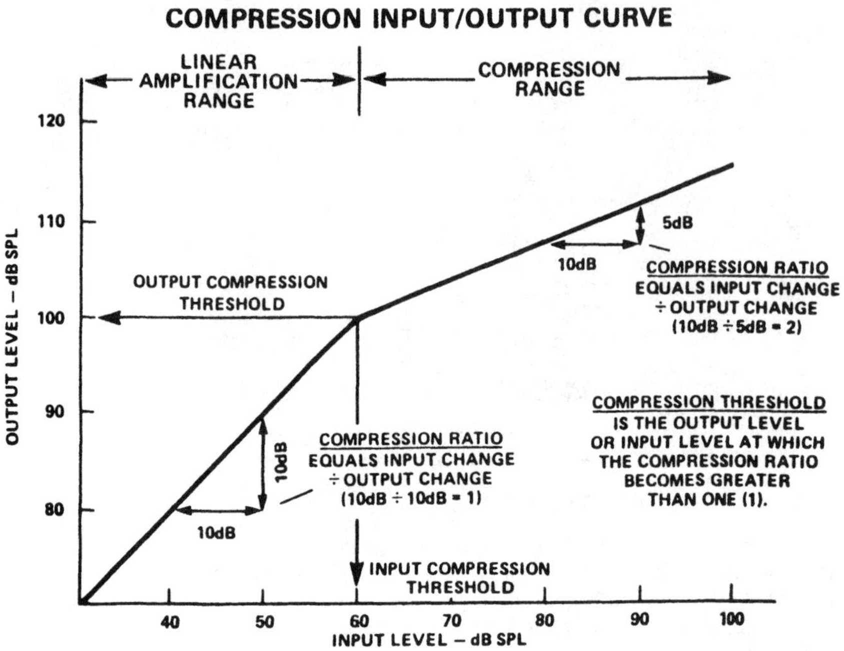

Fig. 37.

ATTACK AND RELEASE TIMES

All compression hearing aids have feedback circuits which automatically sense a change in the input signal and take appropriate action as dictated by their design. Quite simply, compression circuits take time to react. Thus, when a fork drops on a plate or a car door slams, the intense signal enters into the compression circuit, and the output will initially climb to a level above the limiting level. This level can be as high as the saturation output. The compression circuit goes into operation and automatically turns down the gain with the output level decreasing to the limiting level. The time required for the circuit to turn down the gain is called the *attack time*.

Most experts agree that the attack time should be as short as possible to prevent sudden loud sounds being amplified and causing discomfort to the wearer.

When the intense signal which activated the compression circuit is no longer present, the circuit automatically stabilizes. Again there is a brief time period involved which is known as the *release time*. Inappropriate attack and release times can break up a speech

AGC - Input/Output Curve At 60-75-90

Output sound pressure level as a function of the input sound pressure with different positions of the AGC control (g = 40 dB, f = 1000 Hz, PC = off, Tone = N)

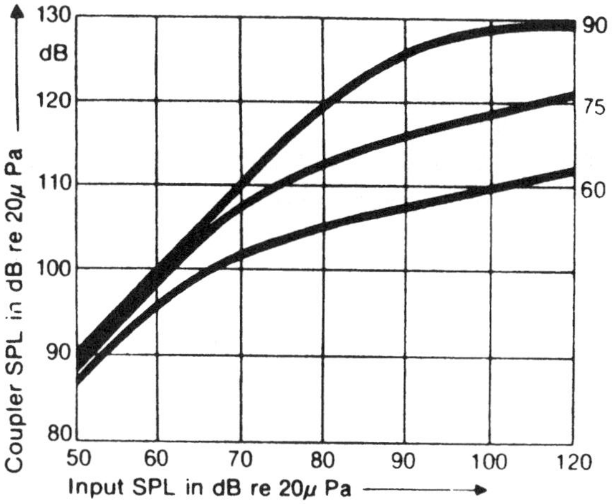

Fig. 38.

pattern because of the varied components in the pattern such as high intensity vowels and weak high frequency consonants. In some cases, some hearing aids may react to the high frequency components unchanged, which may interfere with consonant recognition. *Flutter or pumping action may occur when the release time is too rapid.*

TIME CONSTANTS

The attack and release time constants of an AGC system used to obtain the desired input-output characteristics through the operating range are an important consideration in any sound processing system (Killion, 1979). The proper choice of time constants depends a great deal on the goal set for the compression system of the hearing aid. When the goal is to maximize speech discrimination, for example, the results of Schweitzer and Causey (1977) indicate attack time should be as short as possible, and the release time should be less than 100 milliseconds and perhaps greater than 30 milliseconds.

Killion adds that when the goal is to maximize sound quality, on the other hand, the situation is much less clear. Even under ideal conditions such as found in professional recording studios, the optimum choice of attack and release time for minimum perceived distortion is highly dependent on the program material. Thus, any choice will be wrong at least part of the time. Attack times of 10 msec and release times of 150 msec have found common acceptance in the broadcast industry (Blesser and Ives, 1972). In the absence of reliable research findings on the optimum values for hearing aids (with sound quality as the goal), these values would presumably represent a reasonable first choice for the AGC system of a high fidelity hearing aid.

When the goal is to prevent audible distortion due to amplifier overload, the attack time must be as short as possible. Generally speaking, a separate compression limiting circuit system will be required for amplifier overload distortion.

If the compression limiting is expected to operate only for occasional transient peaks, the release time can also be made quite short . . . perhaps 50 msec . . . since the resulting distortion of low frequency signals will be so brief as to be unnoticed (Killion, 1979). The ideal recovery time in a compression circuit would be that in which information is not lost, but long enough to eliminate any deleterious distortion artifact (Sandlin, 1984). A compression circuit produces an unwanted effect in that it takes a fraction of a second for the signal to be fed back. This slight delay causes a loud attack period at the beginning (overshoot), followed immediately by an undershoot leading to a recovery period. Figure 39 illustrates this type of AGC operation.

INPUT AND OUTPUT COMPRESSION

There are basic families of compression: output and input. Basically, output compression has a feedback loop, after the volume control, which includes the later stages of the amplifier. The feedback loop sends a signal back to the early stages and causes the overall amplification to be reduced by a certain amount. Input compression conversely has the same feedback loop placed before the volume control so as to include only the early stages of the amplifier so that signals are reduced in intensity before they become fully amplified (Curran and Ely, 1979).

Thus the primary differences between input and output compression involves the manual volume control. Output compression has a long tradition in hearing aid manufacture, however, input compression is rapidly increasing in popularity. Output compres-

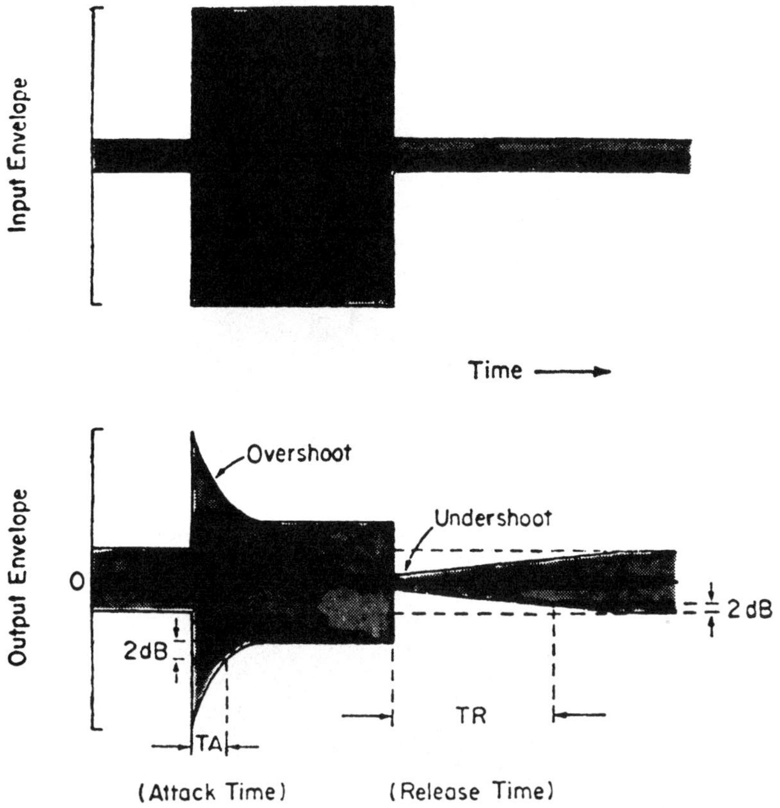

Fig. 39.

sion requires fewer components to manufacture, and is therefore less complex and less expensive.

In input compression, the circuit only starts to work when the signal exceeds a predetermined knee point (generally the level of slightly loud speech) and always stays at the knee no matter where the volume control is set (Curran, 1973). A knee for input signals around 70 dB appears to be optimal for many users; however, higher or lower knees are being used (Sung and Sung, 1982).

On the other hand, for output compression hearing aids, the intensity level where the input signal begins to activate the compression circuit changes as the volume control position is changed. So, if the user turns the volume control down, the threshold of compression (knee) actually goes up. The hearing aid will only compress (reduce gain when very loud sounds enter, perhaps as loud as 90 dB). If the user turns the volume control up to hear a

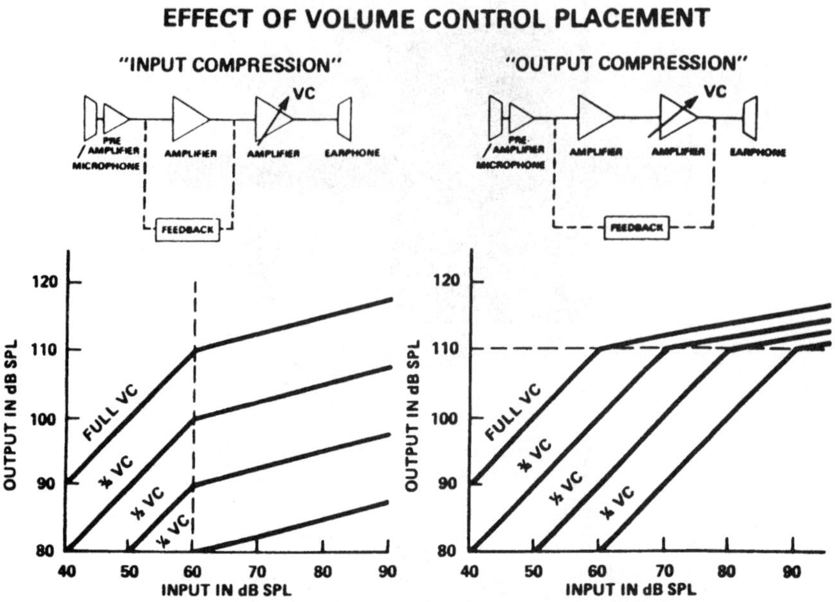

Fig. 40.

soft conversation, the hearing aid may start to compress when those very soft sounds enter the circuit, perhaps 50 to 60 dB (the level of average background noise). This may not be desirable for the hearing aid may be more in compression than not. *Thus the knee of input compression circuits remain at the same level as the volume control is rotated up or down while with output compression, the knee of the compression circuit changes as the volume control setting is changed.*

Walker and Dillion (1982) note that as long as the volume control remains fixed, input and output controlled circuits behave identically, other parameters being equal. Their differences become apparent only when the volume control setting is altered.

Again referring to Figure 40, note that as the volume control is altered, the input-output curve moves vertically for input controlled systems and horizontally for output controlled systems. Thus for input controlled systems, the knee at which compression begins to operate is independent of the volume control position.

Goldberg (1977) notes that input compression amplification has many advantages over linear or output compression. For one, frequency modification can be made within the compression loop. Response changes outside the loop can also be made. The combination of the two gives the designer a broad range of compression controlled responses. When frequency modifications are made outside the loop, after the volume control or prior to the controlled gain stages, the compression function won't change the overall frequency response characteristics. When frequency modifications are made inside the compression loop, the compression function will change the frequency response.

ADAPTIVE COMPRESSION

Adaptive Compression (Variable Release Compression) is an advanced compression circuit, which helps maintain the signal-to-noise ration present at the input by automatically adjusting its compression release time according to the duration of noise in the environment. For short duration noise, in an otherwise quiet environment, limited action occurs and the return to linear operation is rapid. If the noise persists, the release time becomes progressively longer to a maximum of one second. In effect, the hearing instrument reduces the gain for the duration of the noise, ignoring short term fluctuations (Teder, 1987). This eliminates the "pumping and breathing effect", which occurs in conventional signal time compression circuits. (Figure 41A illustrates adaptive compression.)

Fikret-Pasa (1993) investigated the use of adaptive compression with a group of eight sensorineural hearing impaired patients. Her conclusions were that adaptive compression provided an improvement in speech intelligibility and perceived quality over peak clipping.

Telex, Etymotic Research (K-AMP), Starkey, Phonak, and others use some form of adaptive compression or variable release compression in their hearing instruments.

ADDITIONAL COMMENTS

A compression instrument may be classified according to the principal purpose for which it is used on a given hearing aid subject.

1. It may be fitted primarily to prevent and protect the hearing impaired person from being exposed to excessively loud, distorted signals which might otherwise be amplified beyond the threshold of discomfort. Compression aids designed for this purpose have been referred to as *compression limiters*. Compression limiters use an amplitude compressor with a high compression ratio in which the threshold of compression is set so that the compression does not begin to operate until just below the maximum sound pressure level that is intended to

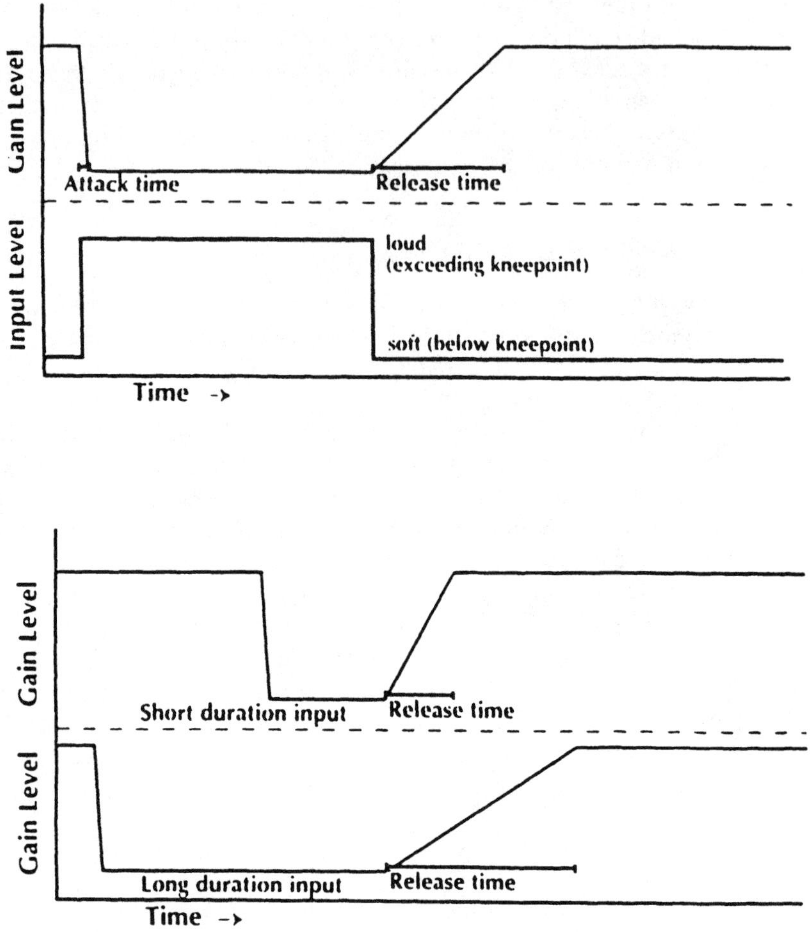

Fig. 41A.

reach the wearer. Compression limiters have found wide use for persons who have low tolerance levels of sound. (Goldberg, 1977).

2. The instruments may be fitted primarily to amplify the normal range of intensities and reproduce them in miniature for subjects having a restricted dynamic range. However, the average long term average presentation level is kept near that corresponding to maximum intelligibility. This type, according to Villchur (1978), can be termed *slow acting, full range amplitude compression.* The compression threshold is made low

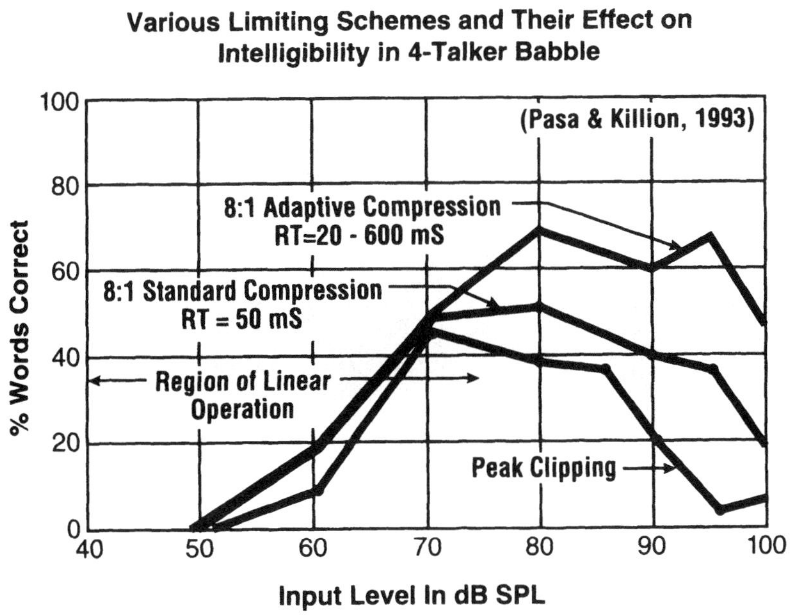

Fig. 41B.

enough so that the compression operates over all or most of the dynamic range of speech, but the response of the compressor is slow, so that it cannot reduce the differences in level among speech elements that succeed one another rapidly.

3. The third type is mainly concerned with altering the short term intensity relationship among speech elements to improve intelligibility. This type of compressor must act rapidly enough to respond to level variations associated with transitions between speech sounds. All the signals of interest to aid the wearer fall within the working range of the compressor. Every possible input level is transformed to a different output level. This type of compression action can be classified as *fast, full range amplitude compression—also known as phonemic or syllabic compression.*

To recapitulate, some compression hearing aids are used chiefly to provide a ceiling to limit at a specific level the signal which reaches the listener's ear. Compression limiting instruments usually achieve this effect without adding an appreciable amount of distortion to the amplified signal (Curran, 1973).

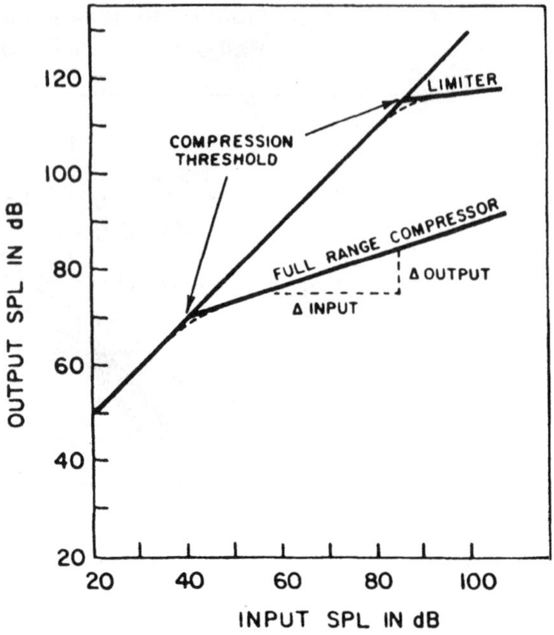

Fig. 42. Relationship between signal input and signal output in compression amplification. The 45° diagonal represents linear amplification with 30 dB of gain. The compression ratio (input/output) of the full range compressor is 3: The compression ratio of the limiter is 10. The output of the full range compressor would normally by subject to further amplification. (With permission E. Villchur, Auditory Management of Hearing Impaired Children, Ross and Giolas Eds. University Park Press, 1978.)

The other two classes, slow acting full range compression and fast acting full range compression perform compression limiting only as a secondary characteristic. Refer to Figure 41.

Goldberg (1977) grouped compression amplification into compression limiting, semi-log compression, and log compression. Compression limiting devices limit the signal at a given level, without adding substantial distortion. Semi-log compression does the same thing, but in a softer manner.

Basically, the limiting action occurs gradually, rather than suddenly, and extends over a larger dynamic range to its upper limit. Log compression amplifiers, which have the greatest dynamic range of all, increase the sound to a definite mathematical relationship. For a compression ratio of .5 an input increase of 10 dB

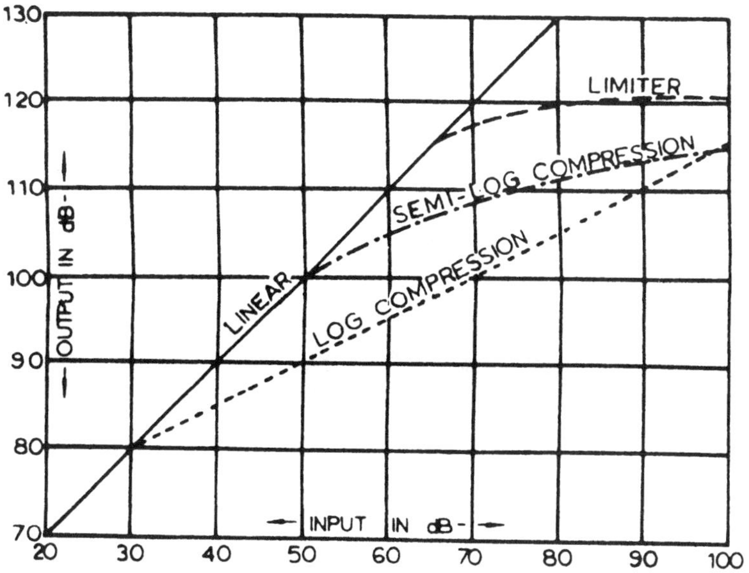

Fig. 43A. Amplifier Input-Output Functions. (With permission Hy Goldberg, 1977.)

will increase the output signal only 5 dB. All log compression amplifiers are basically input compressors with pre-established log functions such as ratios of .7, .5, .4, etc. A .7 ratio translates into a ±10 dB change in input.

Curran (1981) developed a unique input compression function which employs a frequency dependent circuit. Essentially, the system described has a different compression knee for different frequencies. The rationale for a frequency dependent approach to input compression is that an excessive across the board reduction in gain might adversely affect the critical high frequency range which is important to speech intelligibility. Curran hypothesized that since most of the noise in a listener's environment is of higher intensity in the low frequencies, fixing the low frequency thresholds of compression at 60 to 70 dB SPL across frequency tends to cause frequent unnecessary reductions of overall gain in "cocktail party" and similar listening environments when low frequencies predominate.

CLASSIFYING AUTOMATIC SIGNAL PROCESSORS

Killion, Staab, and Preves (1990) proposed a classification system for level dependent frequency response automatic signal processing circuits (LDFR); circuits that automatically change not only the gain, but also the frequency response of the hearing instrument as a function of the input signal. In contrast, the traditional automatic signal processing circuits, ie. the automatic gain control (AGC), or compression circuits, reduce gain at high levels (compression limiting) and/or increased gain at low levels (wide dynamic range compression), but do not change the frequency response of the hearing aid in the process. Well defined terms for fixed frequency response (FFR) automatic signal processing circuits already exist (Figure 43A).

TYPES OF LEVEL DEPENDENT FREQUENCY RESPONSE CIRCUITS (LDRF)

1. BILL (Type 1)

Bass increases at low levels (bass decreases at high input levels). This type of ASP describes the operation of circuits, which provide relatively more bass response for low level inputs than for high level inputs. The BILL circuit is intended for wearers who frequently find themselves in noisy environments, especially when low frequency noise predominates. These hearing aids have been labeled automatic signal processing (ASP) and automatic noise reduction (ANR) to name a few types. BILL hearing aids comprise the majority of commercially available noise reduction hearing aids. An example of a BILL hearing aid is the MANHATTAN Circuit (Preves, Sigelman, 1987). This device is a voltage controlled high pass filter that is activated at approximately 60 dB SPL and becomes more high pass with increasing levels of background noise by varying the filter slope (Figure 43B).

2. TILL (Type 2)

Treble increases at low levels. This type of ASP describes the operation of circuits such as the KAMP, which provide more treble response for low level inputs than for high level inputs. The TILL circuit is intended for wearers with high frequency loss, who typically need more high frequency gain for quiet sounds than they do for loud sounds. An amount of high frequency gain may produce a harsh or shrill sound in a linear hearing aid may become quite acceptable if the treble boost is automatically reduced for high level inputs (Figure 43C).

Killion reported on his design of the KAMP circuit; a four stage compression amplifier to provide high fidelity over a broad range of input levels. This design is based on the premise that hearing impaired subjects have normal growth of loudness for high level

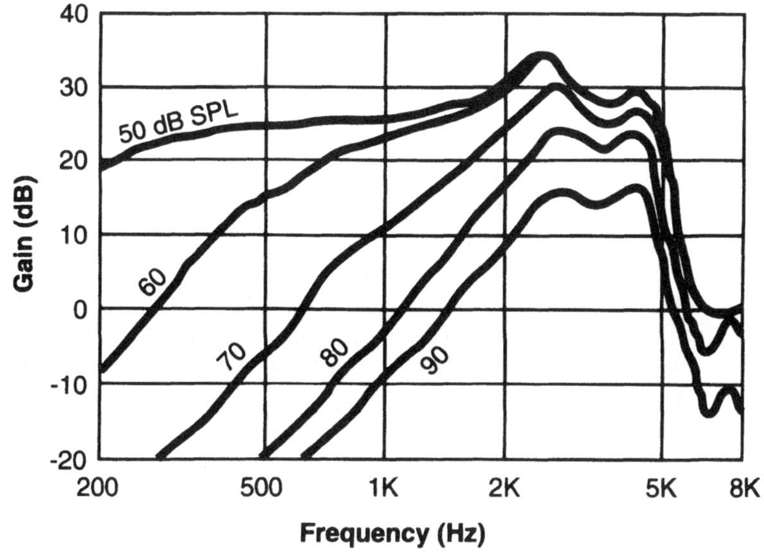

Fig. 43B.

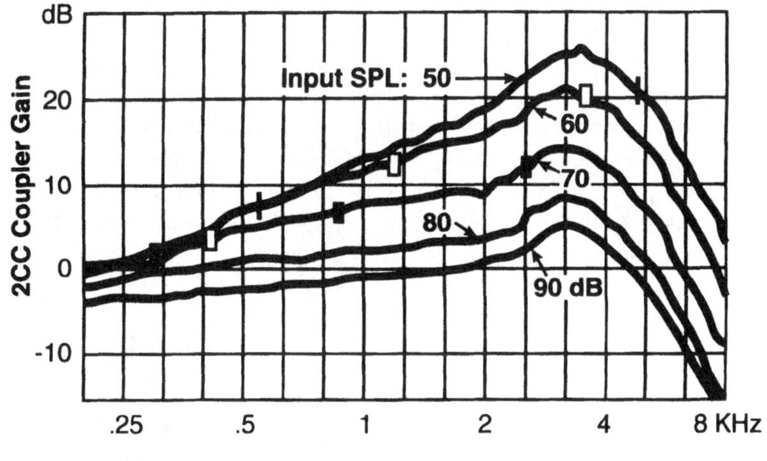

Fig. 43C.

stimuli. Therefore, intense sound should be "acoustically invisible" and, thus, not amplified. RESOUND has produced a programmable hearing aid, which also has a TILL circuit. The K-AMP is appropriate for mild to moderate losses. The RESOUND circuit can be fitted to more severe losses.

3. PILL (Type 3)

(Programmable increases at low levels) is the most versatile; not only can it be adjusted to exhibit either BILL or TILL type processing, but each of its independent processing channels can ignore strong interference in another channel. Some hearing aids can be classified as automatic programmable (increase at low levels) (APILL) (Fabry, 1991). These devices use multi-band compression or frequency dependent compression, and allow the user to program various hearing aid characteristics such as overall gain, high and low frequency cut-off or cross over to arrive at a signal frequency response that is programmed into the hearing aid. Examples are Siemens' TRITON, or the Starkey, RESOLUTION CIRCUIT.

Another group of programmables are the user adjustable programmables; (increases at low levels) (U-PILL). These hearing aids include the THREE M MEMORY MATE, and WIDEX QUATRO.

Worthy of mention is the OTICON MULTI-FOCUS, which is a two channel, adaptive, dynamic range compression instrument, which performs automatically. The instrument provides for linear amplification of the high frequency components of speech, and simultaneously provides for loudness restoration of sounds in the low frequency bands.

Multi-channel technology is available in the ARGOSY 3-Channel Clock Circuitry, which provides versatile in office frequency response shaping without the use of computers, programming boxes, or remote controls. The 3-Channel series can be adjusted to use virtually any frequency response in any of three channels. It is available in K-AMP and Manhattan circuitry (Preves, 1994). (Figure 43D)

The Argosy 3-CHANNEL-K-AMP Hearing Instrument

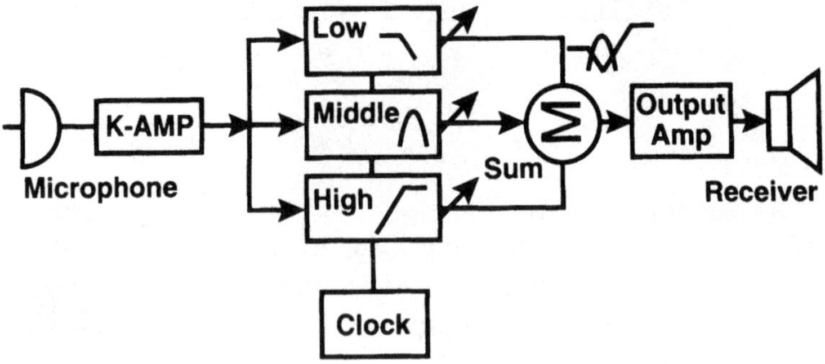

Fig. 43 D

SUMMARY AND DISCUSSION

Hearing aid engineers can design systems having any combination of compression features as has been described in this chapter. It is the responsibility of the hearing aid professional to decide what particular combination of features the client requires. Rational decisions concerning the parameters of hearing aid compression amplifiers can only be made after careful consideration of one's reason for using compression. Let us summarize some of the reasons for using compression.

1. Increased tolerance problems
2. Small dynamic ranges
3. Control of distortion
4. Recruitment problems
5. Impulse noise control
6. Signal to noise improvement
7. Speech intelligibility enhancement

The above reasons for using compression should be related to the following compression options.

1. Compression Threshold (Knee)	High or low?
2. Compression Ratio	Gradual or sharp?
3. Compression Range	Narrow or wide?
4. Attack Time	Fast, moderate, or rapid?
5. Release Time	Fast, moderate, or rapid?
6. Input or output compression	Input or output?

The compression problem is, therefore, a question of selecting the combination of compression characteristics which will provide the most benefit for the individual listener. The research concerned with compression has not been clear as to the benefits of each compression option, and therefore, further research is necessary before firmer conclusions can be reached. However, the following limited recommendations and trends are apparent. Compression should be as unobtrusive as possible and not occur unnecessarily. Loud low frequency sounds should be reduced and generally should not activate the compression circuit to allow the low energy high frequency sounds to pass *comfortably* through. Compression amplification should significantly reduce overload distortion, reduce tolerance problems for loud sounds, reduce excessive manipulation of the volume control, control impulsive noise, and improve the general fidelity of the hearing aid system. It also appears that we are close to improving speech intelligibility in noise, and hopefully improving the problem of recruitment.

HEARING AID HEADROOM & SOUND QUALITY

The sound quality of hearing aids is frequently judged to be inferior to high fidelity audio systems. The problem is partially caused by inadequate headroom resulting from the low voltage battery (1.3 volts) used in hearing aids. Headroom is defined as the difference between the level, at which saturation occurs, and the sum of input level and hearing aid gain (Preves, 1989). Hearing aids with inadequate headroom often have poor sound quality because of the non-linear distortion created by peak-clipping. These distortions, typically occur in high noise level environments. Sometimes the processed speech sound quality is poor, and the listening experience so annoying and fatiguing, that in noisy environments hearing aids are often turned off and removed.

Reducing the gain at high input levels using compression and an adaptive frequency response circuit, can preserve headroom. Another method of preserving headroom is by raising saturation sound pressure levels with push-pull and Class D type output stages (Carlson, 1988). To maximize headroom and improve sound quality, hearing aids of the future will incorporate more compression and adaptive frequency response circuits, and more Class D and Class B output stages (Preves, 1992).

HEARING AID SYSTEMS

BINAURAL AMPLIFICATION

In most research investigations and textbooks, attention is usually devoted to the physiological, neurological, and psychoacoustic advantages of binaural hearing, while little attention is devoted to the actual binaural instruments. Conceivably, the survival of early man depended on his instinctive recognition that both ears contributed to the listening experience. It is plausible that early man used two hands held shells, animal horns, and other contrivances to increase the acoustical signal. From the first electric hearing aid designed by M. R. Hutchinson in 1902, through the evolution of the first vac-

Lesson 17 304-317

uum tubes, to the wearable carbon aids, the devices were generally considered too bulky and heavy to be worn as binaural devices (Johnson, 1980). However, the use of two earphones connected to one amplifier and one microphone, in what was later termed as a Y-cord, was possible. Early transistorized eyeglass instruments were of particular interest for binaural use (and still are) since the mechanical arrangement provided ample space for amplifier, microphone, earphone, and battery for each ear. Electroacoustically, each ear could be fitted independently, yet with the convenience of each hearing aid being joined together as one instrument.

Very early in the development of electric hearing aids, two earphones, one for each ear, were attached to single amplifier output. A single microphone provided the input to the amplifier. In this system shown in Figure 44, two earphones were connected in either parallel or series arrangement to the amplifier output. The arrangement is known as a *Y-cord system*. The acoustic signal from the one microphone and single channel amplifier results in a signal to each of the two earphones which are identical in sensitivity, frequency characteristic, and phase. Therefore, a true binaural experience of localization and spatial orientation does not occur. The Y-cord fitting is also referred to as *pseudo-binaural or bilateral*. The Y-cord system is almost always used with body type hearing aids. Most of the Y-cords today are of the parallel variety. A 3–6 dB drop in output is typical of a Y-cord arrangement.

Despite its limitations, a Y-cord fitting provides for bilateral stimulation in comparison to a monaural fitting. With the development of lightweight wearable headworn hearing aids, came the first opportunity to provide instrumentation more directly related to the two-eared hearing process, one instrument being utilized for each ear. Each instrument has a microphone, amplifier and receiver with no electrical connection between the two instruments. Binaural hearing aid fitting, despite a slow start in the 1950's and 1960's, has gained momentum, and in 1984 amounted to 34% of hearing aid sales in the United States; in 1994 binaural fittings amounted to more than 50% of sales. Historically, it was difficult to demonstrate significant improvement in speech discrimination with addition of a second hearing aid. Binaural users, however, have reported that speech sounded better, or was more natural with the use of two hearing aids. As Pollack (1980) notes, one consistent observation throughout the literature regarding binaural amplification is that while its advantages often cannot be demonstrated clinically, user reports, after a period of experience with two hearing aids, often strongly point to the subjective benefits. The key is an adjustment period. Zelnick (1970) states that the idea of adjustment raises the

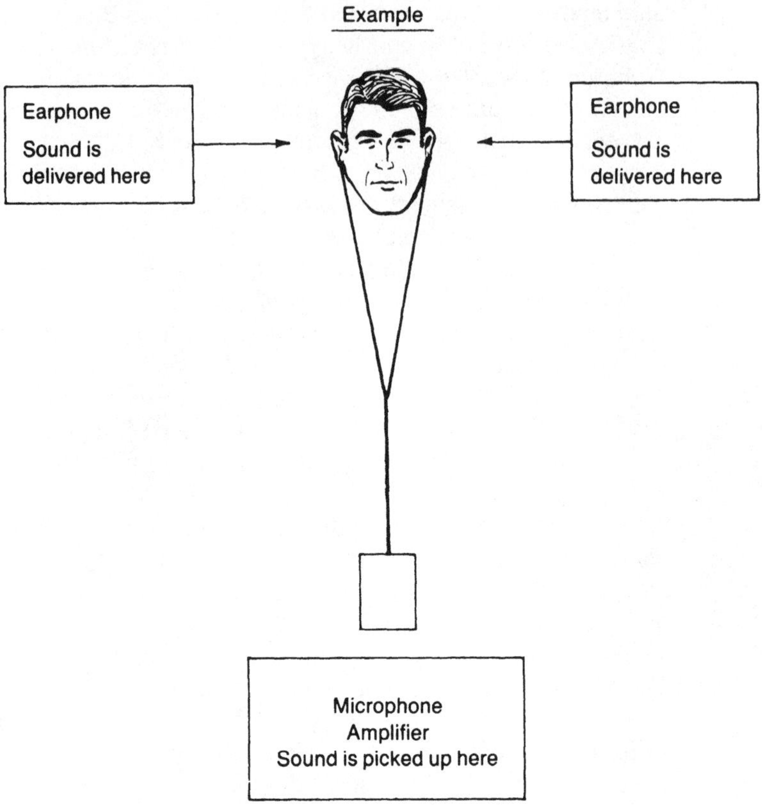

Fig. 44. A Bilateral Output ("Y" Cord fitting) Hearing Aid is a conventional (body type) hearing aid. Sound is picked up byone microphone and then sent to both ears via a "Y" Cord. (With permission James H. Johnson, Binaural Hearing and Amplification, Libby, Ed., Zenetron, 1980.)

argument of whether or not to fit both instruments immediately. Proponents of immediate fitting argue that since the user is going to eventually wear two hearing aids, he should start with fittings that provide the most advantageous hearing aid response. From the start, the user should learn to use and live with binaural amplification.

In concluding this section on binaural hearing aids, consider this quote from Denis Byrne (1980):

> "It is difficult to understand why so many hearing aid professionals seek to deny or minimize the evidence for binaural fitting, especially considering that much hearing aid practice is readily undertaken on the basis of untested, though testable, axioms. I venture to suggest that if all the widely accepted hearing aid practices were examined

critically, comparatively few would be found to have as much scientific justification in terms of rationale and research findings as binaural fitting."

For extensive reading on the subject of binaural amplification covering the rationale and the research, the reader is referred to the two volume "Binaural Hearing and Amplification" by Libby (1980).

CROS AND BICROS

The acronym *CROS* denotes the term *Contralateral Routing of Signals* . . . originally conceived and developed by Harford and Barry (1965). Wullenstein and Wigand (1962) published the results of a similar arrangement but did not pursue the matter. The CROS was developed as an answer to persons with unilateral hearing loss, who complained of major difficulties; the inability to adequately understand speech signals originating on the poorer side of the head, the inability to localize sound, and the significant difficulties of understanding in noise because of the masking influence of the noisy environment (E. Johnson, 1975). Some of these difficulties arise from the *head shadow* effect in which sound originating on the impaired side is attenuated by the shielding effects of the head. The research has revealed that the head shadow effect can reduce the higher frequencies over 2000 Hz by as much as 15–20 dB. This, in turn, influences word recognition negatively. In addition, if there is significant noise, this will tend to mask the signal at the better ear. Harford and Dobbs (1966) concluded that CROS could be used to make communication more effective for individuals who function quite well in many situations, but experience difficulty in some special situations, due to their unilateral impairment.

The application of the CROS principle is shown on Figure 45. A signal originating on the side of the impaired ear is picked up by the microphone routed across the head, by means of wiring or radio transmission, amplified on the side of the better ear, routed through the earphone on that side into the ear canal. The transmission is accomplished by means of an open tubing rather than an occluded earmold.

This allows sound that would normally be heard by the better ear to still be heard on that side, but in addition, the signal from the impaired side is also perceived. This principle can be applied either with eyeglasses or behind-the-ear hearing aids (E. Johnson, 1975).

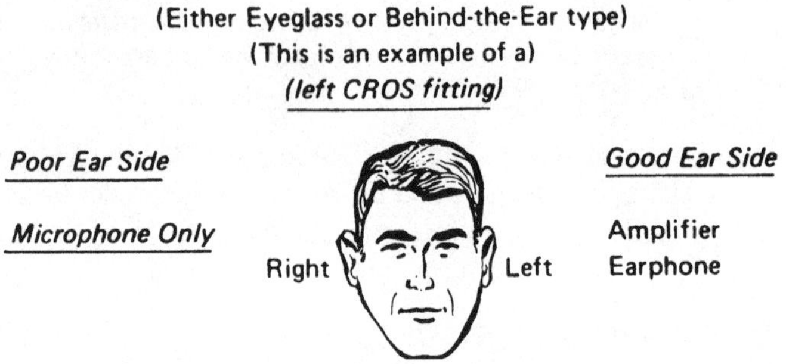

Fig. 45. A CROS (Contralateral Routing of Signals) hearing aid fitting looks like this.

Hodgson (1981) noted that the original purpose of the non-occluding earmold used with CROS was to allow unamplified sound to enter the unilateral's normal ear. However, there are additional dividends: open or no mold fittings (1) reduce low frequency amplification and thereby reduce tolerance problems and the effects of upward spread of masking in noisy situations: (2) retain the useful resonance of the ear canal which is lost when the ear is occluded with a standard earmold and (3) facilitate high frequency amplification. Lybarger (1967) estimated that amplification below 1000 Hz is almost eliminated, and ear canal resonance is retained.

This principle can also be applied to a person with sufficient loss in the better ear to also receive amplification, but with one ear unaidable. This modification of the CROS principle is called BICROS and is illustrated in the Figure 47.

The extra microphone is placed on the side of the unaidable ear, and transmits a signal from that side of the head to the aidable ear. At the same time, amplification is provided in routine fashion for

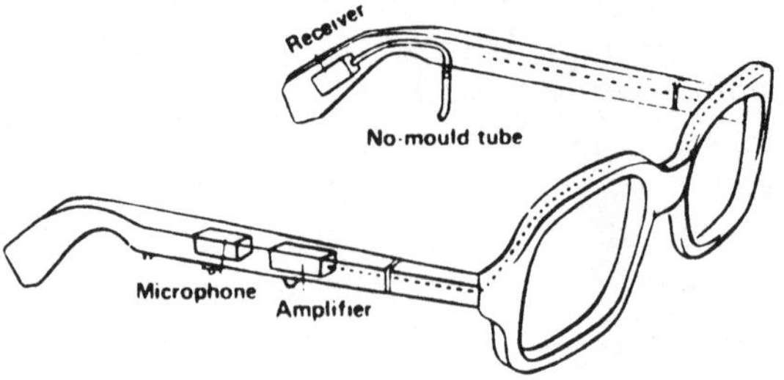

Fig. 46. CROS eyeglass arrangement with no mold fitting.

A *BICROS* Hearing aid fitting looks like this:

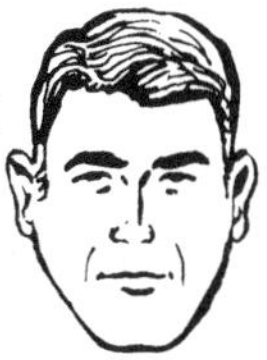

Fig. 47. This type of fitting is sometimes used for a bilateral hearing loss, however, most often you would use a binaural fitting.

sounds reaching the aidable ear directly. BICROS can also be built into eyeglasses, with the off side microphone located in the temple bar on the side of the unaidable ear. The use of an occluding earmold is usually necessary to avoid feedback.

IN-THE-EAR HEARING AIDS

When the first in-the-ear (ITE) instruments were introduced in the late 1960's and early 1970's, component limitations and early ideas in these designs combined with a lack of venting and response modifications collectively limited the effectiveness of these hearing aids. For example, the magnetic microphone, then in use instead of the electret, often presented feedback problems, low gain, and restricted frequency range capabilities. Also, the small 312 and 212 batteries as used in most units, did not always provide an acceptable milliampere-hour capacity (Preves and Griffing, 1976).

While research has not established significant performance superiority of ITE instruments, many people prefer them for their cosmetic and psychological advantages.

ACOUSTIC CONSIDERATIONS OF ITE HEARING AIDS

Lybarger and Baron (1965) noted that a concha microphone location has some advantages over behind the hear and over the ear locations in providing better gain. Berland and Neilsen (1969) also found that the microphone location at the concha is superior. Of course, this fact has implications for ITE and canal hearing aids. Killion (1980) also noted that the method which in some cases would come closest to true directional hearing would be a binaural fitting with matched amplifiers and microphones in the concha

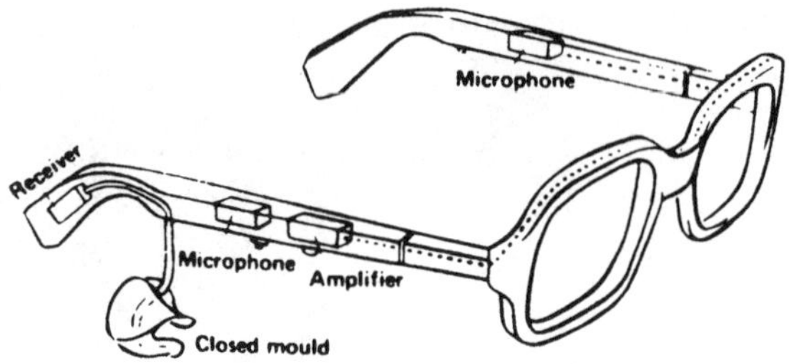

Fig. 48. BICROS eyeglass arrangement.

area of the ear canal. However, the concha should not be entirely filled so that the pinna effect of the outer ear would be preserved. There is some evidence that a hearing aid that uses the focusing and resonance capability of the outer ear provides what can be regarded as greater signal-to-noise ratio for input to the hearing aid microphone. An ITE tends to use the natural physiology of the ear to the benefit of the user. The shorter receiver tubing length of the typical ITE hearing aid results in sensitivity at 2 kHz that is 15–20 dB greater than at 500 Hz. This factor tends to move the primary resonance peak of the ITE closer to 2.7 kHz (which is the primary resonance of the ear). The typical behind the ear (BTE) hearing aid, however, has its primary resonance around 1000 Hz. By external damping procedures and internal acoustic modification, the typical BTE can now easily have its primary resonance peak moved to 2.7 kHz.

CANAL HEARING AIDS

Small, high quality components make construction of this state of the art product available. The cosmetic appeal of the canal aid is undeniably one of its greatest attractions. People who feel they can improve their ability to hear, and yet not have the hearing aid visible, appear to be the interested clients for this type of hearing instrument. (Regan, Hoke et al, 1984).

Besides cosmetic appeal, there are other advantages for canal hearing aids. Less gain and output is typically required for canal aid fittings. Early canal aid fittings, using the same formulas applied to ITE aids, tended to provide too much gain and output. However, it was soon learned that the smaller ear canal cavity, formed by the extension of the sound bore of the aid into the ear canal, resulted in greater sound pressure levels being developed at the eardrum, hence less gain was required to do the job.

Lesson 18
311-317

The canal aid weighs about one-third less than the ITE and has less difficulty with wind noise. Better telephone usage has been reported. Feedback is generally not a problem. The phone can be held in a natural and comfortable position and the clarity of sounds has been reported as good. Using components that are similar to ITE and BTE technology canal aids offer about the same amount of reliability.

The disadvantages are, for one, the higher cost of manufacturing, and this additional cost is passed on to the consumer. However, the cosmetic appeal appears to be powerful enough for many people to be willing to pay the higher price. Longer manufacturing time is to be expected. The constraints of a given individual's ear canal and size and the restrictions of current canal aid technology provide very definite limitations in fitting flexibility. There is obviously less space for more sophisticated circuitry (such as input compression, push pull circuits, etc.), less room for trimpots, as well as markedly reduced options for venting. The client's ability to manipulate the smaller components is certainly a constraint for many elderly individuals.

Another problem is if the ear canal is too small or too shallow, the manufacturer may not have sufficient space to accommodate the required components. If the individual ear canal has a sharp bend, it may be difficult to fit a canal hearing aid. Typical performance characteristics for canal aids are gain ranges from 10 dB to 35 dB and SSPL ranges from 90 to 110 dB. Some loss in the low frequencies may be desirable to help reduce the occlusion effect and feeling of fullness.

In conclusion, Regan (1984) noted that reduction in component size, improvement in component performance, and better application techniques by manufacturers, as well as dispensers familiar with custom products promise to make the canal aid even better in the future.

COMPLETELY IN-THE-CANAL (CIC) HEARING INSTRUMENTS

A recent development is the completely in-the-canal (CIC) hearing instrument. It is the smallest and most cosmetically acceptable hearing instrument ever manufactured. CIC stands for *completely in the canal*; meaning that the visible end of the hearing aid is 1 or 2 mm inside the entrance of the ear canal (Gudmundsen, 1994, Staab, 1994).

A CIC instrument that terminates 1 or 2 mm from the tympanic membrane has been referred to as "peritympanic" hearing aid. The typical CIC instrument terminates 4 or 5 mm from the tympanic membrane and is beyond the second bend of the ear canal (Staab, 1994). The CIC instrument usually includes a set screw volume control. Linear D amplifiers and K-AMP circuits are usually used in the CIC. Removal of a CIC instrument is performed by the use of a thin plastic removal handle.

16 Potential Advantages of CICs (Mueller, 1994):

1. **Increased gain:** A hearing aid that is truly completely in the canal allows the natural acoustic effects of the pinna and concha to occur, which increases the high-frequency input to the microphone.
2. **Increased output:** A deep-fitting CIC hearing aid significantly reduces the residual volumes, resulting in increased ear canal SPL.
3. **Reduced distortion:** Greater real-ear output means that less amplifier gain is required, which can reduce the occurrence of saturation-induced distortion.
4. **Reduction of the occlusion effect:** A secure fit deep in the ear canal reduces the cartilaginous vibrations, thus minimizing the hearing aid occlusion effect.
5. **Reduction of acoustic feedback:** A receiver outlet closer to the eardrum, a secure fit, and minimal venting help reduce acoustic feedback.
6. **Ease of removal:** Its small size and convenient string for extraction make removal of a CIC easier than removal of most in-the-ear or in-the-canal instruments (If the ear canal is relatively straight, insertion might also be easier.)
7. **Improved localization:** Placing the hearing aid microphone in the ear canal allows for more natural pinna effects, thereby improving sound localization.
8. **Reduced wind noise:** A microphone recessed in the ear canal is less affected by wind.
9. **Comfort:** Good impression-taking procedures and precise shell construction usually result in a very comfortable fit (although a short adjustment time may be necessary).
10. **Fewer wax problems for receivers:** A long CIC canal extends beyond the major area of cerumen production and accumulation. (Of course, you need to start with a clean ear canal!)
11. **No volume-control wheel:** Increases high-frequency gain, reduced occurrence of saturation-induced distortion, and au-

tomatic gain-control circuitry help eliminate the need for a volume-control wheel.

12. **Telephone use:** Reduced acoustic feedback during telephone use because less gain is required and because the microphone is recessed deeper in the canal, which results in less shadowing from the telephone receiver. Also, CIC wearers find it more comfortable to place the telephone receiver against their ear.
13. **Listening with headsets:** Like the telephone receiver, other professional or recreational listening devices can be placed on or in the ear with reduced acoustic feedback problems. Even stethoscopes (with special tips) can be used successfully.
14. **Security of fit:** The secure fit of CIC instruments makes them ideal for use in strenuous work or recreational activities.
15. **Use during sleep:** The secure fit, comfort, and reduced acoustic feedback advantages of CIC's allows them to be used during sleep, providing for continued monitoring of speech, environmental sounds, and warning signals.
16. **Cosmetic:** CIC's are barely noticeable in the ear.

ACOUSTIC ADVANTAGES OF CIC INSTRUMENTS:

Miniaturization of hearing aid electronics and power sources, along with a better understanding of hearing aid acoustics, has made possible progressive size reductions for BTE to ITE to ITC hearing instruments.

It only seems natural that the inevitable next step in this progression is a smaller hearing instrument that fits deeper in the ear canal (Agnew, 1994). Not only does this type of fitting provide high cosmetic appeal, but placement of the hearing aid beyond the second bend (deep in the ear canal) provides several major acoustic advantages.

When the canal tip of any hearing aid (or earmold) extends only as far as the fleshy outer part of the ear canal, amplification of low frequency vibrations in the user's own voice in the occluded ear canal produces an echoing, hollow, unnatural sound. This is called the occlusion effect, because it results from partial or total occlusion of the ear canal (Figure 49A).

As the hearing aid is inserted further in the ear canal, the tip of the hearing aid is fitted into the bony portion of the ear canal, thus

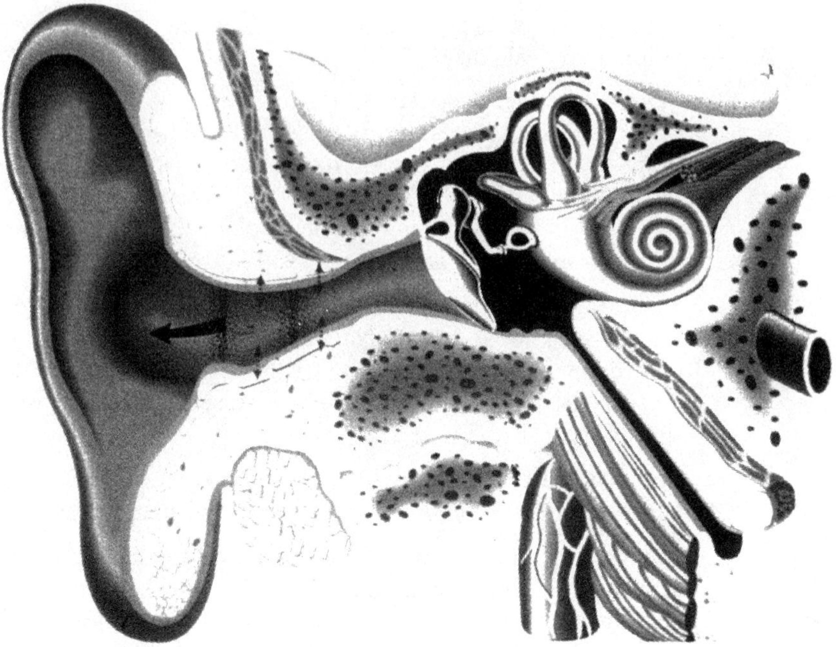

Fig. 49A. The Occlusion Effect

changing the interaction with the ear itself and reducing or eliminating the occlusion effect (Figure 49B).

A second advantage is that the residual volume of air (in the ear canal) between the tip of the hearing aid and the tympanic membrane (V3) is much smaller with a CIC instrument than with a conventional ITE (Figure 49C). This allows the hearing aid to operate at lower acoustic power with resultant lower distortion and sound quality improvement for the user. This results in higher headroom capabilities and lower distortion (Agnew, 1994).

Theoretically every time the V3 is halved, the sound pressure at the tympanic membrane is increased by 6 dB. While the V3, for a typically ITE fitting might be on the order of lcc, it may only be 0.25cc for a deeply inserted CIC hearing aid. This reduces the V3 fourfold, which results in a potential gain increase of 12 dB for the CIC, just due to the V3 cavity size reduction. (Figures 49D, 49E)

Another major advantage of the CIC is the deep placement of the hearing aid microphone in the ear canal. The wearer is better able to use the natural acoustic cues provided by the pinna. As a result, reports show improved speech understanding in the

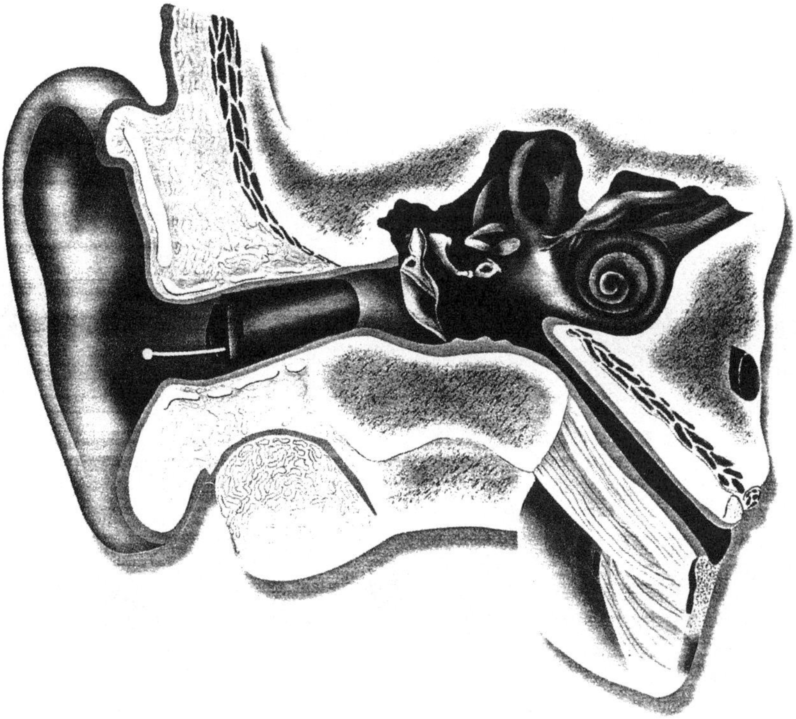

Fig. 49B. Completely-In-The-Canal

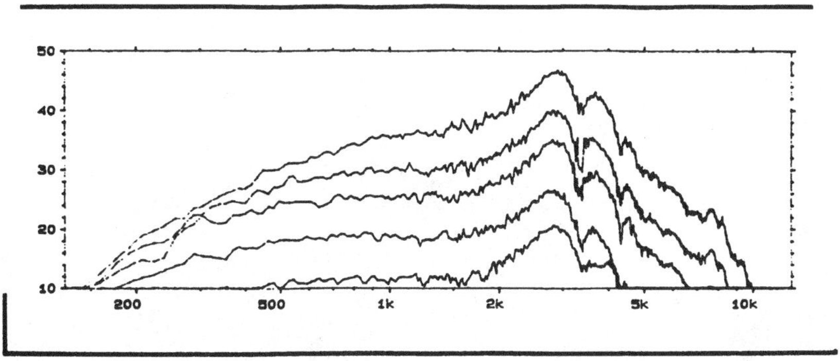

Fig. 49C. The effect of a reduced V3 cavity on a Starkey Tympanette on KEMAR. From lower curve up = 2cc, 1cc, 0.5cc, 0.25cc and 0.12cc.

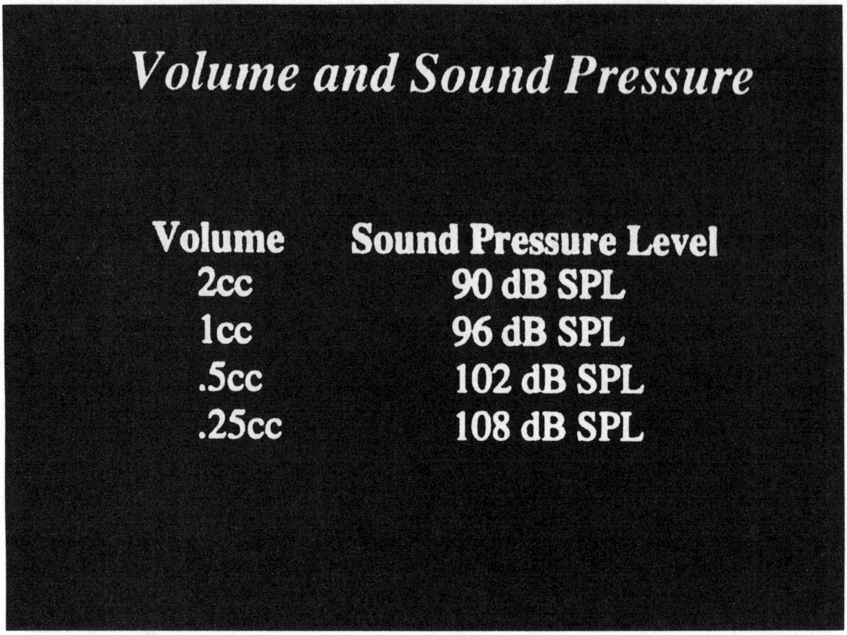

Fig. 49D. Volume and Sound Pressure

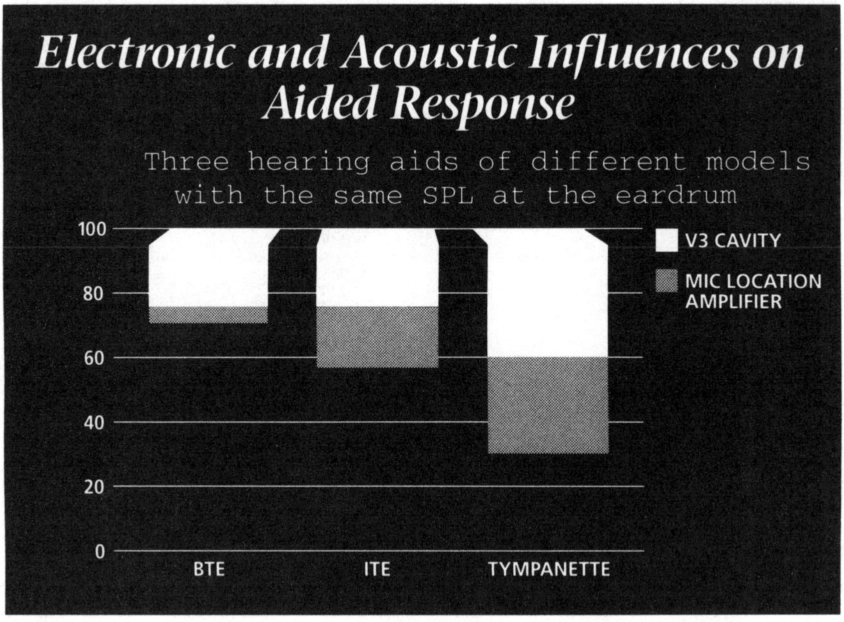

Fig. 49E. Electronic and Acoustic Influences on Aided Response presence of noise, elimination of wind noise, and use of the telephone without feedback (Orchik, 1994, Staab, 1992).

PREDICTING 2cc COUPLER GAIN FOR CIC INSTRUMENTS

Preves, 1994, reported tests which are helpful in predicting the 2cc coupler gain required for a CIC instrument to match prescriptive fitting formulae targets. For a given audiogram, one would expect a CIC hearing instrument to require 14.3 dB less overall gain than an ITE instrument and 8.3 less gain than an ITC instrument in the 2cc coupler. Since much of the increase in output SPL provided by a CIC instrument is in the high frequencies, proportionally less high frequency gain would be required, to provide the required insertion gain for a given audiogram for a CIC instrument than from ITE and ITC instruments.

CONCLUSION

The most important factor in obtaining a properly fitting CIC instrument is to take an accurate impression that extends well beyond the second bend of the ear canal. The constraints of a given individual's ear canal provide definite limitations to fitting flexibility.

If the ear canal is too narrow (or too small), the manufacturer may not have sufficient space to accommodate the required components. There is obviously less space for the volume canal, trimpots, etc. The client's ability to manipulate the smaller components is certainly a limitation for many elderly individuals.

Despite its limitations, the CIC instrument is rapidly gaining in popularity. The only drawback is its cost, about two or three times the price of a conventional hearing aid.

ACOUSTICAL FACTORS AFFECTING THE HEARING AID RESPONSE

There are factors which modify the signal between its source and the eardrum of an aided listener. Byrne (1978) summarized these factors which are usually not taken into account when standard hearing aid measurements are performed. The author of this chapter has modified Byrne's as illustrated in Figure 50.

The responses are divided into *far field effects, near field effects, hearing aid responses, and hearing aid plumbing.* These factors

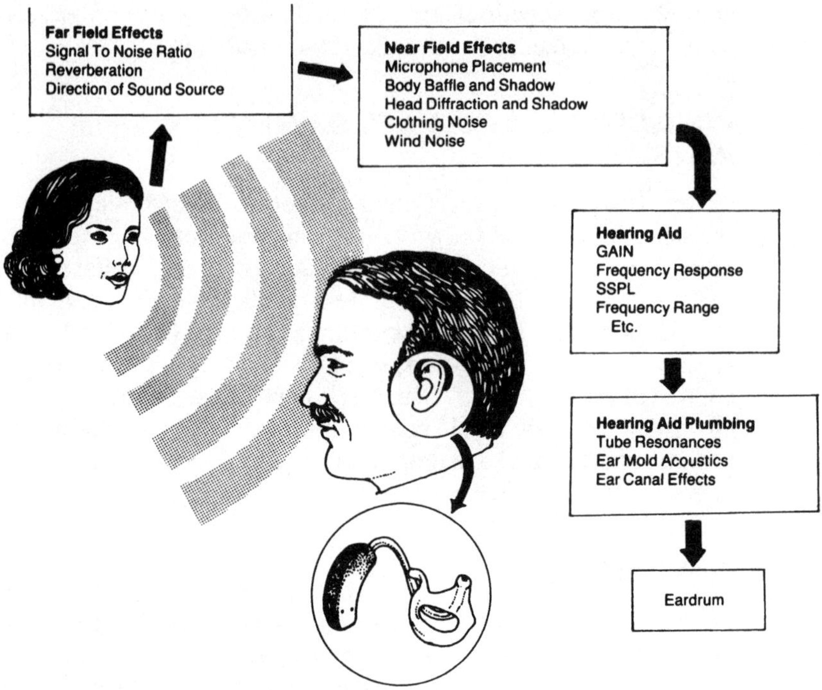

Fig. 50. Acoustical factors affecting the hearing aid response.

tend to alter the gain and frequency response of the hearing aid. To ignore these factors would not be helpful in obtaining the *real ear response* at the eardrum of the listener. The term real ear response is used to differentiate between measurements performed in a test box environment and those measurements performed on a real ear in the ear canal of the listener. These factors modify the output of the hearing aid and thereby influence the maximum output which can be delivered at the eardrum, as well as changing the real ear gain and frequency response. The real ear response is determined in a complex manner by certain physical characteristics of the individual (e.g. shape and size of head, pinna and ear canal, middle ear impedance, etc.) interacting with the characteristic of the hearing aid and its associated "plumbing", the direction of the sound source or sources, and the acoustic properties of the environment (Byrne, 1983).

Far Field Effects

Signal to noise ratio is the relationship between the intensity of the desired signal and the intensity of the background or environmental noise. Perhaps the most important factor is that the hearing aid must ensure the deliverance of a high signal to noise ratio. Hearing impaired listeners require S/N ratios on the order of +20 dB in order to reach maximum intelligibility (Gengel, 1971). Noise levels which have only a moderate effect upon a normal hearing person can severely disrupt word recognition for the hearing impaired person listening to speech through a hearing aid. A sound occurring at one instant of time can mask sounds which closely precede or follow it. There are at least three sources of masking which affect the hearing aid wearer (Byrne, 1983). One consists of environmental sounds which are amplified. Another source consists of noise in the amplifying system, distortion products, and noise associated with hearing aid use (clothing noise, wind noise, etc.). A third source of masking is other components of the speech signal which occur nearly simultaneously (upward spread of masking); amplification of the lower frequencies should be limited to minimize the risk of masking the higher frequencies.

Reverberation is the continued movement of sound pressure waves as the result of repeated reflections after the initiating stimulus has stopped. Perfectly rigid and smooth surfaces reflect most of the incidental sound waves which strike the surface, thus increasing the degree of reverberation (glass, plaster, concrete, etc.). On the other hand, carpet, acoustical tile, drapes, etc. considerably reduce sound reflections by absorbing much of the incident sound energy.

Perhaps the best technique for improving word recognition is to reduce *the distance between the speaker and the listener* (or between the microphone of a hearing aid and the sound source). The closer the listener is to the speaker, the more favorable the listening situation. Important contributions on the subject of Acoustics and Speech Intelligibility are found in the works of Ross (1978) and Finitzo-Hieber (1975).

Near Field Effects—Microphone Placement

Body Baffle Effect (body shadow) is the change produced by the pressure of a body in sound field. Usually refers to the response of a body type hearing aid (conventional, pocket, etc.) when worn on the body, especially under clothing.

Body baffle effects are so substantial that to ignore them amounts to abandoning selective fitting (Byrne, 1978). For example, on the average, body worn aids provide more real-ear gain (gain as actually worn on the person; not test box measurements) at .5 kHz and 10–15 dB less real ear gain between 1.5 kHz and 3 kHz than ear level aids of equivalent technical performance.

Figure 51 illustrates the body baffle effect for sounds directly in front of the wearer (0 degrees incidence) and the body shadow effect, for sounds directly behind the hearing aid wearer (180 degrees incidence). The majority of body worn hearing aids, namely those which have relatively flat or a gently rising frequency response characteristics, provide a low frequency emphasis response to the ear (also because of body shadow, they function as directional hearing aids).

Head Shadow Effect is the difference in reception at each ear created by the interposition of the head, especially when sound waves come from the side. An object the size of a human head will cast a considerable sound shadow above 2000 Hz. Differences have been reported to be as large as 15 dB for a 3200 Hz tone presented in sound field. If speech originates on one side of the head, the sound intensity will be lower at the ear farthest from the sound source (far ear) than at the ear closest to the source (near ear). When measured in sound field with the speaker at a 90° or 270° azimuth relative to the front of the head (facing one ear directly), the near ear SRT will be approximately 6.4 dB better than that of the far ear (Tillman, 1963). If speech is present on the bad ear (or unaided ear for a monaural user), the listener is at a decided disadvantage. The resultant head shadow can result in a substantial loss of word recognition.

Head Diffraction (Head Baffle) deals with the build up of sound from reflection of the head. While head diffraction effects are

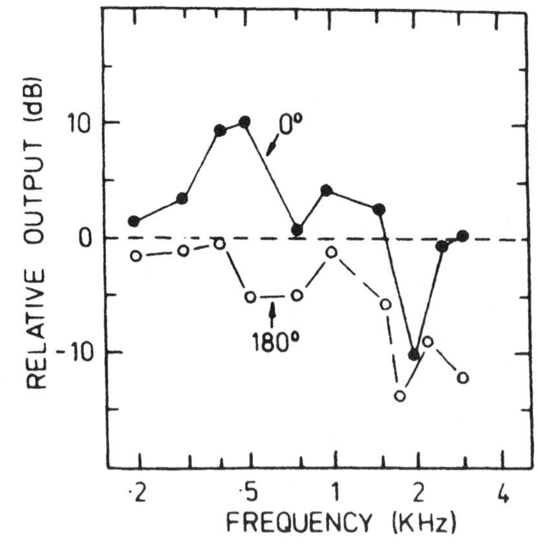

Fig. 51. Differences in output of a hearing aid (body-worn, forward facing microphones) worn on the center of the chest and when suspended in free space (i.e., zero line represents standard frequency response characteristic). Curves show average body baffle (0°) and body shadow (180°) for 4 subjects (measured in an anechoic room). (With permission D. Byrne, Monographs in Contemporary Audiology, 1983.)

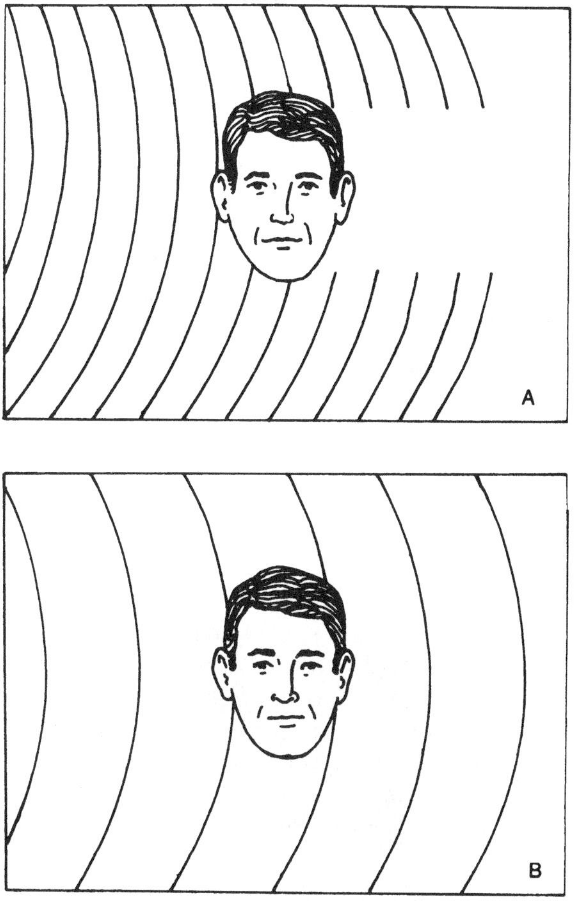

Fig. 52. Head Shadow Effect. Sounds with small wave lengths that encounter large objects will cast a shadow (a) while those with wave lengths that are large compared with the size of the obstacle will readily pass around the object (b).

smaller than body baffle, they nonetheless should be considered. The build up of sound from reflection of the head is greatest around 60 degrees incidence, and head shadow is greatest at about 225 degrees incidence. Refer to Figure 53.

Lybarger and Barron (1965) performed an important experiment with microphone location. The four microphone locations which were examined are illustrated in Figure 54. The results are shown in Figure 55.

The results indicated that a forward up front microphone location is superior to a bottom microphone placement in behind-the-ear

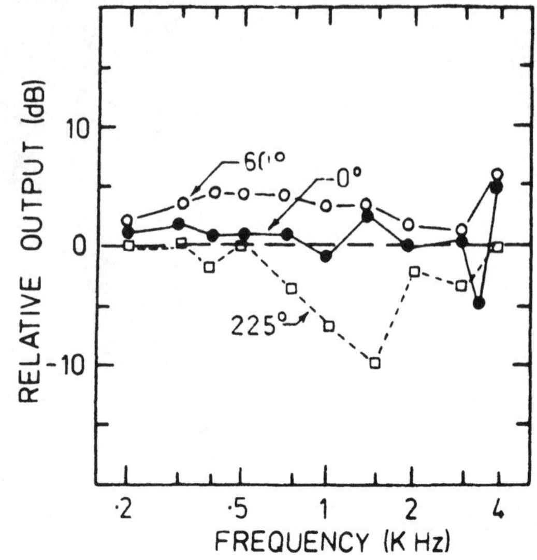

Fig. 53. Differences in output of a hearing aid (BTE, forward facing; non-directional microphone) worn on the head and when suspended in free space. Curves show head diffraction (60°) and head shadow (225°) for 1 subject (measured in an anechoic room). (With permission D. Byrne, Monographs on Contemporary Audiology, 1983.)

hearing aid design. Also the concha microphone location has some advantages over the other microphone locations in providing better gain. Berland and Neilsen (1969) also found that the microphone location at the concha had a number of advantages. The concha microphone location advantages have significant implications for ITE and canal hearing aids.

Clothing noise is present in body type hearing aids and can result in considerable noise and discomfort to the user. Typically, most older type body hearing aids have their microphone opening

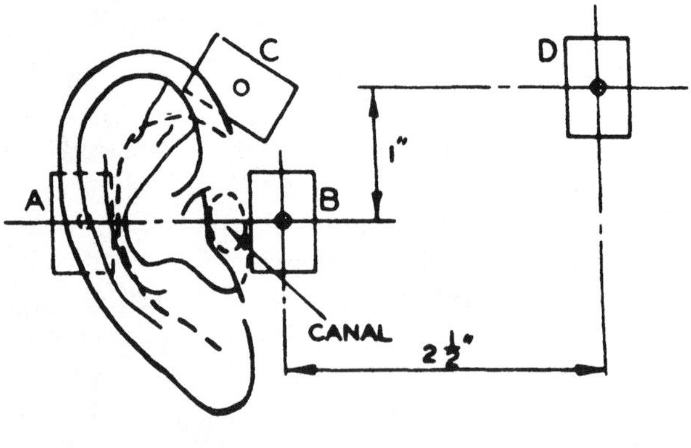

Fig. 54. Experimental microphone placements, S. F. Lybarger and F. E. Barron (1965).

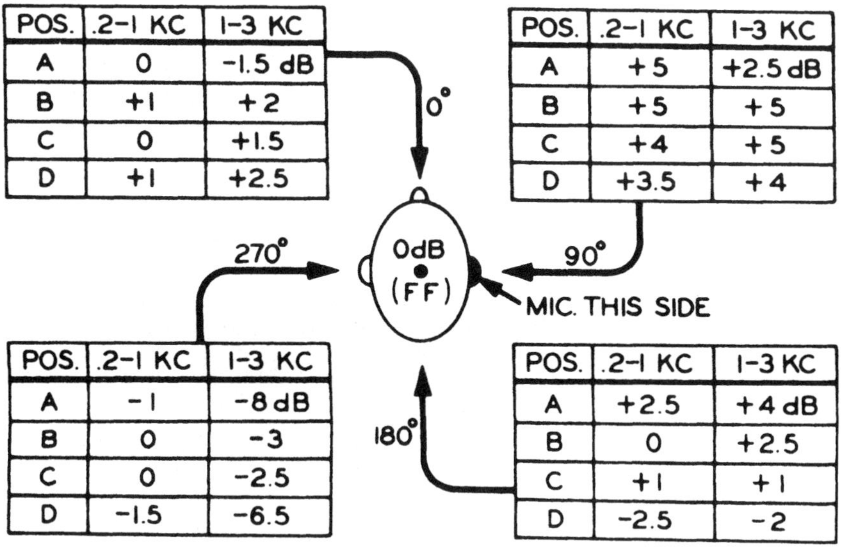

0°:

POS.	.2-1 KC	1-3 KC
A	0	-1.5 dB
B	+1	+2
C	0	+1.5
D	+1	+2.5

90°:

POS.	.2-1 KC	1-3 KC
A	+5	+2.5 dB
B	+5	+5
C	+4	+5
D	+3.5	+4

270°:

POS.	.2-1 KC	1-3 KC
A	-1	-8 dB
B	0	-3
C	0	-2.5
D	-1.5	-6.5

180°:

POS.	.2-1 KC	1-3 KC
A	+2.5	+4 dB
B	0	+2.5
C	+1	+1
D	-2.5	-2

Fig. 55. Relative Responses from Four Microphone Positions, with Sound from Four Different Directions. (S. F. Lybarger and F. E. Barron 1965.)

in the front, usually concealed by the design on the microphone grill. A partial solution has been to place the microphone on the top end of the case, the so-called "top mike". (Berger, 1984). Wearing soft textured and unstarched clothing lessens the problem. Body type aids can also be worn in a harness type arrangement.

Wind noise is a frequent complaint of many hearing aid wearers. This is primarily a problem of ear level hearing aids where the wind can readily create a turbulence around the ear and around the hearing aid itself. Wind noise problems relate primarily to wind velocity, especially where the microphone is not partially covered by the wearer's hair. Locating the microphone opening away from the direct source can often reduce wind noise problems. Wind screens have been developed in an effort to reduce wind noise.

ACTIVE FILTERING

Szosda (1987) pointed out that while revolutionary solutions may be some time away, evolutionary progress in the extraction of the signal in the presence of noise has been steady, due to active filtering. Until recently, low cut and high cut filtering has been achieved with passive components (resistor-capacitor networks); hence, the term "passive filtering". Unfortunately, passive filter networks require a large number of components and as a result are

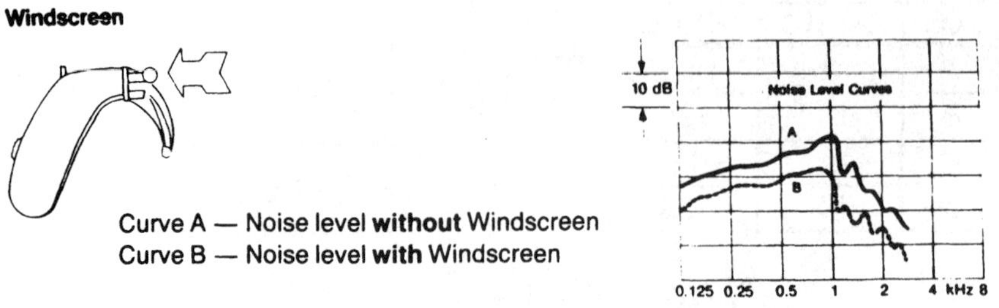

Fig. 56. The curves shown are the **Wind Noise Levels with and without the Windscreen.** It shows the effect the Windscreen has on the wind noise, taken at different frequencies.

quite bulky. Passive filters have fixed characteristics (gain, slope etc.), and as such are not ideal in the dynamic noise environment encountered by the hearing instrument wearer.

In the recent past, the technological move has been from passive to active filters with transistors as the active filter element. An ideal active filter is an integrated circuit (IC), which contains a number of transistors along with other electronic elements. Such integrated circuits have given birth to today's automatic signal processing hearing instruments. While not having the mystique of digital signal processors, they have gained much wearer acclaim.

An active filter network can provide several times greater effectiveness than a network using passive filters. For example, passive controls when used for low frequency modification can achieve an attenuation of 9–10 dB per octave. Active filter controls, on the other hand, can achieve an effective attenuation of 35–45 dB per octave.

THE CONCEPT OF HEARING AID HI-FIDELITY

Tecca and Goldstein (1984) have noted that considerable attention has recently been devoted to the study of listener preference judgments for the evaluation of hearing aid characteristics (Punch 1978, Punch and Beck 1980, Schwartz et al 1979). The increased interest can probably be attributed to the consistent finding that phonetically balanced word lists are insensitive to small differences in hearing aid characteristics, while listener preference judgments have been found to be extremely sensitive. Tecca and Goldstein added that methods based on listener preference judgments have indeed high face validity because they allow clients to choose the instruments they like best.

The knowledge and understanding of the makeup of good quality sound reproduction systems can serve as a base upon which compensation for the person's hearing loss can be added.

Hi-fidelity is largely a personal matter. A commonly accepted definition is that it is reproduced sound with a high degree of similarity to the original sound. Subjective quality responses ultimately set the standards that make sound reproduction "good or bad". The perceived sound quality by the user is responsible for making an "art" out of the science of hearing aid fitting.

A term borrowed from the hi-fidelity industry is *transparency,* which can be defined as an auditory sensation which, when presented to the ear, would result in a faithful representation of the original signal, as if the hearing aid was, in effect, not present. An ideal hi-fidelity system would be acoustically and subjectively transparent.

Three additional terms borrowed from the science of hi-fidelity are pertinent. The term *body* refers to the low frequencies which add depth to the reproduction providing broader bass to the performance. The term *presence* refers to the feeling of realism that

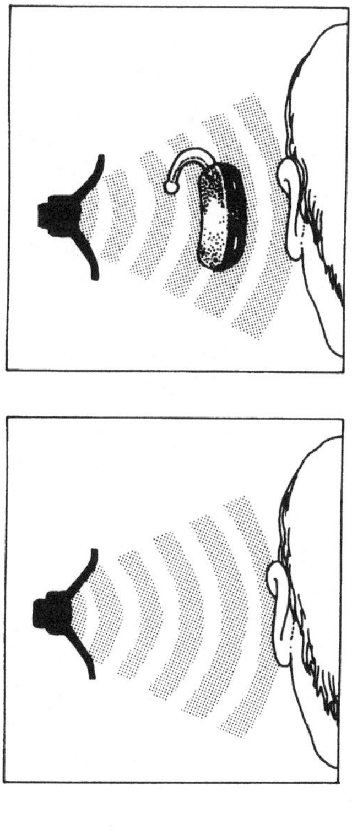

Fig. 57. Transparency can be defined as an auditory sensation which when presented to the ear would result in a faithful representation of the original signal, as if the hearing aid was in effect no present. An ideal hearing aid system would be acoustically and subjectively transparent. The upper figure illustrates a non-transparent condition. The lower figure illustrates the transparent condition in which the patient is not acoustically or subjectively aware of the hearing aid.

the listener is in the presence of the performer. The feeling is created by the mid-range of the reproducing system. When the midrange does not provide adequate amplification, the music or speech seems to have lost its reality, its presence. Many current hearing aid systems provide inadequate mid-range amplification, which detracts from the feeling of presence. The term *brilliance* refers to the feeling of concert hall realism which is created by faithfully adding the high frequencies to the low and middle frequencies, adding a tingle and sparkle to the reproduction.

How can we best achieve a hi-fidelity hearing aid response such as suggested above? Developments in wideband hearing aid transducers, combined with research on new earmold constructions utilizing acoustic horns and predictable damping elements, can result in high fidelity sound quality for speech and music. This viewpoint looks at the hearing aid earmold coupling system as a unit rather than a collection of discrete elements each of which may be varied independently. The new earmold technology informally entitled "earmold plumbing" by Killion combined with wideband, smooth response, low distortion hearing aids can achieve, to a large extent, the philosophical considerations of good sound quality.

Today's sub-miniature hearing aid microphones can be obtained in a wide variety of frequency responses including a nearly flat response from 20 Hz to 20 kHz, with a distortion level well below the limits of audibility.

Wideband Acoustic Modification: At last we have the technology and the tools to modify at the dispenser level the entire frequency spectrum by earmold modification (Killion, 1978) (Libby, 1979). Venting techniques have been used extensively for years. However, venting action is limited to the low frequencies.

We now have additional tools in the form of predictable damping elements and acoustic horn effects, which in conjunction with venting techniques, present a powerful battery for acoustic modi-

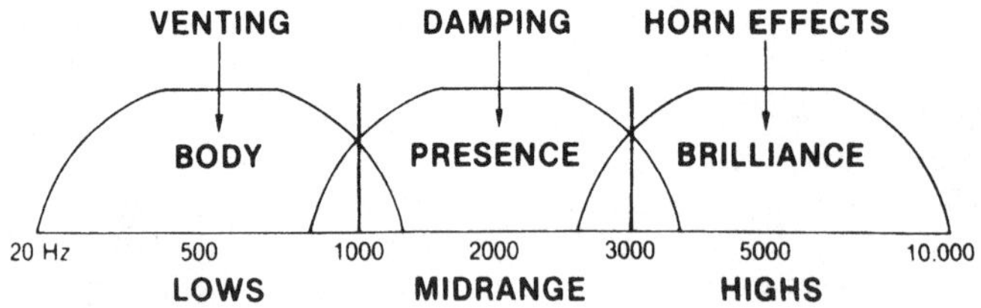

Fig. 58. Wideband predictable earmold modification combining the concept of the body, presence, and brilliance of a high fidelity system. (E. R. Libby 1980.)

fications. Earmold control can be thought of in three frequency regions. Below 1000 Hz, earmold venting is the primary means. In the 1000 to 3000 Hz region, earmold damping is likely to be the primary control means. Above 2000–3000 Hz acoustic horn action (changes in diameter and length of the sound tubing and bore) is likely to be the dominant control means. It should be noted that these modifications are relatively independent of one another and can be performed separately or in tandem. Their main actions, however, are limited to their own frequency region.

THE CONCEPT OF A WIDE, SMOOTH FREQUENCY RESPONSE

Pascoe (1975) and Skinner (1976) have demonstrated that increasing bandwidth resulted in substantial improvement in word recognition. In general, Pascoe and Skinner have noted that the more speech energy between about 200 Hz to 6000 Hz that is audible, the better the ability to understand speech. Fletcher (1942) reported that complete fidelity in the transmission of orchestral music is obtained by the use of a system having a frequency range from 60 to 8000 Hz (Killion, 1979). An 8 kHz bandwidth has been within the capabilities of sub-miniature wideband earphones, but the choice of tubing and earmold required to couple the earphone to the ear is critical if the bandwidth is to be obtained. Mynder's chapter covers the appropriate earmold coupling systems in order to obtain a wide, smooth frequency response.

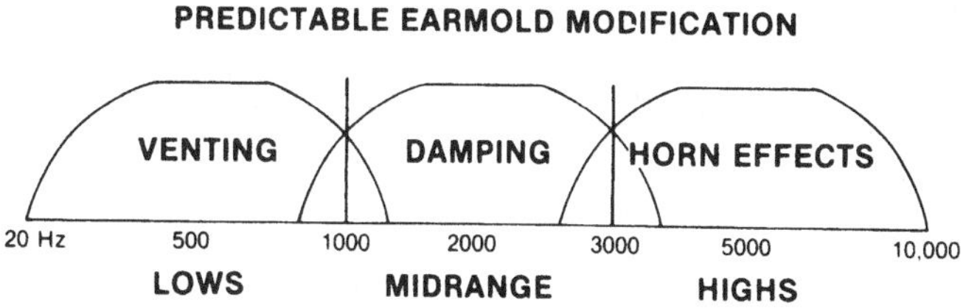

Fig. 59. It should be noted that these modifications are relatively independent of one another and can be performed separately or in tandem. Their main actions are limited to their own particular frequency region. (E. R. Libby 1980.)

DISCUSSION

Consider, however, that the term hi-fidelity itself may have a different meaning for someone with a hearing impairment than for someone with normal hearing. Briefly, we can think of a high fidelity hearing aid as consisting of a sound reproduction system which is hi-fidelity in the conventional sense, in combination with one or more forms of low distortion signal processing, acting to compensate for the hearing impairment. Our primary interest here is the individual with mild to moderate hearing loss who has no difficulty discriminating speech, enjoying full frequency range sound reproduction, etc., provided only that the sound intensity is great enough (Killion, 1979).

Another significant factor is that a hi-fidelity hearing aid design should consider the phenomenon known as *loudness recruitment; abnormal growth of loudness.* Loudness recruitment, according to recent research, is present in practically all individuals with a sensory loss and is not present in conductive or neural involvement.

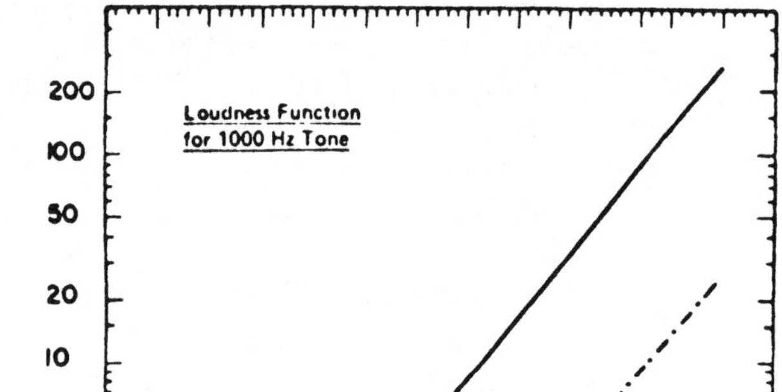

Fig. 60. Loudness of a 1000 Hz tone as a function of loudness level of the normal listener, the typical listener with a cochlear impairment (and recruitment), and the typical listener with a conductive impairment. (With permission B. Scharf, 1978, and Danavox Jubilee Foundation.)

Frequently, in these impairments in which the site of pathology is the cochlea, the person will have a severely diminished dynamic range. The range of sensitivity from threshold to discomfort is decidedly decreased. For this type of person, sounds of low to moderate intensities are inaudible, but sounds of high intensities are at least as loud as with a normal hearing person. In other words, a typical client with a mild to moderate sensory involvement (cochlear) will have trouble hearing low level sounds (whispers and soft speech), but will have no problem hearing sounds of normal or higher intensity levels in quiet. Such users were discussed over four decades ago by Steinberg and Gardner (1947) who observed that many of those with impaired hearing had essentially normal hearing for high intensity sounds, but a loss of normal sensitivity for low intensity sounds. As we mentioned previously, this is due to the recruitment phenomenon and is almost universally present in subjects with cochlear involvement. The chart by Scharf (1978) illustrates this for a typical listener with a 40 dB hearing loss due to cochlear involvement.

Notice how sharply the recruitment phenomenon abnormally increases the loudness growth in a cochlear involvement at or close to threshold and rapidly reaches normal loudness levels at higher intensities. For comparison, in a normal or conductive loss, loudness increases linearly. This phenomenon is the reason why most of the mild to moderate cochlear individuals (which make up most of our hearing aid caseloads) have no trouble conversing with us without a hearing aid and only have problems when we whisper or are in a noisy environment.

THE AMERICANS WITH DISABILITIES ACT (ADA)

The Americans with Disabilities Act (effective January of 1992) requires most businesses to make significant investments in products called, "assistive listening devices" (ALD's) in order to accommodate the hearing impaired. ALD's, such as portable FM or infrared transmitters and receivers, are required in public accommodations and commercial facilities such as hotels, motels, restaurants, theaters convention centers, auditoriums, arenas, retail stores, airports, museums, as well as factories and office complexes.

The ADA law is a civil rights act for the disabled, including the hearing impaired. Failure to comply with the law can result in severe civil penalties and lawsuits by private parties. Courts may impose penalties up to $50,000 for a first violation and up to $100,000 for subsequent violations.

The hearing professional has a valuable role to play relative to the ADA. He or she can be a supplier of the equipment and also be an information resource concerning the various regulations covered under the law.

WHEN A HEARING AID IS NOT ENOUGH

Hearing impaired individuals have relatively more difficulty in word recognition when the acoustical conditions are less than optimal. Such conditions appear to be the rule in theaters, concert halls, houses of worship, and auditoriums; any situation, in other words, in which the primary signal has to traverse a fair amount of acoustical space before being detected by the hearing impaired person (Ross, 1982, Konkle, 1982). These difficulties are experienced not only by individuals wearing hearing aids, but by many elderly people who do not feel the need for amplification in ordinary circumstances. As a result, many of them withdraw from any participation in cultural and social activities.

Fortunately, amplification systems are available which can offer improved communication to hearing impaired persons in public places. The one feature which they all have in common is that the signal is picked up directly at the source stage, sound track, microphones—and transmitted via wires, radio waves, or light beams to the hearing impaired person in the audience. Many of these systems are in daily use in classrooms for hearing impaired children and therefore have been traditionally classified as "classroom" or "group" type instruments.

Currently, there is widespread agreement regarding the negative effect of classroom acoustics upon the speech reception abilities of hearing impaired children. We know that levels of noise and reverberation which may be only mildly disturbing for a normal hearing person may make the comprehension of speech impossible for one who is hearing impaired (Ross, 1982). The relative effects of noise, reverberation, and *distance from the sound source* upon speech can be devastating for hearing impaired individuals. Because of this occurrence, much of the focus of school-based management of hard-of-hearing children involves the use of group educational amplification devices. The basic operation of these systems is such that they by-pass the acoustical conditions in any space by picking up the signal at its source and transmitting it directly via a radio frequency carrier wave to the children.

The adult experiences essentially similar problems in difficult acoustical conditions such as the theater. Such an individual may expend a great deal of energy to comprehend less than his basic auditory abilities would otherwise have permitted. The hearing impaired person requires a signal to noise ratio 10–15 dB greater than a normal hearing person in order to achieve the same word recognition score. It is as if the hearing loss contributed 10–15 dB additional noise to the word recognition process, thus making comprehending speech that much more difficult (Leshowitz and Lindstrom, 1978).

These amplification systems usually provide a much clearer signal to the hearing impaired person with significantly less effort than personal hearing aids. I would like to stress again that personal hearing aids will usually provide substantial benefits when listening in an ideal acoustic environment; but these same hearing aids often fail to improve, and sometimes may be detrimental to communicative function, when used in noisy conditions (Konkle, 1982). Listening problems in public places can be eased considerably with devices currently available. I will describe the various *alternative listening devices* currently available using the classifications of Ross (1982).

ALTERNATIVE LISTENING DEVICES

These devices are classified as *hard wire systems, induction loop systems, AM transmission, FM transmission, and infrared carriers.*

1. Hard Wire Systems

The systems consist of a microphone at the pulpit which delivers the signal by a simple hard wire connection right to the ears of the hearing impaired person. The hardwire system, while useful, has many problems. The person will be restricted to certain seats, and the wire connections are often clumsy and inconvenient to handle.

2. Induction Loop Systems

Another relatively simple arrangement is the induction loop system. This system utilizes a loop of wire which is placed around the circumference of a designated area and delivers the signal from an amplifier. The signal is converted to an electromagnetic field which is received by the telephone coil of a hearing aid.

The intensity of the magnetic field falls off sharply with distance, and variations in intensity are common in different locations in the looped area. It must be remembered that a hearing aid with a telephone coil is necessary in order to interface with the system.

This system is familiar to those who have worked with hearing impaired children. The induction loop system has generally been replaced by the more flexible and efficient FM transmission system in classes for hearing impaired children.

3. AM Transmission

This system employs a low power AM transmitter and AM receiver. The transmitter is usually mounted on a ceiling beam or high on the wall while the ten foot transmitting antenna is connected to adjacent surfaces. The system uses a 480 kHz frequency which FCC regulations permit for this kind of device. A major advantage of this system is that it is inexpensive. Relatively inexpensive fixed frequency receivers are available. The receivers are used with small button earphones and a stock earmold for mild or possible moderate loss for those who do not wear a hearing aid. Individuals with hearing aids can substitute an induction plate instead of the earphone and listen through the telephone coil of their hearing aids. The system has a limited range and is susceptible to electrical interference.

4. FM Transmission

The FM transmission system is the most familiar to those who work with hearing impaired children in regular and special schools. Usually, all that is required is for the speaker to wear the microphone/transmitter and for the listener, the FM receiver/hearing aid combination.

The FM system can be connected directly to various sound systems and then transmitted to personal FM receivers. Many kinds of configurations are possible because of the great flexibility of the system. The range of FM systems is less restrictive than that of the AM systems. The effective indoor range is about 50 to 80 meters, and there is less likelihood of interference from electrical installations within a facility.

FM systems are useful in a number of different situations and are capable of delivering a high quality signal.

5. Infrared Light Carrier

This system is the most recently developed and perhaps the most interesting in its potential. The system transmits audio signals by an infrared light carrier. The light carrier which is invisible to the naked eye, is amplitude modulated by a fixed carrier frequency of 95 kHz, which in turn is frequency modulated by the audio signal. An AM/FM double modulation is the result. A transmitter is plugged into the sound system amplifier or directly to a microphone, which in turn, is led to one or more emitters (radiators) which are situated in advantageous locations for light transmission. The infrared radiation is detected by a photosensitive diode, demodulated, the audio signal amplified, and then delivered to the ears of the listener. The system will transmit through windows but not through walls, and therefore, is usually restricted to the room or theater in which it has its source. A number of systems can be used in adjacent rooms without interference. The infrared radiations can cover a small or large area; it is only necessary to add more emitters when utilizing the system in a large area. Infrared systems will not operate outdoors. Preliminary listening tests have reported the infrared transmission was superior to an FM signal. It appears to be equally effective for those who do and who do not wear hearing aids. The battery life is ample for one single performance, though the batteries are recharged after each one.

CONCLUSION

These special amplifying devices can provide an undistorted signal with a better signal to noise ratio than personal hearing aids in a difficult or noisy acoustic environment. Their wider use should be encouraged by the hearing aid professional. The millions of hearing impaired are potential wearers of these special amplification devices who will, as a result, enjoy fuller participation in the entire gamut of activities our society provides for its members. The reader is encouraged to read the chapters by Mark Ross and Daniel Konkle in the Vanderbilt Hearing Aid Report for fuller explanations of these systems (1982).

SUMMARY

An overview of hearing aid history and development enables the reader to understand the many contributions of current hearing aid technology to meet the needs of the hearing impaired. The type and styles of hearing aid devices utilized have certain design limitations which are related to the classification and degree of hearing impairment to which they are fitted. Basic electronics and simple circuit diagrams serve to acquaint the reader with various hearing aid functions and to help him to understand their application. Amplifiers, transducers, earmolds and various technologies to produce and modify hearing aid response constitute a portion of the information needed by the hearing aid specialist to adequately perform his necessary tasks.

Acoustic devices, beyond the basic hearing aid, include induction loop systems, AM transmission, Fm transmission and infrared carriers. These special amplifying devices provide undistorted signals with a better signal to noise ratio than do most personal hearing aids.

GLOSSARY

An Active Filter an electronic filter circuit, which uses active elements, i.e. tubes, transistors or integrated circuits, in addition to passive elements. An active filter does not necessarily provide an automatic, adaptive, or ASP behavior. "Active" refers to the way a circuit is realized, and not to what it does. In general, an active filter network provides several times greater effectiveness than that of a passive filter network.

Adaptive Compression (Variable Release Compression) a term used by some manufacturers to denote a compression circuit with an automatic variable release time. The length of that release time is controlled as a function of at the compression activating input. Thus, the shorter the time of the compression activating input, the shorter the time release; the longer the compression activating input, the longer the time release.

Adaptive Frequency Response (AFR) the type of hearing aid whose frequency response changes as input level change.

Adaptive Noise Processing the property of signal processing circuits to adapt and change hearing instrument parameters and operating characteristics in response to changes in the environmental noise characteristics and the primary signal.

Adaptive Signal Processing the property of signal processing circuits, which allows them to change their gain and frequency characteristics in response to changes in the signal characteristics and the environment.

AGC (Automatic Gain Control) a non-linear process in which the gain changes as a function of changing signal levels.

AGC-I (Input Controlled AGC) compression amplification whose degree of gain reduction depends on input level and kneepoint.

AGC-O (Output Controlled AGC) compression amplification whose degree of gain reduction depends on the output level and kneepoint.

Analog to Digital Conversion the process of converting an analog signal to digital form.

Analog Hearing Aids hearing aids where the acoustical signal is converted first to an electronic wave form that is a direct analog of the acoustical signal picked up by the microphone. The electrical analog of the acoustical signal is then filtered, amplified, and processed as a continuous wave form.

Attack and Release Time the time required for a dynamic non-linear processor to reach its steady-state value.

Automatic Signal Processing (ASP) a marketing phrase which does not have a precise technical meaning. Thus, ASP is utilized by various manufacturers to denote different types of signal processing, with the implication that the hearing instrument adjusts its behavior in response to the environment. Despite its fluid meaning, the term ASP is increasingly being applied to a newer generation of hearing instruments whose purpose is to enhance desired elements of speech while suppressing the amplification of the undesired elements of speech. Generally, those undesired elements have unwanted noise and reverberation. Most manufacturers use the term ASP to indicate automatic adjustments of the hearing instruments frequency response as the background noise varies.

Bill Bass increases at low levels.

Binaural Listening listening with two ears. Typically, the two ears are receiving different signals.

CMOS a complimentary metal oxide semi-conductor used in newer hearing aid designs.

Coherence the portion of the output signal that is directly related to the input signal. Indicates the total distortion and noise measured at the output of a hearing aid.

Compression Ratio the ratio of the change in output level resulting from a given change in input level in a compression amplifier.

Crest Factor the difference in decibels between the peak sound pressure level and root mean square sound pressure level.

CROS (Contralateral Routing of Signal) a hearing aid for patients with unilateral hearing loss. A microphone is placed near the poorer ear, and the signal is routed to the better ear via an open earmold.

Dichotic binaural hearing with different signals at the ear.

Digital to Analog Conversion the process of converting a digital signal to analog form.

Digital Hearing Aid one in which the acoustic signal picked up by the microphone is first converted to an electronic analog signal and then converted to a digital signal. The digital signal takes the form of a series of binary numbers. The binary numbers representing the audio signals are then processed using digital circuits of the type commonly used in computers. After the digital signal has been processed, it is converted back to an analog electronic signal, which in turn is converted to an acoustic signal by the hearing aid receiver (Levitt, 1991).

Diotic binaural listening with exactly the same signals at the two ears.

Fixed Frequency Response Circuits those with traditional automatic gain control (AGC), which reduce gain at high levels (compression limiting), and/or wide dynamic range compression that increase gain at low levels, but do not change the frequency response of the hearing aid in the process.

FM System an assistive listening device consisting of a microphone, transmitter and receiver.

Full Dynamic Range Compression (FDRC) a feature of an amplification system in which the compression typically occurs over an input range from approximately 45–90 dB SPL.

Harmonic Distortion the addition of spurious harmonic components to a signal. It is expressed as a percentage of the total signal at the point of measurement.

Headroom the difference in SPL between the gain and user settings, and the intensity which causes saturation.

Hybrid the mixture of analog and digital electronics in a hearing aids.

IC (Integrated Circuit) a miniature electronic unit of components and conductors, which is manufactured as a signal module.

Intermodulation Distortion (IM) the distortion of a complex wave form associated with sums and differences amongst frequency components.

Kneepoint (Compression Threshold) the point on an input-output curve at which the slope digresses from unity.

Level Dependent Frequency Response (LDFR) circuits which automatically change gain and frequency response of the hearing instrument as a function of the input signal.

Linear Amplification a hearing aid, or amplification system, for which there is the same gain for input levels until the maximum output of the device is reached.

Non-Linear Hearing Aid a hearing aid, or amplification system, in which overall gain and/or frequency response change as a function of changing input signals.

A Passive Filter an electronic filter, which uses only resistors, capacitors, and inductors (no transistors, tubes, or semi-conductors). It is possible to produce a filter response in a passive filter, however, the bulkiness of the circuit becomes a problem.

Peak Clipping a distortion of a wave form resulting from amplifier saturation.

Reverberation the prolongation of sound by reflection, usually from hard surfaces such as walls. Reverberation time is the time it takes for sound pressure to decrease 60 dB in a room after the initial impulse has stopped. Except for anechoic chambers, every room produces reverberation to some extent. Reverberation can be thought of as a decrease in signal-to-noise ratio.

Saturation the condition caused by peak clipping that prevents an increase in input sound pressure level from causing the same change and output sound pressure level.

Signal-to-Noise Ratio (S/N Ratio) or Message to Competition Ratio (MCR) the ratio of the signal (message) pressure to the noise (competition) pressure, expressed in decibels. For example, if a signal level is 60 dB, and the noise level is 55 dB, the signal-to-noise ratio is 60–55 expressed in decibels or a +5 dB. A signal-to-noise ratio of −5 dB means the noise is 5 dB greater than the signal.

Till treble increases at low levels.

Transducer a device which changes the energy from one form to another. An example: microphone or receiver.

Two-Channel AGC Hearing Aid a hearing aid in which a signal is separated into two frequency bands; each band having a separate AGC circuit.

REFERENCES

AGNEW, J., "Acoustic Advantages of Deep Canal Hearing Aid Fitting,: *Hearing Instruments,* Vol. 45, No. 8, Aug. 1994.

BECK, L. B., LEATHERGOOD, R. W., PUNCH, J. L. "Aided Low Frequency Responses: Speech Quality and Speech Intelligibility," Presented at ASLHA. Detroit, November 1980.

BECK, L. B., "The Veterans Administration Hearing Aid Program: Research Needs in Amplification," Vanderbilt Hearing Aid Report, Upper Darby, PA. *Monographs in Contemporary Audiology,* 6796 Market St., 1982.

BERGER, K. W., "The First Electric Hearing Aids," *Hearing Instruments,* 21, Dec. 1970b, 23–28.

BERGER, K. W., "Western Electric Hearing Aids" *Hearing Instruments,* 23, Jan. 1972, 18, 20, 24.

BERGER, K. W., and MILLIN, J. P., "Hearing Aids," In *Audiological Assessment* (D. Rose, ed). Prentice-Hall, Inc., 2nd ed. 1978.

BERGER, K. W., HAGBERG E. N., and RANE, R. L., "Prescription of Hearing Aids," Herald Publishing Co., Kent, OH. 1977.

BERGER, K. W., HAGBERG, E. N., and RANE, R. L., "Prescription of Hearing Aids," Kent, OH: Herald Publishing House, 3rd ed. 1980.

BERGER, K. W., "The Hearing Aid, Its Operation and Development," National Hearing Aid Society, Detroit, 1984.

BERLAND, O., and NIELSON, T. E., "Sound Pressure Generated in the Human External Ear Canal by a Free Sound Field," *Sound,* 3, 1969, 78–81.

BORNSTEIN, S. P., RANDOLPH, K. J., "Research on Smooth Wide-band Frequency Responses," Current status and unresolved issues. *Hearing Instruments,* Vol 34, No. 12, 1983, 12–16.

BRISKEY, R. J., and WRUK, K., "Acoustic Influence of Vent Inserts," *Hearing Instruments,* 25, Oct. 1974, 12–14.

BRISKEY, R. J., GARRISON, M. J., OWSLEY, P., and SINCLAIR, J., "Effects of Hearing Aids on Deaf Speech," *Aud.* 16, 1967, 173–188.

BRISKEY, R. J., GREENBAUM, W., and SINCLAIR, J., "Pitfalls in Hearing Aid Frequency. Response Curves." Paper presented 13th annual Spring convention. Audio Engineering Society 1966.

BROOKS, D. N., "The Use and Disuse of Medresco Hearing Aids." *Sound,* 6, 1972, 80–85.

BROOKS, D. N., "Pre and Post Hearing Aid Provision Management," Vanderbilt Hearing Aid Report, Upper Darby, PA. *Monographs in Contemporary Audiology,* 1982.

BURKHARD, M. D., and SACHS, R. M., "Anthropometric Manikin for Acoustic Research." *Journal of the Acoustical Society of America,* 58, 1975, 214–222.

BURKHARD, M. D. (ed.), "Manikin Measurements," Industrial Research Products Inc. 1978.

BURNETT, E. D. (ed.), "Handbook of Hearing Aid Measurements," Veterans Administration, Washington, DC. 1978.

BURNETT, E. D., CORLISS, E. L. R., NEDZELNITSKY, V., "Research Problems in Coupler Aid in situ Measurements on Hearing Aids," Vanderbilt Hearing Aid Report (Studebaker and Bess, ed.) Upper Darby, PA. *Monographs in Contemporary Audiology* (1982) 67–74.

BYRNE, D. J., "Some Implications of Body Baffle for Hearing Aid Selection," *Sound,* 6, 1972, 86–91.

BYRNE, D. J., "Binaural Hearing Aid Fitting: Research Findings and Clinical Applications," *Binaural Hearing and Amplification.* Libby E. R., ed. Chicago, Zenetron, 1980.

BYRNE, D. J., "Theoretical Prescriptive Approaches to Selecting the Gain and Frequency Response of a Hearing Aid. *Monographs in Contemporary Audiology,* 1983, Vol 4, No. 1.

BYRNE, D. J., TONISSON, W., "Selecting the Gain of Hearing Aids for Persons with Sensorineural Hearing Impairments," *Scandinavian Audiology* 1976, 5:51–59.

CARVER, W. F., "A Historical and Technical Review (Hearing Aids)." *Handbook of Clinical Audiology,* (Katz, J., ed.) Baltimore, Williams and Wilkins 1978, 479–485.

CHASIN, M., "Using Resistance in Earmold Tubing," *Hearing Instruments,* Vol 34, No 12, 1983.

COLE, N. A., "Prospects for the Application to High Technology of Hearing Aid," *Hearing Instruments,* Jan. 1983.

COX, R. M., "Acoustic Aspects of Hearing Aid-Ear Canal Coupling Systems," *Monographs in Contemporary Audiology,* 1:3, March 1979.

CURRAN, J. R., "CROS Fittings and Open Canal Application," Minneapolis, Dahlberg Electronics, Inc. 1971.

CURRAN, J. R., "Modern Earmold Research," *Hearing Aid Journal,* 28:6, 1975.

CURRAN, J. R., and ELY, W. G., "Clearing the Compression Jingle," *Hearing Dealer,* 24:16, 1973.

DALSGAARD, S. C., and JENSEN, O. D., "Measurements of Insertion Gain with Hearing Aids," 8th International Congress on Acoustics, London, 1974.

DANAHER, E. M., and PICKETT, J. M., "Some Masking Effects Produced by Low Frequency Vowel Formants in Persons with Sensorineural Hearing Loss," *Journal of Speech and Hearing Research,* 18, 1975.

DAVIS, H., and SILVERMAN, S. R. (eds.), *Hearing and Deafness,* Holt, Rinehart & Winston, rev. ed. 1966.

DEBOER, B., "Performance of Hearing Aids from the Pre-Electronic Era," *Median Verlag Audiological Acoustics.* March April 1984.

DELK, J. A., "Comprehensive Dictionary of Audiology," *The Hearing Aid Journal,* 1973.

DODDS, E., and HARFORD, E., "Modified Earpieces and CROS For High Frequency Hearing Losses," *Journal of Speech and Hearing Research,* 11, 204–218.

DUNLAVY, A. R., "CROS: A Review of Applications and Fittings Utilizing Contralateral Routing of Signals," *Hearing Aid Journal,* 21, July 1968, 6–7, 30–32.

DUNLAVY, A. R., "CROS: The New Miracle Worker," *Aud.,* 19, 1970. 141–148.

Duracell International: Packaged Power, 1981. Bethel CT.

DYRLUND, O., and BISGAARD, N., "Acoustic Feedback, Margin Improvements in Hearing Instruments Using a Prototype DFS (Digital Feedback Suppressor) System. *Scandanavian Audiology,* 20, 49–53, 1991.

ELY, W. G., "A Primer on Distortion of Hearing Aids," *Hearing Aid Journal,* 27:10–34, 1974.

FANTEL, H., "Better Listening," New York. Scribners 1983.

FIKRET-PASA, S., "The Effects of Compression Ratio on Speech Intelligibility and Quality." Northwestern Univ., Evanston, Il. 1993.

FINITZO-HIEBER, T., "The Influence of Reverberation and Noise on Speech Intelligibility of Normal and Hard of Hearing Children in Classroom Size Listening Environments," Dissertation, Northwestern University, Evanston, Ill, 1975.

FLECTHER, H., *Speech and Hearing in Communication,* D. Van Nostrand Co. New York, 1953.

FOLWER, E. P., "Bilateral Hearing Aids of Monaural Total Deafness," *Archives Otoloaryngology,* 72, 1960, 57[–]58.

FRENCH, N. R., and STEINBERG, J. C., "Factors Governing the Intelligibility of Speech Sounds," *Journal of the Acoustical Society of America,* 1947.

GERBER, S. E., "Introductory Hearing Science," Phila., Saunders, 1974.

GOLDBERG, H., "Hearing Aid Amplifiers," Dyn-Aura Engineering Labs.

GOLDBERG, H., "Telephone Amplifying Pick-Up Devices," *Hearing Instruments,* 26:19–20, 1975.

GOLDBERG, H., "Hearing Aid Signal Processors and Their Application to the Hearing Impaired," Dyn-Aura Engineering, San Diego, 1982.

GRAUPE, D., and CAUSEY, G. D., "Method and Means for Adaptively Filtering Stationary Noise from an Information Bearing Signal," United States Patent, 4 185-168, 1980.

GRIFFING, T. S., and SHIELDS, J., "Hearing Aid Performance and the Earmold," *Hearing Instruments,* 23, Aug. 1972 6–10.

GRIFFING, T. S., "Cosmetic Appeal and I-T-E Hearing Aids," *Hearing Aid Journal,* October 1976.

GUDMUNSEN, G. I., "Fitting CIC Hearing Aids-Some Practical Pointers," *Hearing Journal,* July, 1994, Vol. No. 7.

HARFORD, E., and BARRY, J., "A Rehabilitative Approach to the Problem of Unilateral Hearing Impairment: The Contralateral Routing of Signals," *Journal of Speech and Hearing Disorders,* 30, 1965, 121–138.

HARRIS, J. D., "The True Goals and Aspirations of Audiology: Harris on Audiology," *Journal of Auditory Research,* 1971, page 441.

HARRIS, J. D., "Psycho-Acoustics and Neurophysiology of Binaural Hearing," *Binaural Hearing and Amplification* (Libby, E. R., ed.) Vol. 1. Chapter II, Chicago, Zenetron, 1980, Page 37.

HAWKINS, D. B., "Signal-to-Noise Ratio Advantage of Binaural Hearing Aids and Directional Microphones Under Different Levels of Reverberation," *Journal of Speech and Hearing Disorders,* Vol. 49, 278–286, August 1984.

HEIDE, J., "Omni Hearing Aid Systems," Dallas TX, 1981.

HIRSH, I. J., "Binaural Hearing Aids. A Review of Some Experiments." *Journal of Speech and Hearing Disorders,* Vol. 15, pp 114–123, 1950.

HODGSON, W. R., SKINNER, P. H., "Hearing Aid Assessment and Use in Audiologic Assessment," Baltimore, Williams and Wilkins 1981.

JOHNSON, E. W., "A Case for Binaural Hearing Aids," *Binaural Hearing and Amplification.* (Libby, E. R., ed.) Chicago, Zenetron 1980.

JOHNSON, J., "Binaural Instrumentation," *Binaural Hearing and Amplification,* (Libby, E. R., ed.) Chicago, Zenetron 1980.

JOHNSON, K. W. and WALKER, W. C., and CUTNELL, J. D., "The Science of Hi-Fidelity," Second Edition, Dubuque, Kendall/Hunt Publishing Co. 1977.

KASTEN, R. N., and LOTTERMAN, S. H., "A Longitudinal Examination of Harmonic Distortion in Hearing Aids," *Journal of Speech and Hearing Research,* 10, 1967, 777[–]781.

KASTEN, R. N., and LOTTERMAN, S. H., "The Influence of Hearing Aid Gain Control Rotation on Acoustic Gain." *Journal of Auditory Research,* 9. 1969, 35–39, Reprinted in *Aud,* 1970, 97–102, and in *Hearing Aid Journal,* 23, Oct. 1970, 16, 31.

KILLION, M. C., "Design and Evaluation of High-Fidelity Hearing Aids," Ph. D. dissertation, Northwestern Un., 1979.

KILLION, M. C., "Transducers, Earmolds and Sound Quality Considerations," In the Vanderbilt Hearing Aid Report (Studebaker and Bess, eds.) *Monographs in Contemporary Audiology,* 1982.

KILLION, M. C., and CARLSON, E. V., "A Wideband Miniature Microphone," *Journal of the Audio Engineering Society,* 18, 1970, 631–635.

KILLION, M. C., and MONSER, E. L., "CORFIG. In Acoustical Factors Affecting Hearing Aids," (Studebaker and Hochberg, eds.) University Park Press, 1980.

KILLION, M. C., "Experimental Wideband Hearing Aid," *Journal of the Acoustical Society of America,* 1976b. 59:S62(a).

KILLION, M. C., "Broadband Hearing Aid Earphones. Acoustical Factors Affecting Hearing Aid Performance," Studebaker and Hochberg (eds.) University Park Press, Baltimore, MD., 1980.

KILLION, M., STAAB, W. J., and PREVES, D. A., "Classifying Automatic Signal Processors," *Hearing Instruments,* 41 (8), 1990.

KILLION, M., "An Acoustically Invisible Hearing Aid," *Hearing Instruments,* 39–44, 1988.

KNOWLES, H. S., "Shocks on Hearing Aid Microphones and Earphones," *ZHA,* 2, 1965, 52–65.

KONKLE, D. F., "Amplification for Specific Needs," Vanderbilt Hearing Aid Report, Studebaker and Bess, eds., 1982, *Monographs in Contemporary Audiology,* Upper Darby, PA.

LESHOWITZ, B., and LINDSTROM, R., "Masking and Speech to Noise Ratio," Proceedings of the Workshop on Prosthetics and Technical Devices for the Deaf, 1978. McPherson, D. E., ed. National Institute for the Deaf.

LEVITT, H., "Advanced Signal Processing Techniques," Vanderbilt Report II. 93–99, *York Press,* Parkton, MD., 1991.

LEVITT, H., and VOROBA, B., "Binaural Hearing," *Introductory Hearing Science,* Phila. W. B. Saunders 1974.

LIBBY, E. R., "The Importance of Smoothness in Hearing Aid Frequency Response, *Hearing Instruments,* 30:4, 1979, 20–22.

LIBBY, E. R., "Smooth Wideband Hearing Aid Responses—The New Frontier," *Hearing Instruments,* 31, Oct. 1980.

LIBBY, E. R., JOHNSON, J. H., and LONGWELL, T. F., "Innovative Earmold Coupling Systems," *Zenetron Monographs* #4, nd (1981).

LIBBY, E. R., "Achieving a Transparent, Smooth, Wideband Hearing Aid Response," *Hearing Instruments,* Oct 1981. Duluth MN.

LIBBY, E. R., "Binaural Hearing and Amplification" (Libby, E. R., ed.) Chicago, *Zenetron,* 1980.

LIBBY, E. R., "In Search of Transparent Insertion Gain Hearing Aid Responses," The Vanderbilt Hearing Aid Report (Studebaker and Bess, eds.) *Monographs in Contemporary Audiology,* 1982.

LIBBY, E. R., and SWEETOW, R. W., "Fitting the Environment-Some Evolutionary Approaches," *Hearing Instruments,* 38 (8), 10–16, 1987.

LICKLIDER, J. C. R., "The Influence of Interaural Phase Relations Upon the Masking of Speech by White Noise," *Journal of the Acoustical Society of America,* Vol. 20 150–159, 1948.

LIPPMANN, R. P., BRAIDA, L. D., DURLACH, N. L., "Study of Multi-Channel Amplitude Compression and Linear Amplification for Persons with Sensorineural Hearing Impairments," *Scandinavian Audiology,* 1976: 5:51–59.

LOTTERMAN, S. H., and KASTEN, R. N., "The Influence of Gain Control Rotation on Non-linear Distortion in Hearing Aids," *Journal of Speech and Hearing Research,* 10, 1967a, 593–599.

LYBARGER, S. F., "The Earmold as Part of the Receiver Acoustic System," Radioear Corp., nd (1958).

LYBARGER, S. F., "Earmold Acoustics," *Audecibel,* 16, Winter 1967, 9–19.

LYBARGER, S. F., "Some Comments on CROS," *Hearing Aid Journal,* 21, July 1968, 8, 33.

LYBARGER, S. F., "Advantages and Limitations of the 'Y' Cord," *Hearing Aid Journal,* April 1973, 6, 34.

LYBARGER, S. F., "Sound Leakage From Vented Earmolds," *Scandinavian Audiology,* supp. 5, 1975, 260–264. Also, *Hearing Aid Journal,* 30:5, 1977, 8, 38–40.

LYBARGER, S. F., and BARRON, F. E., "Head Baffle Effect for Different Hearing Aid Microphone Locations," Paper read at A.S.A., St. Louis, MO., Nov. 1965.

LYBARGER, S. F., "Earmolds. Handbook of Clinical Audiology," (Katz, J., ed.) The Williams & Wilkins Co., Baltimore, MD., 1972.

LYBARGER, S. F., "Selective Amplification—A REVIEW AND EVALUATION," *Journal of the American Audiological Society,* 1978:3:258–266.

LYBARGER, S. F., "In Controlling Hearing Aid Performance by Earmold Design," V. D. Larson, D. P. Egolf, et al., (eds) Grune and Stratton, New York 1979.

LYBARGER, S. F., "Acoustic Feedback Control," Vanderbilt Hearing Aid Report (Studebaker and Bess, eds.), Upper Darby, PA. *Monographs in Contemporary Audiology,* 1982, 87–91.

MADAFFARI, P. L., "Pressure Variation About the Ear," *Journal of the Acoustical Society of America,* 1974.

MAJOR, M., "Acoustical Deviation and Effect," *Hearing Aid Journal,* 22, Jan. 1969, 8–9, 28–29.

MCCANDLESS, G., "Loudness Discomfort and Hearing Aids," Papers presented at 3rd Oticongress, 1973. 39–44.

MILLER, I. D., NIEMOELLER, A. F., PASCOE, D. P., and SKINNER, M. W., "Integration of the Electroacoustic Description of Hearing Aids with the Audiologic Description of Clients," *Acoustical Factors Affecting Hearing Aid Performance,* Studebaker and Hochberg (eds) University Park Press, Baltimore, Md., 1980.

MUELLER, H. G., SCHWARTZ, D. M. and SURR, R. K., "The Use of the Exponential Acoustic Horn in an Open Mold Configuration," *Hearing Instruments,* Vol. 32/No. 10, Duluth, MN., 1981.

MUELLER, G., "Small Can Be Good Too," *Hearing Journal,* Nov., Vol. 7, No. 11, 1994.

MYNDERS, J. M., "Brief Historical Sketch of the Development of Earmolds," *Hearing Aid Journal,* March 1977.

MYNDERS, J. M., "Earmold Style Selection—Some Guidelines for Office Practice." *Hearing Aid Journal,* April 1980.

NABELEK, I. V., "Performance of Hearing Impaired Listeners Under Various Types of Amplitude Compression," *Journal of the Acoustical Society of America,* Vol. 74, No. 3, 1983. 776–792.

NABELEK, A. K., "Temporal Distortions and Noise Considerations," The Vanderbilt Hearing Aid Report (Studebaker and Bess, eds) Upper Darby, Pa. *Monographs in Contemporary Audiology* 1982.

NABELEK, A. K., "Effects of Room Acoustics on Speech Perception Through Hearing Aids," *Binaural Hearing and Amplification,* (Libby, E. R., ed.) Chicago, Zenetron, 1980.

NABELEK, A. K., "Effects of Room Acoustics on Speech Perception Through Hearing Aids by Normal Hearing and Hearing Impaired Listeners," In Studebaker and Hockberg (eds.), *Acoustic Factors Affecting Hearing Aid Performance* (P.P. 25–46), University Park Press, 1980.

NIELSEN, H. B., "A Comparison Between Hearing Aids with Directional Microphone and Hearing Aids with Conventional Microphone," Papers Presented at 3rd Oticongress, 1973, 45–48.

NORTHERN, J. L., and HATTLER, K. W., "Earmold Influence of Aided Speech Identification Tasks," *Journal of Speech and Hearing Research,* 13, 1970, 162[–172.

NUNLEY, J., STAAB, W., STEADMAN, J., WECHSLER, P., and SPENCER, B., "A Wearable Digital Hearing Aid," *Hearing Aid Journal,* Oct. 1983, Vol. 36, No. 10.

OLSEN, W., "Physical Characteristics of Hearing Aids," *Hearing Aid Assessment and Use in Audiologic Habitation,* 2nd Ed. (Hodgson, W. R., and Skinner, P. H., eds.) Baltimore, Williams and Wilkens 1981, 19–44.

ORCHIK, D. J., "Peritympanic Soft Hearing Instrument Fitting in High Frequency Hearing Loss," *Hearing Instruments,* 41 (11), 28–30, 1990.

PASCOE, D. P., "Frequency Responses of Hearing Aids and Their Effects on the Speech Perception of Hearing Impaired Subjects," *Ann Oto Rhino Laryngol.* 1975:84:Supp. 23, 1[–]40.

PIMENTEL, R. G., "Audio Input," *Hearing Instruments.,* June, 1984.

POLLACK, M. C., "Amplification for the Hearing Impaired," New York, Grune and Stratton, 1980.

POLLACK, M. C., "Hearing Aid Feedback," *Maico Audiological Library Series,* 13:35–39, 1975.

PREVES, D., "Obtaining Accurate Measurements of Directional Hearing Aid Parameters. *Hearing Aid Journal* 28:4, 1975, 13, 28.

PREVES, D., "Coupler and in Situ Measurements," Vanderbilt Hearing Aid Report (Studebaker and Bess, eds.) Upper Darby, PA. *Monographs in Contemporary Audiology,* 1982, 74–78.

PREVES, D., and GRIFFING, T. S., "In The Ear Hearing Aids, Parts I, II, III, IV," *Hearing Instruments,* March, May, July, Sept. 1976.

PREVES, D. A., and SIGELMAN, J., "A New Signal Processor for ITE Hearing Aid Fittings," *Hearing Instruments,* 37 (10), 52–59, 1987.

PREVES, D. A., "Real Ear Insertion Gain Provided by CIC, ITC, and ITE Hearing Instruments," *Hearing Journal,* Aug. 1994.

PREVES, D. A., "The Headroom Problem in Hearing Aid Performance," *Hearing Journal,* 42 (10): 21, 1989.

Preves, D. A., "Future Trends in Hearing Aid Technology in Strategies for Selecting and Verifying Hearing Aid Fittings," Valente, M., Thieme, NY, NY, 1994.

PUNCH, J. L., and BECK, E. L., "Low Frequency Response of Hearing Aids and Judgments of Aided Speech Quality," *Journal of Speech and Hearing Disorders,* Vol. 45/Mo. 3, August 1980.

REGAN, R., HOKE, M., SIGELMAN, J., and OLSEN, N., "Canal Hearing Aids 1984," *Hearing Instruments,* Vol. 35, No. 4, 1984.

RINTELMANN, W., "Hearing Assessment," Baltimore, MD., University Park Press, 1979.

ROSS, M., "Classroom Acoustics and Speech Intelligibility," *Handbook of Clinical Audiology* (Katz, J., ed.) 2nd Edition Baltimore, MD., Williams and Wilkins, 1978.

ROSS, M., "Communication Access," Vanderbilt Hearing Aid Report, Studebaker and Bess eds., 1982. *Monographs in Contemporary Audiology,* Upper Darby, PA.

SACHS, R. M., and BURKHAD, M. D., "Making Pressure Measurements in Insert Earphone Couplers and Real Ears," *Journal of the Acoustical Society of America* 51, 140 (a), 1972.

SANDLIN, R. E., "Advances in Hearing Aid Technology," *Hearing Disorders in Adults.* (Jerger, J., ed.) San Diego, College Hill Press, 1984.

SCHARF, B., "Sensorineural Hearing Impairment and Hearing Aids," (Ludvigsen and Barfod, ed.), *Scandinavian Audiology,* Supp 6, 1978.

SCHWARTZ, D., and WALDEN, B. E., "Zenetron Munich-Salsburg Symposium on Hearing Health Care," *Excerpta Medica,* 1980.

SCHWARTZ, D. M., MONTGOMERY, A. A., PUNCH, J. L., WALDEN, B. E., and PROSEK, P. A., "Quality Judgements of Hearing Aid processed Speech by Hearing Impaired Listeners," Presented as ASLHA Convention, Atlanta GA., 1979.

SCHWARTZ, D. M., "Hearing Aid Selection Methods: An Enigma," The Vanderbilt Hearing Aid Report (Studebaker and Bess, eds.) Upper Darby, PA., *Monographs in Contemporary Audiology,* 1982.

SCHWEITZER, H. C., "Tutorial Paper: Principles and Characteristics of Automatic Gain Control Hearing Aids," *Journal of the American Audiological Society,* 5, 84–94, 1979.

SEDACCA, Y. C., "Basic Audio Information for Hearing Aid Consultants," *Hal-Hen Widex, Inc.,* nd. Also, *Hearing Aid Journal,* 15, 1962, issues 4 and 5.

SKAFTE, M., and CRANMER, K., "Hearing Aid Dispensing—1984," *Hearing Instruments,* May 1984.

SKINNER, M. W., "Speech Intelligibility in Noise-Induced Hearing Loss: Effects of High Frequency Compensation," Ph.D. thesis,. Washington U, St. Louis, MO., 1976.

SKINNER M. W., KARSTAEDT, M. M., and MILLER, J. D., "Amplification Bandwidth and Speech Intelligibility for Two Listeners with Sensorineural Hearing Loss," *Audiology (in press).*

SHAPIRO, B., "What You Can Do to Fight Mercury Pollution," *Hearing Instruments,* 22, Feb. 1971, 24.

SHAW, E. A. G., "Diffuse Field Sensitivity of External Ear Based on Reciprocity Principles," *Journal of the Acoustical Society of America* 1976:60: S102(a).

STAAB, W. J., "CROS and Open Canal Fitting," *Telex Audiological Reports,* XII:5, 1972.

STAAB, W. J., "Limiting Systems in Hearing Aids," *Auditone Technical Reports,* 4, October, 1982.

STAAB, W. J., "Hearing Aid Handbook," Blue Ridge Summit, PA., Tab Books, 1978.

STAAB, W. J., "Clarifying the CIC Mystique," *Hearing Review,* Aug. 1994, Vol. 1, No. 7.

STAAB, W. J., "The Peritympanic Instrument Fitting Rationale and Test Results," *Hearing Journal,* 45 (10), 21–26, 1992.

STAAB, W. J., "Hearing Aid Compression Amplification," *Hearing Aid Journal,"* 25:12, 1972.

STEINBERG, J. D., and GARDNER, M. B., "The Dependence of Hearing Impairment on Sound Intensity," *Journal of the Acoustical Society of America,* 9, 11–23 1937.

STEVENS, A. E., "The First 'Wearable' Aid," *Hearing Instruments,* Dec. 1959, 13.

STOKER, R., "An Audiometer Telephone Interface," *Hearing Instruments,* Vol. 33, No. 6, 1982.

STUDEBAKER, G. A., and ZACHMAN, T. A., "Investigation of the Acoustics of Earmold Vents, *Journal of the Acoustical Society of America,* 47, 1970, 1107–1115.

STUDEBAKER, G. A., "Fifty Years of Hearing Research: An Evaluation of Progress, Ear and Hearing," Vol. 1/No. 2, March-April 1980, page 57.

STUDEBAKER, G. A., COX, R. M., FORMBY, C., "The Effect of Environment of the Directional Performance of Head-Worn Hearing Aids," *Acoustical Factors Affecting Hearing Aid Performance,* Baltimore, MD., University Park Press 1980.

SUNG, G. S., SUNG, R. J., and ANGELLELI, R. M., "Directional Microphone in Hearing Aids: Effects on Speech Discrimination in Noise.," *Arch. of Otol.,* 101, 316–319, 1975.

SUNG, R. J., and SUNG, G. S., "Low Frequency Amplification and Speech Intelligibility in Noise," *Hearing Instruments,* 1:20–47, 1982.

SZOSDA, M. E., "Active Filtering for Hearing Aids," *Hearing Journal,* 40 (4), 1987.

TECCA, J. E., and GOLDSTEIN, D. P., "Effect of Low Frequency Hearing Aid Response on Four Measures of Speech Perception." *Ear and Hearing,* Vol. 5/No. 1, 1984.

TEDER, H., "Noise and Speech Levels in Noisy Environments," *Hearing Instruments,* 41 (4), 32–33, 1990.

TEDER, H., and SMRIGA, D. J., "Personal Communication," 1984.

TILLMAN, T., KASTEN, R., and HORNER, J., "Effect of Head Shadow on Reception of Speech," Paper Presented at ASHA, Chicago, IL, Nov. 1963.

VEIT, L., "Hearing Aids with Automatic Volume Control (AVC) and Related Problems of Circuitry," *ZHA,* 12, 1973, 186–200.

VICTOREEN, J. A., "Hearing Enhancement," Charles C. Thomas, 1960.

VILLCHUR, E., "Signal Processing to Improve Speech Intelligibility in Perceptive Deafness," *Journal of the Acoustical Society of America,* 1973:53:1646–1657.

VILLCHUR, E., "Signal Processing. Auditory Management of Hearing Impaired Children," Ross and Giolas (eds.) University Park Press, Baltimore, MD., 1978.

WALKER, C., and DILLION, H., "Compression in Hearing Aids: An Analysis, A Review of Some Recommendations," *NAL report 90.* National Acoustic Laboratories, Australia, 1982.

WULLENSTEIN, H. L., and WIGAND, "Uber Horhilfe zum Beidseitigen Horen fur Einseitig Ertaubte und ihre Voraussetzungen (A Hearing Aid for Single Ear Deafness and its Requirements)" *Acta Oto-Laryngologica,* 54, 1962, 136–142.

ZELNICK, E., "Options in the Fitting of Binaural Hearing Aids," *Hearing Aid Journal,* 1970.

ZELNICK, E., "Binaural Hearing Aids for Infants," *Hearing Aid Journal,* 26:7, 1973.

ZELNICK, E., "Effectiveness of Binaural Hearing Aids," Second Annual Oticongress, Copenhagen, 1971.

Zenith Hearing Aid Corp. "Hearing Aids and Their Components," (1968).

APPENDIX

American National Standard, Specification of Hearing Aid Characteristics, ANSI S3.22-1987

DEFINITIONS

3.1 Reference Sound Pressure Level
Throughout this standard, all sound pressure levels are referred to 20 uPa.

3.2 Input Sound Pressure Level
For non-directional hearing aids, the input sound pressure level is the sound pressure level at the microphone opening of the hearing aid. For directional hearing aids, the input sound pressure level is the sound pressure level in a progressive sound field adjacent to the microphone openings of the hearing aid.

3.3 Acoustic Gain
Acoustic gain is the difference between the output sound pressure level in an earphone coupler and the input sound pressure level.

3.4 Gain Control
A gain control is a user operated control for the adjustment of gain.

3.5 Saturation Sound Pressure Level for 90-dB Input Sound Pressure Level
The saturation sound pressure for a 90-dB input sound pressure level is defined as the sound pressure level developed in 2-cm earphone coupler when the input sound pressure level is 90-dB, with the gain control of the hearing aid full-on. The abbreviation for this term is SSPL90.

3.6 High-Frequency Average (HFA) Saturation Sound Pressure Level
The HFA saturation sound pressure level is defined as the average of the 1000, 1600, and 2500-Hz values of SSPL90 (abbreviation HFA-SSPL90).

3.61 Sound Purpose Average (SPA) Saturation Sound Pressure Level (SPA SSPL90)
The SPA saturation sound pressure level is defined as the average of the SSPL90 at the special purpose frequencies selected by manufacturer (refer to Sec. 3.15).

3.7 Full-On Gain
The full-on gain is the acoustic gain when the gain control of the hearing is at its full-on position.

3.8 High Frequency Average (HFA) Full-On Gain

The HFA full-on gain is defined as the average of the 1000, 1600, and 2500-Hz values of full-on gain (refer to Sec. 6.4 for measurement conditions).

3.81 Special Purpose Average (SPA) Full-On Gain

The SPA full-on gain is defined as the average of the full-on gain at the special purpose frequencies selected by the manufacturer (refer to Sec. 3.15).

3.9 Reference Test Gain Control Position

The reference test gain control position is defined as the setting of the hearing aid gain control so that the average of the earphone coupler sound pressure levels at 1000, 1600, and 2500 Hz, or at the three special purpose frequencies, with a pure-tone input sound pressure level of 60 dB, is 17 dB less than the HFA-SSPL90 or the SPA-SSPL90, respectively (refer to Sec. 3.15). If the gain available does not permit this and for AGC aids, the reference test gain control position is the full-on position of the gain control.

3.10 Reference Test Gain

The reference test gain is defined as the acoustic gain of a hearing aid when its gain control is set to amplify a 60 dB sound pressure level input signal to a level in the coupler that is 17 dB below the SSPL90 value for the hearing aid. If the gain available will not permit this, and for AGC hearing aids, the reference test gain is the HFA full-on gain or SPA full-on gain of the hearing aid. Gain and saturation values are determined on the basis of the average of 1000, 1600, and 2500 Hz values or the values at the special purpose average frequencies (refer to Sec. 3.15 and 6.6).

3.11 Automatic Gain Control Hearing Aid

A hearing aid incorporating means (other than peak clipping) by which the gain is automatically controlled as a function of the magnitude of the signal being amplified is defined as an automatic gain control hearing aid. The abbreviation for automatic gain control is AGC.

3.12 AGC Knee Point

The knee point is the point on the input-output curve of an AGC hearing aid at which the curve first departs by 2 dB on the output sound pressure level scale from the extension of the linear portion of the input-output curve that exists at input levels below the compression or limiting portion of the curve.

3.13 AGC Control

An AGC control is any control that affects the steady state operation of the AGC function excluding the user operated gain control, any tone control, or a peak clipping control.

3.14 Directional Hearing Aid

A hearing aid in which the microphone sensitivity is dependent on the direction of sound incidence when measured under free-field conditions is a directional hearing aid.

3.15 Special Purpose Hearing Aid

A special purpose hearing aid is an instrument whose full-on gain at 1000, or at 1600 Hz, or at 2500 Hz is less than the maximum full-on gain minus 15 dB.

If an instrument is found to meet the requirement for being a special purpose hearing aid, the manufacturer may substitute three 1/3 octave frequencies (ANSI S1.61976, R1984) each separated by 2/3 octave, for formulating special purpose averages (SPA). The special purpose frequencies shall be specified and used for all measurements.

V

ACOUSTIC COUPLERS

JOEL M. MYNDERS, BC-HIS

INTRODUCTION

Hearing aid amplification is one form of hearing loss management. It differs from the other options of surgery and medicine, in that instruments must be individually adapted and fitted for correction. In the fitting concept, both physical and acoustical adaptation combine. Traditionally, for most of the history of electrical hearing aids, the earmold was *the* acoustic coupler. However, today a majority of hearing instruments fitted to patients are the "custom" type that place the electronics completely in the external ear or canal. Thus the shell of these styles of hearing aids replaces the earmold used with behind-the-ear, eyeglass and body aids. The information in this chapter will have application for both earmolds and the shells of custom-type aids.

Current digital-programmable hearing aids have compression and filtering technologies electrically adjustable by the hearing aid clinician via computers. Thus the potential for *electrical* modifications, in contrast to *acoustical* modifications, of hearing aid response has multiplied a hundred-fold and more. The goal of the newer technologies is improved signal-to-noise performance. In the past, some earmold options such as drilled belled canals, CFA molds, Libby Horns and resonator-"style" molds all aimed at improved signal-to-noise ratio as well.

Digitally programmable hearing aids allow the hearing professional to electronically modify the frequency response, output, and in certain instruments, the release time, compression ratio and crossover frequency for two or three independent bands. Given this high degree of computer-assisted adjustment, it brings into question the usefulness of traditional earmold acoustic options. Are earmold acoustics still valid?

Some manufacturers report that half of the programmable aids fitted are the behind-the-ear type. In these units, earmold considerations such as pressure relief venting, earmold and material selection all remain part of the fitting process. Advances in materials and design now enable the hearing health professional to maximize the impedance match between the hearing aid and ear. The appropriate coupling between receiver and ear canal, in many instances will determine the smoothness of the aided response, the effective real ear high frequency gain, and in the final analysis, the patient's acceptance of the hearing aid.

This chapter will bring together in one place detailed information about past earmold practices with the idea that as technology changes, the role of the acoustic coupler will be altered. However, past practice may offer insights and possible reapplication and modification of past practices for current fitting problems.

Clinicians find themselves in the enviable position of having a very wide range of *acoustical* (through earmold technology) and *electrical* (through computer assisted applications) fitting options and choices to maximize a patient's fitting. Clinical findings show that a combination of these acoustical and electrical control options often give the best amplification results for patients. Thus the question, "Are earmolds acoustics still valid?" is answered in the affirmative.

In this chapter, the historical review, the functions of earmolds, the impression process, the measurement process and the modification process will apply to either earmolds or shells for custom hearing instruments. Since 12–15% of the instruments currently fitted use earmolds, chapter sections on the selection process, and the counseling process apply to these fittings.

CHAPTER OBJECTIVES

At this point, the reader will have a reasonable overview of applied hearing aid amplification. This chapter will review the history, the general theories, the impression process, the selection process, the electro-acoustic measurement process, the counseling process about earmolds and the modification process. Since earmold usage has been drastically reduced over the past ten years, many clinicians have limited experiences regarding earmold acoustics and options. This chapter contains practical information about fitting hearing impaired patients. The information may not be used every day, based upon the patients and clinicians preference for "custom" type hearing instruments. However, in the course of dispensing hearing aids, the clinician must have knowledge of coupler choices and their effects.

HISTORICAL REVIEW

The first hearing aids didn't use earmolds. They used a headset similar to that of an audiometer. With the development of miniature receivers, it was possible to create a snap-on earmold. Figure 1 shows early hearing aids with different receiver types. The one at the left has an earmold attached.

The first earmolds were made from galvanized rubber in five "standard" sizes. They "approximated" the shape of a person's external ear. The first custom earmold is credited to a New York dentist, Mayer B. A. Schier, in 1922. He used dental material to make

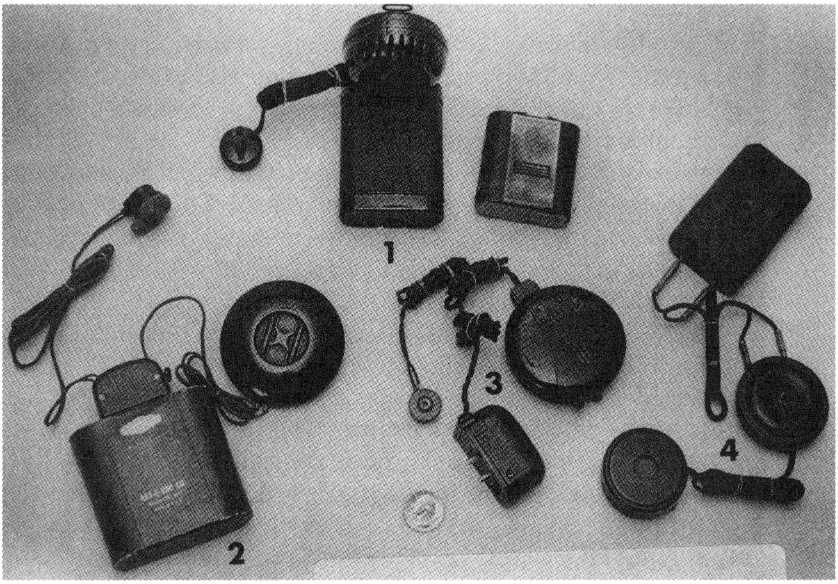

Fig. 1. Early Electric Hearing Aids

an impression of the pinna, concha and ear canal. From this impression, an individualized earmold was fabricated from lucite. The main purpose of these early earmolds was comfort, permitting the hearing aid to be worn for extended periods. Earmold acoustics, as a hearing aid science, had not yet begun. In the 1920–40's there were no measurement techniques that could assess the effect of an earmold.

The first textbook on hearing aids, published by Watson & Tolan (1949) was entitled *Hearing Tests and Hearing Instruments.* There is a short part concerned with earmolds:

> DESIGN OF INDIVIDUALLY MOLDED EAR INSERT
>
> The individually molded ear insert should follow good acoustic practice. Molded ear inserts in which a section of the channel is narrowed, definitely reduce the effectiveness of the aid. Such constriction of the insert channel has the effect of reducing the high frequency response. Grossman notes that bone conduction transmission is provided through the individually molded ear insert with little or no tip extension into the ear canal for types of deafness where high frequency emphasis is required with the more conventional type of ear insert having an extension into the ear canal reserved for conductive types of deafness and those not requiring marked high frequency emphasis.
>
> Avoiding narrowing channels in ear inserts in order to assure better high frequency reproduction would appear to be advisable from experimental studies. (P. 360).

This 1949 reference was subsequently validated by earmold researchers. (First Symposium on Earmolds held in Philadelphia in 1974) This was followed by the first book on earmolds published, arising from the Danavox Symposium, 1975.

A second important milestone in early earmold development was the "vent". The vent is basically a channel drilled through the body of an earmold to reduce acoustic pressure. Dr Schier is credited with this development, which he called a "side branch orifice", which is shown in Figure 2.

The original purpose of this vent was to produce comfort not acoustic performance. The pressure and "stuffed-up" feeling patients experienced when wearing custom fitted earmolds could be relieved, if the side-branch orifice was drilled.

There was not much new in earmolds during the Great Depression and World War II. In fact, there were no measurement standards for the hearing aids themselves. In the late 1950's to early 1960, the first agreed upon performance standards were implemented. One of the early hearing aid engineers was Samuel Lybarger (1967) who published an article entitled *Earmold*

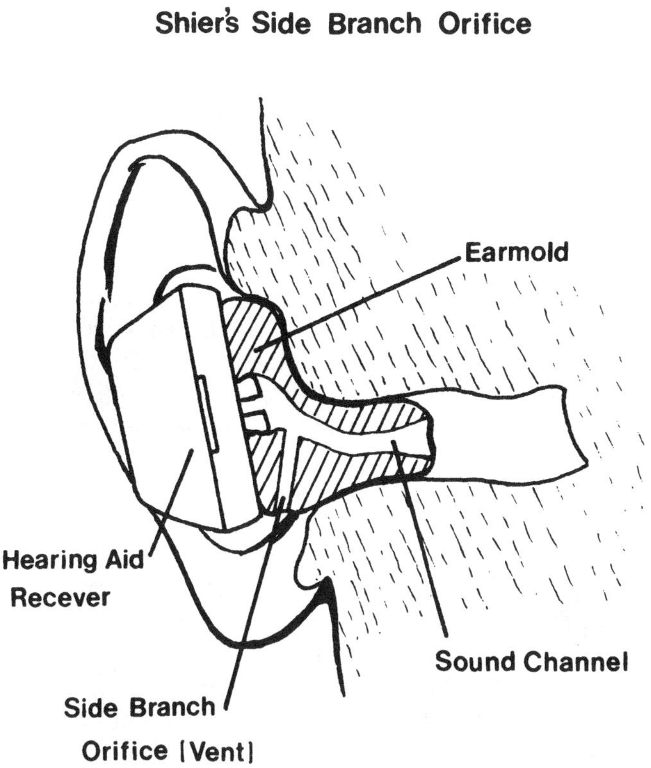

Fig. 2. Earliest Type of Vent with Button Receiver

Acoustics. Efforts were made to measure the effects earmolds had on the hearing aid's acoustic output. Venting was examined and explained. This period of rapid growth in knowledge continued into the 1980's. The hearing aid trade journals and the audiology journals had frequent articles about earmold inventions developed by hearing aid specialists, earmold laboratories, university clinics and some manufacturers.

Lewis and Plotkin (1962) developed an earmold for the Zenith Hearing Aid Corporation called the "Acoustic Modifier". The mold was characterized by a short canal with a wide bore and a vent covered with a felt-like material. Many dispensers used this modified earmold. In the early 1970's, there were three new *venting systems* presented to dispensers to ease the problems of vent drilling. These were the Variable Venting Valves (V.V.V.), the Positive Venting Valve (P.V.V) and the Select-A-Vent (S.A.V.). Green and Mynders (1974, 1975) reported on their results with these venting systems.

A final category of earmold development was the development of "resonator" type earmolds that employ a version of the Helmholtz resonator effect. It was first developed by Rubein Johnson, a hearing aid dispenser in Oklahoma. Mynders (1979) reported on the Johnson invention called the "Gold Crown Earmold". It was cast from gold with resonating chambers and an opening in the bore of the canal. Other resonator molds were the F.G.M., developed by a dispenser in California; the C.F.A. developed by Pacific Coast Labs; the Macrae molds developed at the National Acoustic Labs in Australia. They were all sophisticated but never gained wide acceptance and use.

With increasing markets for in-the-ear and in-the-canal style of hearing aids, by 1993 only 14% of hearing aids dispensed in the United States were non-custom types. Earmold usage had declined drastically. There are still occasionally some innovative developments from individuals and labs, but not with the same force as were the rapid developments of the 70's and 80's.

Preves (1980) noted that the shells of custom aids were influenced by existing earmold acoustics. In other words, venting, dampers and horn effects were often tried for in-the-ear and in-the-canal fittings with varying degrees of success. A major factor with shells as the coupler was the receiver location which was not in the canal portion of the aids. This changes the "acoustics" that still exist for behind-the-ear, eyeglass and body aids. The transmission effects of connector, tubing and earmold cavities are of no consequence with in-the-ear, in-the-canal and completely-the-canal instruments.

FUNCTIONS OF HUMAN ACOUSTIC COUPLERS

To understand any device, you must know what its purpose is. The human acoustic coupler is either an earmold or the shell of a custom hearing aid. What is an acoustic coupler? Basically it is a device, either an insert or a shell which attaches a hearing aid to the human ear. They are made from hard or soft plastics, after an impression of a patient's external ear canal has been taken.

The functions of acoustic couplers include:

1. To COUPLE the hearing aid to the ear.
2. To RETAIN the BTE aid on the outer ear.
3. To SEAL the ear acoustically to prevent feedback.
4. To acoustically MODIFY the gain, frequency response and output of the hearing aid.

5. To be physically COMFORTABLE for long periods of time.
6. To be AESTHETICALLY ACCEPTABLE to the patient.

For particular cases, the hearing aid clinician may use some or all of these functions listed. Functions 5 and 6 should never be underestimated relative to their value. Lack of attention to these two non-acoustic functions will be causes for patient rejection of hearing aid use.

ACOUSTICS OF EARMOLDS

Acoustics factors are involved when measuring the degree and type of hearing loss by audiometry. There are acoustics involved in measuring actual hearing aid performance and earmold acoustics. Finally, there are acoustics involved in measuring the effects of an earmold on ear canal resonance.

Research in the area of speech acoustics has yielded valuable information for hearing aid development. For example, high frequency formants of many consonants are important to the understanding of speech. The frequency range from 2500–3500 Hz is critical to word recognition function.

Much of the speech energy occurs from 50–1000 Hz, but much of the speech intelligibility occurs from 1000–8000 Hz. Thus hearing aids must reproduce audible high frequencies, in order for clients to achieve maximum intelligibility. Studies of insertion loss demonstrated that some earmolds did not allow extended high frequency response, because they were not designed to do so.

Current earmold technology encompasses "control areas" for acoustics generated in the hearing aid and earmold. The graph below, Figure 3, clearly shows the relationships by frequency and sound quality judgment, with an overlay of an actual hearing aid's response.

Earmold acoustics is a marriage between the human acoustic coupler and the science of acoustics. For many years, measurement of acoustical events occurring in an earmold, or at the eardrum, was not possible due to the physical size of the measuring devices. With the advent of the probe microphone assembly, it became possible to measure more precisely acoustics within the ear canal. The human ear canal, by its size and shape, acts as a natural resonating cavity, which boosts certain sounds significantly. The greatest gain occurs at approximately 2600 Hz in the adult ear.

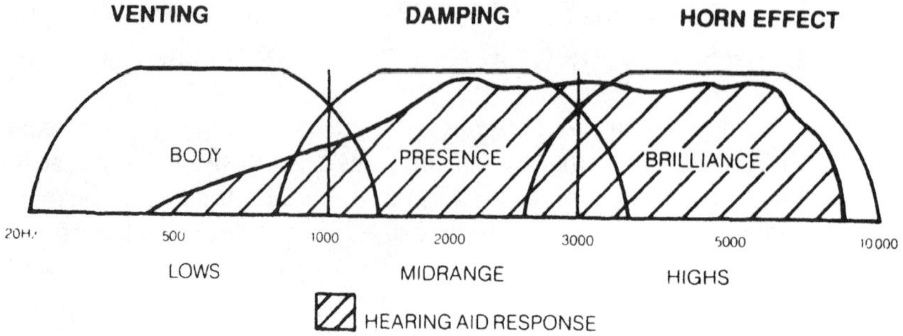

Fig. 3. Control Areas of Earmold Acoustics

Figure 4 shows how accommodating "nature" is. Where the natural acoustic energy of speech declines, nature gives a boost in the form of "natural" ear canal resonance.

Ear canal resonance is necessary for listeners to hear naturally. Hearing impaired individuals still have "natural" ear canal resonance. However, their hearing loss diminishes its contribution. With the hearing impaired, another item which alters ear canal resonance effectiveness is the earmold. The earmold creates an "insertion loss" or a loss of hearing sensitivity. Figure 5 presents a pictorial of insertion loss.

Earmold acoustics require an understanding of a specialized vocabulary associated with acoustical physics and the physical phenomena of the science that relates to earmolds. A monograph by Cox (1979) served as the major resource for the following:

The new words you should understand are 1) acoustic impedance—the opposition of the flow of acoustical energy through a system, 2) acoustic inertance—occurs when a volume of air is made to oscillate and is not compressed to any significant extent,

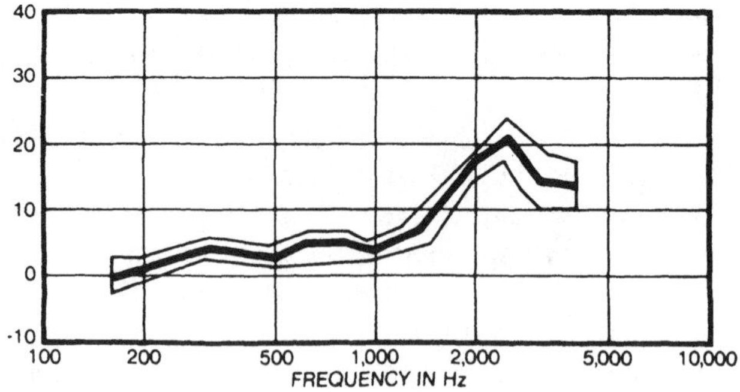

Fig. 4. Natural Ear Canal Resonance

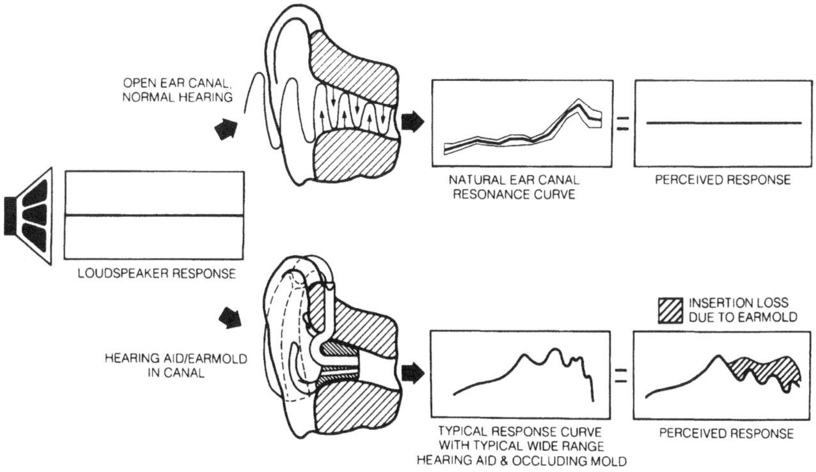

Fig. 5. Representation of Insertion Loss

3) acoustic compliance—occurs when aid is enclosed in a cavity with rigid walls, 4) acoustic resistance—occurs whenever acoustic energy is dissipated by frictional loss due to collision of air particles, 5) acoustic transformer—occurs by gradually increasing the final opening of a sound tube which maintains the high frequency response due to wavelength resonances in the sound channel, 6) resonance—the basic or natural frequency of vibration that is unique to an air filled cavity, and finally 7) Helmholtz Resonance—occurs in a hearing aid coupler when a length of tubing is adjacent to a cavity with a volume of air enclosed in it.

Basically, in earmold acoustics, one is concerned with the transmission of sound from the hearing aid's receiver to the human eardrum.

To describe the acoustical terms defined above, let us begin with acoustic impedance. This is the opposition to the acoustic flow of energy. It occurs in two forms, (a) one that temporarily changes the acoustic flow (e.g. a resonating cavity drilled in an earmold) or, (b) one that dissipates some of the energy (e.g. a sintered metal pellet in the tube or earhook).

There are two types of acoustic impedance; resistant and reactive. Resistant acoustic impedance is relatively constant from frequency to frequency. Reactive acoustic impedance is determined by acoustic mass and compliance.

The acoustic mass of a human acoustic coupler is the air from the hearing aid's receiver to the eardrum. The impedance of a mass of air in hearing aid tubing is directly proportional to the length of the tube and inversely proportional to the diameter of the tube. It is known that low frequencies travel through hearing aid tubing with little resistance. It is the high frequency sounds that encounter opposition in an acoustic coupler.

Acoustic compliance is air enclosed in a cavity with rigid walls. This situation exists in the walls of the earmold itself, but only partially in the ear canal and not at all at the eardrum, which moves in and out as a function of sound pressure changes. The value of acoustic compliance in a rigid-walled cavity is proportional to the volume of the cavity. When the volume of air is increased, as in using a belled bore or a shorter canal length in an earmold compliance is increased. This is important because in physical systems, highly compliant materials offer less opposition to high frequency sound transmission.

Acoustic resistance occurs when air particles collide with each other, (e.g. in earmolds, in the tubing or at the location of dampers). When there is an acoustic resistance, there is always some acoustic energy dissipated as heat.

Acoustic resonance occurs when the total impedance of the acoustical system is determined by the acoustic resonance. Unfortunately, there is not a simple acoustic situation in earmold acoustics.

Quarter-wave resonance in tubing usually occurs in tubing sections where there are convolutions and identations in the tubing wall. There are half-wavelength resonances existing in many fittings when the internal hearing aid receiver has a large volume of air in front of the diaphragm of the receiver and is then attached to a long earmold tubing.

The various resonant peaks seen in Figure 6 can be due to wavelength resonances.

The quarter-wavelength resonances that occur with the wideband receivers are due to an impedance mismatch resulting from high-impedance characteristics of the wide band receivers and low impedance characteristics of the eardrum.

Acoustic transformer phenomenon will be recognized among hearing health professionals by its more popular name of "horn effect". For years, those who made musical brass instruments have known that flaring the end of a brass horn produces a big effect on the acoustical quality of the sound produced. It was not until the 1970's that "belled" bores (i.e. horn effect) were used by large numbers of hearing aid clinicians. The effect of a belled canal in the earmold was to maintain high frequency performance.

The following outline details parts of the earmold system that are involved in the various acoustical phenomena.

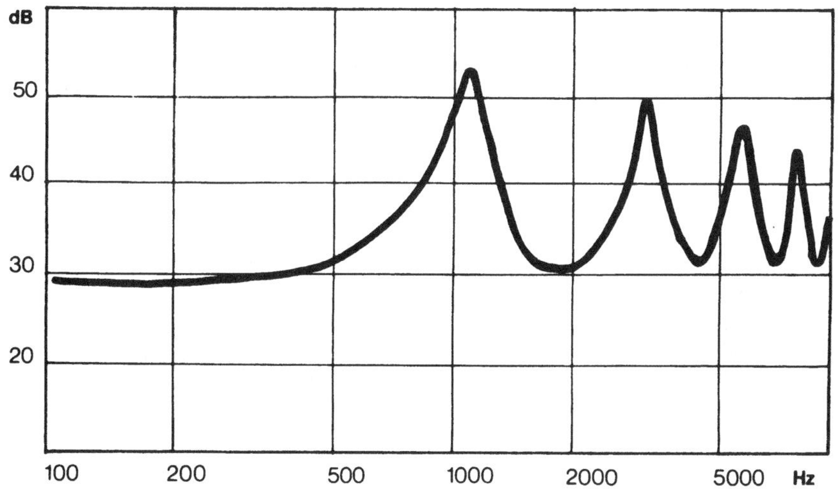

Fig. 6. Wave Length Resonances

I. ACOUSTIC INERTANCE
   a) Tubing
   b) Bore at a Vent

II. ACOUSTIC COMPLIANCE
   a) Air inside and in front of the receiver
   b) Hearing aid receiver's diaphragm

III. ACOUSTIC RESISTANCE
   a) Knowles Dampers
   b) Sintered metal pellets
   c) Lamb's wool
   d) Star Dampers

Earmold acoustics came about as a result of component developments. Figure 7 shows the profound changes in frequency response as a result of the use of wide band receivers.

For years hearing aids were basically low fidelity devices with typical frequency ranges of 325–3900 Hz. Today's receivers make possible ranges from 90–9500 Hz and beyond. The acoustic contribution of the earmold in preserving this acoustic gain for the patient is critical.

Killion (1976) found that by using stepped bore tubings in earmolds, large changes in acoustic frequency response could be

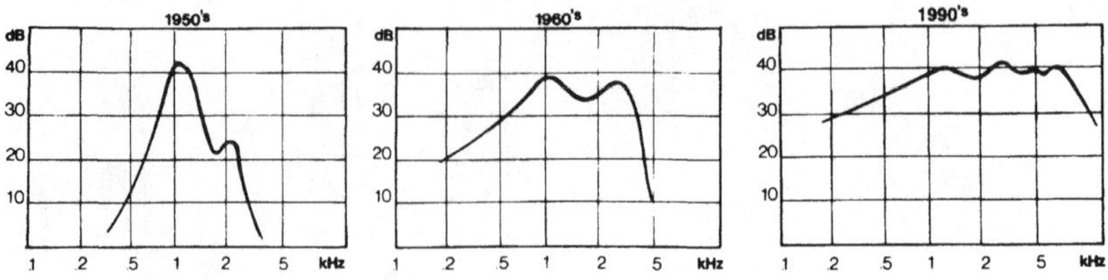

Fig. 7. Expanding Frequency Response Range in Hearing Aids from the 1950's to the 1990's.

obtained. His research resulted in a family of earmolds that were "acoustically tuned" for certain acoustic effects. This series of options incorporate venting, damping and horn effects. Most of the earmolds are characterized by two sizes of tubing cemented together and precisely positioned dampers in that tubing.

The Killion System (1980) uses numbers and letters to designate the different style earmolds. The number refers to the frequency involved, while letter or letters refers to the effect. A final number refers to decibels. For example:

8CR means 8000 Hz "Canal Response"

6AM means 6000 Hz "Acoustic Modifier"

"B" means "BOOST"

"C" means "CUT"

6B10 means 6000 Hz BOOST—10dB higher at 6000 Hz than at 1000Hz

6C5 means 6000 Hz CUT—5 dB lower at 6000 Hz than 1000 Hz

Figure 8 details the Killion System of "acoustic control" through acoustic tuning accomplished by specific venting, damping and the use of belled bases.

The important point in Killion's invention of "earmold plumbing" was that with behind-the-ear hearing aids with wide band receivers the hearing aid clinician could actually cancel the improvements created by the wide-band receivers. In other words, a high-fidelity hearing aid could become low fidelity by the incorrect earmold selection.

Earmold technology offers hearing aid clinicians considerable control over specific frequency responses. The technology allows the fitter to control one frequency area independently or a combination of all three simultaneously. What does this mean in everyday dispensing practice? It means that the fitter has several options in maximizing the client's fitting with behind-the-ear aids.

	APPLICATION	LOW-FREQUENCY (VENTING)	MID-FREQUENCY (DAMPING)	HIGH-FREQUENCY (HORN EFFECT)
Killion 6R12 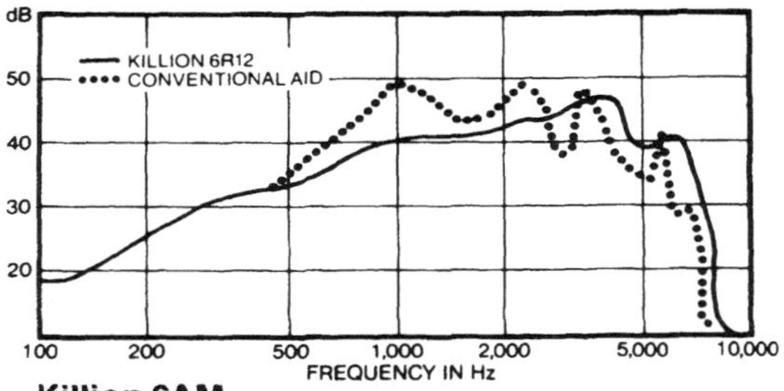	Client has mid-freq. tolerance problems or limited needs in mid-freq. with extended hi-freq. compensation required.	Venting effects will be determined by vent diameter, location and length.	Eliminates first two typical peaks just below 2.7kHz; does not compensate for earmold insertion loss.	6kHz cut-off with maximum boost just below 6K with 5dB increase between 4–6K.
Killion 6AM 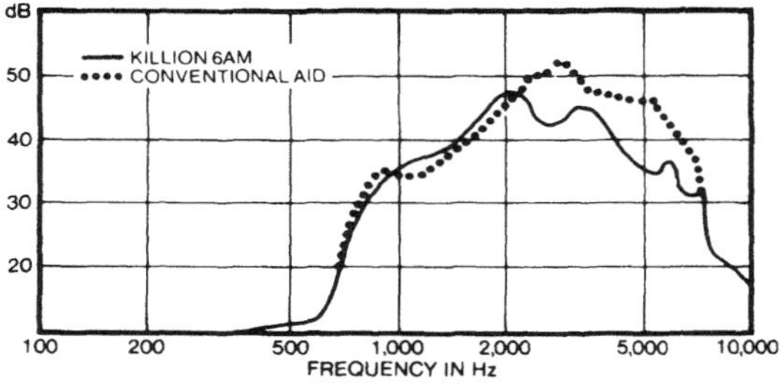	Client requires no low-freq. amplification but requires extended hi-freq. compensation.	Vent design similar to Acoustic Modifier concept with significant low-freq. reduction.	Eliminates first two typical peaks just below 2.7kHz; does not compensate for earmold insertion loss.	6kHz cut-off with maximum boost just below 6K with 5dB increase between 4–6K.

Fig. 8. Killion's System for Control of Earmold Acoustics

Killion 8CR

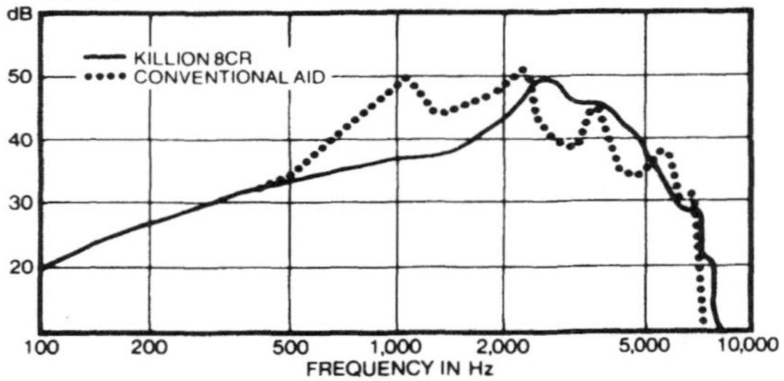

	APPLICATION	LOW-FREQUENCY (VENTING)	MID-FREQUENCY (DAMPING)	HIGH-FREQUENCY (HORN EFFECT)
Killion 8CR	Client has good tolerance and requires a steady hi-freq. increase. Improved noise discrimination is needed.	Venting effects will be determined by vent diameter, location, and length.	Boost at 2.7kHz compensates for insertion loss with a flat insertion gain and smooth mid-freq. response out to 8kHz.	8kHz cut-off with boost at 8K to give extended hi-freq. energy beyond 8K.
Killion 6B0	Client needs mid-freq. modification but no extended or increased hi-freq. needs.	Venting effects will be determined by vent diameter, location and length.	680 ohm — 10dB Reduction re. 1K 1500 ohm — 18dB Reduction re. 1K 3300 ohm — 22dB Reduction re. 1K 4700 ohm — 26dB Reduction re. 1K	Provides almost no hi-freq. boost. Basically a conventional earmold with mid-freq. damping.

Killion 6B0

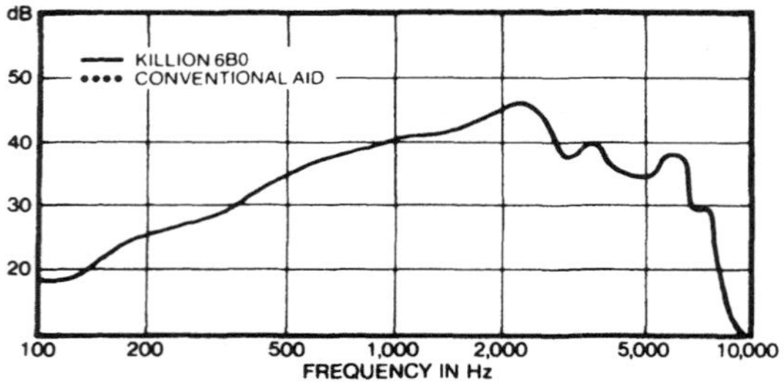

(Fig 8. continued)

FREQUENCY IN Hz

Killion 6B5

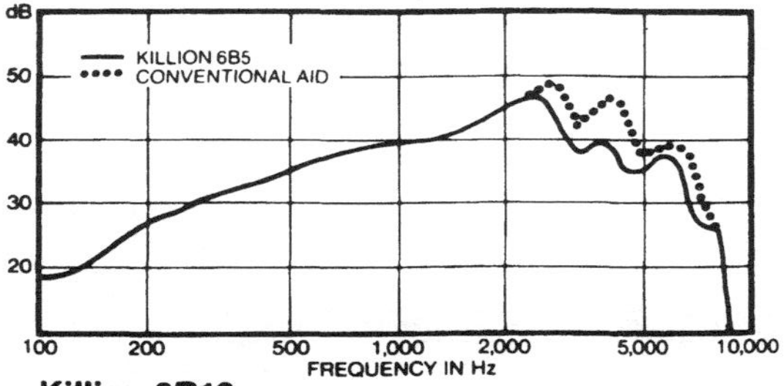

Client needs mid-freq. modification and slight hi-freq. increase.	Venting effects will be determined by vent diameter, location and length.	680 ohm—10dB Reduction re. 1K 1500 ohm—18dB Reduction re. 1K 3300 ohm—22 dB Reduction re. 1K 4700 ohm—26dB Reduction re. 1K 0 ohm—Conventional earmold resp.	Provides 5dB boost at 6kHz relative to 1K. Starts at 2.5-3kHz and extends to 6 kHz.

Killion 6B10

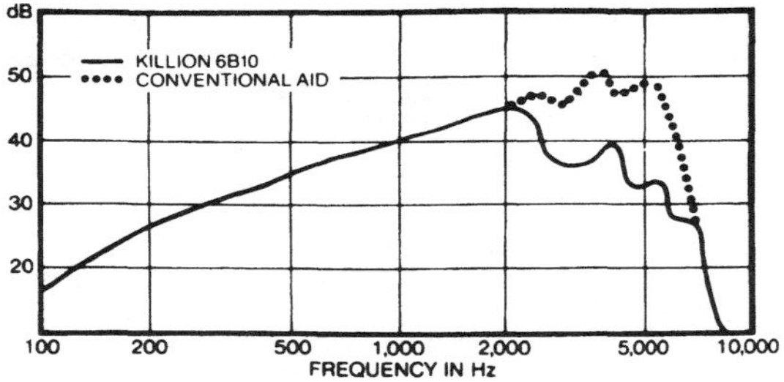

Client needs mid-freq. modification and moderate hi-freq. increase.	Venting effects will be determined by vent diameter, location and length.	680 ohm—10dB Reduction re. 1K 1500 ohm—18dB Reduction re. 1K 3300 ohm—22dB Reduction re. 1K 4700 ohm—26dB Reduction re. 1K 0 ohm—Conventional earmold resp.	Provides 10dB boost at 6kHz relative to 1K. Starts at 2.5-3kHz and extends to 6kHz.

(Fig 8. continued)

Killion 6C5 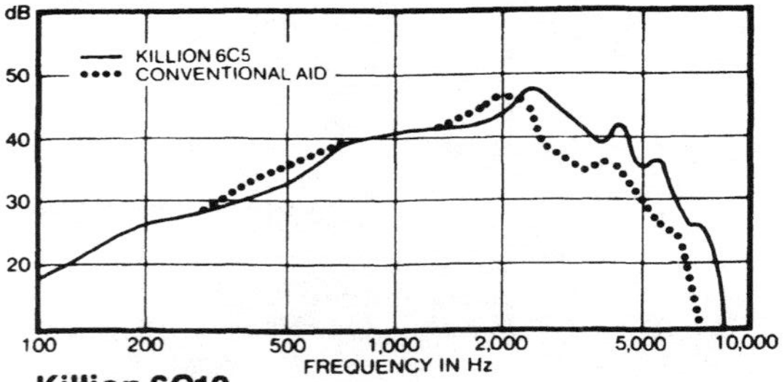	Client needs mid-freq. modification and slight hi-freq. attenuation.	Venting effects will be determined by vent diameter, location and length.	680 ohm—10dB Reduction re. 1K 1500 ohm—18dB Reduction re. 1K 3300 ohm—22dB Reduction re. 1K 4700 ohm—26dB Reduction re. 1K 0 ohm—Conventional earmold resp.	Provides 5dB cut at 6kHz relative to 1K. Starts at 2.5-3kHz and extends to 6kHz.
Killion 6C10 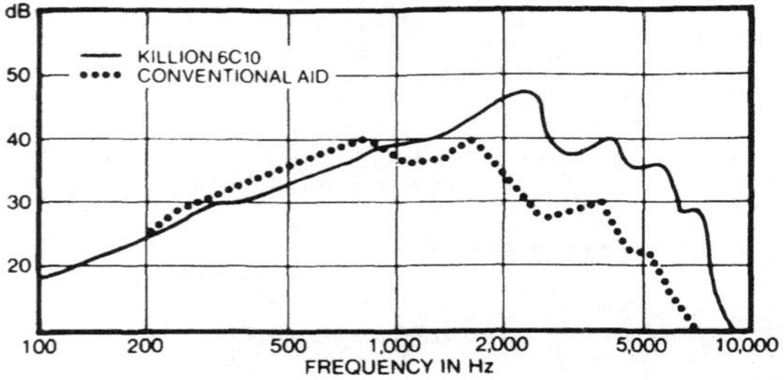	Client needs mid-freq. modification & slight hi-freq. attenuation. This design for emphasis in the mid & low freq.	Venting effects will be determined by vent diameter, location and length.	680 ohm—10dB Reduction re. 1K 1500 ohm—18dB Reduction re. 1K 3300 ohm—22dB Reduction re. 1K 4700 ohm—26dB Reduction re. 1K 0 ohm—Conventional earmold resp.	Provides 10dB cut at 6kHz relative to 1K. Starts at 2.5-3kHz and extends to 6kHz.

(Fig 8. continued)

Killion's earmold system inspired further system developments by Bakke (1983), Bennett (1978), Goldberg (1977), Johnson (1979), Libby (1980), Schlaegel (1983), Macrae (1983) and others. The essence of these systems is expanded discrete acoustic control via the earmold, for maximum benefit from applied amplification—in other words, IMPROVED HEARING.

For researchers and hearing aid specialists, earmold technology has some basic philosophic considerations as summarized by Libby (1980). They are: (a) to preserve the balance acoustically between the high frequencies and low frequencies in the normal speech spectrum, (b) to preserve normal eardrum free field transfer, (c) to extend high frequencies in wearable hearing aids, (d) to minimize and/or eliminate the usual 1000 Hz resonant peak in mild to moderate loss fittings, (e) to create a smooth slope in the overall frequency response of an aid and finally (f) to keep the output of the aid within the client's dynamic range.

Shells have seen changes in the past few years. Research done by Philips in the Netherlands resulted in the development of a new hearing instrument technology called "peritympanic". The Philips research showed that the position of the shell/case created significant differences in the following areas: (1) gain increase, (2) frequency response, (3) the occlusion effect and (4) cosmetics. The new peritympanic hearing aids required a whole new impression technique. Clinicians fitting these instruments had to be specially trained and certified. The Philips discovery germinated two new case/shell creations. These are the "C.I.C." completely-in-the-canal and the Micro-Canal style of instruments. Figure 9 shows canal positioning of the new shell designs.

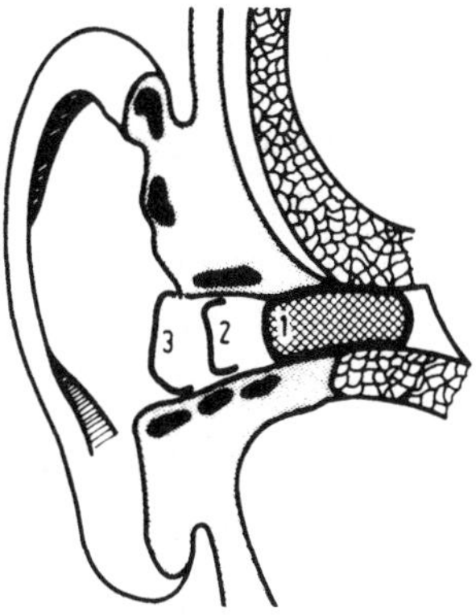

Fig. 9. Shell Positions of Instrument Styles - (1) Peritympanic, (2) Completely-in-the-Canal and (3) Micro Canal

THE IMPRESSION PROCESS FOR EARMOLDS & SHELLS

A good impression is a prerequisite for a well fabricated earmold or a comfortable custom instrument. Earmold laboratories report that the impression quality is THE major factor in earmold fittings. It has been estimated that 9.5% of all impressions sent to labs have to be remade. This means that out of every 100,000 impressions 9,500 will have to be remade, causing delay to the patient and possible loss of confidence in the clinician.

If the ear impression is inaccurate or flawed, the mold or shell of custom instruments will have built-in problems with fit or acoustic feedback. This underscores the need for a standardized detailed protocol for this area of fitting hearing aids.

Area One in this impression process is knowing the anatomy of the EXTERNAL ear. The anatomy that directly affects earmold or custom instrument usage and impression adequacy are as follows: the external auditory canal, the concha and tragus.

The Vagus Nerve has a branch which passes near the external auditory canal. When this nerve is irritated by pressure or a rubbing action of the earmold against the bones of the external auditory canal, pressure is transmitted to the nerve causing a cough reflex.

The fatty tissue lining the auditory canal is a thin layer of fat stretched over the bone and covered by the dermis. The dermis is the sensitive layer of inner skin which is covered by the epidermis. Because the epidermis is thin, the skin in the bony portion of the canal is one of the most sensitive areas of the human anatomy.

The fatty tissue lining the external cartilaginous portion of the auditory canal is very soft, moveable, and has the property to stretch greatly.

Figure 10 shows the anatomical features of the External Ear. For good communication with earmold or hearing aid labs, it is suggested to clinicians to use the medical terms that define location. These terms are listed here.

SUPERIOR—of or toward the HIGHER POSITION

INFERIOR—of or toward the LOWER position

ANTERIOR—of or toward the FRONT

POSTERIOR—of or toward the REAR

MEDIAL—of or toward the CENTER

LATERAL—of or toward the OUTSIDE

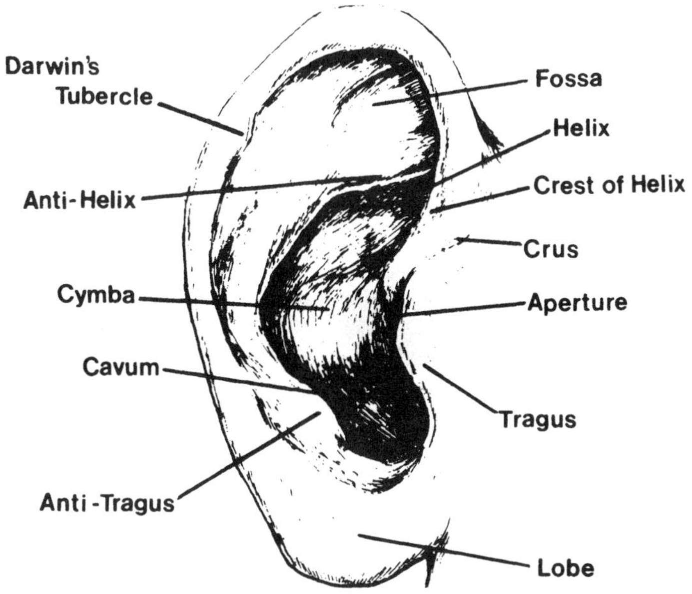

Fig. 10. Anatomy of the External Ear

Figure 11 shows three styles of earmolds with the names of the parts that reflect anatomical location.

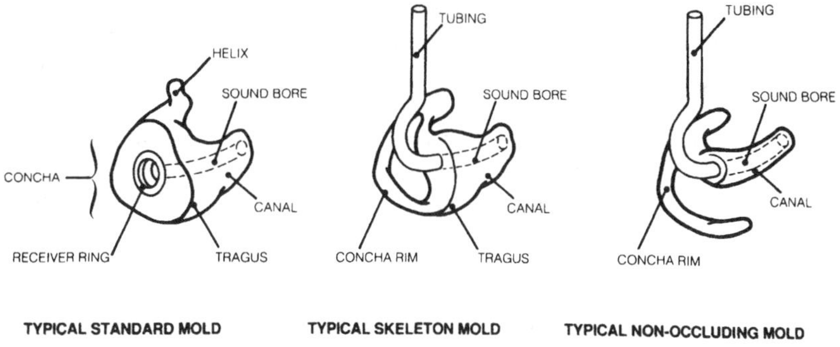

Fig. 11. The Anatomy of Different Earmold Styles

Area Number Two in the impression process is preparation and tools. Hygiene is a primary factor. Hands and tools must be clean. Perform these tasks in front of the patient. In this manner, the patient is aware of your concern for safety and hygiene. Precautions must be taken when taking impressions of patients with communicable diseases such as AIDS, exzema, dandruff, etc. Surgical gloves are suggested. The tools needed are:

- Medical Otoscope
- Earlight
- Impression Material
- Impression Material Measures
- Tweezers with Blunt End
- Impression Syringe
- Foam or Cotton Ear Blocks
- Dental Floss

After arranging tools and cleaning your hands and the tools, the next preparatory step is to counsel the patient about what you are going to do.

A major part of hearing aid dispensing is the professionalism with which you manage your clients. This includes not only common courtesy, but also careful counseling. Explain every aspect of the procedures you are going to perform. People sometimes fear the unknown. Inform the client that you are going to take an impression of the ear using a soft, plastic material similar to that which dentists use. The material, once packed, must set-up for ten minutes. Tell your client that if the impression you are taking is not perfect, you will be making a second or third one to ensure success and comfort of the fitting.

Before taking the impression, ask your client if he/she has had ear surgery or ear infections, and if there is any soreness or swelling now present, consultation with their doctor should take place before making the impression.

Area Three of the Impression Process is the OTOSCOPIC Examination. This part of the hearing aid clinician's role is very important because it is here that potential problems are observed. It is also the point where, if medical conditions exist, referrals are made before proceeding with fitting the hearing aids. Knowledge based on careful attention to the otoscopic exam is essential to good clinical management.

The examination includes scrutiny of the pinna and surrounding area before using the otoscope.

Your inspection should reveal the following to you:

1. The approximate size of the impression needed.
2. The length and course of the external canal.
3. The shape and convolution of the canal, concha and helix areas.
4. The presence of wax, possible trauma and other disorders, and the integrity of the eardrum.

Figure 12 shows the proper insertion of the otoscope. It is important to note that there will be significant differences in canal size, direction and shape in adults, children and infants. Figure 13 shows a cut-away of generalized differences.

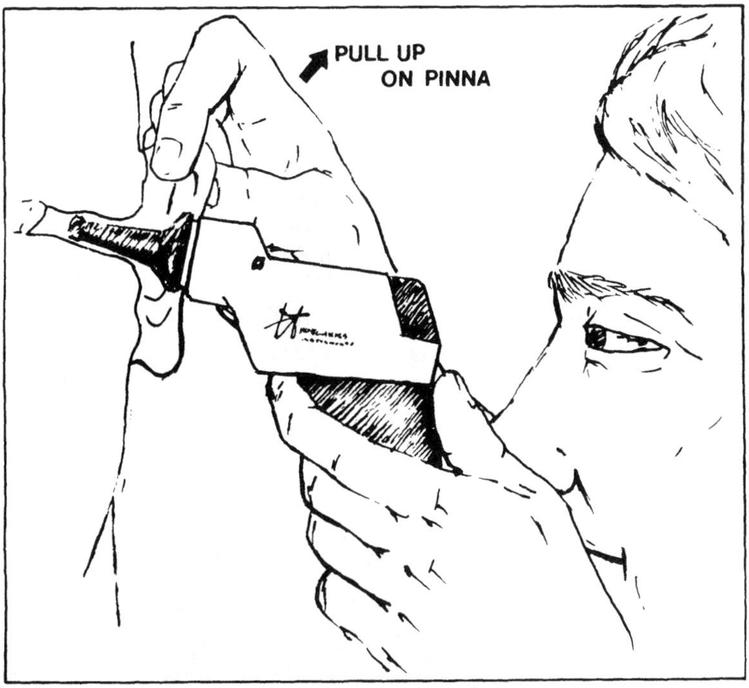

Fig. 12. Looking Through an Otoscope

With otoscopic examinations, practice makes perfect. This is truly a skill acquired by practice. There are some training videos and manuals available that give views of different conditions that can be seen during otoscopic examinations.

The following list from Microsonic (1994) describes some typical otoscopic examination findings.

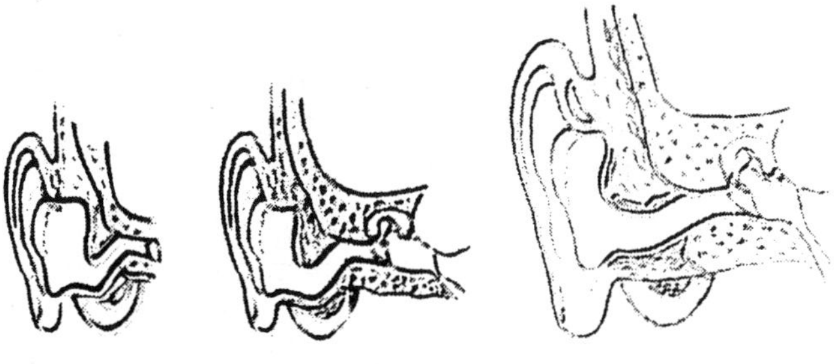

Fig. 13. Anatomical Shape Differences Due to Age

a. Atresia or Stenoses. This involves complete or partial closing of the ear canal. In extreme cases there may be no pinna at all or closure of the canal to the point where the drum is not visible.

b. Impacted wax or cerumen. Wax creation is a normal phenomenon. The amount varies from patient to patient. Otoscopically it can range from dry to wet. Colorwise it ranges from light yellow to orange, to red to black. If the drum is not visible due to wax, it is considered "impacted" and should be removed. If there are lumps of wax but the drum is visible, it should also be removed. Cerumen management technique is then indicated. This is the most common finding by hearing aid clinicians when performing otoscopic examinations.

c. Aural Discharge. There may be, occasionally, fluid coming from the external ear canal. Presence of any liquid should act as a red flag for the dispenser. The client should be referred to an otologist before attempting an impression.

d. Bony Growths. Unusual bony growth of the ear canal is cause for referral to an otologist.

e. Inflammatory Conditions. A bacterial or fungal infection in the ear canal may make the ear red and sensitive. A pimple in the pinna or ear canal may also be sore. Both require medical attention prior to making an impression.

f. Prolapsed Canal. This refers to a flap of tissue that occludes the external canal. Lift the pinna back and the flap will open up. The foam plug should be inserted in the canal past the second bend before taking the impression. With this condition, be ABSOLUTELY sure to allow the impression to set for a full TEN MINUTES before removing.

g. Enlarged Canal. This is usually due to past ear surgery. EXTREME caution should be exercised by the clinician with this type of client. Often there will be no drum or ossicles, and the canal skin will usually be very sensitive. Prior to the impression process, an enlarged canal will usually require multiple otoblocks.

h. Foreign Objects. If the otoscopic examination reveals a strange color or shape, there may be a foreign object lodged in the ear canal. Examples are pencil erasers, insects, cotton, peas, etc. Medical referral is necessary for removal.

i. Eardrum Distention. This is most often due to fluid behind the drum, with the drum appearing to be ballooned out. Medical management is indicated.

j. Eardrum Retraction. When middle ear problems cause eustachian tube dysfunction, normal pressure equalization of the drum does not occur. Abnormal middle ear pressure can cause the eardrum to retract and stretch back over the ossicles. Medical management is essential.

k. Eardrum Perforation. If a tear or perforation in the eardrum exists, medical management is essential. In this case, a patient should HAVE MEDICAL CLEARANCE for an impression to be made.

The otoscopic examination will indicate whether or not there is excessive hair growth in the ear canal. If this condition exists, the hair must be cut before the impressions are taken.

Area Four is sizing the otoblocks. Canal blocks are currently of two types, cotton or foam. Figure 14 shows the differences.

The function of the blocks is to prevent impression materials from reaching the eardrum. They act as a "safety" catch if the impression material lodges in the canal. Finally, they provide a good cross-sectional fullness to the impression. The clinician is CAUTIONED to carefully size the blocks. Have several sizes available.

If necessary, trim or add to the block for best sizing. The block should be placed beyond the second bend of the canal. You must look in the ear again to see if placement is correct. CAUTION: too small a block will allow impression material to flow beyond the second bend and may encroach upon the eardrum. This situation could cause major problems. Figure 15 shows impression material passing the block. Sizing the block is a critical safety factor.

Area Five is TAKING THE IMPRESSION. Historically there have been three methods of taking an ear impression: the hand packing method, the tamper method and the syringe method. Morgan (1994) states the syringe method is today the preferred method because the impressions done by this technique are more often

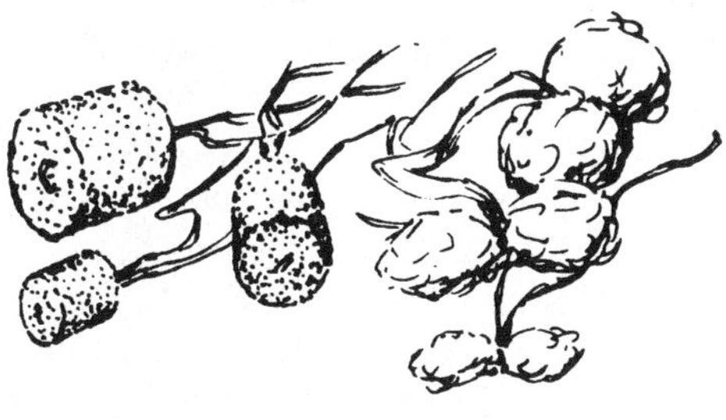

Fig. 14. Earblocks: Foam & Cotton

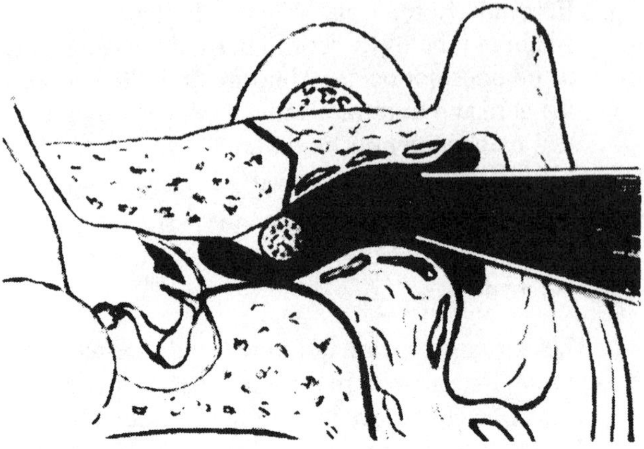

Fig. 15. Impression Passing Block

successful. Figure 16 and text from Microsonic (1994) outline and describe the whole impression process.

Additional Points in Impression Taking

- If the client wears glasses or dentures, make sure these are in place while taking the impression.
- NEVER flatten or smooth out the finished impression with the palm of your hand while impression material is in the client's ear.
- Children are sometimes fearful and can be hard to work with. Let the child watch you take an impression of mother's ear to alleviate his fears. Let him play with a piece of the "dough". NOTE: It is difficult to use a block with SOME children. The impression may be better formed without it in these cases.

DEEP CANAL IMPRESSIONS

European Research by Philips developed a deep canal hearing aid impression technique that differed from common practices. This system used a newly designed syringe, as shown in Figure 17 that automatically mixed a newer free flowing, highly accurate dimensionally stable silicone material. Because the new deep canal hearing aids were built to sit ¼″ from the eardrum, the impression taking methodology had to change. The new impression technique has been called the "peritympanic technique". This differs from the traditional impression technique in that the impression material is very fluid so that it will flow down to the eardrum. An

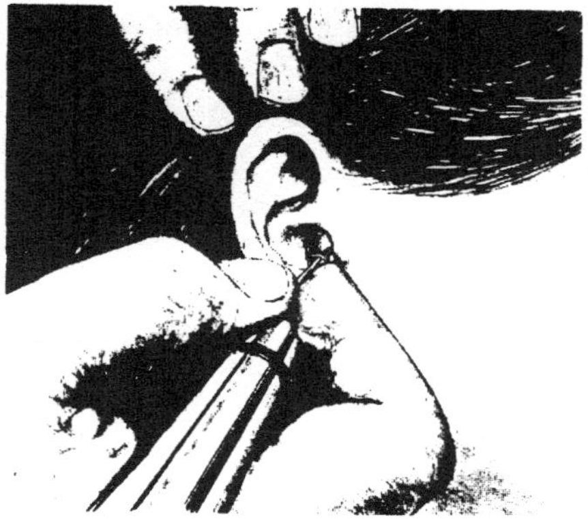

STEP 1
A cotton or foam block is an ABSOLUTE NECESSITY when using the syringe. Set a tight block just past the second bend. Foam blocks MUST be compressed to insure proper results. Be sure to use the correct size foam block even though it may appear to be larger in diameter than the ear canal.

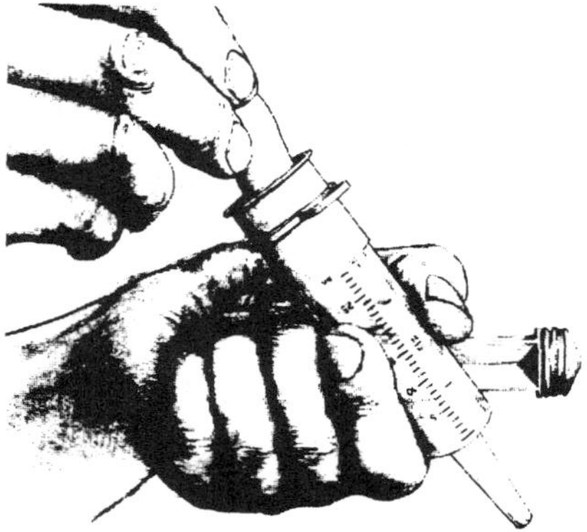

STEP 2
Mix the impression material according to instructions and place in the barrel of the syringe. The quicker you can use the material the better the impression.

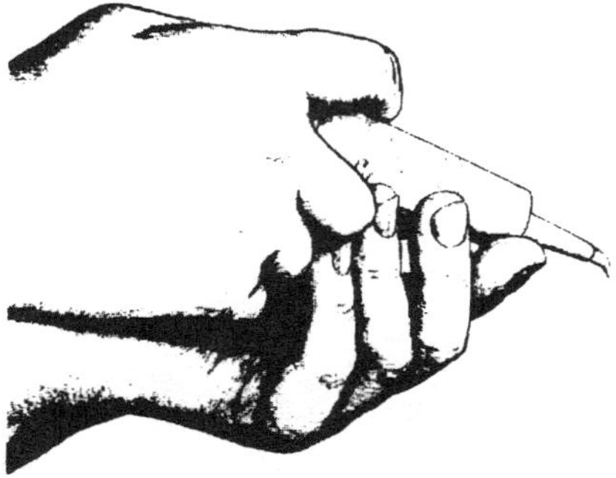

STEP 3
Insert the plunger and gently push the material into the nozzle to remove air pockets.

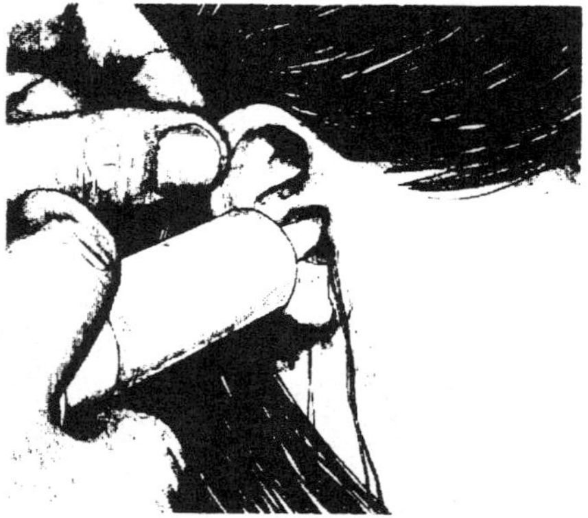

STEP 4
Place the nozzle into the canal and fill the canal.

Fig. 16. The Whole Impression Process

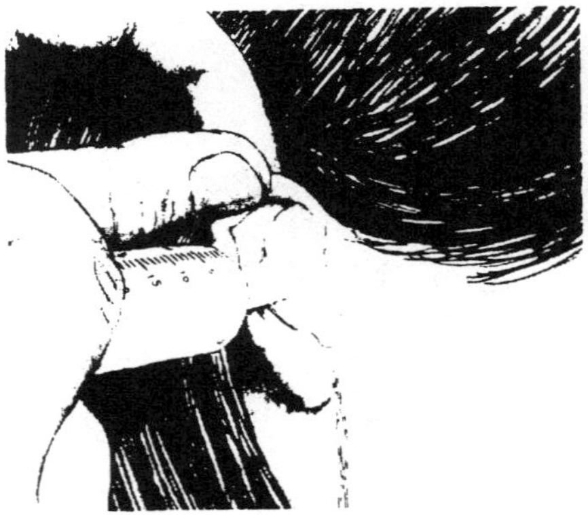

STEP 5
As the material fills the canal, slowly withdraw the syringe and fill the helix and concha areas completely. Then cover the tragus.

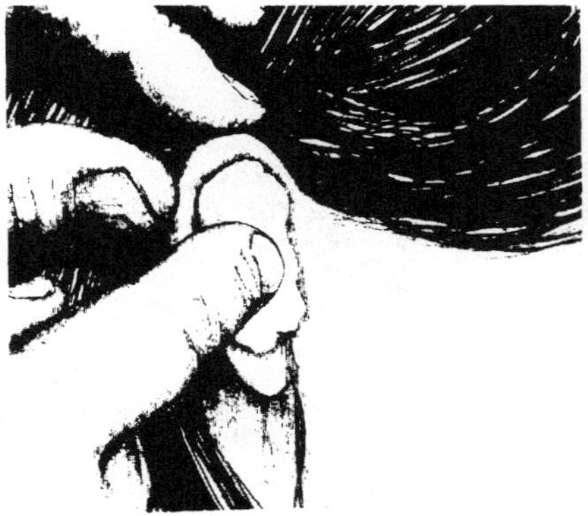

STEP 6
When the external ear has been filled completely, press your finger GENTLY in the concha and helix areas. BE CAREFUL NOT TO PRESS HARD AS IMPRESSION WILL DISTORT.

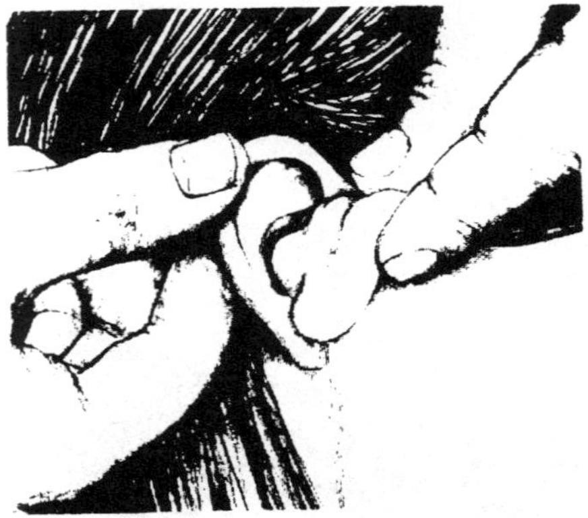

STEP 7
Allow a FULL 10 MINUTES of curing time before removing. The impression can be distorted if removed too soon. To remove, gently press ear away from the impression. Remove helix curl slightly. Bring impression straight out while holding thread. Take your time. Don't strain the impression with a long steady pull.

HELPFUL TIPS FOR BETTER IMPRESSIONS

- If the client wears glasses or dentures, make sure these are in place while taking the impression.
- NEVER flatten or smooth out the finished impression with the palm of your hand while impression material is in the client's ear.
- Ask your client to talk and chew after the impression material is in place. This is to help assure a comfortable fitting custom earmold which will not unseat when the jaw muscles constrict the ear canal.
- Children are sometimes fearful and can be hard to work with. Let the child watch you take an impression of mother's ear to alleviate his fears. Let him play with a piece of the "dough". NOTE: It is difficult to use a block with SOME children. The impression may be better formed without it in these cases.

(Fig. 16. continued)

"umbrella" style flange with an aerating tube is lubricated and placed down on the eardrum. A hull is also used for sizing and positioning of the face plate. The step by step technique must be learned. Certification is currently required for these protocols. This new syringe technique takes earmold/custom instrument impressions quickly and easily with consistent uniform results. The viscosity and set-up time are preset. Some hearing aid clinicians have adopted the original Philips protocols and use a block. The current completely in-the-canal style custom hearing aids could use this technique. It could also be used for problem feedback cases, due to differences in the impression material itself.

Figure 17 shows the gun syringe with cartridges and tips. The steps in using the free-flowing impression material and syringe are described by Microsonic (1994):

STEP 1: The Ready-Press syringe has two preassembled component parts—a handle and a plunger. Hold the release back in the handle.

STEP 2: Slide the cartridge onto the handle. The cartridge flange will fit directly behind the retainers on the handle. Lock it in place with the hinged retainer.

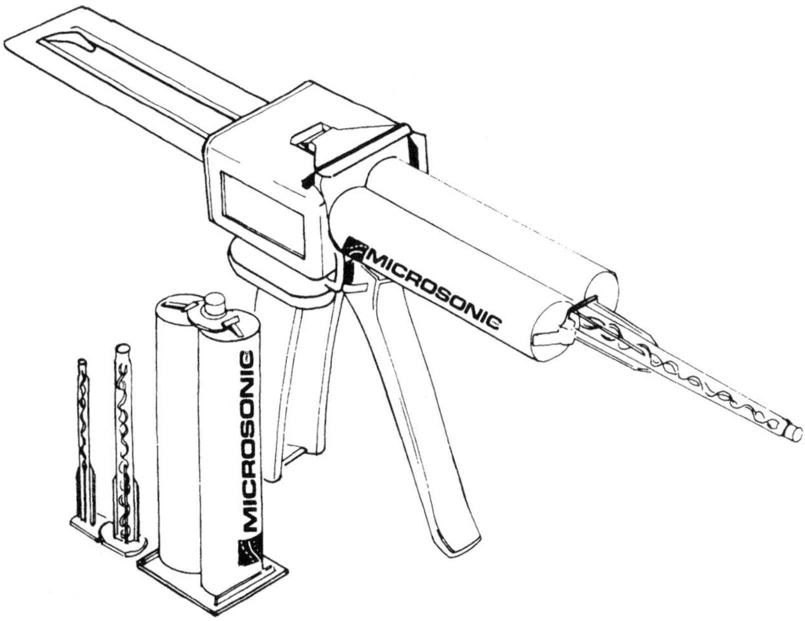

Fig. 17. The Impression Gun

STEP 3: Twist the cap at the end of the cartridge and remove.

STEP 4: Press the plunger forward to fit into the cartridge. (If the plunger does not enter the cartridge, check to see that the cartridge is properly aligned.)

STEP 5: For best results, after placing a cotton or foam block, lightly coat the client's ear with baby oil or earmold lubricant using a cotton swab before proceeding with the impression.

STEP 6: Squeeze out enough material to be sure that the material is flowing uniformly from both openings.

STEP 7: Place the proper size tip (small for children and small ears, or large for adults) where the cap was and twist lock into position.

STEP 8: Squeeze out and discard approximately ¼″ to ½″ of the impression material through the end of the tip to insure that it is mixing properly.

STEP 9: Within 30 seconds, fill the entire ear canal as far as the block, making sure to also fill the tragus, concha and helix areas. DO NOT UNDERFILL. After 4 to 5 minutes, test the outer surface of the silicone material by indenting or scratching the surface. If the material does NOT retain the indentation, it is ready to be removed.

Area Six is IMPRESSION MATERIAL choices. There is a debate described by Sandlin (1993) about that which is the best impression material to use. The questions posed are (a) which is most efficient? (b) which is the easiest to use? and (c) which is the most professional? The types of impression material available are ethyl methacrylate and addition-cured silicone in two formats; the hand-mixed type and the free-flow automatic type. The ethyl methacrylate is a powder and liquid is measured by the clinician, mixed together in a bowl, transferred to the syringe and used. The mixture amount is critical to set-up time and impression clarity. Temperature is a variable factor with this material. The stability of the powder/liquid format has been challenged in the past. The silicone hand-mixed type is very stable once it has set. There is, however, some expansion of the material during set-up. The newer free-flow automatic silicone has absolute minimal expansion and thus is an improvement over the hand-mix type silicone. Advocates of the powder/liquid system state that if the variables of mix and temperature are carefully monitored by the clinician, the accuracy of the powder/liquid system has years of effective fittings to support its usage. Currently many earmold labs have pre-mixed powder and liquid materials to solve the mix-amount problem. There is no simple answer. The thoughtful hearing aid clinician should be prepared to use whatever impression material he or she works well with but has another material available for problem fittings.

Area Seven in the process is IMPRESSION CRITIQUING. Earmold laboratories and hearing aid manufacturers state that a good impression is essential for them to perform their part of the hearing aid fitting process. Many fitting problems can be avoided, if the clinician doesn't send the lab impressions that do not meet standards. This assessment of impression quality includes the following questions to be answered by the clinician for each impression.

- Is the impression smooth and complete?
- Is the canal portion long enough to show the beginning of the canal's second bend?
- Is the helix portion of the impression clearly defined?
- Is the concha complete?
- Are there weld marks (caused by impression material drying too quickly)?
- Are the edges of the folds in the ear's concha rounded and not sharp which is due to mashing the material in the concha against the skull?

Special attention should be given to canal length and diameter. For mild losses, the canal portion of the impression may be short and reach just the first bend in the canal. For moderate losses, the canal portion should go beyond the first bend. The diameter should accommodate any special acoustic options you may order. In severe losses, the canal portion may need to be long and extend beyond the second bend. The diameter should always be full. Too much canal length on an impression is never a problem for the lab; too little is.

Remember, too, that in most cases the acoustic seal of an earmold occurs at the aperture of the canal, not deep within the canal. Too great a canal length can be uncomfortable for the wearer, and can make the mold very difficult to insert and remove. Correct canal length depends entirely on the requirements of the individual client and the hearing aid style being fitted.

Because these steps require visualization of acceptable or unacceptable impressions, there is a series of drawings shown in Figure 18 relative to problem impressions compared to an "ideal" impression. The clinician's goal should always be an "ideal" impression.

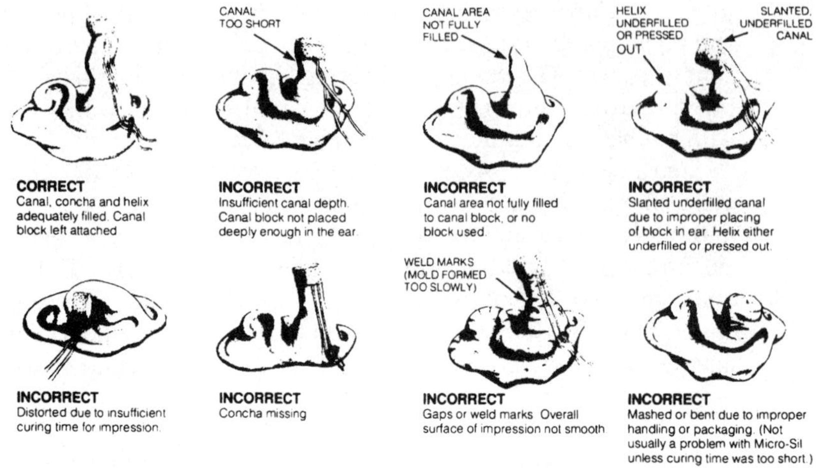

Fig. 18. Drawings for Impression Critiquing

For the manufacturers of custom hearing aids, the impressions give them vital visual information necessary to make the hearing aids. Benzinger (1993) states that critiquing your impressions does include the following for "custom" instrument fittings.

a) *Canal size.* Will it accommodate the hearing aid receiver?

b) *Length of canal.* Longer is better past second bend and necessary for CIC and deep canal fittings.

c) *Second Bend Definition.* For power in-the-air aids the second bend can be critical to the fit.

d) *Horn or Reverse-Horn Canal Shape.* This impression can cause lab problems due to venting, receiver size and fit comfort.

e) *Restricted area between Tragus and Antitragus.* Space needed for components and trimmer options can be a problem.

f) *Helix Area.* This area allows lab possible extra room for components.

THE SELECTION PROCESS FOR EARMOLDS

The hearing aid clinician's skills are put to the test in this particular area. The accomplished clinician will use visual analysis of the outer ear and an analysis of the patient's manual dexterity in handling the earmold or shell of a custom instrument to select the PHYSICAL options of the mold or style of custom shell. The second area for the clinician is ACOUSTIC options. It is in this area that analysis of the audiogram and recommended target gain and output are analyzed to select the acoustic effects that couplers provide. The third area of selection is tubing and earhook options. The fourth area is earmold materials. Historically there have been hard or soft earmold materials. However, advances in plastics have expanded the clinicians choices. In this selection area, the clinician must keep abreast of what the earmold laboratories and hearing aid manufacturers offer.

The fundamental goal of coupler selection in the fitting of hearing aids is effective correction and client satisfaction. Errors, or lack of knowledge, in clinical choice often is the reason for client rejection of hearing aid amplification. This would result in failure to meet habilitation or rehabilitation goals. The fitting flexibility described here relates to behind-the-ear and eyeglass hearing aids. It, secondarily, relates to custom hearing aids.

The naming of the physical choices follows the NAEL (National Association of Earmold Labs) terminology (1970). For some styles there is no agreement, so a descriptive generic name is used.

In making style selections, do not underestimate the patient's attitude about the cosmetics of the earmold. While it is not always possible to give a patient what is wanted cosmetically, the majority can be satisfied without sacrificing fitting goals.

PHYSICAL STYLE OPTIONS/OCCLUDING

This is a popular style of earmold because it effectively seals the canal while leaving an open space in the concha to enhance appearance. This style can be made from most materials and can be ordered with most available acoustic options. This style is also chosen by many dispensers since it can be easily converted to other styles if necessary.

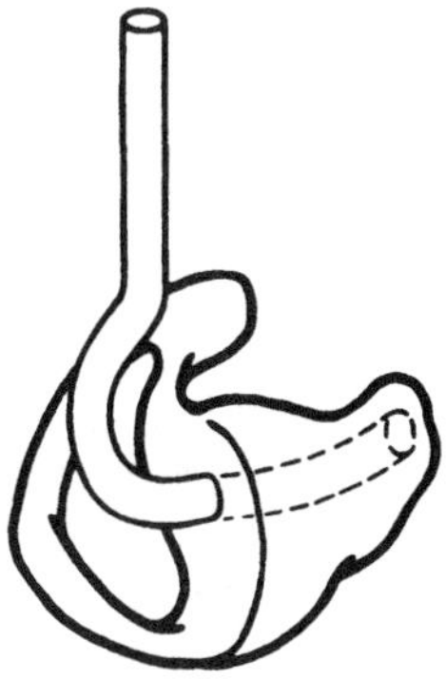

Fig. 19. Skeleton

This style can be ordered with different positions in the earmolds anatomy removed e.g. ¾ of a skeleton, ½ of a skeleton for the areas to be removed. The more that can be retained, the greater the acoustic seal.

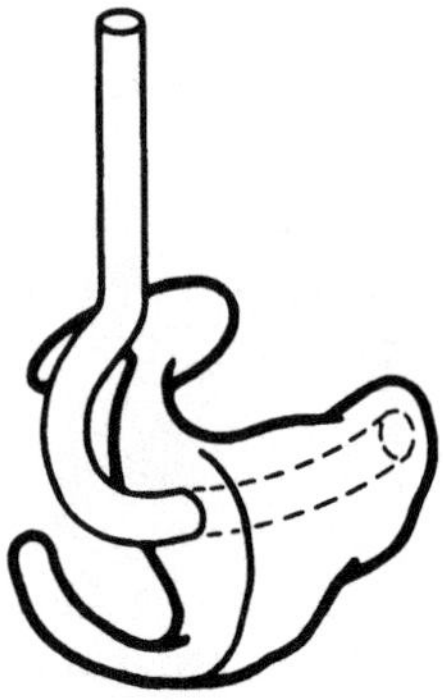

Fig. 20. Semi-Skeleton

This type of earmold uses only the canal portion of the impression, with the helix and concha areas removed. Experience indicates that a canal style earmold should have a long canal. New materials now allow canal style molds to be used with power behind-the-ear hearing aids.

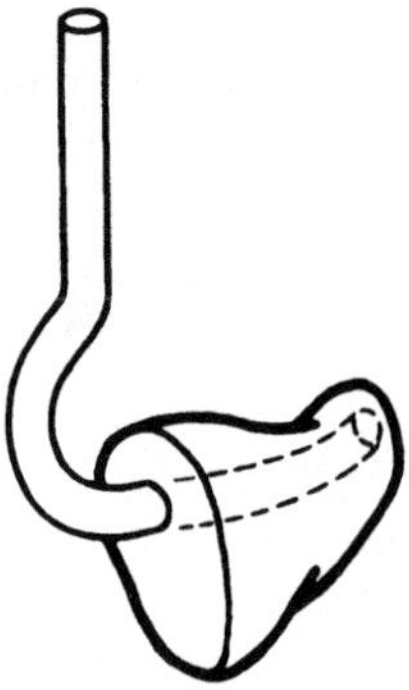

Fig. 21. Canal

When canal shape or concha abnormalities make retention of the standard canal style not possible or desirable, this style can be used. A finger-like projection along the bottom of the concha holds the mold in place. This earmold is easy for the wearer to insert and remove.

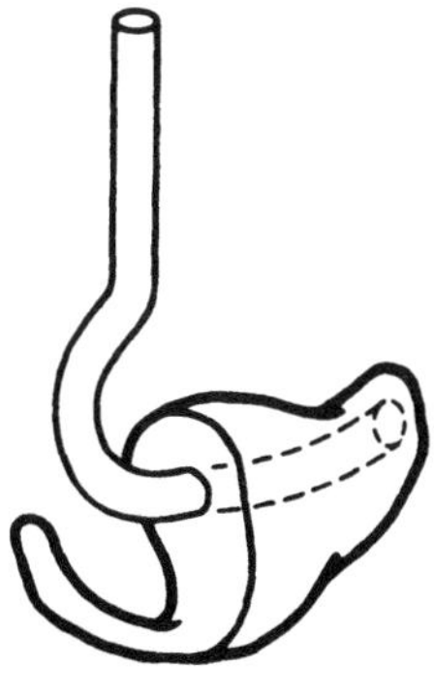

Fig. 22. Canal-Lok

The addition of a helix to the canal-lok mold provides additional retention without sacrificing the cosmetic advantages of canal-lok style.

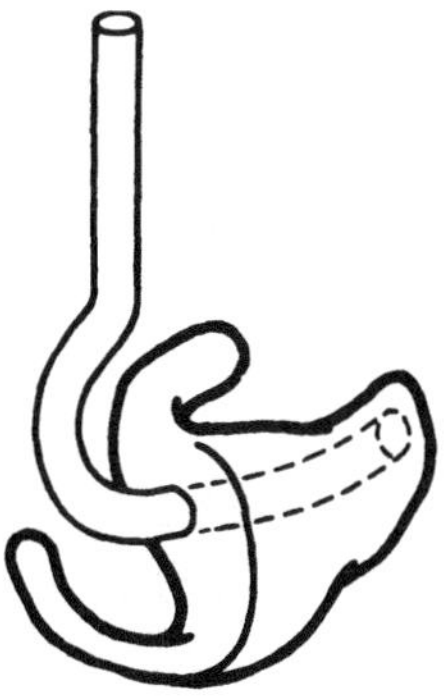

Fig. 23. Canal-Lok with Helix

This mold style may be the most commonly used now since so many moderate gain aids are of the "custom" type. This style was designed for higher gain and output instruments. Because there is

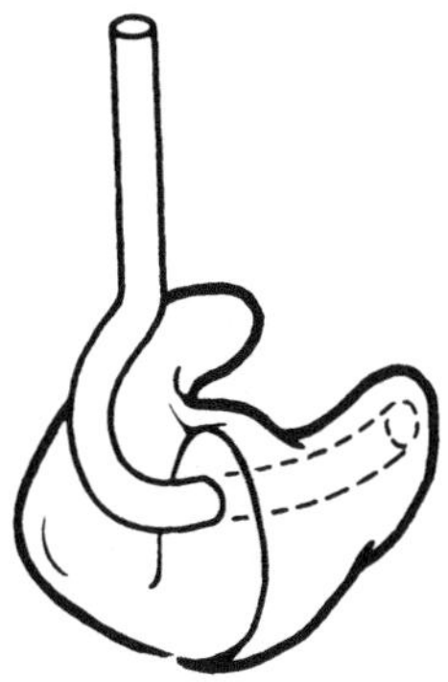

Fig. 24. Shell

greater contact in the concha bowl and helix, the seal is tighter. There are many acoustic and material options.

This style improves physical appearance and patient comfort. The molds are pressure molded to eliminate shrinkage, and are hollowed out in the concha and helix area to improve the cosmetics and reduce the weight of the mold. Available ONLY in Poly Methacrylate and Poly Ethyl Methacrylate combinations. Also available in Micro-Canal configuration.

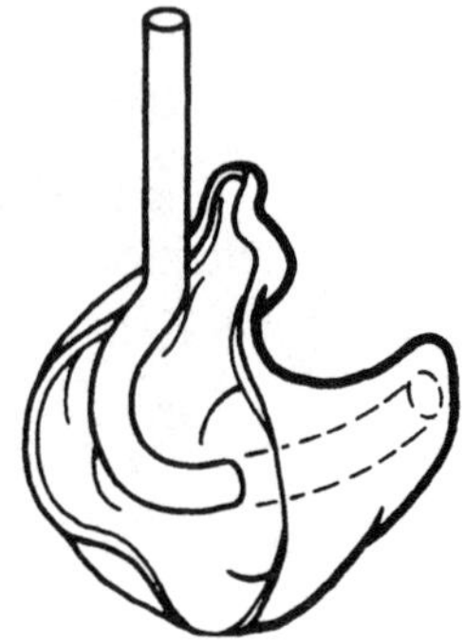

Fig. 25. Micro-Shell

This mold is a reduction of the standard shell style. It is indicated when a patient's ability to work the helix part of the mold into that part of the ear is in question. Many manual dexterity problems can be solved by selecting this style.

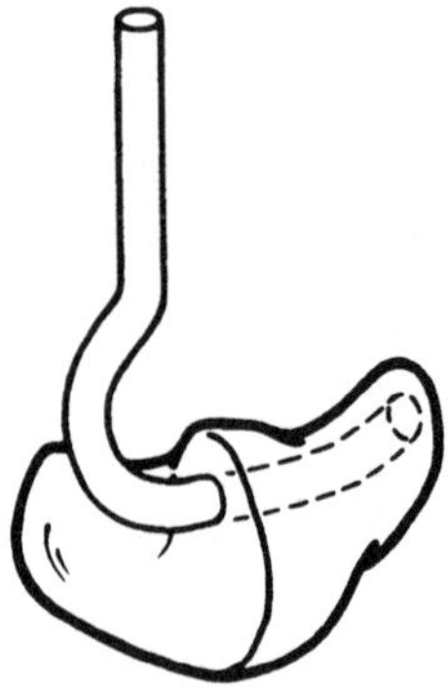

Fig. 26. Regular with Tubing

Regular style earmolds are used with hearing aids that have an external receiver that is snapped into the earmold (usually body-type aids). Historically, this was the earliest type of custom earmold. Regular style earmolds have three receiver ring options:

standard, D-90 and 4404. The standard receiver ring is available in metal or plastic, and the earmold can be made in both hard and soft materials.

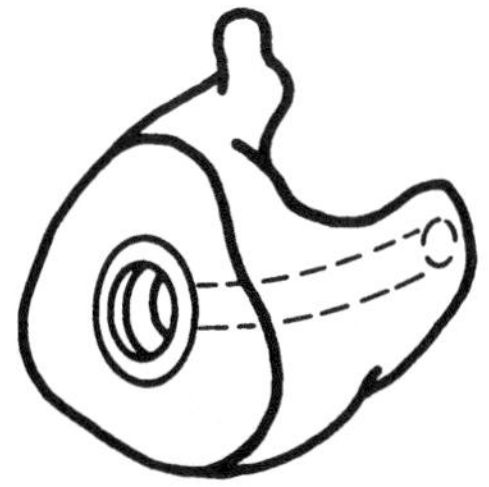

Fig. 27. Regular

This earmold style was developed to provide support on small and/or soft pinnas that use an external hearing aid receiver. The wire is embedded in the body of the regular earmold.

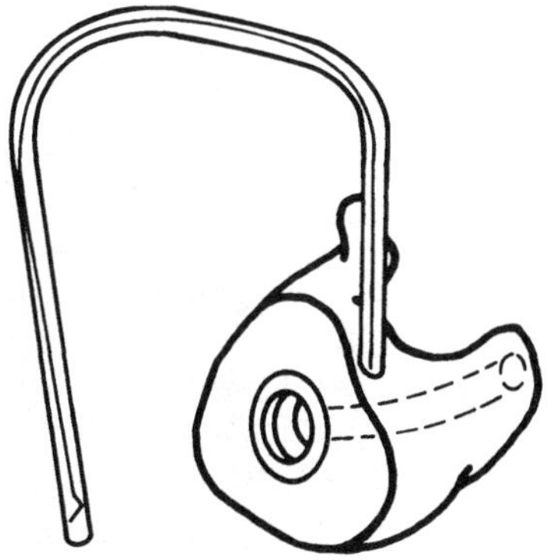

Fig. 28. Regular with Wire Hook

Because the majority of behind-the-ear hearing instruments are high power (52-68dB HFA-Gain) and ultra high power (69dB HFA Gain and above), the need for better sealing earmolds has become tantamount. Another factor affecting a good seal in hearing aid fittings is jaw bone deterioration in the 85–100 year old age group. This group also experiences cartilaginous and skin changes in the canal.

THE PHYSICAL STYLE OPTIONS

This mold reduces feedback by changing the design of the canal portion of the mold. The design is useful in fittings in which jaw movement is the cause of feedback, and it becomes necessary to

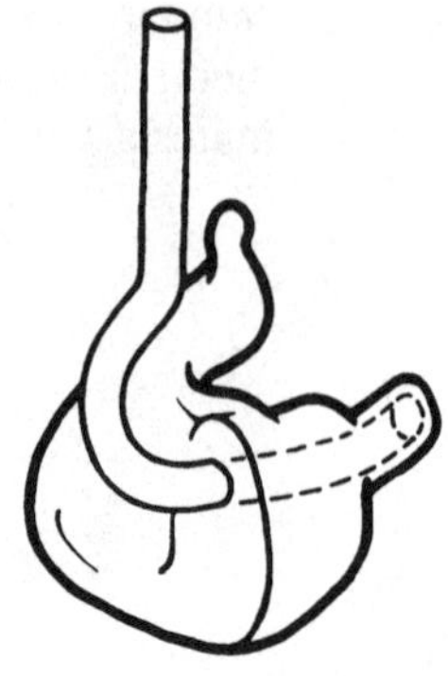

Fig. 29. Power Mold

eliminate the portions of the earmold's canal that is affected by the movement.

One of the most common occurrences in fitting higher gain aids is the presence of feedback. Microsonic Lab developed an answer in 1975 in an earmold option called the Tragus Mold. This tragus configuration can be ordered with most physical styles and does not preclude using additional acoustic options. The Tragus Mold increases the girth of the canal portion at the tragus while carrying a lip over the usual termination point of the mold at the outside of the tragus. This results in a tighter seal at the tragus and in the canal. Because the tragus is flexible and can be expanded without discomfort to the client, this configuration gives the best acoustic seal. Tragus molds do require a change in standard impression technique, in that one must cover the entire surface of the tragus with impression material. "A GOOD IMPRESSION IS ESSENTIAL FOR A TRAGUS MOLD" OTHERWISE THIS APPLICATION WILL NOT BE EFFECTIVE.

A listing of other anti-feedback control options that are individually described later on in this chapter are:

1. Shell Mold with Hard Body and Soft Canal
2. Soft Shell Mold

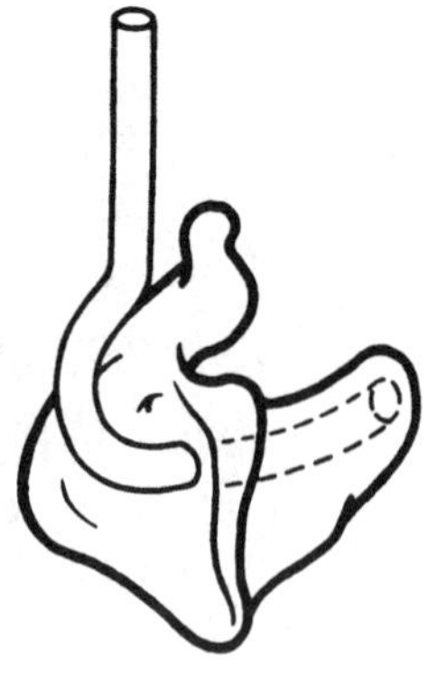

Fig. 30. Tragus Mold

3. Macrae Anti-Feedback Resonator Mold
4. Other Resonator Effect Molds
5. E-Compound
6. Patriot Mold (A soft canal configuration)
7. Dipping Custom-aid's shells in soft coating material.

SHELL MOLD WITH SOFT CANAL

This mold option uses a change of material to create a tighter seal. The shell mold gives a good seal normally. The soft canal expands with body heat to create a tighter seal. The thick walled tubing reduces the possibility of mechanical feedback through the tubing wall.

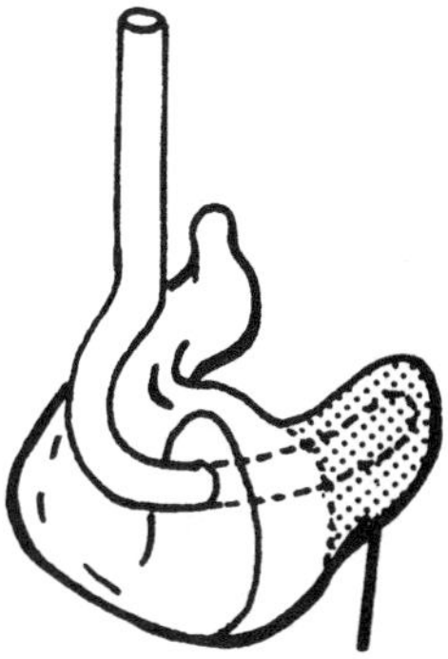

Fig. 31. Shell with Soft Canal

MACRAE ANTI-FEEDBACK

The mold is characterized by a hollowed out shell with a glued on face-plate. There is a small vent hole near the helix. Tube #1 carries the sound from the aid directly to the sealed ear canal. There is a Tube #2 which carries the sound into a larger resonator cavity

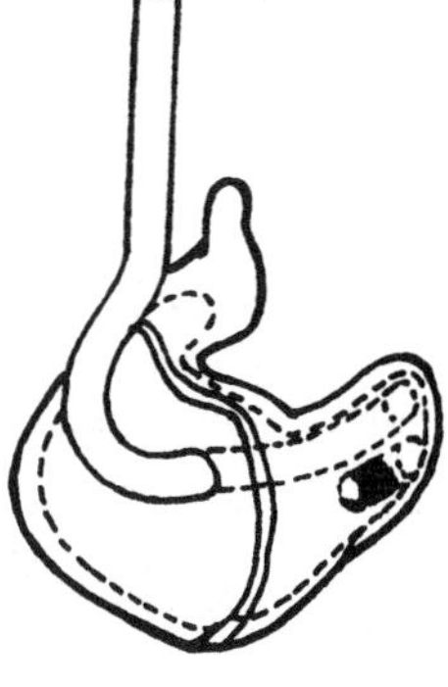

Fig. 32 Macrae Anti-feedback

through an acoustic damper. As long as the ear is effectively sealed, the client can get higher volume without feedback.

A second category of Physical Style earmold options is the family of non-occluding earmolds. The primary objective of this style option is to reduce the occlusion effect while acoustically "bleeding" off the low frequency response of the hearing aid. Patients reported more "natural" sounding amplification when fitted with earmolds of this type. In effect, non-occluding molds provide an overlay of amplification in that sound still enters the ear canal on its way to the drum and bypasses the earmold. Occluded earmolds force all the sound to be processed through the hearing aid, since the canal is sealed off. Patients who report great problems with the occlusion effect should be offered the choice of a behind-the-ear fitting with "non-occluded" earmolds instead of "custom" instruments. Three non-occluding earmold designs are shown in Figure 33 from Microsonic (1994).

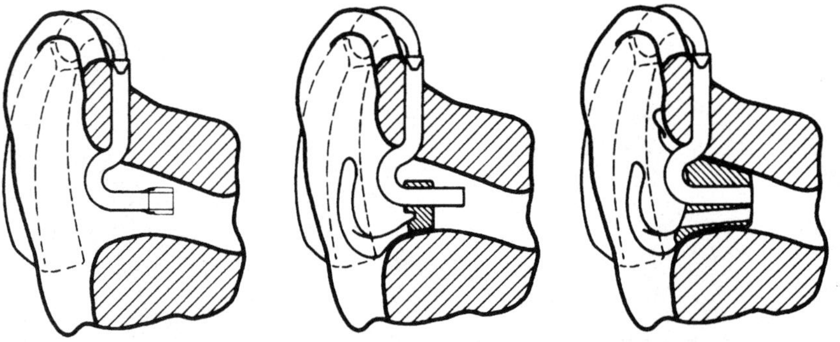

Fig. 33. Examples of Three Non-Occluding Earmolds

The applications for non-occluded earmolds are:

- unilateral hearing loss, i.e. CROS and IROS fittings
- maximizing the reduction of the "occlusion effect!"
- Use with patients who have a chronic drainage problem since aeration of the ear canal is possible with non-occluded types.

The actual physical style option of the non-occluding family is described. Non-occluding earmolds were originally developed for unilateral hearing losses in conjunction with CROS type hearing aids. When these earmolds are used for a single aid (behind-the-ear or eyeglass), the fitting is referred to as IROS. Non-occluding molds are also referred to as "open" molds.

The CROS type of mold is good for CROS and many IROS fittings. Lucite is recommended for these mold styles. The drawings in Figure 34 show the differences.

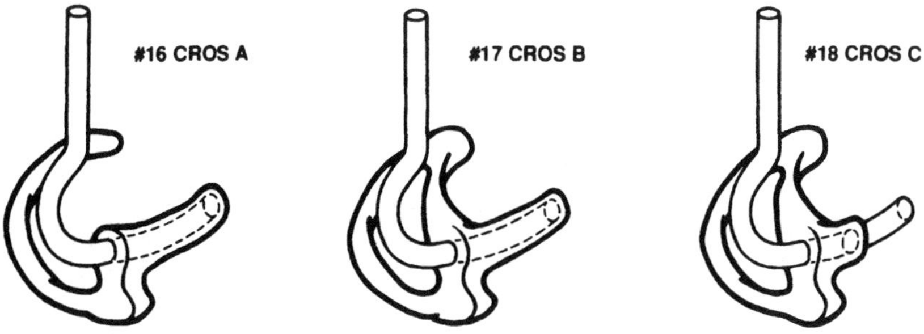

Fig. 34. The CROS Family Earmold Styles

With the CROS-C mold the tubing that projects into the ear canal can be changed in insertion depth. Figure 35 shows changes in low frequency response as a result of different tubing length into the canal.

Using non-occluded earmolds can create an acoustic feedback problem. As a result labs created various styles of "Free Field" earmolds to help control feedback when using non-occluded molds.

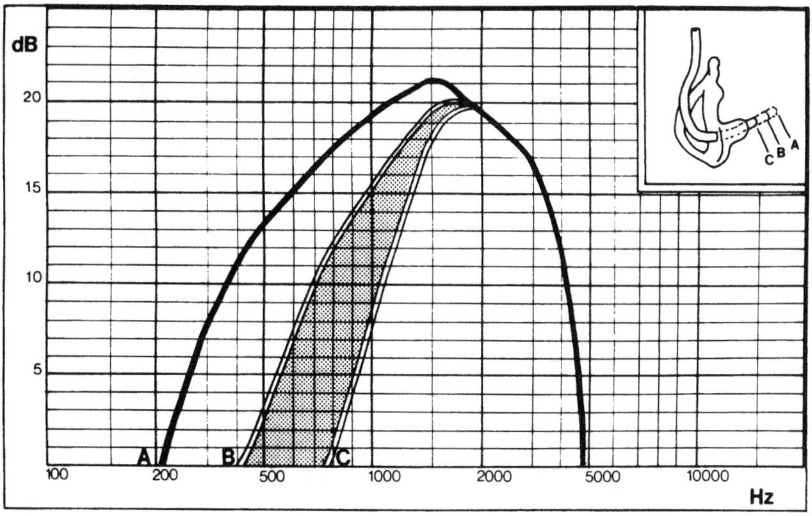

Fig. 35. Frequency Response Changes Caused by Tubing Length

The Free Field mold is the predecessor of the Janssen. It differs from the CROS mold in that it is more reduced in the concha ring and bridge area. Non-occluding earmolds present certain fitting restrictions. Since there is no seal, there is always the possibility of increased incidence of feedback.

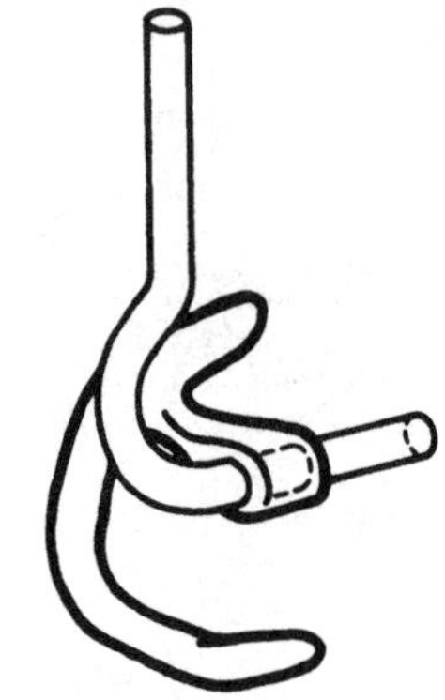

Fig. 36. Free Field

Developed by Microsonic Lab, the Advanced Design Free Field was created to assist dispensers in using more non-occluded molds without encountering acoustic feedback. It seals the canal entrance while leaving the canal itself unoccluded. An SAV vent system allows dispensers to change the acoustic characteristics as required.

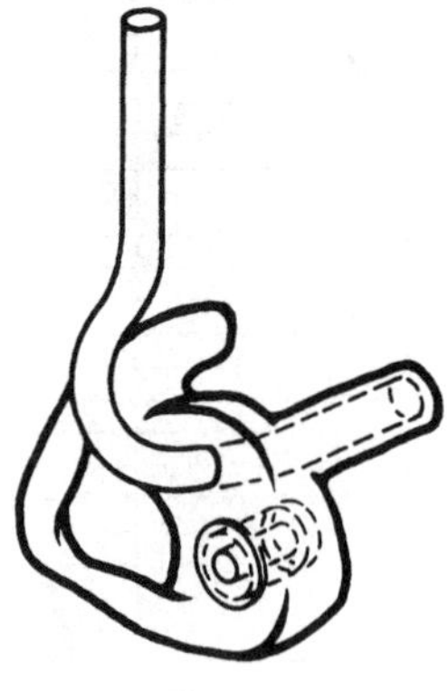

Fig. 37. Advanced Design Free Field

This style was developed by Janssen, a dispenser. This mold was developed for tube fittings. However, tube fittings require a high level of manual dexterity on the part of the hearing aid specialist. The Janssen mold incorporated unique features:

1. the canal is made of vinylflex so it can be bent by the fitter and trimmed and drilled according to tube size needed.
2. tubing is molded around the tragus
3. the canal portion of the mold rests in the top part of the canal
4. the length of the canal is as long as possible

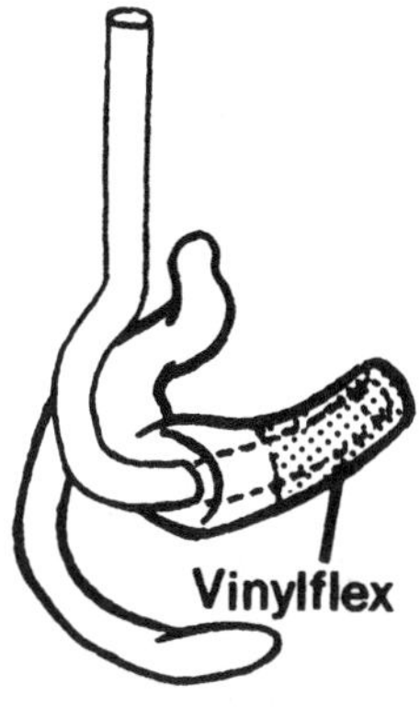

Fig. 38. Janssen Mold

In addition to the physical style options described so far there are also some unique and specialized Non-Occluded options that deal directly with specific acoustic goals. These are described below:

Based upon Horn-theory in earmold acoustics. This style enhances the range from 5–9 Hz. A contra-indication for this style is size and curves present in the ear canal. If the belled portion occludes too much of the canal much of the non-occluded effect is lost.

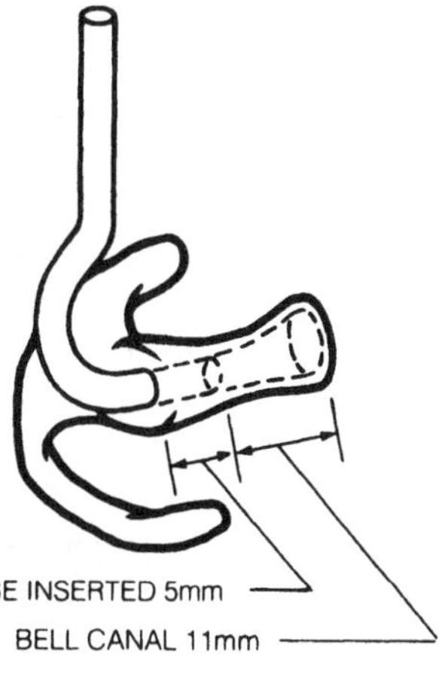

Fig. 39. Janssen with Belled Canal

Lybarger's Dual-Diameter System employs a center section of 1/32 diameter tubing in a non-occluding earmold to produce a resonator that provides an average of 12 dB additional gain in the range from 4000 to 7000Hz. This configuration is designed for losses that are normal out to 1500–2000Hz and then drop off sharply. This style of earmold combines the maximum effect of venting and the benefits derived from the resonator type earmold used with extended high frequency hearing aids.

Special earhooks may be used with a Lybarger mold to smooth the response and inhibit acoustic feedback.

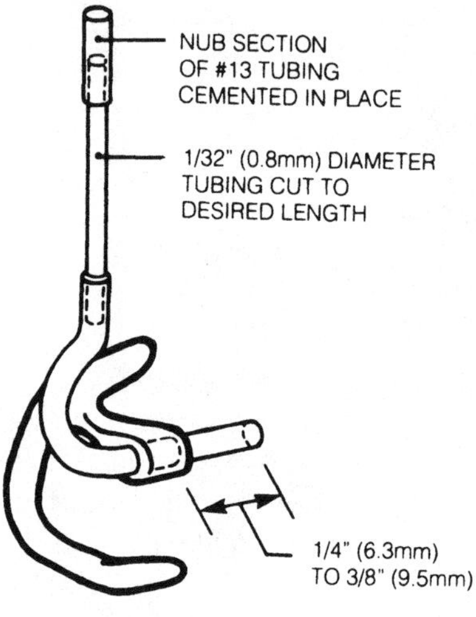

Fig. 40. Lybarger Mold

ACOUSTIC OPTIONS

The second selection area is ACOUSTIC Options. To conceptualize the range and effects of practical earmold acoustics, examine the graphs in Figure 41 presented by Libby (1980).

The control areas are relatively independent of one another and can be used separately or collectively.

There are three independent variables of acoustical control. Venting is the first and it affects frequencies from 1000Hz and below. Damping is the second and more markedly affects frequencies between 1000–3000 Hz. The third is Horn Effect which affects frequencies from 3000 Hz and above.

Figure 42 lists the dispensers options for acoustic modifications using the earmold.

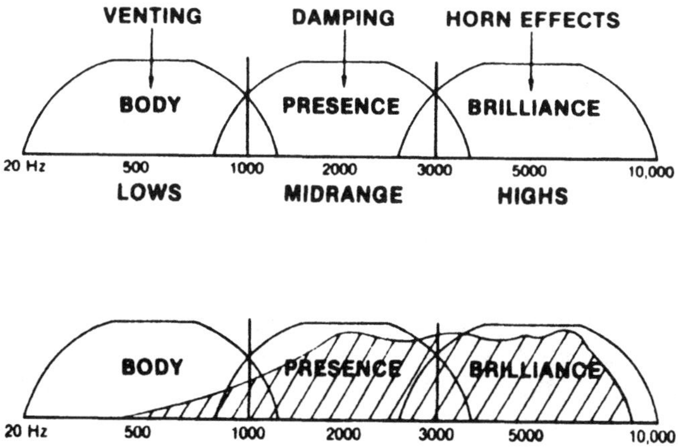

Fig. 41. Acoustic Control Areas

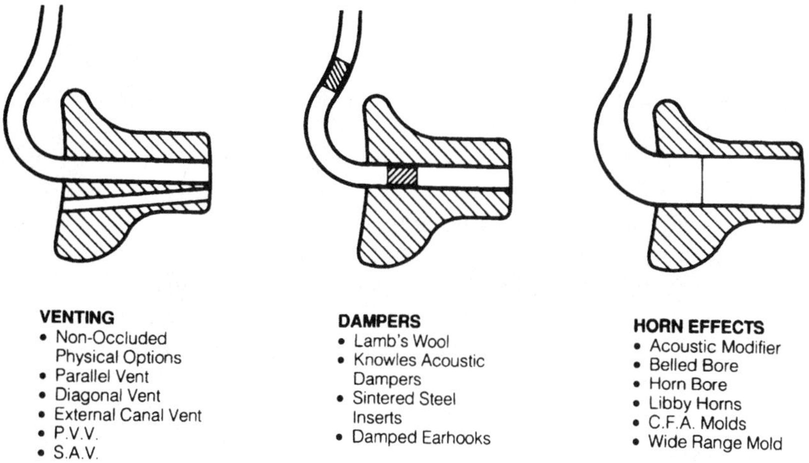

Fig. 42. Dispenser Options in Earmold Acoustics

Lybarger (1979) stated that earmold modifications practice developed over the years from a state akin to mysticism to a somewhat more orderly understanding of the acoustic processes involved.

As acoustical modification knowledge has grown, there evolved two methods of classifying the acoustical differences created in earmolds. The first was Lybarger's chart, which divided the final response of the hearing aid/coupler system into three areas: Low

Frequency—concerned with 800–2000 Hz and below, Primary Peak Response—concerned with 800–2000 Hz, and finally Secondary Response—concerned with frequencies above 2000 Hz.

With this classification, it was possible to measure the variables in acoustical response created by tubing diameter, tubing length, length of earmold canal, bore diameter, bore length, and filter effects. As newer earmold configurations, such as variable venting systems, non-occluding earmolds and an open vent earmold were developed, they were accurately described.

The oldest acoustical response option is earmold venting. What is earmold venting? It is a bored opening in an earmold from the tip of the earmold in the canal to the outside atmosphere. These vents can be big or small, short or long, and anywhere in between.

What is the purpose of venting? There are three basic functions of a vent. They are (a) to reduce the feeling of fullness caused by the earmold, (b) to reduce a resonant effect the client describes as "hearing in a tunnel", and (c) to improve speech clarity through better frequency response.

Lybarger's list for earmold venting includes 1) for static pressure equalization, 2) for moderate low frequency reduction, 3) for strong low frequency reduction, 4) for extreme low frequency reduction and 5) for adjustability.

Lybarger (1979) states that the traditional view is that venting reduces low frequency response. He states, however, that for in-the-ear and canal hearing aids, a vent can increase low frequency response within a restricted frequency region.

Earmold vents have three basic configurations, (1) a channel along the outside of the earmold, referred to as an external vent, (2) a diagonal vent and (3) a parallel vent construction. Figure 41 shows venting placement options using a cross-sectional view. It has been demonstrated that the parallel vent is preferred to maintain acoustic integrity. The diagonal vent can cause a higher incidence of feedback and, subsequently, a reduction of high frequency gain. The parallel vent will modify low frequency response and not affect high frequency response. The diameter and length determines the acoustical response.

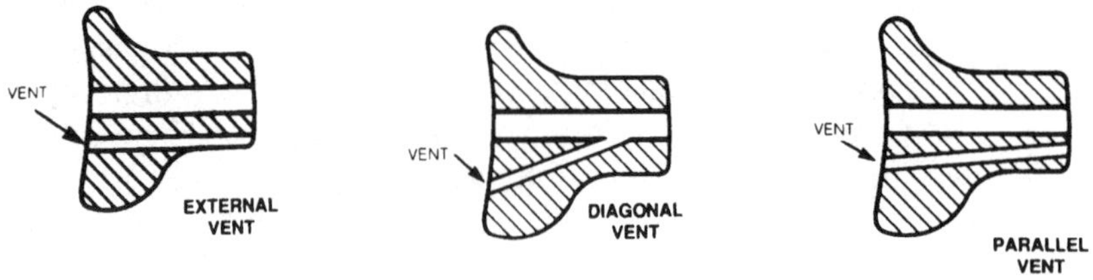

Fig. 43. Venting Configurations

Parallel venting is an effective method of modifying the low frequency response of an amplification system without having any effect on the high-frequency area. In the 1970's, research was focused on the acoustic effect of various vent sizes. It was found that effects on the frequency response are determined by the location, diameter and length of the vent as shown in Figure 44.

A dispenser may order a specific length and diameter vent in any earmold.

CUSTOM VENT EFFECT
FREQUENCY CUT-OFFS DETERMINED BY
DIAMETER AND LENGTHS

FREQUENCY	DIAMETER	LENGTH
250	.042	.7"
250	.030	.35"
250	.021	.175"
500	.085	.7"
500	.060	.35"
500	.042	.75"
750	.120	.7"
750	.090	.35"
750	.063	.175"
1000	.168	.7"
1000	.120	.35"
1000	.084	.175"
1000	.0588	.0875"

Fig. 44. Effect Table for Custom Venting

Diagonal venting is not recommended because of possible influence on the high-frequency response and introduction of acoustic feedback. In some cases a diagonal vent may be required due to physical size restraints.

Often, if acoustic feedback occurs as a result of traditional venting techniques, an external vent may be required. This is simply an external channel that runs partially down the length of the canal and into the body of the mold. Early dispensers drilled their own vents on a trial and error basis, supplemented by experience. Today, labs will drill a vent at the dispenser's request. If a vent is drilled too big or too short, the earmold may be worthless. To simplify the application of the desired measured effects of venting, several venting systems were developed by earmold labs.

The first of these was described by Qualitone, reported by Griffing & Shields (1972). The system is called the Variable Venting Valve or V.V.V. as shown in Figure 45. The rationale for the invention was to give the patient control of the hearing aids frequency response.

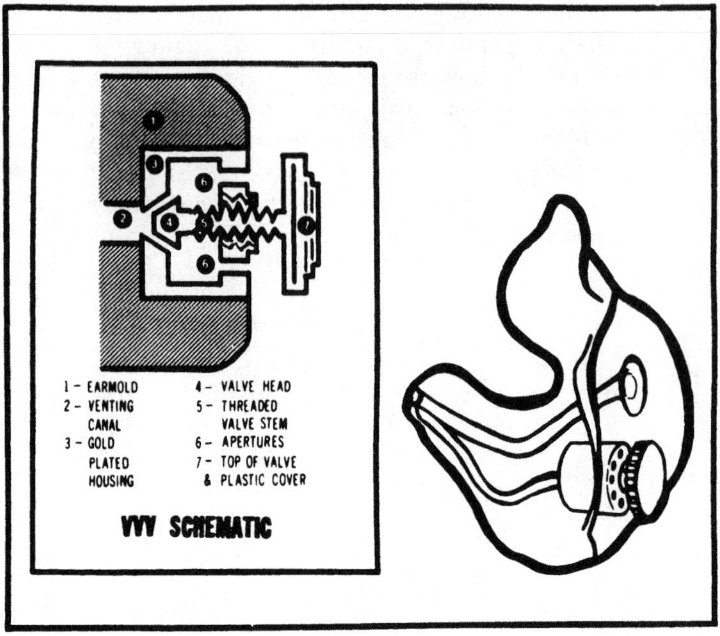

Fig. 45. Variable Venting Valve (V.V.V.)

The next two venting systems are the Positive Venting Valve described by Blue (1972) and the Select-A-Vent system. The concept is the same in both systems. The drawings and graphs below show the location of the vents, the vent hole sizes and acoustic effect of different vent sizes.

Figure 46a shows the P.V.V. vent by cut away drawing.

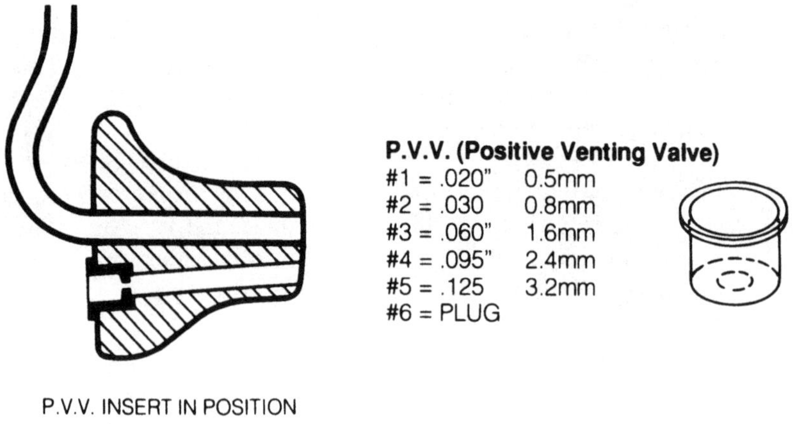

Fig. 46a. Positive Venting Valve (P.V.V.) System and

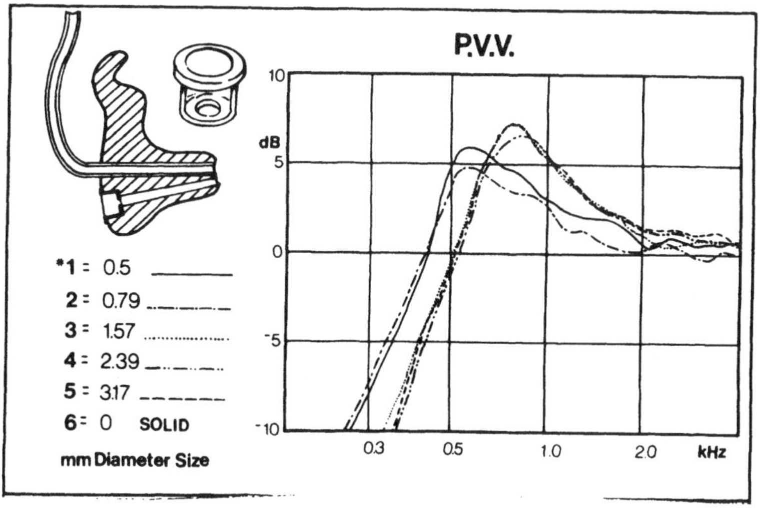

Fig. 46b. Effects Chart

Figure 46b shows the effects of the P.V.V. vent plugs.

Reports by Mynders (1975) on the value of these venting systems show little if any relationship between the size of the vent hole and speech clarity. The clinicians must evaluate the effects of various vents to find the best result for the patient.

Figure 47a shows the same type of cut-away of the S.A.V. vent for comparison purposes.

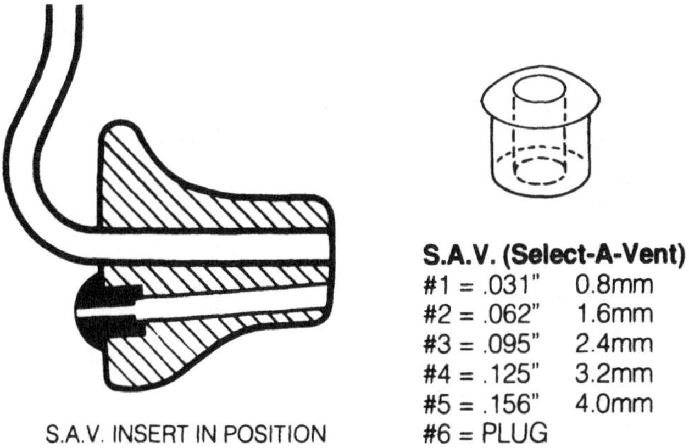

Fig. 47a. Select-A-Vent (S.A.V.) System and Effects Chart

As in Figure 47b, the acoustic effects of thedifferent sized S.A.V. vents are graphed for comparison again.

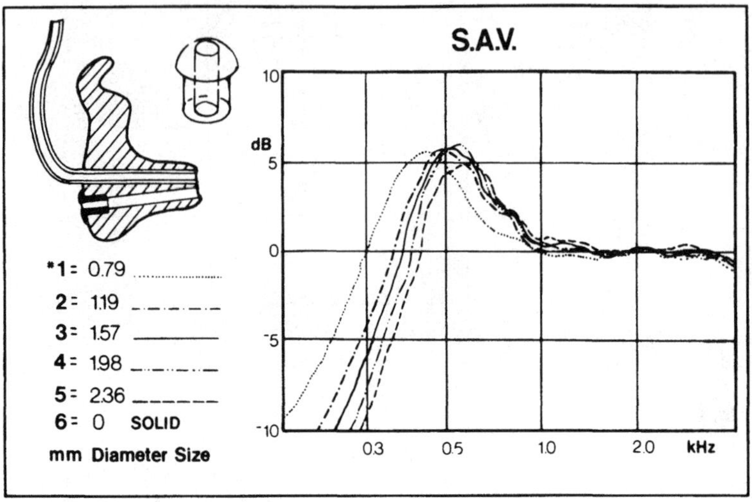

Fig. 47b.

Referring to Figure 41 entitled "Control Areas of Earmold Acoustics", you will see that dampers are the devices that control the midrange area.

A damper causes acoustic resistance to the sound passing from a hearing aid. The purpose of using dampers is to smooth the frequency response in the mid-frequency range from 1000–3000Hz. Originally, dampers were used in the external receivers of body aids, but now most are used in the tubing or earhook of behind-the-ear aids. Research has shown that the placement of the damper in the tubing and earhook makes a considerable difference in which specific frequencies are damped. Figure 48 shows the effect of damper placement.

The clinical choices for damper types are shown here with their acoustic effects.

LAMB'S WOOL

Lamb's wool in Figure 49 is the oldest acoustic damper used with hearing aids. The density of the lamb's wool, once inserted, determines the damper effect. It is effective but not easily controlled. The lamb's wool is carefully placed into the earhook or the tubing.

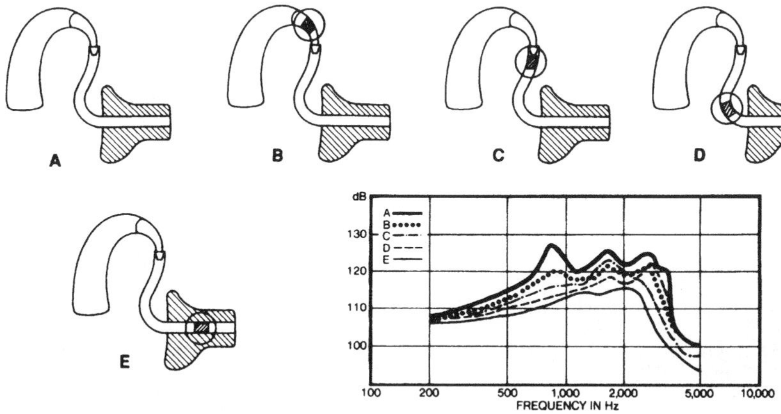

Fig. 48. Damper Locations and Effects

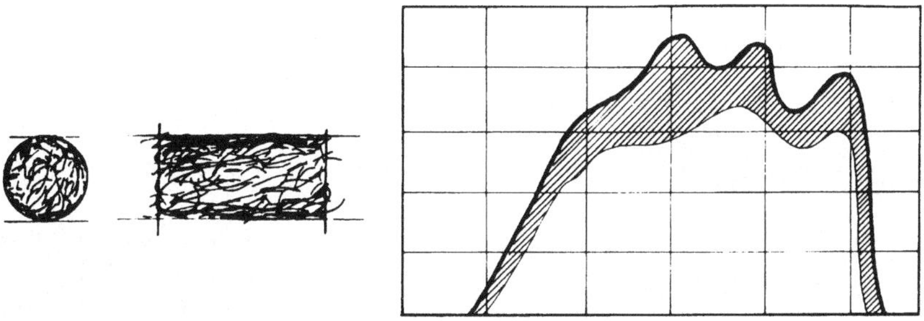

Fig. 49. Lambs Wool Damper

SINTERED STEEL INSERTS

A series of pellets with different degreese of porosity which give different levels of acoustic resistance. See Figure 50.

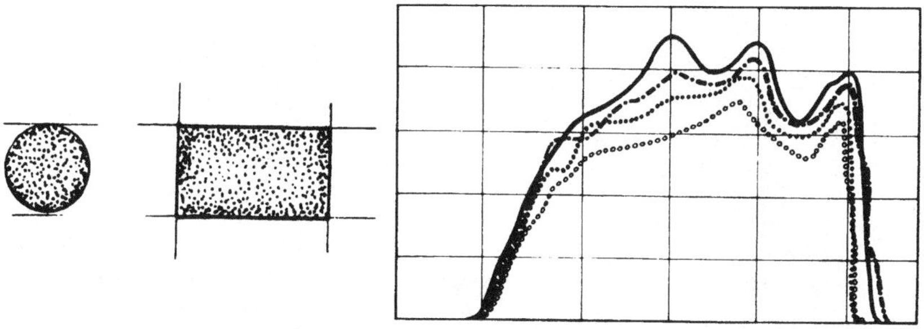

Fig. 50. Sinter Steel Damper

STAR DAMPER

Star damper is an addition to damper options. This is made from silicone material and has little mositure build-up problems. Must be cut to different lengths and measured in order to know exact effects.

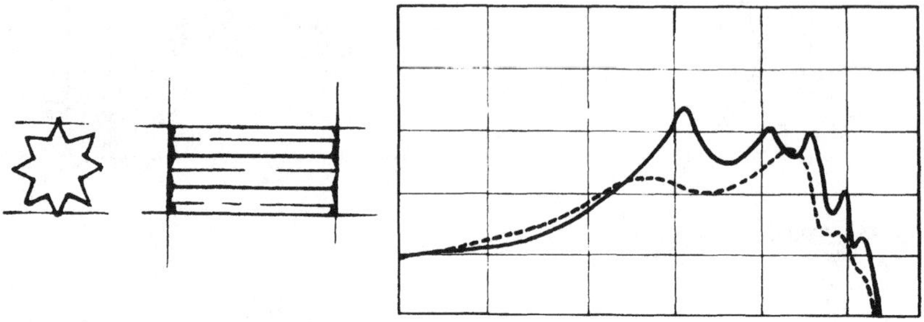

Fig. 51. Star Damper

KNOWLES ACOUSTIC DAMPERS

Knowles Acoustic Dampers are a refinement of acoustic control. These dampers are in a metal housing with a color-coded plastic mesh screen at one end. See Figure 52. There are six different Knowles dampers available: 680, 1000, 1500, 2200, 3300 and 4700 in Ohm values. The Knowles dampers are probably the most convenient damping system. PLEASE NOTE: The description of the various dampers is in Ohms *not* frequency. Moisture collection can be a problem.

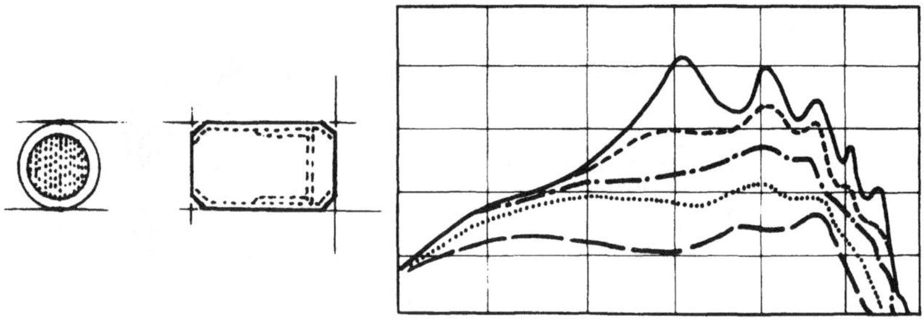

Fig. 52. Knowles Acoustic Dampers

In musical acoustics the "belling of a tube will ENHANCE high frequency signals passing through that tube. The reverse is also true, in that the narrowing of the end of a tube will REDUCE the high frequency components.

With many of today's hearing instruments reproducing high frequency signals out to 7000–9000Hz, it is particularly important that the tube and earmold not restrict the resonance in the sound channel and cut off high frequencies. Incorporating a horn of some type is critical to achieving a successful fitting.

In some cases, audiograms showing an upward audiometric curve slope in the higher frequencies need to be reduced instead of enhanced. In these cases the reverse horn must be used.

In addition to the two horn effect options reviewed in Figure 53, the clinician has many more to choose from.

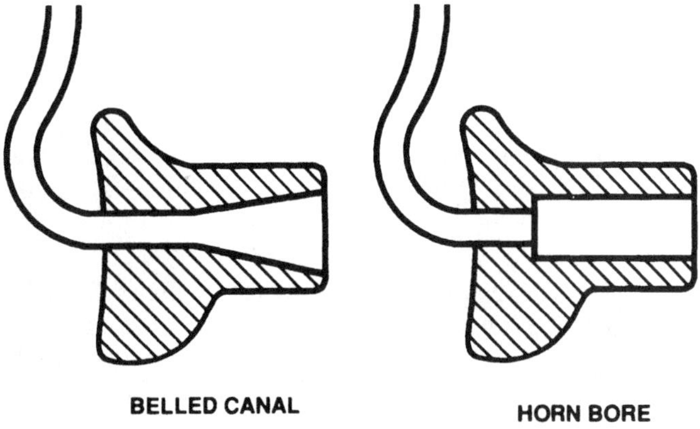

Fig. 53. Horn Effect Molds

The most basic of horn effects are the laboratory belled bore canal and the simple horn bore. These are options in any earmold style and are especially important with wide band receiver aids to preserve the high frequency signal.

The horn effect was first applied to earmolds in the late 1950's with the development of earmolds called the "Acoustic Modifier" or High Frequency Short Canal/Wide Bore earmolds. This mold can be easily altered by the dispenser, which allows variable control over the high frequency response in any given fitting. For best results it is suggested that a S.A.V. or P.V.V. venting system be used with this earmold.

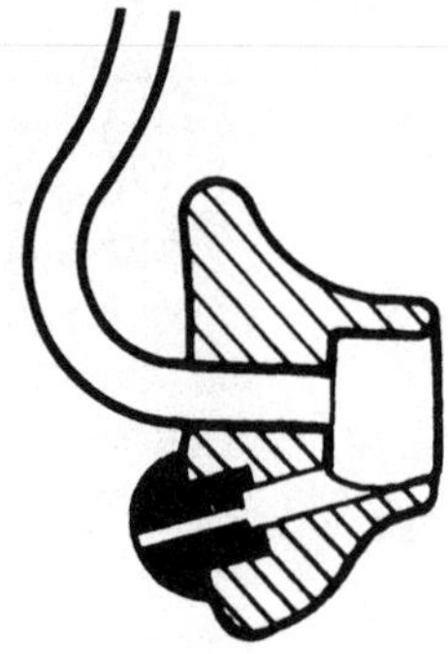

Fig. 54. Acoustic Modifier Mold

Dampers can be used for those clients who demonstrate tolerance problems.

Dampers create "acoustic resistance". Acoustic resistance creates a reduction in energy and produces heat as a by-product. This situation may cause moisture build-up in the tubing which is seen as condensation on the interior tubing wall. Sometimes moisture build-up is so great that it may block the tubing completely.

Damper positions were chosen because of wave length resonance. Libby, Lybarger and others recommend that dampers be positioned in the earhook or connector of an aid rather than in the tubing itself. Libby recommended that by changing damper location it is necessary to use a Knowles damper with a higher acoustic resistance (Ohms):

When using acoustic damping material, don't double damp! What does this mean? Some new aids had damper elements internally installed or installed in the earhook. If a fitter then selected a mold or earhook that incorporated a damper in the sound transmission system, "double damping" occurred with a resulting decrease in gain, output, and frequency response. The clinician must consult the specification sheet to see if a damping element is included.

Referring back to Figure 41, the final area of earmold acoustic control is Horn Effects. Horn Effect is an area of earmold technology needing further clarification. In acoustics, narrowing the sound channel outlet will reduce the high frequency spectrum of a complex signal. Conversely, if one widens the outlet of the sound channel, the high frequency spectrum will be enhanced. Fundamentally, this is due to the ease with which air particles flow out of the sound channel. See Figure 55.

There is a final area in Acoustic Options. It combines some of the three areas of acoustic control. The molds are referred to as Resonator Earmolds. See Figure 56.

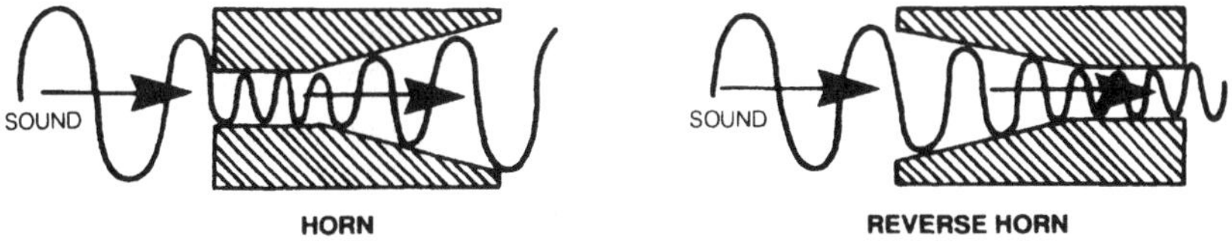

Fig. 55. Horn Effects

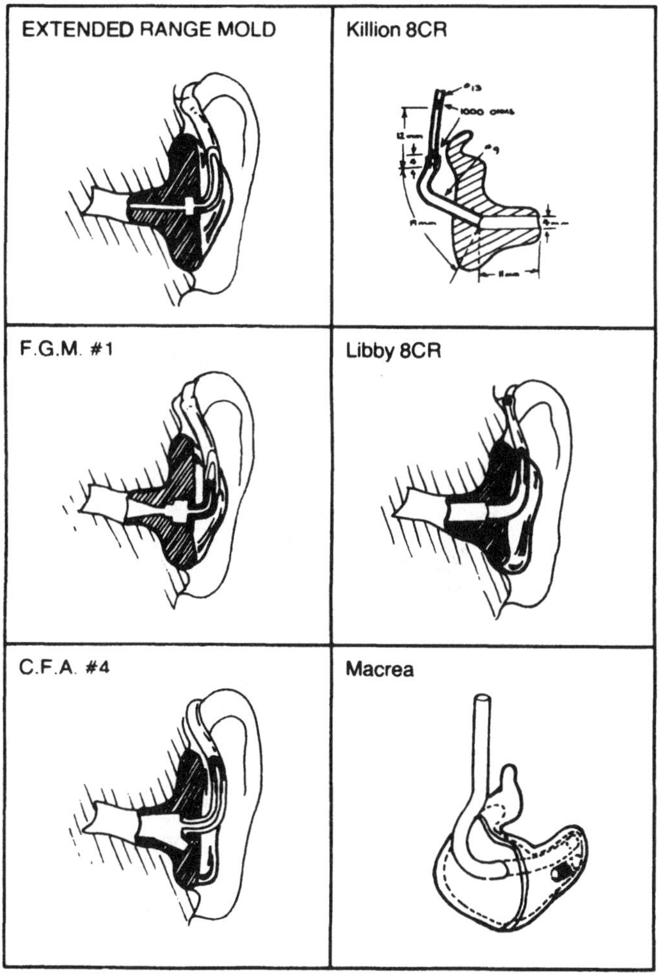

Fig. 56. Resonator Mold Choices

Resonator function is not new, but its application to earmolds in a controlled manner is. In a Helmholtz Resonator, the resonant frequency is directly proportional to the square root of compliance. The resonant frequency is also inversely proportional to the square root of the mass.

Resonator Theory is part sound and part acoustics. Using a Helmholtz-type resonator in an earmold takes a given amount of sound energy passing through the hearing aid's sound transmission tube and re-arranges it by frequency.

This acoustical phenomenon does not really change the total energy present. The design of the Helmholtz Resonator in earmolds has as its goal to dampen low frequency output and boost high frequency performance. Because of the amount of this "acoustic boost", the hearing aid client often turns down his volume control and thus obtains a better signal-to-noise ratio than before the resonator earmold was applied.

In order to simplify the selection process, there are two earmold systems that accomplish different acoustic objectives. System #1 is the CFA System as shown in Figure 57. It incorporates a standardized tube and elbow that attaches to various drilled bores in the mold to accomplish desired acoustic effects.

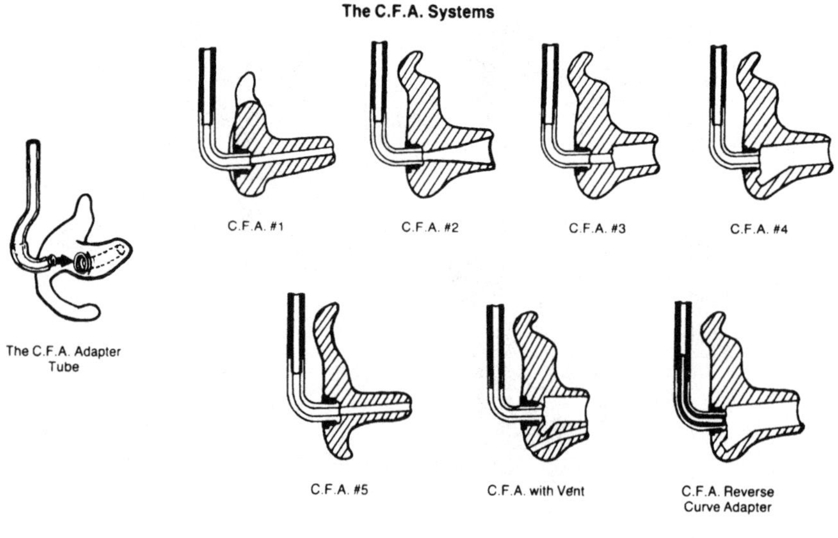

Fig. 57. C.F.A. Earmold Options

The Second System is the Libby Horn System as shown in Figure 58. Each of the Libby Horn Molds utilize a stepped bore tubing. The design follows aspects of the Killion designs.

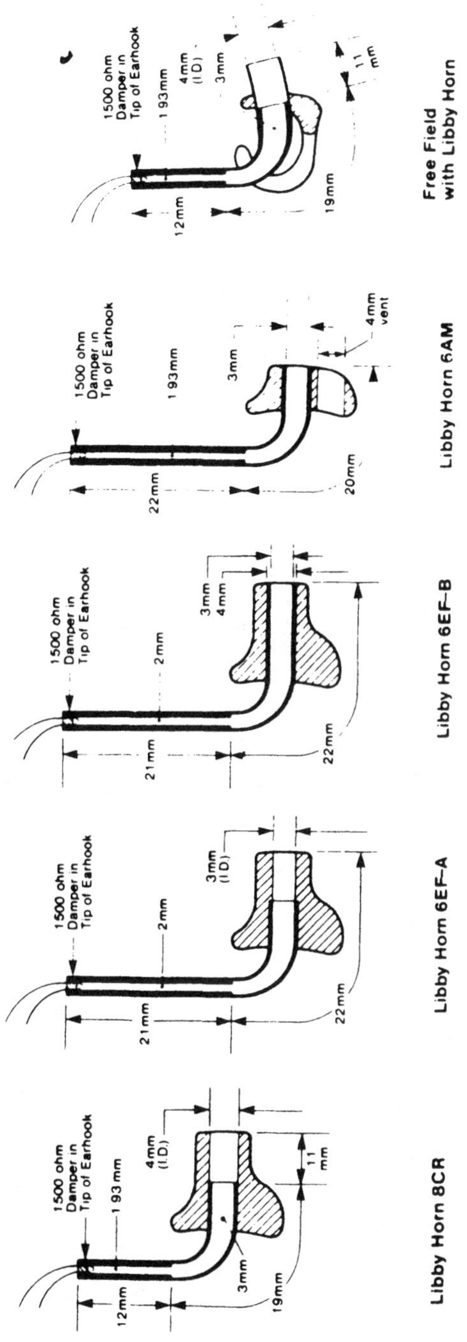

Fig. 58. Libby Horn Options

Affecting the passage of sound through the channel that leads to the eardrum will have acoustic effects as were described on the Acoustic of Earmolds section of this chapter. Tubing affects acoustic inertance. Dampers in the tubing and ear hook affect acoustic resistance. The National Association of Earmold Labs standardized tubing interior and exterior diameters and coded these with a Tubing Size Number. See Figure 59.

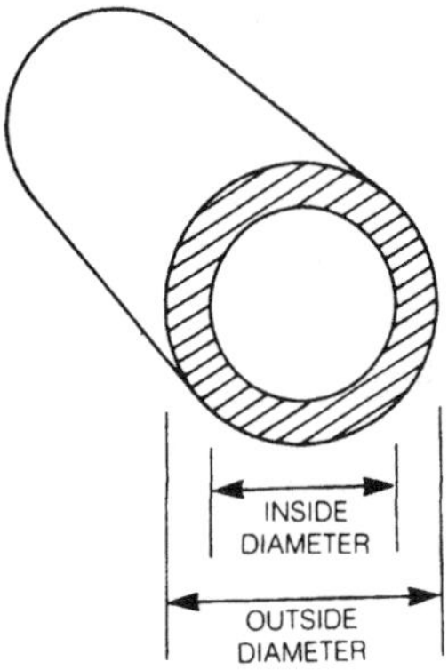

Standard N.A.E.L. Tubing Sizes

SIZE TYPE	INSIDE DIAMETER		OUTSIDE DIAMETER	
9	.094"	2.4mm	.160"	4.1mm
12	.085"	2.2mm	.125"	3.2mm
13 Standard	.076"	1.9mm	.116"	2.9mm
13 Medium	.076"	1.9mm	.122"	3.2mm
13 Thick Wall	.076"	1.9mm	.130"	3.3mm
13 Double Wall	.076"	1.9mm	.142"	3.6mm
14	.066"	1.7mm	.116"	2.9mm
15	.059"	1.5mm	.116"	2.9mm
16 Standard	.053"	1.3mm	.116"	2.9mm
16 Thin	.053"	1.3mm	.085"	2.2mm

Fig. 59. NAEL Tubing Sizes

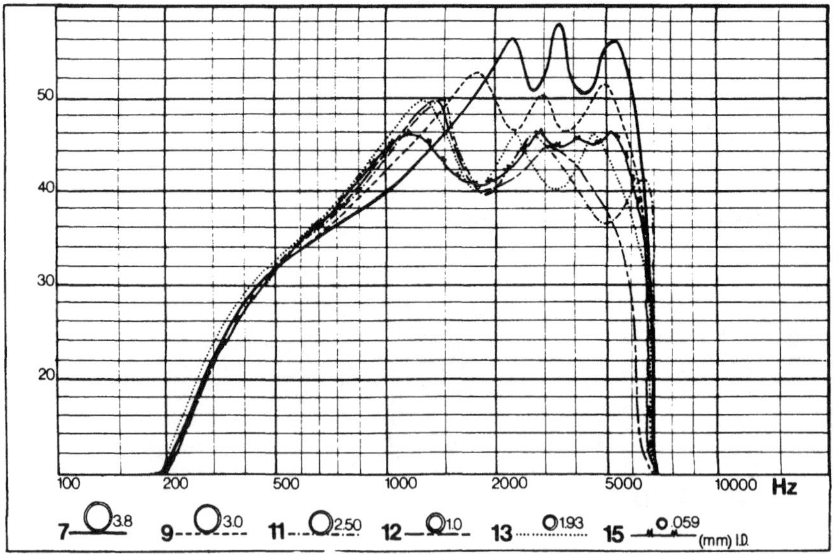

Fig. 60. Acoustic Effects of Tubing Diameters

Tubing diameter is a time-honored method of changing frequency response. There are ten tubing sizes standardized by the National Association of Earmold Labs (N.A.E.L.), although only six of them reflect differences in the inside diameter (only the inside diameter affects acoustic performance).

SPECIALIZED TUBING OPTIONS

This darkened area is a hard plastic elbow with a male part that snaps into a female ring in the mold. The interior diameter is constant. The mold is drilled for different acoustic effects.

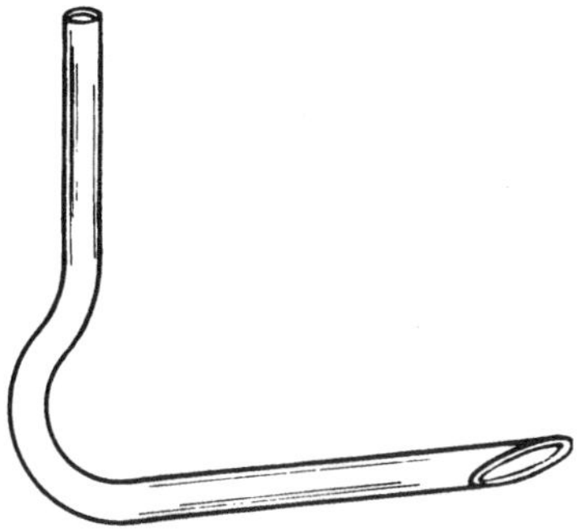

Fig. 61. CFA Tubing

The darkened area is a stepped bore construction. It comes in 3mm and 4mm horn sizes.

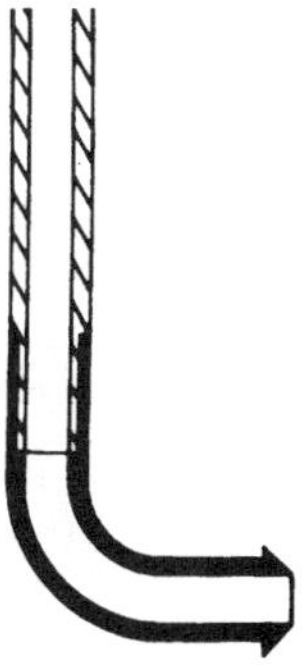

Fig. 62. Libby Horn

This is a standard tube with a gold flange to retain the tubing in soft molds. No cement is necessary.

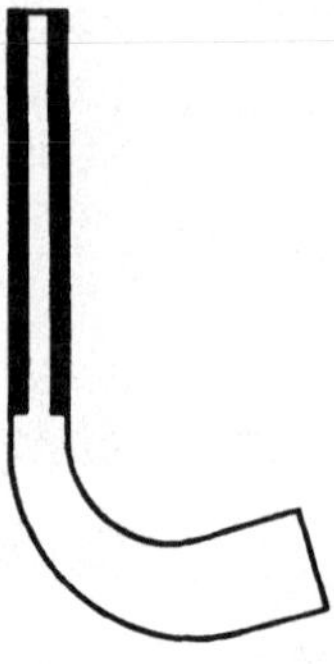

Fig. 63. Tube-Lock

Moisture condensation is common in earmold tubing. Dri-Tube is a denser plastic used for the tubing with greater resistance to the temperature changes that cause the condensation.

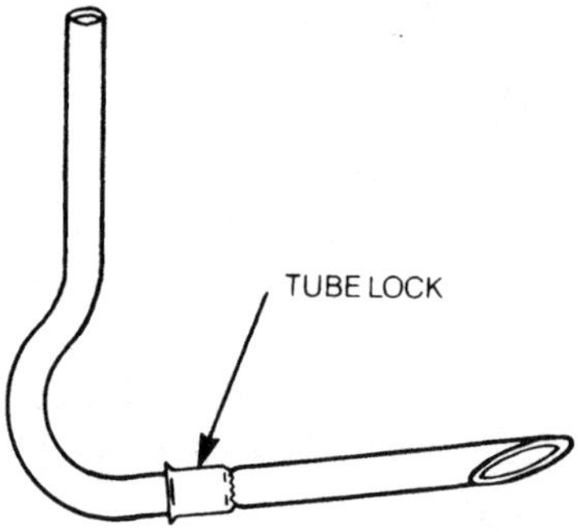

Fig. 64. Dri-Tube

Many manufacturers of behind-the-ear hearing instruments have ear hook options that acoustically change the responses of their aids. There are, however, some unique audiometric configurations that pose a challenge to the clinician when confronted with them. Entymotic Research the developer of the K-Amp circuitry, developed several specialized ear hooks that adapt to most behind-the-ear type aids. The effects are specific band reject 2Hz Notch Filter, High Pass Filter and a Low Pass Filter.

Killion's 2kHz Notch Filter Earhook is used with a conventional earmold, and provides the equivalent of Macrae's special notch filter mold. It can be evaluated easily without the need for special molds or test tips.

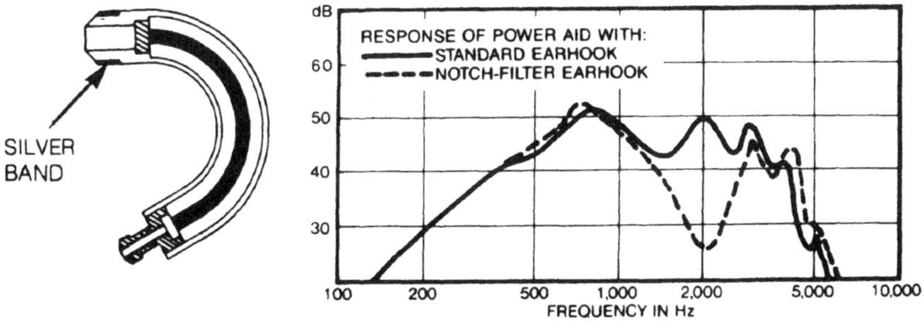

Fig. 65. 2K Notch Filter Earhook

The High-Pass Earhook is a versatile took adaptable to certain high frequency applications. Used with Lybarger molds in an open canal, it changes a wide band aid into a high-pass aid with greatly reduced output below 3kHz. This hook can also be used with other types of open canal tubes, and with closed canal fittings. In standard open canal applications, the output below 2kHz will be reduced to a level well below the natural sound entering the open ear. Thus, amplification will be heard only above 2kHz. In closed mold situations, the High-Pass Earhook provides high frequency boost above 2kHz which is not otherwise available, although some amplification below 2kHz will normally be audible.

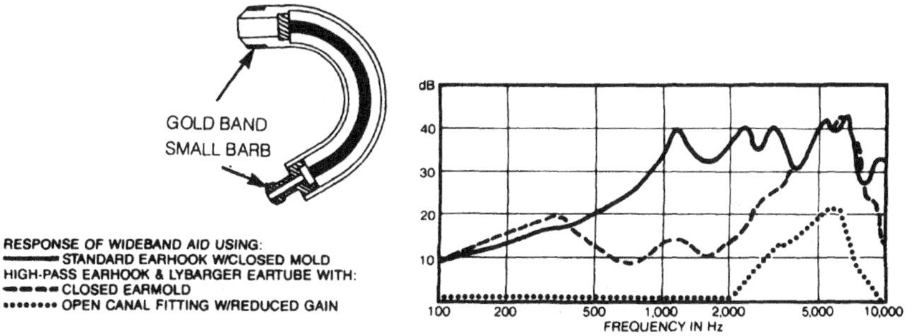

Fig. 66. High Pass Earhook

The Band-Reject Earhook helps in cases where the hearing loss is greater in the low and high frequencies and less in the mid ranges (reverse "cookie bite"). The audiogram shows typical projected improvement in the thresholds at various frequencies when this earhook is used in conjunction with an open earmold.

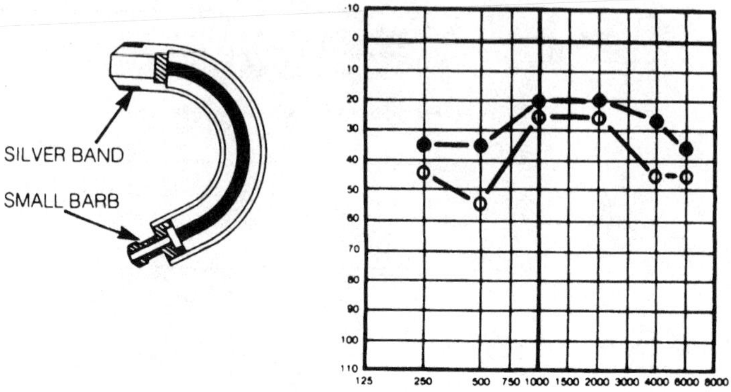

Fig. 67. Band Reject Earhook

The ER 12-1 Low-Pass earhook is used for both reverse slope and "cookie-bite" audiogram configurations, and works best with the 1.5 LP earmold style option.

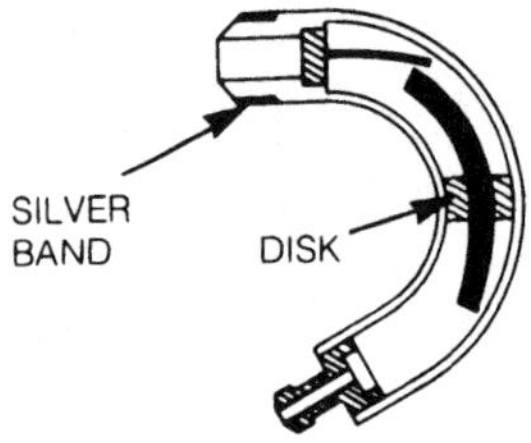

Fig. 68. Low Pass Earhook

EARMOLD MATERIALS

Plastics used in earmolds come in many formulations. All plastics are defined and measured by an organization called the American Society of Testing and Materials or ASTM. The two properties that ASTM is concerned with in earmold fabrication are water absorption and toxicity. The general variations in plastics include density, water absorption, clarity, toxicity, hardness and tensile strength. Earmold plastics are regulated by the FDA.

A confusing factor in clinician selection of earmold materials is that there is not standardization of name of materials from one lab to another. To assist clinicians in overcoming this problem chemical names will be used here to describe the various earmold materials.

Poly Methyl Methacrylate	A fine grade dental acrylic, lucite is available in clear, translucent tint, opaque beige or brown colors.
Poly Methyl Methacrylate	This is an extra find grade of lucite that is good for most allergy cases. Is available in clear or opaque pink.
Poly Methyl Methacrylate and Poly Ethyl Methacrylate	This is a combination of hard and semi-soft material in the same mold.
Poly Ethyl Methacrylate	This is a heat cured semi-soft vinyl plastic that will soften with body temperature. It comes in clear, beige, or translucent tint, and can be used for any application.
Thermoplastic Polyvinyl Chloride	This is a soft, proven thermoplastic that can be used for most earmold styles. This material is excellent for children and for improved acoustic seals in high gain hearing aids. It provides many advantages of silicone but at a lower cost, and is available in translucent tint, brown, opaque beige or clear.
Silicone #1	This material is a flexible inert silicone from which most earmold styles can be fabricated. Most allergy problems can be solved with clear silicone. This material is available in opaque clear, translucent pink, opaque beige and opaque brown.
Silicone #2	The softest, most comfortable silicone available. M-2000 earmolds are proven in power aid applications. Canal or canal-shell styles are often sufficient to overcome acoustic feedback, and require less bulk in the client's ear. Available in tint, opaque clear, beige & brown.
Dual-Durometer Silicone	Featuring a super-soft silicone canal combined with a special, firmer silicone body, this product permits easy use of Tube-Lock. Available in tint, opaque clear, beige and brown.
Polyethylene	This hard material is appropriate for severe allergy cases, and is available in opaque pink.

A major reason for selecting a hard or soft mold is comfort of seal. The table from Microsonic (1994), Figure 69, describes the material and gives a description of hardness of each material option.

The clinical aspects of material selection require evaluation of the individual patient's case. The considerations are:

- Is there an existing or past allergic reaction history? The clinician must ask the patient. The reaction that occurs with earmolds, ear hooks, tubing and hearing aid cases is contact dermititis. In some cases you and the patient won't know until the condition presents itself, often for the first time.
- Is the pinna soft or hard? This factor is critical because the insertion ease of the earmold can depend upon the material selected. The soft materials are used with hard ears most often.
- What is the power range of the aids to be fitted? High gain and high output hearing aids all require a good acoustic seal to prevent feedback and loss of benefit from the hearing aids. The anti-feedback style options should be used here.
- What about earmold cosmetics? The color choices are clear translucent pink, brown and opaque beige. It is also possible to get brown tubing. Involve the patient in selection process. Don't underestimate the importance of cosmetics to your patients.

The delivery of a hearing aid system is a rehabilitative process. The fitter must explain to the client what he or she must know and

HARDNESS TABLE OF EARMOLD MATERIALS:
Shore "A-2" (Hand-held) Durometer Tester #67977; ASTM D-2240

MATERIAL	Shore A Durometer		NOTES
	Canal Tip	Base	
Lucite	—	Hard	>A and D scale reading
Super Alerite	—	Hard	>A and D scale reading
Lucite w/Vinyflex I	A-94	Hard	>A and D scale reading
Synth-A-Flex II	—	A-48	
Vinylflex II	—	A-88	
Medi-Sil	—	A-48	
M-2000	—	A-28	
M-2000 Plus	A-28	A-78	
Micro-Lite II	—	A-50	
Polyethylene	—	Hard	>A and D scale reading
Lucite Body w/Synth-A Flex II	A-48	Hard	

Fig. 69. Hardness Table of Earmold

do to achieve satisfaction with the hearing instruments. Part of the client information must include the care and management of the earmold or custom shell.

The first point to cover with the patient is insertion of the ear-mold or custom aid. A suggested format follows:

1. Have the aid turned off to eliminate feedback when inserting it.
2. Show the position of the mold or custom aid when inserting it. It should be held between the thumb and forefinger.
3. Slide the mold or custom shell into the ear canal. Use a rocking motion until the client feels the mold or the custom aid pop into place. Pull down on the ear lobe gently to facilitate insertion.
4. Demonstrate "incorrect" insertion by having the client view this in a mirror.
5. Place the mold or custom aid into the patient's ear several times explaining the steps each time. The repetitions are helpful with the hearing impaired in the event they have not heard all you have said.
6. Stress to the client that *positioning* is what he or she is learning. Custom earmolds and custom aids do fit, but they must be correctly positioned by the client to make insertion easy.
7. Inform the client that most people require a few days to learn insertion technique. This statement will reassure the client who has difficulty with this part of the hearing aid delivery procedure.

Explain and demonstrate to your client that wax may form in the earmold or custom instrument's canal bore and that it should be wiped with a tissue lightly dampened with an antiseptic solution. Stress that alcohol should NEVER be used to clean them.

The second area of care for the earmold is tubing change. If the tubing becomes cracked, yellow or stiff, it must be replaced. Another factor in earmold care is moisture development in the tubing. If moisture does develop, a silica gel dehumidifier kit should be used and/or the Dri-Tube Tubing.

CAUTION: Zinc-Air batteries should NEVER be placed in a dehumidifier kit as it will affect the active chemicals and cause short battery life.

Earmolds and well fitting shells of custom hearing instruments are critical to effective hearing aid performance. If the electronics are working well, but the mold/shell isn't sealed well, the result may be poor aided performance and possible acoustic feedback.

Several conditions dictate earmold replacement or shell recasing to the hearing aid clinician.

1. Patient's weight has changed 6 lbs or more.
2. Physical growth in both children and adults pinnas.
3. Hearing thresholds have changed.
4. Damage and discoloration of the earmolds.
5. Changes in the ear tissue due to wearing earmolds or custom shells.
6. Earmold Innovations that offer Improvement for a given fitting.

PATIENT COUNSELING ABOUT REPLACEMENT

Advise patients if their hearing aid uses an earmold, the mold is an expendable item as are batteries. In general, a *soft mold* should be changed every year. A *hard mold* should be changed every two years. In the case of custom aids, consider every two or two and half years for "recasing".

THE MEASUREMENT PROCESS

Measuring acoustic effects of the human acoustic coupler has been done for years. Originally, hearing aid test sets were used to show coupler (earmold) effects. The concept of measuring the overall effects of targeting prescriptive gain objectives has become more prevalent clinically with the development of small user friendly real-ear measurement systems. The protocol and rationale for real-ear measurement is covered in Chapter VIII in this book.

Below is the procedure for evaluating acoustic effects of earmolds on the hearing aid's response, using a 2 cc coupler in an Electro-Acoustic Hearing Aid Analyzer. See Figure 70 as reported by Frye (1976).

The procedure for evaluating the earmold system's effect upon the hearing aid is as follows:

1. Mount the earmold to the coupler by using modeling clay rolled into a donut shape.
2. With the microphone removed from the coupler, check the positioning of the bore of the mold.

Lesson30 415-425

3. Slide the microphone into the coupler.
4. Place the aid, mold and coupler into the sound chamber at the reference spot for the aid's microphone.
5. Run a standard test set battery of gain at full on with 60dB input level, output at 90dB and frequency response at Reference Test Gain.

It should be stressed here again that the responses obtained through hearing aid test sets are not exactly what will be found in the real ear. However, they are repeatable and do give a good indication to the fitter of the compilation effect of earmold acoustic variables.

THE MODIFICATIONS & SERVICE PROCESSES

Modifications are performed by the hearing aid clinician in his or her office as part of the "fitting" of hearing aids. Modifications can be divided into two general categories. First, there are problems of fit that have to do with physical size or feel of the earmold or custom aid. Secondly, there are problems that have to do with sound quality.

To modify earmolds or the shells of custom aids, the hearing aid clinician must have a motor driven grinder and buffer. For in-office locations, bench-type grinder/buffer motors are best. For in the field earmold modifications, the dispenser will need a hand-held grinder/buffer motor.

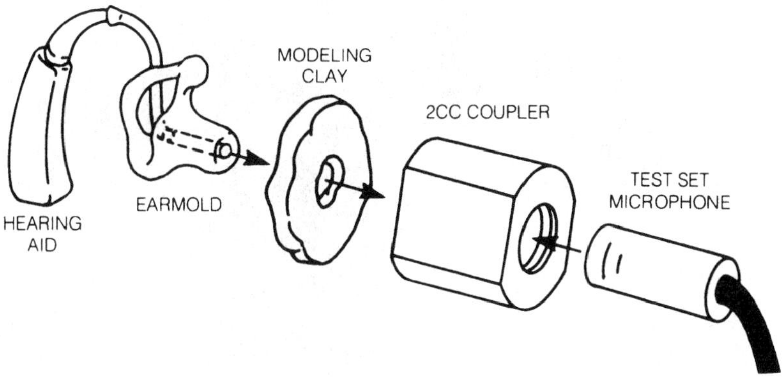

Figure 70 Set-Up for Electro Acoustic Analysis of a Hearing Aid

Physical modifications performed at the dispensing level include:

a) Reducing/Removing the helix area

b) Reducing Canal Length

c) Creating a "slit-leak" vent effect

d) Drilling vent holes

e) Removing high points that cause discomfort

f) "Belling" a canal

g) Changing by reduction one earmold style to another (e.g. shell to canal shell).

REMEMBER: A hearing aid shell or earmold that is not comfortable to wear for extended periods *will not be worn!*

An electro-acoustic hearing aid test set for a dispensing practice includes an electronics module to generate the source signals, and provides a read-out of gain, output and distortion percentages. A quiet test chamber provides the interface between hearing aid and test set. Below is Figure 71 showing such a test set.

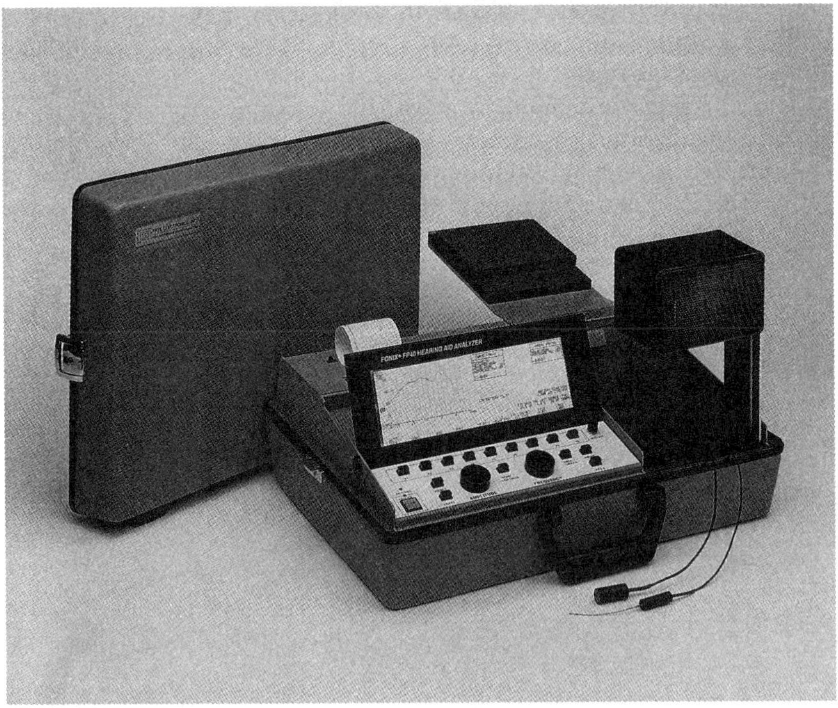

Figure 71 Electroacoustic Hearing Aid Analyzer

Grinding and polishing speeds for the different grinders have been published. Figure 72a shows a bench grinder with a mold being buffed. The most common grinder motors are made by Red Wing or Baldor. Figure 72b is a table developed by Microsonic Labs that defines the different earmold materials and the RPM speeds for effective grinding and polishing.

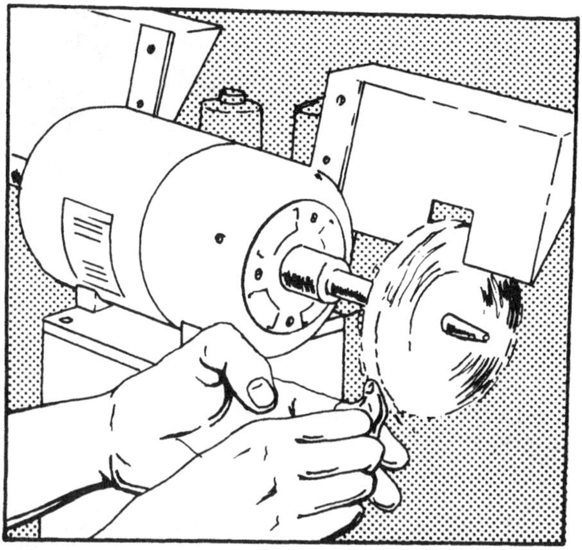

Fig. 72a. Grinding an Earmold on a Bench Grinder.

BENCH GRINDER
(RED WING OR BALDOR MOTORS)
WITHOUT HIGH SPEED ATTACHMENT

MATERIAL	GRINDING		POLISHING	
	Speed R.P.M.	**Tool-Stone**	**Speed R.P.M.**	**Buffing Compound or Solvent**
Lucite & Alerite	3,450	smooth	3,450	buffing compound*
Vinylflex II	3,450	coarse	3,450	buffing compound*
Polyethylene	3,450	smooth	3,450	buffing compound*
Micro-Lite II	3,450	very smooth	—	solvent
Synth-A-Flex II	3,450	coarse	—	solvent
Medi-Sil II, M-2000, M-2000 Plus	highest possible	very coarse	—	—

* Use with felt tool or buffing wheel.

Fig. 72b. Table of Speeds and Materials

Since not all patients can be seen in offices there is a hand tool grinder as seen in Figure 73a used for house call patients. The grinding and polishing table in Figure 73b shows the differences that using this type of grinder makes.

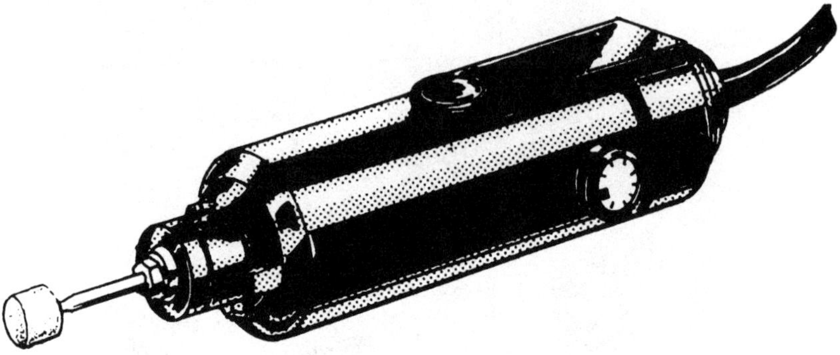

Fig. 73a. Dremel Hand Tool for Earmold Grinding and Table for Speeds and Materials.

VARIABLE SPEED MOTO-TOOL 370 OR
DREMEL MOTO-TOOL M270-5
use with Dremel Solid State Motor Speed Control

MATERIAL	GRINDING		POLISHING	
	Set Motor Speed On	Tool-Stone	Set Motor Speed On	Buffing Compound or Solvent
Lucite & Alerite	6	smooth	3-4	buffing compound*
Vinylflex II	5	coarse	3	buffing compound*
Polyethylene	4	smooth	3-4	buffing compound*
Micro-Lite II	4 to 5	very smooth	—	solvent
Synth-A-Flex II	5 to 6	coarse	—	solvent
Medi-Sil II, M-2000, M-2000 Plus	6	very coarse	—	—

* Use with felt tool or buffing wheel.

Fig. 73b. Dremel Hand Tool for Earmold Grinding and Table for Speeds and Materials.

PRIOR to trimming or buffing custom type instrument shells, either ITE, ITC or CIC, BE SURE TO INSTALL A BATTERY to reduce circuit problems due to static electricity.

Earmold modification techniques must be learned by experience. There is no formula indicating how much to reduce the helix or canal portion of an earmold or custom aid to achieve a comfortable fit. Once you grind down a mold or custom aid, you cannot restore easily what you grind away. If the ground area feels sharp or rough, grind and buff it more. The skin tissue of the external ear canal is sensitive to abrasion or pressure points. A modified earmold or custom shell, which has not been sufficiently smoothed, can cause a lesion or sore.

To acoustically modify the earmold, you can do the following:

(a) reduce the mold's canal length; thus the output can be reduced,

(b) change variable venting plugs for maximum venting possibilities,

(c) insert dampers, lamb's wool, sintered steel pellets, star dampers or Killion Dampers into the tubing,

(d) change tubing thickness,

(e) bell the canal bore.

Each of these adaptations has a measured effect, but still require the hearing aid clinician's experience to create the desired effect.

MODIFICATIONS & SERVICE PROCESSES

Acoustic modifications should be based on patient complaints about their fitting. The following situations may be solved by the following:

PROBLEM	ANSWER
1. Aid sounds tinny.	1. Drill vent hole. Use dampers.
2. Aid sounds harsh.	2. Reduce volume. Drill vent. Shorten canal.
3. Aid sounds hollow.	3. Increase vent size. Shorten canal. Bell canal.
4. Doesn't like sound of own voice.	4. Shorten vent. Enlarge vent. Bell canal.
5. Not loud enough.	5. Reduce vent size.
6. Feedback all the time.	6. Close vent entirely. Build-up canal.
7. Hears sound, but doesn't understand with aid.	7. Reduce low Hz. Enlarge vent. Shorten canal.

CLASSICAL MODIFICATION AND EFFECT CHART

	Modification	Effect on Low Frequencies (Below 750 Hz)	Effect on Frequencies Between 750 and 1500 Hz	Effect on Frequencies Between 1500 and 3000 Hz	Effect on High Frequencies (Above 3000 Hz)
TUBING DIAMETER	Larger I.D. Tubing & Horn Tubing	Negligible	Moves peak to higher frequency	Increases height of peak and moves to higher frequency	Increases
	Smaller I.D. Tubing	May reduce below 1 KHz	Moves peak to lower frequency	Reduces height of peak and moves to lower frequency	Reduced by large decrease
TUBING LENGTH	Longer Tubing	Increases	Moves peak to lower frequency	Moves peak to lower frequency	Negligible
	Shorter Tubing	Slightly Decreases	Moves peak to higher frequency	Moves peak to higher frequency	Negligible
LENGTH OF EARMOLD CANAL	Longer Earmold Canal	———	Increases level of response curve ———	———	———
	Shorter Earmold Canal	———	Decreases level of response curve ———	———	———
BORE DIAMETER	Larger Diameter Bore Through Earmold Canal*	Negligible	Moves peak to higher frequency	Moves peak to higher frequency	Increases
	Smaller Diameter Bore Through Earmold Canal*	Negligible	Moves peak to lower frequency	Moves peak to lower frequency	Decrease
BORE LENGTH	Longer Bore Through Earmold Canal*	Slightly Increases	Moves peak to lower frequency	Moves peak to lower frequency	Decreases
	Shorter Bore Through Earmold Canal*	Slightly Decreases	Moves peak to higher frequency	Moves peak to higher frequency	Increases

Fig. 74 Classical Earmold Modification and Effects Table

VENTING	Small Vent (.031"/0.8mm)**	Negligible	Negligible	Negligible	Negligible
	Medium Vent (.064"/1.6mm)**	Decreases	Increases peak height	Negligible	Negligible
	Large Vent (.094"/2.4mm)**	Decreases	Increases peak height	Negligible	Negligible
NON-OCCLUDING MOLD	Non-Occluding Mold	Eliminates	Moves peak to higher frequency and increase height	Increases peak height	Negligible
OPEN VENT MOLD	Open-Vented (High Frequency) Mold	Decreases	Reduces peak height	Negligible	Negligible
FILTER INSERTS	Filter Insert at Hearing Aid Nub	Negligible	Reduces peak height	Reduces peak height	Negligible
	Filter Insert at Earmold Tip	Slightly Decreases	Large Reduction	Large Reduction	Decreases

NOTE: Because of wide variation in earphone types and internal acoustical systems in hearing aids, this chart must be considered as a guide for average conditions.

* Applies to earmolds for conventional earphones.

** Vents of short lengths are more effective in reducing low frequency response. Gain must be limited with larger size vents to avoid feedback.

(Fig. 74. Continued)

The next chart details probable intervention effects on the frequency response of hearing aids.

The table below reported by Microsonic (1994) details the classical modifications and effects of changing earmold plumbing.

A qualified hearing aid clinician is one who develops a range of modification interventions to solve fitting problems. That range includes conventional modifications described in this section, plus computer/software adaptations available in programmable hearing instruments. It is usually a combination of conventional and high tech modifications that result in satisfied, well-fitted patients.

SERVICE FOR EARMOLDS

Earmold service begins at the first fitting session. Earmolds come with a long tubing that must be sized (cut) to required lengths. The connector/ear hook of the behind-the-ear aids should often be "angled" as well. Not adjusting this connector/earhook can make wearing the aids uncomfortable. Figure 75 shows the tubing fitting process. With the hearing aid placed behind the patient's ear, mark the tubing ¼″ to ⅜″ above the connector/earhook termination point. Then cut the tubing and attach the mold to the aid. This simple procedure, if not done correctly, causes pain and discomfort when wearing the instrument.

A common earmold service problem is the collection of ear wax in the canal and on the outer surface of the mold. Surface wax can be wiped off, but you or your client will have to use a wax loop to

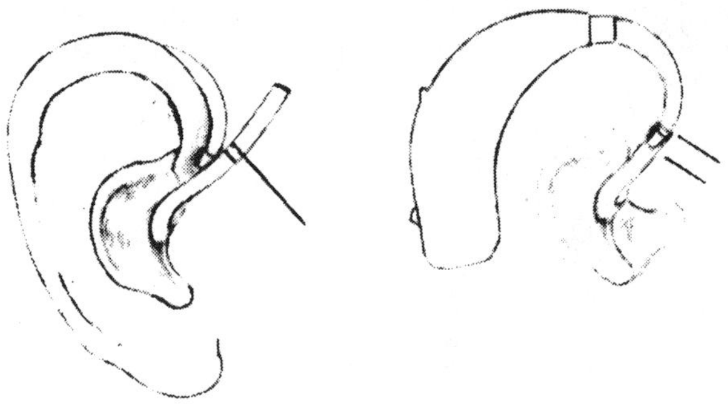

Fig. 75. Fitting Tubing

remove the wax from the canal. The most important service item for "tubed" earmolds is tubing change. It should be emphasized that tubing WILL deteriorate. It has to be changed. One recommendation is to change it every six months. This will eliminate emergency situations caused by deteriorated tubing. The technique for tubing change is shown below:

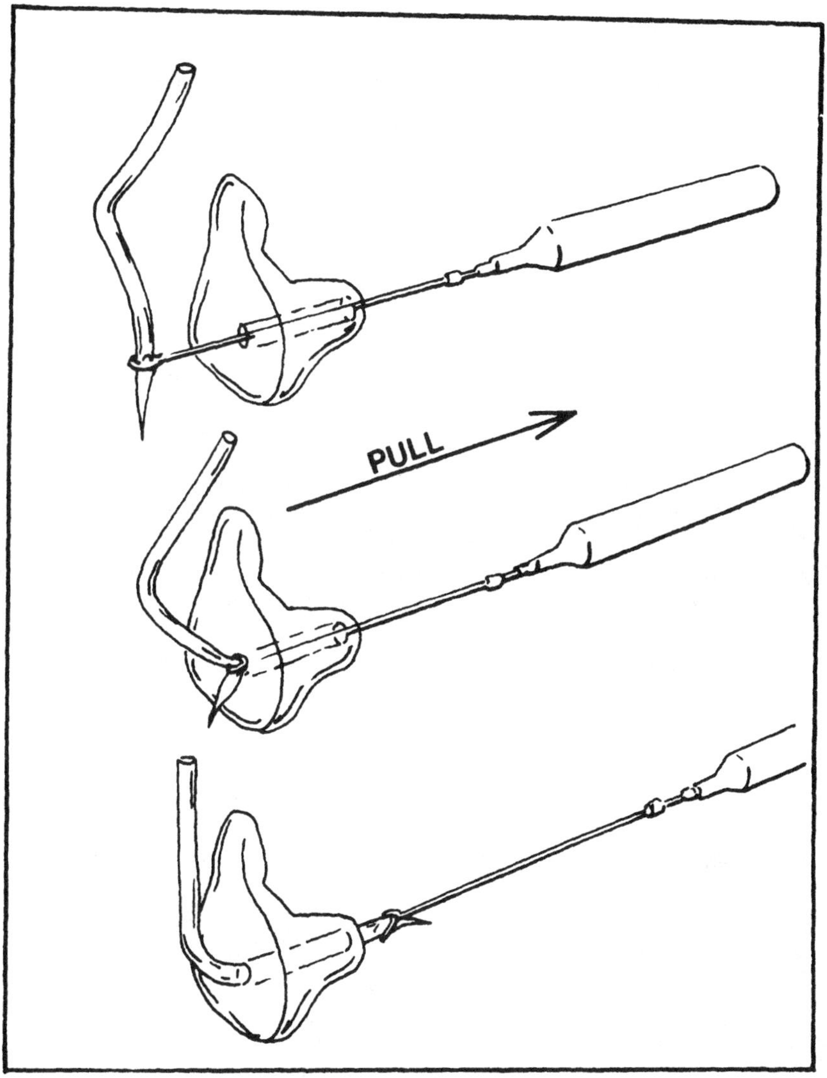

Figure 76 Tubing Change Procedure

SUMMARY

In summary, the human acoustic coupler as it relates to hearing aids has an important history and a changing future. The change from behind-the-ear, eyeglass, and body aids to "custom" type instruments has radically affected the utilization of the accumulated knowledge about earmolds.

In striving to be an effective hearing aid clinician, one must know about the most effective earmold choices in order to maximize fittings even though the percentage of instruments using earmolds is very limited today. Digital and digital programmable hearing aids now perform many of the acoustical modifications accomplished in the past through earmold technology.

GLOSSARY

Acoustic ohm unit of measurement of resistance to the flow of sound pressure waves through a medium. The unit is equal to a pressure amplitude of one degree per square centimeter per second of flux amplitude.

Allergen any substance which produces an allergic reaction e.g., the case material of a hearing aid, a lucite earmold.

Antifeedback is the goal for a hearing aid clinician whose patient's hearing aids have a whistling problem. There are procedures and lab options that are referred to as "antifeedback".

Bony Portion refers to the anatomy of the ear canal after the second bend in the canal. With deep canal hearing aids and molds, this anatomical area has become critical to a "good" fit and patient comfort.

Completely-in-the-Canal refers to a newer style of hearing instruments that fit just as the name implies.

Concha the shell-like cavity of the outer ear in which the entrance of the external ear canal is located.

Coupler any device by which one portion of an acoustical system is joined to another e.g., an earmold is the "coupler" for a hearing aid.

Damper a mechanical device that decreases the amplitude of amplified signals in hearing aids.

Dual Durometer Silicone is one type of earmold material characterized by a softer canal and firmer bowl portion of the fabricated mold.

Earmold vent a hold drilled into an earmold to relieve pressure or alter the acoustic output of a hearing aid e.g., drilled types, S.A.V., P.V.V., etc.

Feedback the oscillation (whistling sound) a hearing aid may make. Earmolds that do not seal can be one cause of feedback.

Helix the incurved ridge at the edge of the external ear above the concha.

Horn theory an acoustic horn structure which will transfer the high pressure at the narrow end of the horn to lower pressure at the mouth of the horn. This system helps preserve high frequency response in hearing aid signals.

Insertion gain the difference between the sound pressure level at the eardrum produced by a hearing aid and the sound pressure level at the eardrum **without** the hearing aid.

Insertion loss the loss that occurs when the earmold occludes the ear canal and destroys the natural ear canal resonance.

Lesion any pathological or traumatic change of tissue.

Non-occluding earmold a family of tubing earmold styles that leaves the ear canal open to outside aid e.g., C.R.O.S., Janssen, Free-Field, etc.

Poly Methyl Methacrylate is a dental grade of lucite used in the making of earmolds, a common name for this material is lucite.

Prolapsed Canal a flap of tissue that occludes the external canal. It can cause problems during the impression process or further into a fitting.

Resonator any structure, material or device which can be set into vibration by sound pressure waves of its natural frequency originating in another vibrating body.

Resonator Molds are a group of different earmold options that create a resonator effect as the amplified sound passes through the earmolds tubing and cavities. The result is often a boost in high frequency amplification.

Tragus the small stiff ridge in front of the external ear canal's opening.

REFERENCES

"Acoustically Tuned Earmold—General Reference Data" American Research & Design Group, Technical Report, 1980

AGNEW, J, "Ear Impression Stability." Hearing Instruments, Vol. 37/12, pp. 8–12, 1986

AUSTIN, C. D., KASTEN, R. N. & WILSON, H. "Real-Ear Measurements of Hearing Aid Plumbing Modifications," The Hearing Journal, Vol. 43/7, pp. 30–35, 1990

BENNETT, HARRY, Personal Correspondence to the author concerning F.G.M. Earmold Design, Western Hearing Research, Fresno, CA, 1978

BENZIGER, L. "Make a Perfect (Ear) Impression," Hearing Instruments, Vol. 44/12, pp. 18–22, 1993

BERANEK, L. L, "Acoustics," McGraw-Hill Co., New York, 1954

BERGENSTOFF, HANS, "Earmold Design and its Effect on Real Ear Insertion Gain," Hearing Instruments, September 1983

BERGER, K. W. "The Hearing Aid: Its Operation and Development." (2nd Edition) National Hearing Aid Society, Livonia, MI 1984

BERLAND, OLE, "No Mold Fitting of Hearing Aids," Oticon Electronics, A/S, Copenhagen, Denmark.

BLUE, J. V., "Positive Venting Valve Concept," The Hearing Dealer, 23, 1972

BRISKEY, R., and WRUK, K., "Acoustic Influence of Insert Vents," Hearing Instruments, 25:12–14, 1974

BUERKLI-HALEVY, O., "Response-Modifying Earhooks—Special Fitting Solutions for Hard-To-Fit Losses," Hearing Instruments, Vol. 39/4, pp. 44–47, 66 1988.

CAINE, MYRON, "Plastics & Materials Used in Earmolds," Hearing Instruments, December, 1974.

CHASEN, MARSHALL, "Using Acoustic Resistance in Earmold Tubing," Hearing Instruments, Vol. 34, No. 12, 1983.

COX, ROBYN M., "Acoustic Aspects of Hearing Aid-Ear Canal Coupling Systems," Monographs in Contemporary Audiology, Vol. 1 No. 3.

CURRAN, J. R., "CROS Fittings & Open Canal Amplification." Monograph from Dahlberg Electronics, Inc., Minneapolis, 1971.

DALSGAARD, STIG C., "Earmolds & Associated Problems," The Almqvist & Wiksel Periodical Company, Stockholm, Sweden, 1975.

DURRANT, J. D. & LOVRINIC, J. H., "Bases of Hearing Science," Williams & Wilkins Company, Baltimore, MD, 1977.

EWERTSEN, H. W., IPSEN, J. G. & NIELSON, S. S., "On The Acoustical Characteristics of the Earmold," Acta Otolaryngol, 47, 312–317, 1957.

FRYE, GEORGE J., "The Earmold-Again," Audecibel, Spring 1976.

GOLDBERG, H., "Earmold Technology-Application Notes," Audiology & Hearing Education, August/September, 1977.

GREEN, D. S., "Non-Occluding Earmolds with CROS & IROS Hearing Aids," Arch. Otolaryng, Chicago, 89, 96–522, 1969.

GRIFFING, T. S., "Proposed: A Safety Protocol for Taking Ear Impression," The Hearing Journal, Vol. 45/2, pp. 28–29, 1992.

GRIFFING, T. S. & SHIELD, JUDITH, "Hearing Aid Performance and the Earmold," Hearing Instruments, 1973.

GRIFFING, T. S. "Variable Venting of Earmolds," Hearing Dealer, December, 1971.

HICKOK, MS, R. L. MCSPADEN-HICKOK, MS DANA & MCSPADEN, PH.D J. B. "A Venting We Will Go!" - Part III, Audecibel, July, Aug.

JANSSEN, G. & ROWLAND, R., "Hearing Device Retainers," Hearing Instruments, Vol. 38/9, p. 28, 1987.

KILLION, M. C., "Earmold Options for Wide Band Hearing Aids," JSHD, No 46, February, 1981.

KILLION, M. C., "Earmold Plumbing for Wideband Hearing Aids & Experimental Wideband Hearing Aids," Journal Of The Acoustical Society of America, Vol. 59, 1976.

LEWIS, E. & PLOTKIN, W., "The Role of the Acoustic Coupler in Hearing Aid Fitting," paper presented at ASHA Convention, Chicago, 1962.

LIBBY, E. R., Innovation Earmold Coupling Systems—Rationale, Design and Clinical Applications, Zenetron, Inc. Chicago, 1980.

LIBBY, E. R., "The Importance of Smoothness of Hearing Aid Frequency Responses," Hearing Instruments, 4:20–22, 1979.

LYBARGER, S. F., "Earmolds" (Chapter 44), in Katz, J. (Ed.), "Handbook of Clinical Audiology" (3rd Ed.), Williams & Wilkins, Baltimore, 1985.

LYBARGER, S. F., "In Controlling Hearing Aid Performance by Earmold Design, *Acoustical Factors Affecting Hearing Aid Performance,* Grune & Stratton, New York, 1979.

LYBARGER, S. F., Specification of Measures of Hearing Aid Performance, Symposium on Amplification for Sensorineural Hearing Loss, Twin Peaks, California, July, 1971.

LYBARGER, E. F., "Earmold Acoustics," Audecibel, Winter, 1967.

LYBARGER, S. F., The Earmold as a Part of the Receiver Acoustic System, Canonsburg, Pennsylvania, Radioear Corp., 1958.

MACRAE, JOHN, "Vent for High Powered Hearing Aide," The Hearing Journal, January, 1983, Vol. 36, No. 1.

MCDONALD, F., DOUGLAS & STUDEBAKER, G. A., "Earmold Alteration Effects as Measured in the Human Auditory Meatus," Journal of The Acoustical Society of America, 48, 1970.

MCCOLLOM, H. and MYNDERS, JOEL M *Hearing Aid Dispensing Practice,* Interstate Printers, Danville, IL 1984.

MEDING, M. D., B & RINGDAHL, A., "Allergic Contact Dermatitis from the Earmolds of Hearing Aids," Ear & Hearing, Vol. 13, No. 2, 1992.

MORGAN, R., "The Art of Making a Good Impression", The Hearing Review, March, 1994.

MYNDERS, JOEL M. (Editor) *Custom Earmold Manual - Revised 5th Edition,* 1994 Published by Microsonic, Inc., Ambridge, PA 15003

MYNDERS, JOEL M., (Editor), "Professional Products Catalog" Earmold & Research Labs, Wichita, KS 1986.

MYNDERS, JOEL M., "C.F.A. Adapter System," The Hearing Journal, Vol. 36, No. 5, May, 1983.

MYNDERS, JOEL M., "The F.G.M. Earmold Field Report," The Hearing Journal, August, 1983.

MYNDERS, JOEL M., "The Continuous Flow Adapter Systems; Field Report," The Hearing Journal, 1983.

MYNDERS, JOEL M., "New Earmold Technology; Earmold Plumbing and Resonator Theory Join Forces at the Coupler," Hearing Aid Journal, Vol. 34, No. 5, March, 1981.

MYNDERS, JOEL M., "Earmold Style Selection—Some Guidelines for Office Practice," Hearing Aid Journal, April, 1980.

MYNDERS, JOEL M., "A Preliminary Field Report of a Patented Earmold Invention," Hearing Aid Journal, April, 1979.

MYNDERS, JOEL M., "Brief Historical Sketch of the Development of Earmolds," Hearing Aid Journal, March, 1977.

MYNDERS, JOEL M., "Hearing Aids: A Current Overview," The Otolaryngologic Clinics of North America, Audiology, October, 1978, W. B. Saunders Co., Phila., PA.

NAEL Standard Terms for Earmolds, The Hearing Dealer, 22:11, 1971.

NORTHERN, J. and HATTLER, K. W., "Earmold Influence of Aided Speech Indentification Tasks," Journal of Speech and Hearing Research, 13, 163–172, 1970.

POLLACK, M. C., Hearing Aid Feedback, Maico Audiological Library Series, 13:35–38, 1975.

PREVES, D. A., "Effects of Earmold Venting in Coupler Manikin & Real Ears", Hearing Aid Journal, March 1977.

RAAS, M. H. and BLOOMGREN, M., "Earmold Modification Techniques," Hearing Instruments, Vol. 41/1, pp. 20–23, 1990.

SANDLIN, PH.D. ROBERT, "Some Thoughts on Impression Taking Techniques to Reduce Hearing Aid Returns," Sound Waves, Spring, 1993, published by Widex Hearing Aid Company.

SCHLAEGEL, N & JELONEK, S., "Selecting the Right Earmold for a High Frequency Fitting." The Hearing Journal, Vol. 44/3, pp. 15–18, 1991.

SHAW, E. A. G., "The External Ear," *Handbook of Sensory Physiology,* W. D. Keidel and W. D. Neff (eds.), Springer-Venleg, Berlin, Germany, Vol. V/1, Chapter 14.

SNEYD, ALEC, *Emtec Earmould Handbook* published by Emtec Labs, Letchworth, U.K. 1985.

STAAB, W. J., "The Peritympanic Instrument Fitting Rationale and Test Results", Hearing Aid Journal, October, 1992, Vol. 45, No. 10 p. 21.

STAAB, W. J., Hearing Aid Handbook, Tab Books, Blue Ridge Summit, PA 17214, 1978.

STAAB, W. J. CROS and/or Open Canal Fittings, Telex Audiological Reports, Section XII, Topic Five, 1972.

STUDEBAKER, G. A. and ZACHMAN, T. A.. "Investigation of the Acoustics of Earmold Vents," Journal of The Acoustical Society of America, 47, 1107–1115, (1970).

SULLIVAN, E. J., "Fine Tuning," Audecibel Fall, 1976.

Sullivan, E. J., "Anatomy of the Ear—as it Pertains to An Earmold," Hearing Aid Journal, February, 1975.

Sweetow, R. W., "The Truth Behind 'Non-Occluding' Earmolds," Hearing Instruments, Vol. 42/16, p. 25, 1991.

Weatherton, M. A., and Goetzing, C. P., "The Effects of Various Modified Earmolds on Hearing Sensitivity," Journal of Auditory Research, 11"25–32, 1970.

Lesson 17
431-484

VI

SELECTING AMPLIFICATION SYSTEMS

Wayne J. Staab, Ph.D.

INTRODUCTION

Hearing aids are not fitted based on the degree of hearing loss necessarily, but on the degree of hurt—and only when that hurt is great enough, whether socially, economically, financially, or psychologically, does the individual become a candidate for hearing aids. It is only after any, or all, of these "hurts" have been recognized by the patient, that the hearing aid selection process truly begins. Realize also that the magnitude of the difficulties are not such that they may be immediately or completely resolved. As Lybarger (1981) suggested in a somewhat tongue-in-cheek, but not altogether untrue, manner:

> A hearing aid is an ultra-miniature electro-acoustical device that is always too large.
> It must amplify sound a million times, but bring in no noise.
> It must operate, without failure, in a sea of perspiration, a cloud of talcum powder, or both.
> It is a product that one puts off buying for ten years after he needs it, but cannot do without it for thirty minutes when it has to be serviced.

In a more straight-forward manner, a hearing aid is intended to amplify sound energy and present it to the ear as effectively and as naturally as possible. Therefore, a properly selected and fitted hearing aid or aids should allow, at a minimum:

1. the client to wear hearing aids at a comfortable loudness level,
2. little unnecessary overamplification of loud sounds,
3. improved communicative ability of the normal conversational speech level range,
4. better hearing aided than unaided,
5. fit and modify changes, and
6. a means to evaluate the selection.

To accomplish these goals, the hearing aid performance must be shaped to compensate for the loudness, frequency, and temporal changes resulting from impaired hearing.

CHAPTER OBJECTIVES

This chapter presents critical elements and events in the history of hearing aid amplification system selection. The reader is presented with approaches that have been intended to enhance the selection process. The irony is that technological advances are occurring at such a rapid pace that they often seem to make the selection process more difficult because of the number of parameters under the dispensers' or manufacturers' control. The chapter also identifies hearing aid measurement criteria which assist in the selection process. The dispenser should understand the rationales of the selection procedures presented and how each relates to the determination of appropriate hearing aid amplification systems and their subsequent acceptance by those who use them. Additionally, hearing aid selection involves more than just the hearing aid and its function. The patient's age, profession, activity level, residual hearing, and acceptance of the hearing impairment are as important as any other consideration in the hearing aid fitting process. The hearing aid must interface with the needs of the hearing impaired in terms of the magnitude, type, and duration of the hearing deficit, as well as with the environments in which listening takes place. Realize also that the hearing aid selection process is not a static event ("*the* appropriate amplification system"), but an ongoing process subject to constant changes and decisions. Also, until such time that there is consensus agreement on ***the*** appropriate hearing aid selection procedure, directions will continue to reflect the divergence in underlying philosophies. It might be said that until such time, the procedure that is best is that which the dispenser understands and that appropriately meets the patient's needs.

HEARING AID CANDIDACY—AUDIOLOGICAL FACTORS

Potentially, every individual with a hearing impairment may be a candidate for hearing aid use. And, although concepts that dictate hearing aid candidacy on the basis of specific levels or types of losses should be discarded, generalizations might still be applied, but should remain, generalizations. The emphasis should be on the ***handicap*** and the problems a particular hearing loss presents.

PATHOLOGY

Conductive hearing impairments often respond favorably to medical and/or surgical treatment. When these can be utilized, and the client wishes to enact them, these are the recommended choices. However, for a number of reasons, a person with a conductive loss may wish to remedy the situation with hearing aids instead. When this happens, good success can generally be expected.

Most hearing instruments fitted today are fitted to those with sensorineural, and to a lesser extent, mixed hearing impairments. Their prognosis is not as good as for conductive losses, and are less when the pathology involves the central auditory nervous system (CANS). Still, hearing aids are considered as the primary rehabilitative treatment for these losses to date.

DEGREE OF HEARING IMPAIRMENT AND HEARING AID EXPECTATIONS

The hearing loss classification identified in Figure 1, along with the ranges, is arbitrary and varies among authorities. Although the hearing loss levels are based on the pure-tone average of 500, 1000, and 2000 Hz, a person's hearing thresholds may easily overlap several categories.

Near Normal/Borderline (<25 dB). Most often this is considered to be "normal" hearing. Hearing handicap is questionable. Still, a number of individuals believe that they experience difficulty, especially if listening demands are critical to their work or learning environment. Amplification, if accepted, will seldom involve more than part-time use. These are not usually candidates for amplification.

Hearing Loss Classification

Hearing Classification*	Hearing Threshold in dB**
Normal Hearing	< 20 dB
Near Normal/Borderline	21 – 25 dB
Mild Hearing Loss	26 – 40 dB
Moderate Hearing Loss	41 – 55 dB
Moderately-Severe Loss	56 – 70 dB
Severe Hearing Loss	71 – 90 dB
Profound Hearing Loss	91 dB >

* Near Normal, Mild, Moderate, Moderately-Severe, and Severe Hearing Losses are considered to be Hard-of-Hearing. The Profound Hearing Loss category is considered as being deaf.

** These ranges are arbitrary and vary among authorities.

Fig. 1. Description and range of hearing impairment. Descriptions such as this are arbitrary and vary among authorities. (Adapted from Stabb, W. J. Hearing Aids: A User's Guide. Phoenix: Wayne J. Staab, 1991, p. 30.)

Mild Hearing Impairment (26–40 dB). This is a slight handicap for some—significant for others. Some may have difficulty hearing faint and/or distant speech but are likely to "get along" in most situations. Sustained attention, however, is frequently difficult for many with this degree of loss. Speech and language is learned normally and monitored via the traditional auditory feedback mechanism. Depending upon communication requirements, and acceptance that a hearing handicap exists, candidates may or may not need amplification with hearing aids. Most will find that hearing aids are too noisy unless some type of open canal fitting is employed or some unique noise suppression/cancellation approach is used. If hearing aids are worn, they most likely are not worn constantly.

Moderate Hearing Impairment (41–55 dB). Persons having this level impairment understand conversational speech at relatively close distances without great difficulty. Under normal conditions speech may have to be repeated often. Speech may show articulation problems (omissions, substitutions, and distortions of speech sounds). Moderate hearing impairments may benefit well from hearing aid use.

Moderately-Severe Hearing Impairment (56–70 dB). These persons would understand conversational speech only if it were loud and/or close in proximity. Considerable difficulty would be expected in group or noisy situations. They appear "not to pay attention." Enough hearing is present to learn or maintain present language and speech through the auditory feedback mechanism when amplification with hearing aids takes place. Excellent benefit from hearing instruments can be expected.

Severe Hearing Impairment (71–90 dB). These persons may hear sound or loud voice close to the ear. They identify environmental noises, and may distinguish vowels but not consonants. They seem to be "ignoring" communication. Hearing aids enable this degree of hearing impairment to become relatively functional for ordinary purposes of life. Language and speech will not develop spontaneously in a youngster and may deteriorate significantly if the loss occurs over time, as with an adult.

Profound Hearing Impairment (91 dB>). These individuals do not rely on hearing as their primary avenue of communication. Speech and language must both be developed through careful and extensive training since these cannot be learned by ear alone, even with amplification. Hearing levels in this category are often identified in the "deaf" range. Hearing aids are intended to allow the user to maintain contact with the environment and to allow the utilization of any auditory clues that might be presented. Many of the individuals in this category do not utilize amplification, but rely on manual communication.

SLOPE OF HEARING LOSS

The contour of hearing threshold levels (slope), as seen on the audiogram, allows for the following generalizations, without much change in expectations since these generalizations were written (Berger and Millin, 1968):

- Most favorable: Flat, gradually rising, or gradually falling
- Less favorable: Steep falling, deep saucer-shaped, or irregular dips and peaks
- Least favorable: Sharp drop at any lower frequency, islands of hearing only, reverse slopes, or remnants of hearing at lower frequencies only

SPEECH PERFORMANCE

Word Recognition (Speech Discrimination)

Unaided word recognition scores (formerly referred to as speech discrimination scores) provide one indicator of successful prognosis with amplification. True today, as during earlier years, the following expectations of successful hearing aid use are indicated when using the CID 2-22 word lists (Berger and Millin (1971):

- 90% and higher: Suggests probable good results with amplification
- 70–90%: Suggests mild difficulty, even though results are not that bad
- 50–70%: Suggests substantial difficulty—poor results
- 50% and lower: Suggests the probability that amplification will not be entirely successful

However, this is all relative. If the user has a 40% aided score, it may be a very significant improvement over a 10% unaided word recognition score. In other words, the hearing aid fitting may be successful if the person cannot function without hearing aids, but can with the units. Exceptions to the generalized rules suggested are common.

DYNAMIC RANGE (DR)

The dynamic range is identified as the dB range between the threshold of sensitivity and the uncomfortable loudness level (UCL). It represents the range of usable hearing. One of the goals of the hearing aid selection process is to provide amplification that provides sufficient gain to be heard, but which does not have output levels that exceed the uncomfortable listening level. As such, the dynamic range identifies the upper and lower limits of amplification.

The dynamic range is significantly reduced for individuals with sensorineural hearing impairments because the thresholds are shifted toward the upper limits of hearing comfort. Additionally, the upper limit of the dynamic range may be significantly lowered as the result of recruitment. In general, greater success with amplification can be expected for those individuals having greater dynamic ranges.

HEARING AID CANDIDACY—PSYCHOLOGICAL/MOTIVATIONAL FACTORS

As opposed to audiological factors of hearing aid candidacy, which can be measured readily and fairly accurately, psychological/motivational measurements of hearing handicap are more difficult to assess. As was stated in the introduction to this chapter,

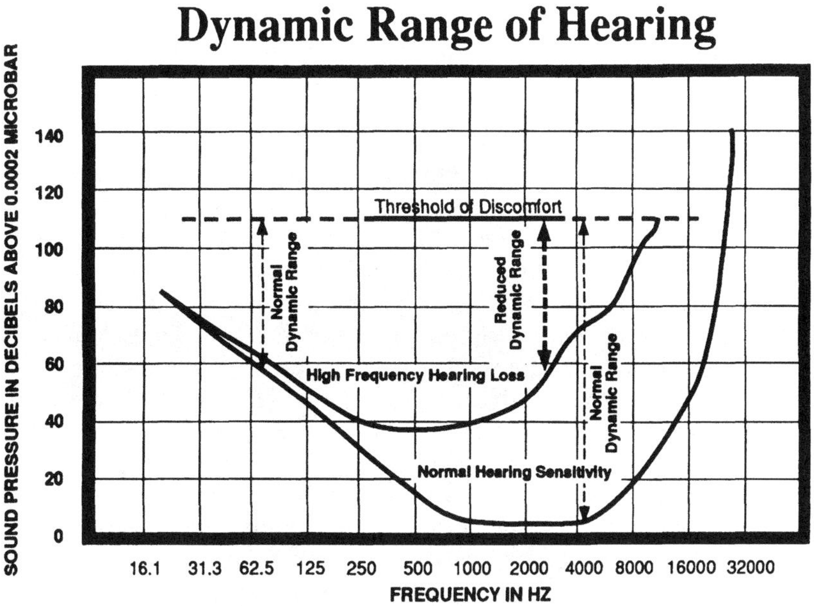

Fig. 2. The dynamic range (DR) of hearing is identified as the dB difference between the individual's thresholds of sensitivity and discomfort. In this example, the DR at 4000 Hz is approximately 105 dB for the "normal" hearing curve, but only about 40 dB for the "high-frequency hearing loss" patient. The DR varies with frequency.

hearing aids are not fitted necessarily based on the degree of hearing loss, but on the degree of "hurt." It is the responsibility of the dispenser to be aware of the perceived need for amplification ("hurt") by the client. The issues that follow are intended to provide insight. A more complete understanding can be found in a manual devoted to the hearing impaired client by Staab (1991).

LOSS RELATED TO ONSET

A person who loses hearing suddenly might have little difficulty in using hearing aids from the start—providing use begins fairly early after the incident. On the other hand, if the hearing impairment is congenital or becomes gradually worse over a period of years, the adjustment period is generally longer.

GENERAL ATTITUDE OF THE USER

Most generally, the potential hearing aid client is unhappy because the loss was not correctable by medical and/or surgical treatment. While the aids may adequately satisfy the needs, complete acceptance depends upon the motivation of the client and also on an understanding of what constitutes successful hearing aid use.

MOTIVATION

The motivation to wear hearing aids depends largely on the need and acceptance for hearing assistance. The greater the need, the greater the motivation, and the greater are the chances for successful use. (Motivational factors are more easily identified with adults than with children. The prognosis with children often is more dependent on audiological factors). Some individuals feel considerable bitterness, frustration, and resentment toward their handicap. As a result, they may tend to be more "on guard" than usual about themselves and their interpersonal relationships.

Some hearing impaired persons attempt to deny or "cover" their disability and are perceived by others as being immature, indifferent, hostile, or stubborn. Friends, family, and coworkers often see the hearing impaired person as inattentive, disinterested, or preoccupied.

In addition to expected difficulties in verbal communication associated with hearing impairment, the following self-feelings are often reported: loneliness, isolation, fear, inadequacy, inferiority, negative self-worth, rejection, helplessness, hopelessness, hypersensitivity, submissiveness, and apathy.

The attitude of the client is also partly influenced by the age at which the handicap occurs. The following generalization can be stated: the earlier in life the hearing handicap, the greater the social handicap and the less the psychological implications. The later in life, the greater the psychological implications and the less the social difficulties. This relationship is diagrammed in Figure 3. Specific approaches used to determine the degree of handicap, its acceptance, and prognosis are provided later in this chapter under self-report procedures or hearing handicap inventories.

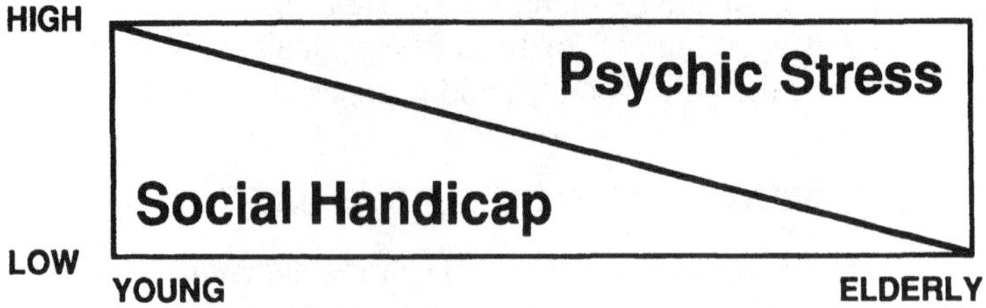

Fig. 3. Diagrammed relationship between age, handicap, and stress.

SUCCESSFUL HEARING AID USE

When considering whether hearing aid use will be successful or not, a number of considerations should be kept in mind.

- How much of the time are the hearing aids used?
- Have the needs of the user been fulfilled?
- How satisfied is the user with the hearing aids?

Assessing the value of hearing aids by determining the amount of time they are worn or by how satisfied the client is with them is not necessarily an indication of how well the client's needs have been fulfilled—either partially or completely. Take, for example, the person who lives alone and only wears aids when visitors are present. These aids might not be used often, but the satisfaction and the fulfillment of a need may have been met.

Likewise, a client may wear hearing aids many hours per day but may still not be satisfied with them—but they fill a need. Or, the need for amplification may have been met but the client is neither satisfied nor are the aids worn as often as they should be.

The medium of success obviously must be achieved by meeting a combination of the considerations just identified. For some clients the hearing aids become inseparable companions, a means of remaining in or re-entering the hearing world. To others, they are burdensome and are rejected or discarded after a short trial period. It is suspected that the majority of users lie somewhere between.

Good information of a longitudinal nature or on large samples is not available to determine accurately the degree of success the hearing impaired have with amplification. Survey questions, and therefore the responses, tend to be influenced by the intent of the developer. Still, data from various studies present information that can be used to make assumptions about successful use.

WHAT IS THE EXTENT OF HEARING AID USE?

This can refer to the actual number of hours the aids are worn throughout the day, where they are worn, or might be more accurately defined as the percent of time the aids are worn during the person's demands on listening skills.

Successful Use Based on Actual Hours Used

The number of hours a person wears the aids can be recorded. Care must be exercised when using these data because the degree of hearing impairment and the listening demands come into play. Therefore, these data are somewhat questionable in determining

Table 1. Hours per day hearing aids are used.

Study	<5 hrs daily (or never)	5-8 hrs daily (occasionally)	>5 hrs daily (all the time)
Carstairs (1973)	35%	40%	25% (8+ hrs)
Stroup (1977)			62% (6+ hrs)
Plomp (1978)	5-10%	5-30%	60-90% (studies' summary)
Slusser (1981)		31%	69%
Maxwell (1981)			62% (8+ hrs)

successful hearing instrument use. Summarized data in Table 1 from various studies show that hearing aids are worn for a large part of the day by those who need them.

Successful Use Based on Use For Various Activities

Figure 4 shows the extent of client satisfaction for various activities. Those who did not take part in an activity are excluded from the table (Carstairs, 1973). Those not involved in the activity in question, or who could manage without their aids, were not included in the figures indicating satisfaction.

If generalizations could be made about the results indicated in Figure 4, it might be said that almost all users are satisfied when speaking to only one person, and very few when talking to two or more. Greater satisfaction might be expected when alone in the house or while shopping, and fairly high for public meetings. Satisfaction might be expected to be low for work and travel.

Successful Use as a Percentage of Time Used During Listening Demands

The data that follows in Figure 5 shows the percentage of time hearing aids were used during a person's demands on listening skills (from interpretations of studies by Kodicek and Garrad (1955), Brooks (1972), and Carstairs (1973):

If successful use of hearing aids is measured by the number of persons who wear the aids all the time, only a small portion will have been helped. As was pointed out, however, this may not be the appropriate way to evaluate successful use. The demands on listening, and the desirability to utilize the potential benefits of amplification during those times, must be taken into consideration.

Successful Use on Having Fulfilled the Needs of the Client (Benefit)

From the previous information it might be estimated that a fairly high percentage of the users' hearing needs are fulfilled. Even though, this still leaves a sizable number unfilled. Of the unfulfilled

Use and Satisfaction of Hearing Aids For Specified Activities

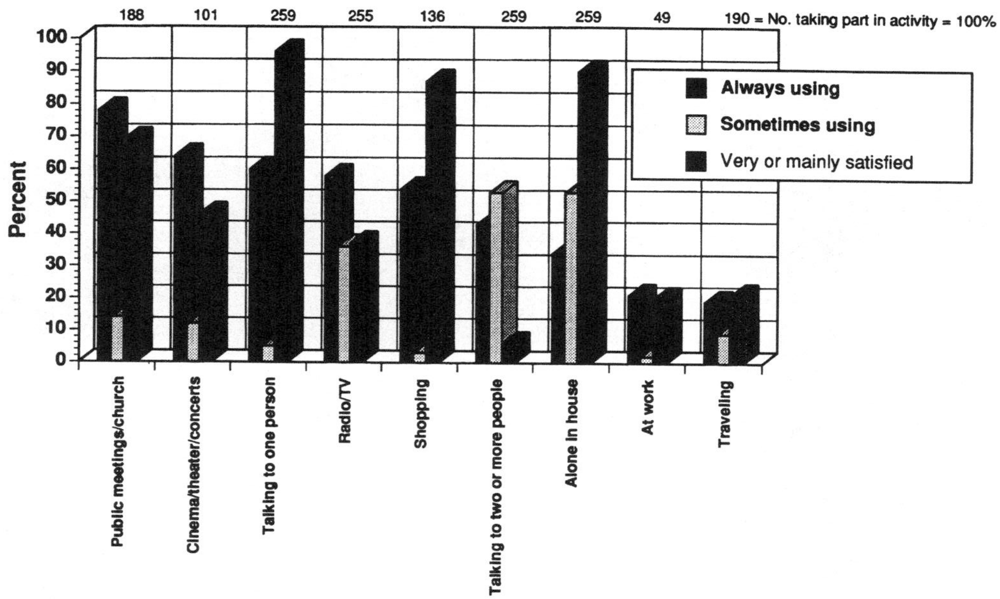

Always using	78	64	60	58	54	43	34	21	19
Sometimes using	14	12	5	36	3	53	53	2	9
Very or mainly satisfied	69	46	96	37	87	6	90	20	21

Fig. 4. Patient use and satisfaction of hearing aids for specified activities. (Graphed from data by Carstairs, V. Utilization of hearing aids issued by the National Health Service. Audiology. 1973;7:72–76.)

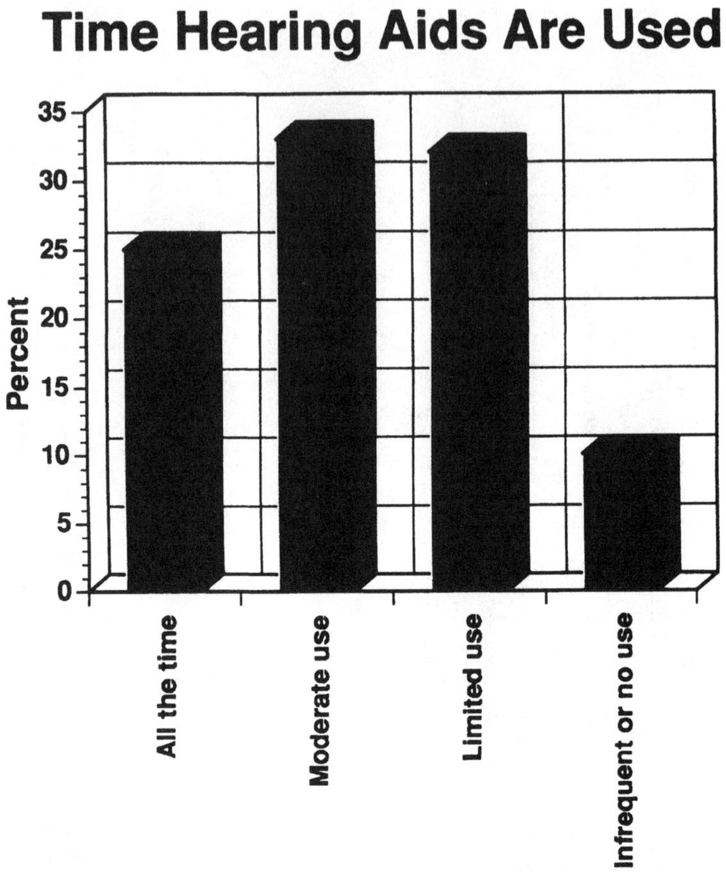

Fig. 5. Successful hearing aid use as a percentage of time the aids are being worn.

needs, it might be speculated that about one half of the wearers are most likely not satisfied because they are not using their hearing aids advantageously or in the proper environments. Reasons given in support for these nonsatisfactions include:

- Minor technical problems relating to inability to manipulate the controls properly, improper earmold fit, understanding batteries, etc.
- Occupational setting conflicts that often have individuals wearing hearing aids in noisy environments or while performing manual labor.
- Some have been told by close associates that wearing hearing aids would make their hearing poorer (reassurance based on solid factual information is needed).

- Lack of understanding from close associates.
- Inadequate instructions in the use of hearing aids.
- Hearing aids were of no help (especially in understanding speech).
- Hearing aids amplified background sounds as much or more than speech.
- Hearing aids made some sounds too loud.
- Hearing aids were uncomfortable to wear.
- Hearing had recovered sufficiently so hearing aids were no longer necessary.
- The embarrassment of wearing aids (too bulky, unattractive, or conspicuous).
- Generalized dissatisfaction with the hearing aid experiences.
- Someone told them that they did not need to wear hearing aids.

Many of the problems may be apparent only on visiting with the patients and observing their domestic circumstances. Much of the dissatisfaction and inadequate understanding of hearing aid experiences may be a mixture of valid and invalid complaints. In many cases, the source of the complaint may come not from the aids but from feelings of inadequacy, strong personal commitments, or exaggerated pride. Moreover, if measures of benefit are to accurately reflect that derived from a hearing aid in the real world, measures should sample various communication situations in which hearing aid users would like to use their hearing aids. Benefit estimates based on functional gain improvements or probe microphone measurements of a "target," aided SRT and word recognition scores, or audibility (articulation) indexes continue to be open to question.

Successful Use Based on Client Satisfaction

Satisfactory use of hearing aids can be considered as making the lives of the hearing impaired easier or more enjoyable. Based on this premise, studies by Hughson and Thompson (1944); Kodicek and Garrad (1955); Northern, Ciliax, Roth, and Johnson, 1969; Brooks (1972); Cunningham, Merle, and Drake (1978); Slusser, 1981; Hughes, Arthur, and Weinstein (1982); and Oja and Schow (1984) indicate that "success" may be as high as 80 to 90%. The extent of satisfaction with hearing aids for specified activities is shown in Figure 4 along with hearing aid use (Carstairs, 1973). Because ratings of satisfaction are rather subjective, and therefore difficult to quantify, there is great disparity in definitions of satisfaction, and in the ways it has been measured.

HEARING AID SUCCESS: SUMMARY

In all the preceding, the data and interpretation must be viewed somewhat cautiously. Any subjective assessment of performance depends to some extent on the patient's expectations about what the hearing aids will do. If complete restoration of normal hearing function is expected, there will be no great satisfaction. If goals are set lower, greater satisfaction will result, even though they might fall short of the goal of complete rehabilitation.

In conclusion, it might be said that persons benefit from hearing aids when they can communicate better with the aids than without them. This will depend on how well the aids reproduce sound, the kinds of everyday listening the client is in, the peculiarities of the client's hearing impairment, and user expectations.

FACTORS INFLUENCING RECOMMENDATION AND CHOICE OF HEARING AIDS

Frequently, hearing aids are selected on the basis of cost, weight, size, cosmetics, and convenience. While these issues must be taken into consideration, they should assume importance commensurate with other considerations. As stated earlier, the eventual goal in recommending hearing aids is for the client to function better with amplification than without amplification. However, this recommendation is good only if the client will accept the aids. If the client will wear amplification and be satisfied with it only if certain cosmetic or other personal wishes are fulfilled, then these can take on as important a role as any performance consideration.

AGE

The recommendation and choice of hearing aids for children suggests special considerations. The difficulty is in determining if the child needs aids, which aids, and if the aids are functioning adequately once they have been fitted. Close cooperation between the various specialties involved is needed to determine the benefits and approach to amplification for children. Early, effective amplification is a prerequisite if the intent is to avoid a delay in speech and language development, or to achieve relatively normal language capability.

The elderly, at the other extreme, frequently show a general slowing of auditory interpretation capacity along with a loss in hearing sensitivity and the communication difficulties associated with it. Such an individual will find the aids difficult to use in noisy or chaotic environments. These limitations must be recognized and accepted if satisfaction is to be achieved. It is very difficult to predict the ability of the presbycusic to benefit from amplification.

WHO SUGGESTED AMPLIFICATION?

If the impetus for the evaluation and recommendation originated outside the user, prognosis is poor until he or she is convinced that amplification is needed and that it improves his or her performance under everyday conditions. Recommendations for amplification by a physician are more likely to be accepted than from other hearing health care providers.

COSMETIC CONSIDERATIONS

Cosmetic aspects of hearing aids must be considered frequently—especially for those persons who are aware of and respond to reactions of others to the sight of their hearing aids. Alpiner (1967) has reported that even persons confined for life to an institution (in their 80's and 90's) of both sexes insisted upon "inconspicuous" aids. Such culturally-determined attitudes are not easy to change and must be considered in the recommendation.

The primary question should be whether the client will wear the type of hearing aids recommended, especially when in the company of others. If they won't be worn, they do no good. It may be better to obtain less than what is felt to be optimum performance for the sake of at least some performance.

DEXTERITY

Dexterity, whether it be due to very young age, physical handicap, or because of advancing age, must be considered in hearing aid recommendations. Arthritic fingers may have (not necessarily will have) considerable difficulty with a barely protruding, narrow, or small volume control. Likewise, the telephone switch (if present) must be located and manipulated easily by the user. When difficulties are anticipated, the choice might be directed toward recommending hearing aids with larger and more accessible controls, or even remote controls. Dexterity is also an issue during insertion of the earmold or hearing aid into the ear, replacing the cell, and adjusting any of the other controls the hearing instrument might be equipped with, including remote controls.

PART-TIME OR FULL-TIME USE?

This depends on the degree of loss and the potential client's requirements for better hearing. If the loss is mild, part-time use may be considered. Assistance may be needed only in certain situations—perhaps a boost in church, conferences, with TV, etc. The demands on hearing will vary from time to time and with activity.

If part-time use is recommended, logic should dictate when the hearing aids will be worn. If the potential user's demands require efficient communication, full-time use should be considered.

During these first contacts with the potential user, be extremely careful not to promise too much. Some dispensers feel that a certain degree of pessimism rather than optimism about expected performance with the hearing aids leads to more satisfied users. The client may then feel that the hearing aids are performing better than were expected, rather than having a feeling of disappointment in their performance because of what was promised, but not delivered. Regardless, the real issue is to ensure that ***realistic*** expectations are conveyed to the patient.

PRESELECTION OF AMPLIFICATION

HEARING AID STYLE—BY MANNER OF PLACEMENT

The degree and characteristics of the hearing impairment, the environment(s) in which the aids will be used, user dexterity and mobility, life styles, expectations about what hearing aids can do, the referral source, previous hearing aid use, costs, user expectations and cosmetics, and numerous other issues determine this preselection issue. Still, in general, most users want the smallest, most cosmetic instrument that will perform the task. Figure 6 illustrates the trends in hearing aid style in the U.S. over the past several years. This trend is typically followed in other countries as well. Generally, instruments fitted at the ear level, and especially those that penetrate into the ear canal, are the most secure. A decision must be made also about the option for remote control of hearing aid function. Additional decisions relative to electroacoustic features should be reserved for the actual hearing aid evaluation, and not identified here in the preselection process.

Ear Level Hearing Instruments

A number of styles comprise this category. What they have in common is that they all have complete electronics at the level of the ear, either over the ear, or to varying degrees within the external ear itself.

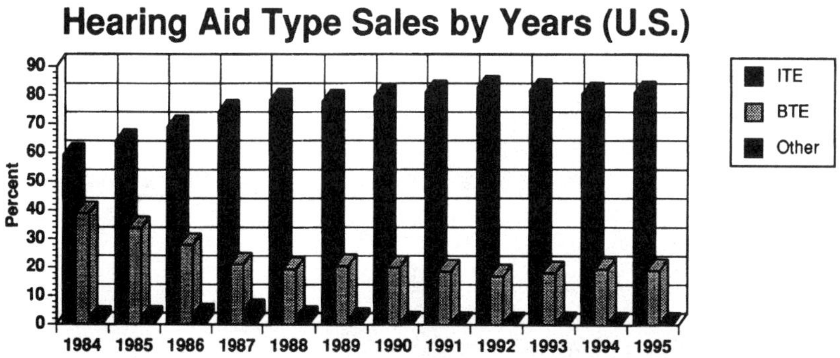

Fig. 6. Percent of hearing aids sold by type (ITE, BTE, and Other) in the U.S. from 1984 through 1995. Data collected from the Hearing Industries Association (HIA) Statistical Data Reports over that time period.

In-The-Ear (ITE) Hearing Aids. These seem to be used most successfully between pure-tone averages of 35 dB to about 70 dB. Listeners with hearing levels better than 35 dB generally have fairly good low-frequency hearing and have difficulty in noticing significant benefit. This benefit is minimized further if large vents are used to attenuate low frequencies, due to increased feedback. Beyond about 70 dB success is reduced, primarily due to feedback (Wernick, 1985). The choice of ITE variations (full concha, low profile, half concha, etc.) is determined largely by the component demands of the instrument.

In-The-Canal (ITC) Hearing Aids. Although more limited in gain and output than ITE aids, the microphone pickup location and slightly deeper insertion provide for additional overall SPL and therefore, require less amplifier gain (about 5 dB) than for outside the ear microphone pickup locations.

Completely-In-The-Canal (CIC) and Peritympanic Hearing Aids. These instruments fit entirely within the ear canal. They continue the advantages of the ITC by providing additional overall SPL, especially in the high frequencies. The greatest advantages occur when the microphone pickup location is inside the aperture of the ear canal, when the residual volume between the end of the instrument and the tympanic membrane is smallest, and when full contact is made by the end of the instrument with the bony canal (Staab, 1989; 1992). They appear to function best for high-frequency hearing losses, even those of a precipitous nature (Staab et. al., 1992). These instruments require about 10 dB less gain than ITC hearing aids, for the same level of hearing impairment.

Behind-The-Ear (BTE) Hearing Aids. Also commonly referred to as over-the-ear or postauricular hearing aids, these are designed to fit behind or over the pinna, and with an earhook and earmold, secure their position. They fit the widest range of hearing losses (from mild to profound), are available in a variety of sizes, and provide the greatest number of electroacoustic options available among hearing aids.

Eyeglass Hearing Aids. The fitting range of these instruments is essentially the same as for BTE instruments, but because of the difficulty of matching optics with the hearing aid, their use has fallen to an insignificant share of the market.

Body-Worn Hearing Instruments

Their primary use is with individuals whose hearing levels are so severe that gain and output cannot be controlled unless there is separation of the microphone and receiver of the aid. These instruments provide a hard wire separation of the hearing aid receiver which is worn at the ear level from the remainder of the instrument, which is worn usually on the torso. The body-worn aid is also used with individuals who have difficulty manipulating the controls on smaller hearing aids.

Inplantable Hearing Instruments

These instruments have not yet achieved extensive usage, and for the most part, have been limited to the post-lingually deafened adult, and more recently, to children.

Special Feature Hearing Instruments

At times the nature of the hearing impairment requires something other than traditional hearing aids.

CROS (Contralateral Routing of Off Signals) Hearing Instruments. The CROS hearing aid and its variations should be considered for individuals who have no aidable hearing on one ear and normal or aidable hearing on the apposite ear. Additional decisions must be made as to if the signal from the poor ear side should be routed to the better ear by RF (radio frequency) wireless transmission or if a hard wired system will suffice. Figure 7 illustrates some of the more common CROS variations.

Bone-Conduction Hearing Instruments. These are most often reserved for situations in which chronic discharge from the ears renders fitting earmold-type hearing instruments impossible.

Auditory Trainers. These special hearing instruments provide for maximizing the signal-to-noise ratio from the speaker (often a teacher) to the listener. Although they can be used in a variety of environments, they are most often found in schools.

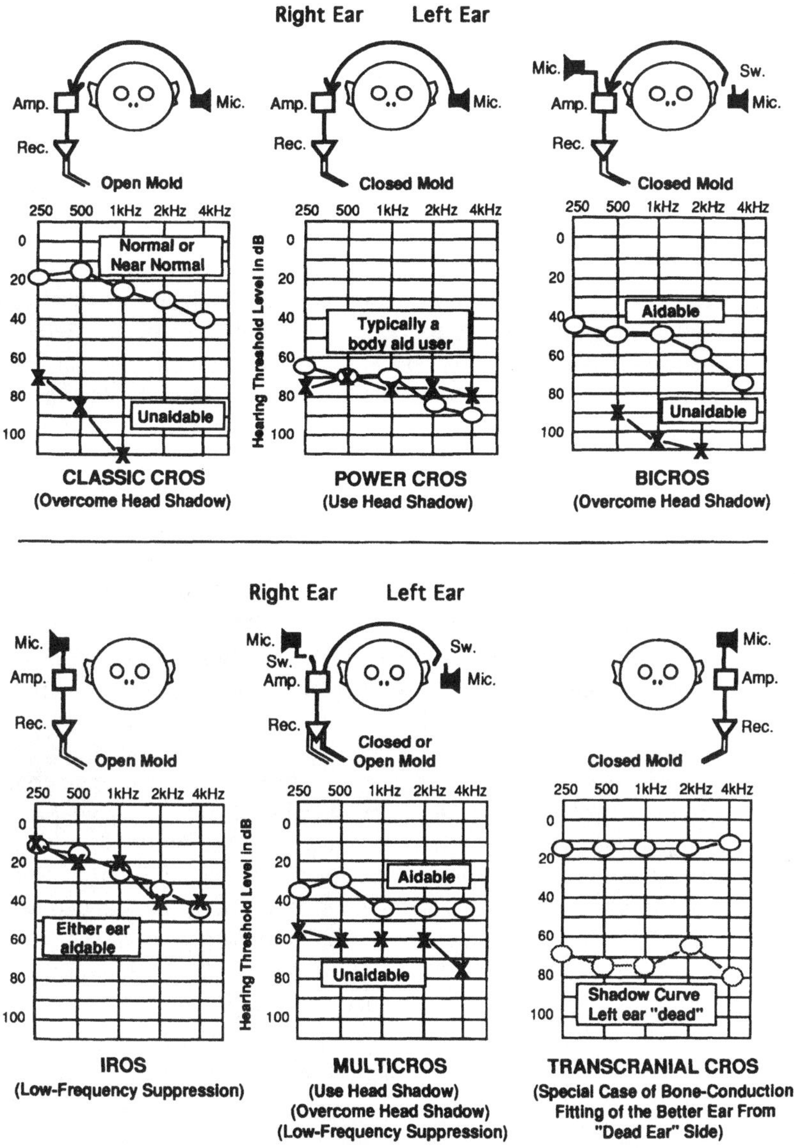

Fig. 7. Major types of CROSS type hearing aids. Sound transmission can occur by either wires connecting the two sides or by radio frequency (RF) transmission with no wires. (With Permission Staab, W. J., and Lybarger, S. F., in Katz, J. (Editor). Handbook of Clinical Audiology, Fourth Edition. Baltimore: Williams & Wilkins, 1994, p. 662.)

BINAURAL vs. MONAURAL AMPLIFICATION

General agreement exists that, unless significant contraindications exist, binaural amplification is the arrangement of choice. Instead of generally defining the criterion for binaural candidacy, clients should be given the opportunity to experience a complete system before decisions are made about which half of the fitting is not necessary.

The real advantage of amplified binaural hearing is not that the two ears are made the same, but that dichotic hearing occurs. Dichotic hearing refers to a condition in which two complete, but independent hearing aid systems, are presented to each ear—compatible with the use of both ears for normal hearing. The sound presented to one ear, however, differs from the sound presented to the other ear in frequency, phase, time of arrival, duration, bandwidth, sound pressure, or other acoustical or temporal characteristic.

Collectively, the effects of dichotic hearing provide for improved sound localization (Stevens and Newman, 1936); the elimination, reduction, or better utilization of the sound shadow caused by the head (Olsen and Carhart, 1967); binaural summation to increase the apparent loudness of sound; binaural loudness squelch effect, or the improvement in signal-to-noise ratio when two ears are involved rather than one (Carhart, 1965); and masking level differences—the ability to separate primary sounds from background or unwanted sounds (Hirsh, 1948).

An additional issue surrounding the use of binaural amplification involves "late-onset auditory deprivation" (Silman, Gelfand, and Silverman, 1984). This can be identified as reduced word recognition scores in the unaided ear following a period of asymmetrical stimulation, and was found in 40% of the monaural hearing aid wearers in their retrospective study. It is because of this, and the well-documented advantages of binaural amplification, that when monaural amplification is elected when binaural was recommended, a "binaural waiver" is often requested. This document, signed by the client, is the client's confirmation that a monaural selection was made contrary to the advice given.

Although little solace can be found in generalized criterion for binaural candidacy, some basic tenants are assumed. For example, for binaural amplification to work, it is projected that there is a correctable impairment in both ears. It has been suggested that binaural amplification may be best if thresholds are within 15 dB of each other and if word recognition scores are within 8 to 12% of each other (Briskey, 1980). The thought is that too great a discrepancy between the ears may result in the poorer ear reducing the performance of the better ear. Still, it would be wrong to eliminate binaural amplification as a consideration, even if greater discrepancies occur. On the other hand, even when the previous criterion are met, certain life styles (i.e., physically challenged, home bound, etc.) may make the use of two instruments more difficult to manage than one.

When one ear only is to be amplified, the decision is often difficult, and may have little to do with hard and fast rules. Instead, decisions may be made on selecting the ear with the widest dynamic range, the best word recognition score, or ear preference (Dempsey, 1994).

It has been estimated that the number of individuals who can benefit from binaural amplification is 70% to 85% (Briskey, 1980; Erdman and Sedge, 1980). Some hearing impaired individuals also require a period of adjustment before the benefits of binaural amplification can be demonstrated (Nábelek and Pickett, 1974). Hearing aid sales practice reports indicate that in 1983, 27.4% of hearing aid sales in the U.S. were binaural (Cranmer, 1983), and in 1992, the percentage was 55.4% (Cranmer-Briskey, 1994).

GENERAL DESCRIPTIONS OF HEARING AID SELECTION PROCEDURES

To satisfactorily recommend hearing aids for a particular loss based upon hearing performance is no simple task. As evidence of this, myriad and divergent procedures have been employed since the late 1930's to select, verify, and monitor wearable amplification systems, with no single technique emerging as an accepted standard. Instead, what has emerged for the most part over the years are revisions or minor improvements of previous approaches, presented under the auspices of "new" approaches. It seems evident that a lack of knowledge about the impaired auditory system, specific requirements for appropriate amplification, and means to involve meaningful psychoacoustical measures have contibuted to the plethora of hearing aid selection procedure. In spite of these barriers, it does seem clear, however, that certain basics describe the ***general*** approaches used. These serve as the foundation for the classifications that follow and are identified to assist the hearing aid specialist in evaluating the various hearing aid selection procedures. In turn, the hearing aid specialist must justify the selection rationale based on one or more (or combinations) of these approaches. As long as appropriate justification for the rationale can be given, this author believes that no procedure is "right" or "wrong." In general, no attempt will be made to support or degrade a given hearing aid selection approach.

Two philosophies of hearing aid selection involve (1) non-selective amplification approaches, and (2) selective amplification approaches.

NON-SELECTIVE APPROACHES TO HEARING AID AMPLIFICATION

These are also referred to as non-comparison techniques and ascribe to the following philosophy: no differences in amplification requirements exist among the hearing impaired, and therefore, there is no need to make a comparative evaluation. As such, these approaches are not hearing aid selection techniques because no rational approach is used to identify or select specific electro-acoustics, and there is no actual comparison of aided performance or comparisons to projected performance.

EMPHASIS ON COUNSELING

The goal of this approach is to counsel the client relative to his/her hearing problem and the ***expectations*** of hearing aid use. It is believed that counseling is the most important contributor to successful hearing aid use and not the specific hearing aids selected (Resnick and Becker, 1963). Although many dispensers would have difficulty endorsing this approach, experience and documentation weighs in favor of hearing aid users being able to adapt to almost any type amplification.

"FLAT" AMPLIFICATION

This approach suggests that amplification should be provided equally to all frequencies in the speech range, regardless of the audiometric configuration. It assumes that a flat hearing aid frequency response is preferred by the hearing impaired. This assumption is yet to be supported. To the contrary, most hearing aid selection approaches follow a concept of "selective amplification".

SLOPE EXPRESSED IN dB PER OCTAVE

These approaches suggest that a certain slope per octave is best for a given group of individuals. Most notable of these procedures are those of Davis, et. al., (1947) and of the Medical Research Council of the United Kingdom (1947).

The Davis, et. al., (more commonly known as the Harvard Report) study and subsequent comments was interpreted by many as suggesting that a flat, or 6–8 dB/octave rise in the frequency response of a hearing aid, would perform equally as well as or better than selective amplification, regardless of the audiometric configuration. In reality, the Report does not exactly recommend such a procedure, but instead states that a *range* of slope between 0 and + 6 dB/octave, along with various other recommended parameters, is desirable. It should be noted that a rather substantial difference exists between aids having 0 and 6 dB/octave slope. For a 250 to 4000 Hz bandwidth, a 6 dB/octave slope hearing aid would have 24 dB more gain than would the aid having 0 dB slope. Therefore, in spite of the suggestion against selective amplification, the Harvard report contains substantial support *for* selective amplification! (The Harvard Report did conclude that low-pass slopes of −6 dB and −12 dB had unacceptable properties). Figure 8 shows the 6 dB/octave master hearing aid response of the Harvard study along with two other high-pass responses that were used in the study.

The United Kingdom Medical Research Council (1947) study resembled the Harvard study but was less complete. Their "optimum frequency responses" are shown in Figure 9. The basic curve, based on Articulation Index calculations, has an upward slope

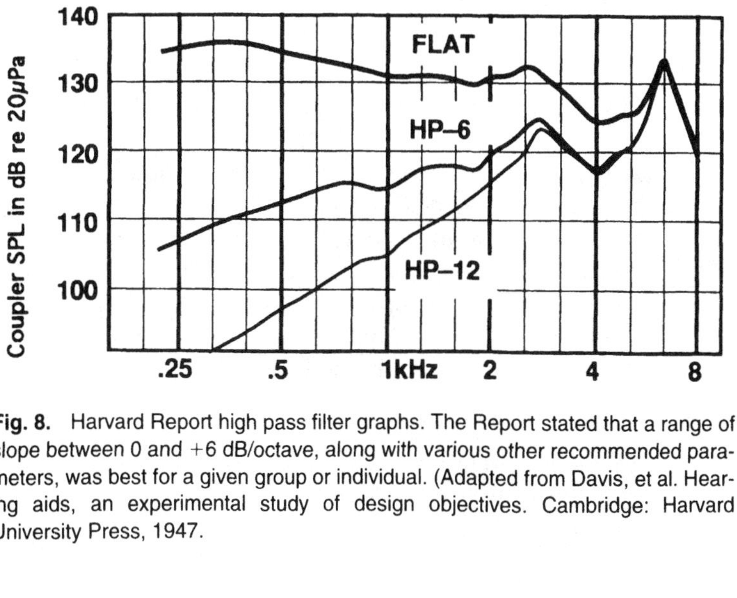

Fig. 8. Harvard Report high pass filter graphs. The Report stated that a range of slope between 0 and +6 dB/octave, along with various other recommended parameters, was best for a given group or individual. (Adapted from Davis, et al. Hearing aids, an experimental study of design objectives. Cambridge: Harvard University Press, 1947.

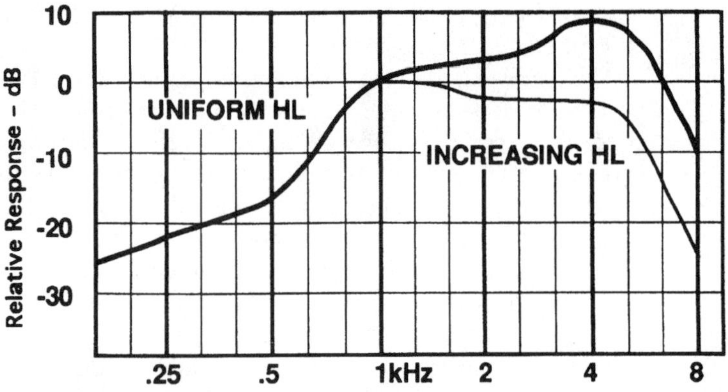

Fig. 9. Recommended "optimum frequency responses" of the United Kingdom Medical Research Council. (Adapted from Medical Research Council Special Report No. 261, Hearing aids and audiometers, London: His Majesty's Stationery Office, 1947.

averaging about +7 dB/octave. With a hearing loss greater in the high frequencies, a reduction in gain was proposed (lighter line).

Basic concerns about non-selective amplification hearing aid procedures include: (1) no attempt to measure aided performance, (2) no defined (repeatable) clinical procedure, (3) no verification of the aided response, (4) too simplistic and casual an approach, (5) the client may purchase an aid based on coast and not on performance, (6) the professional abdicates his/her clinical fitting responsibility, (7) blame is on the manufacturer for user failure, and (8) the dispenser does not contribute to performance selection.

SELECTIVE AMPLIFICATION HEARING AID APPROACHES

Selective amplification includes those hearing aid fitting approaches that are designed to determine the optimum hearing aid performance for the client. These procedures assume that (a) differences in hearing aids exist, (b) differences in amplification requirements for patients exist, and (c) that these differences are sufficient to be measured. These assumptions may be based on any, or a combination of, the listener's:

- Pure-tone or speech thresholds
- Word recognition scores or ability to understand or differentiate some aspect of speech
- Comfort levels

- Some aspect of the dynamic range of hearing, or
- Loudness judgments
- Or other features/measurements

In other words, selective amplification refers to the assumption that some unique combination of hearing aid performance characteristics exists that provides for optimal listening for a given individual. Some of these approaches provide for an actual aided ***comparison*** of hearing aids, while others attempt to ***predict*** aided hearing aid performance. Some procedures use a combination of the two; prediction and comparison. Comparative approaches focus on the *auditory experience* (comparison methods after-the-fact, retro-comparative techniques, and trial and error methods), whereas predictive approaches focus on *auditory potential.* Regardless of how selective amplification is accomplished, a variety of procedures have been used.

PRESCRIPTIVE (PREDICTIVE: FORMULAE) HEARING AID SELECTION APPROACHES

Predictive procedures based on pure tones have flourished because of the inconsistency found in word recognition-based hearing aid selection procedures. Prescriptive hearing aid selection approaches assume that if average conversational speech is amplified to the listeners' comfortable loudness level, the fitting will result in user satisfaction by providing acceptable sound quality, clarity of speech, and comfort (McCandless, 1994). As opposed to word recognition-based hearing aid selection procedures (which can demonstrate whether the aids selected are or are not adequate, but only "after the fact"), predictive selection procedures allow specific electroacoustic characteristics to be calculated to suggest optimum aided word recognition. Within the framework of pre- scriptive procedures, two general philosophies have emerged with which to calculate the prescribed gain. One approach is to prescribe sufficient gain to amplify speech to a comfortable listening level based on ***threshold data.*** The other approach is to prescribe sufficient gain based on ***suprathreshold data*** to place the average speech spectrum within the user's MCL or preferred listening range. Prescriptive approaches assume that hearing aid electroacoustics can be determined through the clinical assessment of the auditory system. The major purpose is to ensure detection of speech signals to maximally enhance word recognition.

Prescriptive Procedures Based on Audiometric Pure-Tone Threshold Measures

Use of Audiometric Pure-Tone Threshold Data. The use of pure-tone audiometric threshold data for hearing aid selection continues to be used more frequently than any other type measurement. Because pure-tone data forms the bases for many hearing aid selection approaches, its historical contribution will initiate the discussion of hearing aid selection approaches that subscribe to selective amplification.

With hearing aid selection procedures based on pure-tone thresholds, MCL is ***predicted,*** not actually measured. Calculations to a preferred listening level (MCL) based on thresholds, infers that the gain required can be specified accurately to perform this task. Arguments for using threshold data to predict MCL include the reasons why MCL-based approaches are *not* as desirable: (1) reported poor reliability of MCL measurements, (2) the difficulty of obtaining MCL measurements with children, the elderly, or with those having language and/or verbal problems, and (3) that MCL measurements are time consuming.

Considered *advantages* of hearing aid selection procedures based on pure-tone thresholds include: (1) they are efficient, (2) the gain required can be easily calculated, and (3) thresholds can be obtained on the widest variety of clients (readily available). A basic concern is that these procedures are based on formulae in which the gain prescribed increases as a constant with increased hearing loss—that calculations from threshold do not consider individual differences in the amount of gain required. There is an assumption that the gain prescribed will deliver speech at a comfortable loudness level. The question is, are the calculated gain predictions appropriate to restore the average speech spectrum to MCL for the pathological ear?

Inverted Audiogram (Direct Mirror Fitting)

This approach is also known as "audiogram fitting" or "mirror fitting of the audiogram" (Watson and Knudsen, 1940). The objective of this hearing aid selection approach is to set the frequency response of the hearing aid to mirror the image of the hearing loss. The pure-tone sensitivity curve on the audiogram is provided an amount of gain at each frequency that is identical to the dB loss at that frequency (to move the aided threshold to "normal" or to essentially 0 dB). Figure 10 illustrates a fairly common pure-tone audiometric configuration and how this approach is used to attempt to restore the pure-tone thresholds. For example, a 50 dB pure-tone threshold at 500 Hz would require 50 dB gain from the hearing aid

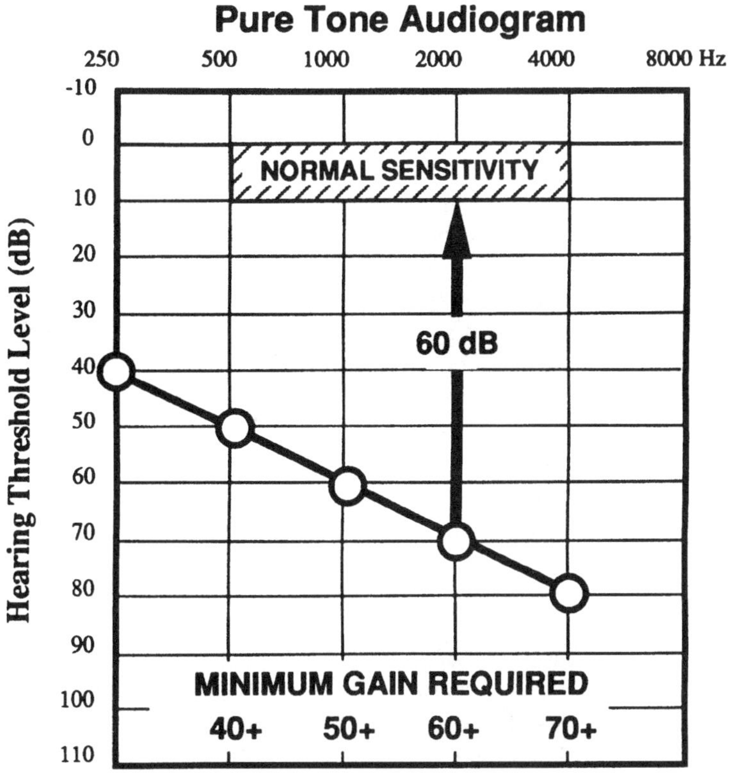

Fig. 10. Example of a hearing loss and the gain that would be required to restore the pure-tone thresholds to "normal" in a direct mirror fitting of the audiogram.

at 500 Hz; 70 dB of hearing aid gain would be required to overcome the 70 dB pure-tone loss at 2000 Hz, etc. As a result, this approach might be better identified as ***"direct mirror fitting"*** to separate it from later approaches that could be described more accurately as ***"fractional mirror fitting,"*** and which serves as the foundation upon which almost all threshold-based hearing aid formulae are based.

A basic problem reported with direct mirror fitting is that it assumes a subject utilizes speech at threshold, rather than at a suprathreshold level, as normally occurs. Insisting upon amplification that places speech at or near normal sensitivity levels would overpower a listener easily because the gain required confuses physical sound intensity (dB gain) and subjective loudness acceptance (dB HTL). The problem is especially acute for a hearing loss that increases with frequency (Lybarger, 1978). Additionally, the fact that equal loudness contours tend to flatten at suprathreshold levels strongly suggests that gain requirements based on a 1:1 dB ratio between gain and HTL will lead to over-amplification. Aside from this, if normal conversational speech is assumed to be between 65–70 dB SPL at 1 meter, and if this input level is coupled with the gain requirements suggested in Figure 10, the output at 1000 Hz would be 125 to 130 dB for normal conversational speech (65 + 60 = 125; or 70 + 60 = 130), and this without any consideration for reserve! It would be a rare hearing instrument user that would tolerate this output level routinely for normal conversational speech, much less for loud sound! This procedure assumes that SPL (hearing aid output as measured in a 2cc coupler) and HTL (audiometric level) can be compared directly, which they cannot. Additionally, the effects of earmold coupling and potential effects of upward spread of masking are not taken into consideration with mirror fitting.

Therefore, sufficient evidence exists to support the contention that direct mirror fitting, while seeming to have face validity initially, is not a reasonable approach. Still, it is undeniable that most approaches to the selection of hearing aids use the concept of mirror fitting at least to some extent.

Adjusted Audiometric Pure-Tone Data (Fractional Mirror Fitting)

These approaches use the audiometric hearing threshold levels as a starting point but adjust the gain levels recommended according to some pre-determined criteria.

Gain Proportional to, But Not Equal to the Loss at Each Frequency. This approach is similar to the direct mirror fitting inverted audiogram except that the gain required is less by about 10 to 15 dB, or some other constant value, at each frequency. A variation of this is to select hearing aid components that roughly reflect the slope of the patient's pure-tone hearing loss (Reddell and Calvert, 1966; Pascoe, 1975). They found that aided performance using this approach was superior to that of hearing aids based on a uniform slope concept, both for word recognition scores in quiet and noise and for subjective patient preference.

"Use Gain" Estimates (Formation of the Half Gain Rule). These approaches attempt to relate the average gain required in the hearing aid to the average gain used for a given loss. Also called "operating" and "functional" estimates of gain, initial approaches did not attempt to provide information about the frequency response required from the hearing aid (gain by frequency), although most current procedures do. Introduced initially by Lybarger for the Radioear Hearing Aid Company (Radioear 'One-Half Rule' for Maximum Gain, 1944), he proposed a formula to select maximum output level (what is called maximum gain) and also "use", or "preferred" gain (operating gain). The latter was based on the assumption that the optimum hearing aid response curve is the mirror image of about one-half the audiogram curve in dB. This initiated the birth of the half gain rule that forms the basis for most hearing aid formulae calculated from hearing threshold levels. It is because the half gain procedure forms the bases for so many hearing aid fitting formulae that it is explained in such detail.

Using the half-gain rule philosophy as a basis, the "use" gain approach projects a rough estimate of the actual gain a person will use (require) from the hearing aid (Lybarger, 1944, 1953, 1963). It relates the average gain to the average air-conduction hearing loss. The formula is based on restoring average conversational speech (65 dB SPL) to within the listener's MCL range. The half-gain rule provides greater gain as the hearing loss increases, providing gain of approximately one-half the average hearing loss, at least for mild and moderate hearing levels. This relates the average maximum gain (average of 500, 1000, and 2000 Hz) to the average air-conduction hearing loss (Lybarger, 1955). It is not based on gain that is essentially half the hearing loss, but on an average maximum gain that increases one-half as fast as the hearing loss, starting at a predetermined level. The *use gain* formula as described initially by Lybarger (1944) for a monaural fitting is as follows:

$$\mathbf{MG = MG_o + 1/2(HL - HL_o) + K_1\ dB}$$

Where:

MG = Desired average maximum gain for a given loss

MG_o = A base maximum gain that applies for an average loss of HL_o (predetermined to 40 dB)

HL = Average air-conduction hearing loss (.5, 1, 2 kHz)

HL_o = Gain required for the air-conduction hearing loss (predetermined)

K_1 = Correction that depends on the amount of conductive hearing loss present. It's function is to reduce the saturation output level for sensorineural losses, and to increase it for any conductive portion of the loss. A suitable formula for K_1 is:

$$K_1(dB) = 1/4(HL_{ac} - HL_{bc} - 20)$$

The correction factor depends on the conductive loss. For example:

Air-bone gap = 0 = −5.0 dB
10 = −2.5 dB

Table 2. Recommended Maximum Gain (MG) in dB for Average AC-BC Hearing Loss Difference of:

Avg. A.C. Loss–dB	0 d B or less	10	20	30	40 dB or more
30	35	37.5	40	42.5	45
40	40	42.5	45	47.5	50
50	45	47.5	50	52.5	55
60	50	52.5	55	57.5	60
70	55	57.5	60	62.5	65
80	60	62.5	65	67.5	70
90	65	67.5	70	72.5	75
100	70	72.5	75	77.5	80

$$20 = 0 \text{ dB}$$
$$30 = 2.5 \text{ dB}$$
$$40 = 5.0 \text{ dB}$$

For a transistor hearing aid the basic formula is:

$$\mathbf{MG = MG_o + 1/2(HL - 30) + K_1}$$

Assuming a 40 dB average hearing loss, having no air-bone gap:

$$MG = 40 + 1/2\,(40 - 30) + (-5 \text{ dB})$$
$$MG = 40$$

A table was developed that eliminated the need to perform the calculations (Table 2). Note that the gain increases 1/2 as fast as does the air-conduction loss.

In 1953 Lybarger modified this formula for *maximum gain* by relating it to one-half the hearing threshold level in the speech frequencies, retaining the constant, the correction factor for the air-bone gap, and the plus 5 dB. New, was the inclusion of a 15 dB reserve gain. A 1963 formula version was for *operating gain,* and also recognized that 15 dB was too much reserve gain for ear-level hearing aids. The 1963 formula version, based on a monaural fitting, was as follows:

$$\textbf{Use, Operating, or Functional Gain} = \frac{\mathbf{A}}{\mathbf{2}} + \frac{\mathbf{(A - B) + 5}}{\mathbf{4}}$$

(Actual gain person will use)

Where: A = Average air/conduction hearing threshold (.5, 1, and 2 kHz)

B = Average bone/conduction hearing threshold (.5, 1, and 2 kHz)

$A - B/4$ = Correction factor for the air-bone gap
$+5$ = Constant

For *maximum gain* a reserve of 15 dB is added to the operational gain. Also, the +5 constant in the formula is changed to −10 dB for a binaural fitting. (Additionally, with the change at about that time from the ASA to ISO (ANSI) audiometer calibration, the +5 dB was omitted, rendering the results almost identical).

Based on this formula, an average 50 dB loss monaurally, having no air-bone gap, would require an *operating gain* of 30 dB. It's *maximum gain* would be 45 dB.

Average air/conduction thresholds (500, 1000, and 2000 Hz) = 50 dB

Average bone/conduction thresholds (500, 1000, and 2000 Hz) = 50 dB

Monaural			Binaural	
50/2	= 25		50/2	= 25
50 − 50/4	= 0		50 − 50/4	= 0
25 + 0 + 5	= 30 dB	operating gain	25 + 0 − 10	= 15 dB
30 + 15	= 45 dB	maximum gain	15 + 15	= 30 dB

Figure 11, adapted from Pascoe (1990), illustrates how the half-gain rule relates to restoring average conversational speech (considered to be 55 dB HL when presented in the sound field) to MCL, at least up to hearing threshold levels of about 60 dB. For losses greater than 60 dB, slightly greater gain is required as the loss becomes more severe. This tends to support clinical practice procedures that select initial frequency/gain characteristics on the half-gain rule.

A ***simple variation of "use gain" estimates*** that has been used is as follows: For speech MCLs (in SPL), 65 dB is subtracted (this latter number approximates the level of normal conversational speech). The resultant number represents the *minimum* gain requirement. This practice has been used with many Master Hearing Aids. For example:

Use Gain	= **MCL**	95 dB SPL
	− **normal conversational speech level**	65 dB
	= **Use Gain**	30 dB

POGO (1983). An acronym for Prescription of Gain and Output, this fitting formula provides a fairly straightforward approach to defining hearing aid requirements for gain and output across the frequency range for a closed earmold system (McCandless and Lyregaard, 1983). The goal of the prescription is to amplify speech

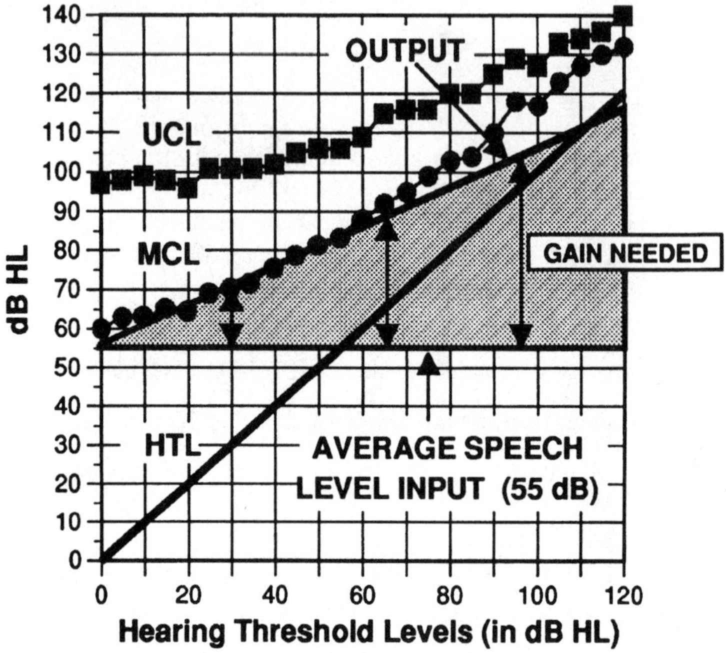

Fig. 11 Average MCL and UCL (LDL) levels as they relate to varying levels of hearing loss (in HTL). This shows support for the half-gain rule for losses at least up to about 60 dB, providing the intent is to raise a 55 dB SPL input level of speech to the MCL. (Adapted from data by Pascoe, D.P. Clinical measurements of the auditory dynamic range and their relation to formulas for hearing aid gain, in Presbyacousis and Other Age Related Aspects. 14th Danavox Symposium, 1990, pp. 129–147.)

to MCL. Because the application of the half gain rule was believed to provide too much amplification at the low frequencies (leading to a decrease in speech recognition in noise, possibly due to an upward spread of masking), POGO reduces the gain at low frequencies from the half gain rule by −10 dB at 250 Hz and by −5 dB at 500 Hz. A 10 dB reserve gain is added to help in selecting hearing aids from the manufacturers' 2-cc full-on acoustic gain curves. Hearing thresholds are obtained under earphones.

The *gain* portion of the formula for POGO is as follows:

Frequency in Hz	**250**	**500**	**1000**	**2000**	**3000**	**4000**	**6000**
Multiply HTL by:	**0.5**	**0.5**	**0.5**	**0.5**	**0.5**	**0.5**	**0.5**
Correction factor:	**–10**	**–5**					
Reserve:	**+10**	**+10**	**+10**	**+10**	**+10**	**+10**	**+10**

The hearing aid *output* requirement under POGO is equal to the average UCL for 500, 1000, and 2000 Hz in HTL. To correct for

2cc coupler measurement in dB SPL, a 4 dB correction factor is added to this value. Additionally, correction factors are applied for earmold modifications, such as vents and horns.

$$\frac{\textbf{UCL 500 Hz + UCL 1000 Hz + UCL 2000 Hz}}{\textbf{3}}$$

The aided performance is recommended to be verified by either (a) real-ear probe-tube microphone measurements or (b) by sound-field functional gain measurements (McCandless, 1988).

Libby One-Third Gain Rule (1986). Libby (1986) reported on a formula based on an assumption that the gain in mild-to-moderate hearing losses more closely approximates a one-third gain rule than a one-half gain rule. Libby suggested that mild hearing losses used very little amplification in real life situations and therefore, the prescription should reflect the amount of gain *actually* used. For hearing losses greater than moderate (severe and profound) he suggests a two-thirds gain rule. Corrections at the lower frequencies are intended to prevent too much amplification and possible upward spread of masking effects.

Libby Target Real Ear Gain (One-Third Gain Rule) =

Frequency in Hz	**250**	**500**	**1000**	**2000**	**3000**	**4000**	**6000**
HTL multiplied by:	**0.33**	**0.33**	**0.33**	**0.33**	**0.33**	**0.33**	**0.33**
Correction:	**–5**	**–3**					

Use of Audiometric Pure-Tone Threshold Data Adjusted for the Speech Spectrum

A number of approaches to hearing aid selection provide prescriptive gain formulae that mirror the long-term average speech spectrum by adjusting the pure-tone threshold data, after applying the half gain rule and making adjustments, as set forth by Lybarger (1944). An historical perspective of these follows.

Lybarger Half Gain Rule, Accounting For Frequency Differences (Radioear Formula, 1944). Lybarger (1944) filed a patent application and was the first to suggest the use of audiometric HTL multiplied by a frequency-dependent factor. He adjusted the hearing threshold level values to arrive at an optimum hearing aid response curve that was the mirror image of about half the audiogram curve in dB. To arrive at this "half gain rule," he multiplied thresholds by a factor between 0.3 and 0.7, before mirroring, depending upon the expected contribution for different frequencies. In general, high frequencies were given more importance, and the multiplication factors were chosen to account for the importance of the high-frequency speech spectrum information. This approach formed the basis for literally all hearing aid fitting formulae today that are based on pure-tone thresholds. An example for a 50 dB hearing loss follows:

Optimum Hearing Aid Response Curve (Gain):

250 Hz		**1000 Hz**	
HTL	**= 50 dB**	**HTL**	**= 50 dB**
50/2	**= 25**	**50/2**	**= 25**
25 × 0.3	**= 7.5**	**25 × 0.7**	**= 17.5**
7.5 + 25	**= 32.5 dB**	**17.5 + 25**	**= 4.25 dB = gain required**

(***Radioear One-Fourth Rule for Output***). It should be recognized that although most formulae relate primarily to the prescription of gain, the "Radioear Basic Fitting Procedure" (Lybarger, 1955) provided for the selection of the saturation output ***before*** the selection of gain, using the Radioear "one-fourth rule". The one-fourth rule relates the average saturation output to the average air-conduction hearing thresholds as follows:

$$SO = SO_o + \tfrac{1}{4}(HL - HL_o) + K_1 \quad \text{(dB re } 20\mu\text{bar)}$$

A suitable formula is: $SO = 115 + \tfrac{1}{4}(HL - 40) + K_1$

Where: SO = Desired average saturation output for a given average hearing loss (Average = Average of 500, 1000, and 2000 Hz)

HL = Average air-conduction hearing loss

SO_o = Average saturation output that applies for a given loss (Table 3)

HL_o = Average air-conduction hearing loss (for the client)

Table 3. Recommended Saturation Output (SO) in dB re 20μPa for Average AC-BC Hearing Loss Difference of:

Avg. A.C. Loss–dB	0 d B or less	10	20	30	40 dB or more
30	107.5	110	112.5	115	117.5
40	110	112.5	115	117.5	120
50	112.5	115	117.5	120	122.5
60	115	117.5	120	122.5	125
70	117.5	120	122.5	125	127.5
80	120	122.5	125	127.5	130
90	122.5	125	127.5	130	132.5
100	125	127.5	130	132.5	135

K_1 = Correction that depends on the relative amount of conductive loss present. K_1 has the same function as in the case of the maximum gain in the half-gain rule.

Example: Client HL average = 60 dB

- $SO = 115 + \frac{1}{4}(HL_{ac} - 40) + K_1$
- $SO = 115 + \frac{1}{4}(60 - 40) + K_1$
- $SO = 115$ dB SPL

Notice that the recommended saturation output increases one-fourth as fast as the hearing loss for a given AC-BC difference. This is an average value, to be matched to the same frequency *average* data for the hearing aid measured in a 2-cc coupler.

Slide Rule Approaches

In the mid 1970s a number of hearing aid manufacturers published their fitting formulae via the use of slide rules (Figure 12). Other manufacturers during that time period, especially those that pioneered prescriptive fittings to their dispensers, kept their fitting prescriptions secret or applied their concepts to master hearing aids. (The latter are discussed later in this Chapter).

Pure-Tone Thresholds Used to Predict the Desired Hearing Aid Slope A variety of approaches have been used to help determine the hearing aid amplification slope to provide for the best speech recognition (Lybarger, 1955; Berger, 1976; NAL, 1976). At least one of these (Lybarger, 1955) was used when gain-by-frequency was not a part of fitting formulae.

Radioear "One-Fourth Slope Rule" (Lybarger, 1955)

This method was an early approach to using the pure-tone threshold data to determine the desired slope of the hearing aid frequency response curve that would yield the best discrimination scores. The rule assumed that the slope of the frequency-response curve should be corrected in the low frequencies for body-baffle at a rate of +3 dB/octave from 250 to 1000 Hz, and +3 dB/octave in the high-frequency region (1000 to 4000 Hz) for essentially a "flat" audiogram. *Departures* from this slope are made on the basis of one-fourth of the departure of the audiogram slope from a flat audiogram in both the low- and high-frequency regions. Low-frequency slope is determined by drawing a line from the loss at 1000 Hz through the half-octave between 250 and 500 Hz (at 354 Hz). The high-frequency slope is determined by drawing a line from the loss at 1000 Hz through the quarter-octave between 2000 and 2800 Hz (at about 2400 Hz).

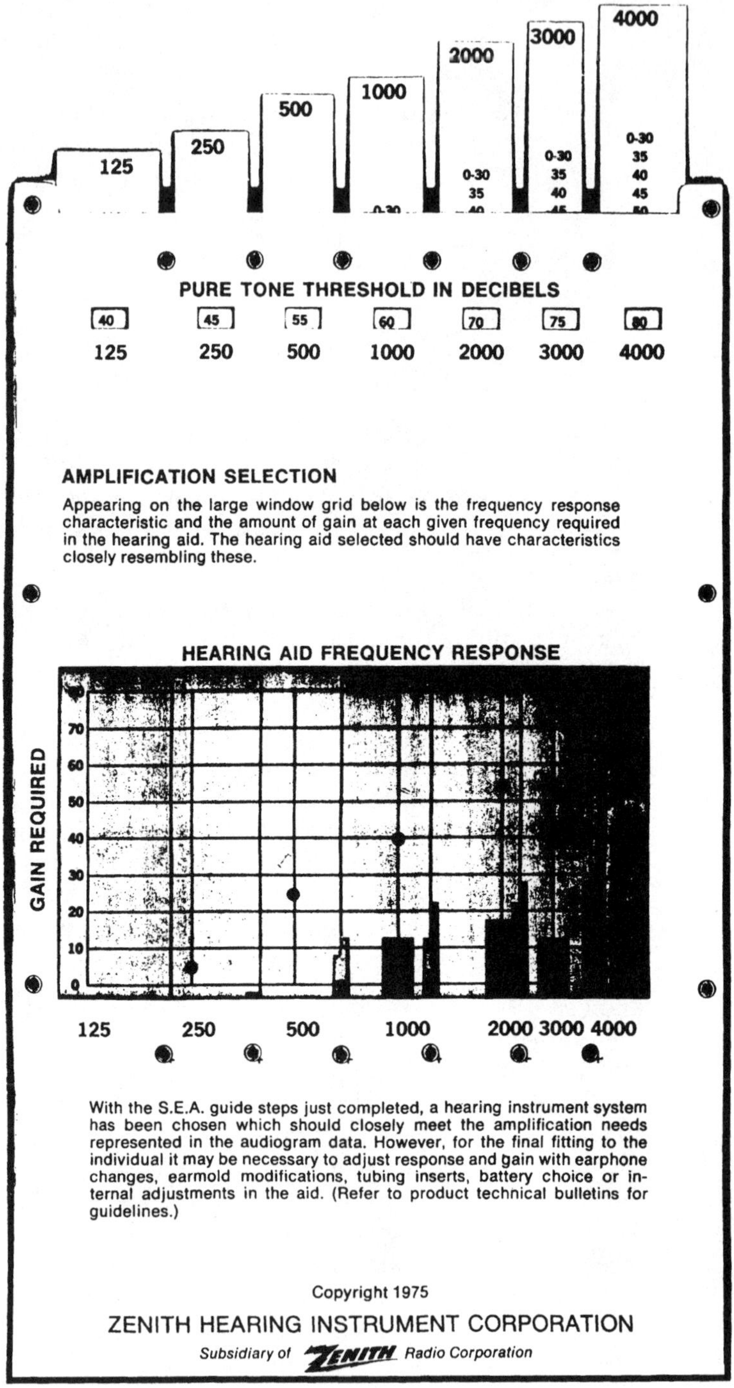

Fig. 12. Example of a slide rule used as a guide to hearing instrument selection. From audiogram data, the gain by frequency is determined. The threshold for the various frequencies shown at the top of the slide rule is moved to fit into the boxes. The gain recommended is identified by the dots at those frequencies shown in the large rectangle. The guide also provides suggestions for SSPL90 and earmold selection (not shown). (Zenith S.E.A. Guide to Hearing Instrument Selection, Zenith Hearing Instrument Corporation, 1975.)

Figure 13 shows an audiogram and a hearing aid response curve (trend lines only), and Table 4 provides a quick means of determining the recommended hearing aid slopes for the low and high frequencies.

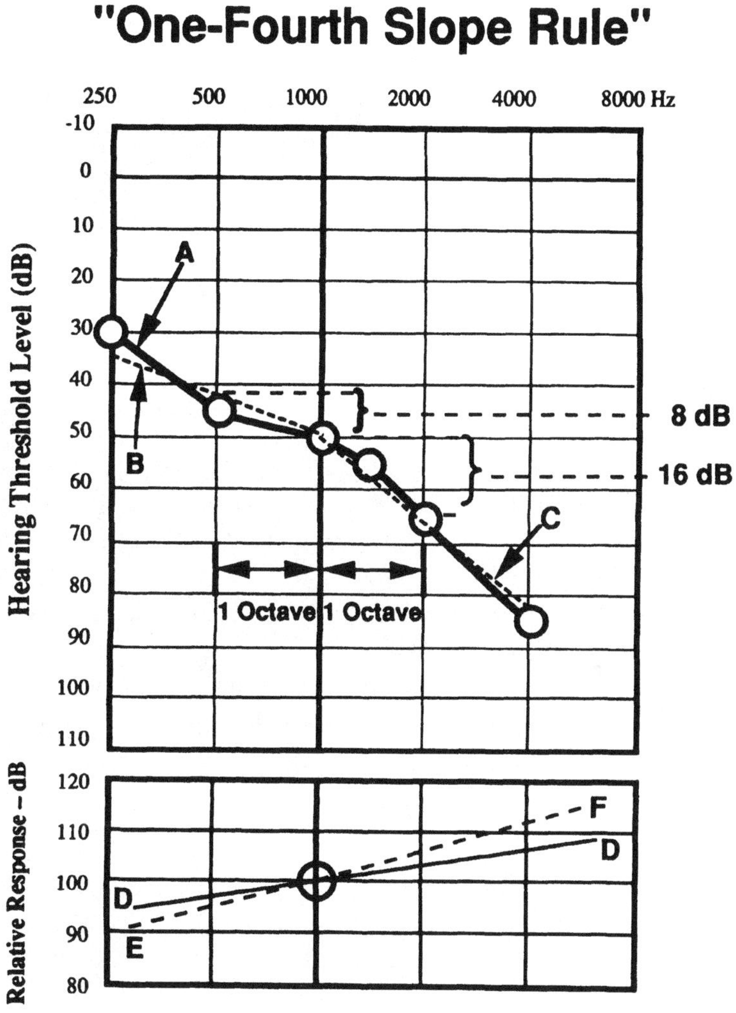

Fig. 13. Utilization of the "one-fourth slope rule." The slope in the low frequencies is determined by drawing a line from the loss at 1000 Hz through the half-octave between 250 and 500 Hz, and the high-frequency slope by drawing the line from the loss at 1000 Hz through the quarter-octave between 2000 and 2800 Hz. (Adapted from Lybarger, S. F., Radioear basic fitting procedure (condensed form for clinical use), Radioear Corporation, Original written June 14, 1955, Revised July 10, 1957.)

Table 4. The Desired Slope of the Hearing Aid Frequency Response Curve can be Obtained From This Table, With Threshold Levels From the Audiogram (Radioear "One-Fourth Slope Rule")

Audiogram Classification	Audiogram Slope (dB/Octave)	Recommended HA Frequency Response Curve Slope (dB/Octave)
Sharply Falling	−20	+8
	−16	+7
	−12	+6
	−8	+5
	−4	+4
Flat	0	+3
	+4	+2
	+8	+1
	+12	0
	+16	−1
Sharply Rising	+20	−2

This table applies to low-frequency (LF) and to high-frequency (HF) regions.

Berger Formula (1976, 1989). The Berger formula was prompted, in part, by the poor performance of speech recognition tests in selecting an appropriate hearing aid. It is based on the following postulates:

- Aided performance should show improved word recognition at conversational levels
- Gain should be slightly greater than one-half the pure-tone levels
- Low-frequency ambient noise is detrimental (if amplified)
- Less gain is needed at 500 Hz than at higher frequencies
- Speech sounds higher than 4000 Hz are relatively unimportant for speech

Berger's formula is based on applying the half gain rule to thresholds obtained under earphones at specific frequencies, and then dividing (or multiplying) the hearing threshold level at that frequency by values that reflect the importance of speech for those frequencies. Figure 14 diagrams the approach. At 500 Hz and 6000 Hz, the threshold is multiplied by 0.5. At 1000 Hz the threshold is multiplied by 0.63; 2000 Hz by 0.67; 3000 Hz by 0.59; and 4000 Hz by 0.53. These values provide the operating gain of the hearing aid (which in turn is used to predict the targeted aided performance). A reserve gain of 10 dB is added at each frequency to provide the maximum gain required by the hearing aid for each frequency. Ad-

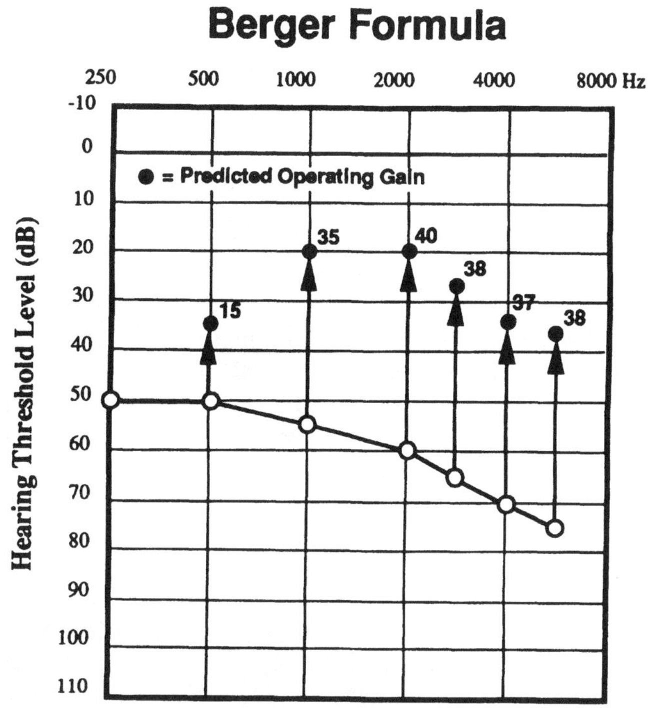

WORKSHEET

	.25	.5	1	2	3	4	6k Hz
HTL	50	50	55	60	65	70	75
X by	–	0.30*	0.63	0.67	0.59	0.53	0.50
Operating Gain		15	35	40	38	37	38
Reserve Gain		10	10	10	10	10	10
Maximum Gain		25	45	50	48	47	48

* 0.50 for a 50 dB HTL

Fig. 14. Diagram concept of the Berger formula for hearing aid prescription. The predicted operating gains are the "target" to be achieved through functional gain or mic-probe real ear measurements.

ditionally, correction factors for conductive and mixed losses, monaural versus binaural, as well as for hearing aid microphone pickup locations (BTE, ITE, ITC and Body-Worn aids—Berger, 1988), can be applied. The "target" (operating) gains at each frequency provide dispensers with an "objective" measurement of hearing aid performance in that the aided sound-field performance of the hearing aid could be compared to the operating gain, and adjusted if necessary, to more closely match the target.

The recommended saturation output for the hearing aid is based on sound-field pulse tone UCLs at 500, 1000, 2000, and 4000 Hz, converted and recorded in SPL. The recommended saturation output is approximately 4 to 6 dB above the UCL. When the dynamic range is restricted, the Berger fitting approach includes provisions for AGC-type output limiting systems.

NAL (1976, 1986). Originally presented as the NAL (National Acoustics Laboratory of Australia) formula for hearing aid selection, based on approximating the half-gain rule (Byrne and Tonnison, 1976), the revision—NAL (R) or NAL Revised (Byrne and Dillon, 1986)—is a commonly-used formula for selecting real-ear (insertion or functional) by the frequency band of a hearing aid. The original formula was changed because it was not deemed to meet the goal of amplifying all frequency bands of speech to an equal loudness. The revised version goal is an attempt to amplify all frequency bands of speech to equal loudness, specifically to a 60 phon equal loudness contour. This was accomplished by restoring a greater amount of desired amplification in the lower frequencies. Thresholds are obtained under earphones. The formula uses a half-gain rule combined with a one-third slope rate to control for excessive gain in the high frequencies for steeply-sloping hearing losses (thresholds are multiplied by 0.31 at each frequency to correct for variations in audiometric slopes). Speech spectrum corrections are factored in for frequency, and a gain constant is applied to each frequency as well. The gain constant value is 0.05 times the summed HTL at 500, 1000, and 2000 Hz for the client.

NAL (R) Target real ear gain (insertion gain or functional gain) =

Frequency in Hz	**250**	**500**	**750**	**1000**	**1500**	**2000**	**3000**	**4000**	**6000**
HTL multiplied by:	**0.31**	**0.31**	**0.31**	**0.31**	**0.31**	**0.31**	**0.31**	**0.31**	**0.31**
Speech spectrum correction	**−17**	**−8**	**−3**	**+1**	**+1**	**−1**	**−2**	**−2**	**−2**
Add calculated constant:	**+X**	**+X**	**+X**	**+X**	**+X**	**+X**	**+X**	**+X**	**+X**

(X = 0.05 (HTL 500 Hz + HTL 1000 Hz + HTL 2000 Hz)

How closely the hearing aid meets the target insertion or functional gain is best measured by probe-tube microphone systems (Byrne and Dillon, 1986), but functional gain measures, although not recommended, can also be used.

A formula is also provided for deriving 2cc coupler gain but is beyond the scope of this chapter. The reader is encouraged to refer to the original article.

DSL Method (1988). The Desired Sensation Level (DSL) method has been developed for hearing aid selection and fitting of preverbal children (Seewald and Ross (1988) in order to apply a more uniform and valid approach to fitting this population. Major issues addressed by this procedure are that: (1) the selection and fitting of amplification to children is based on relatively limited information, (2) the acoustic properties of the ears of young children are quite different from those of adults, and (3) amplification to learn speech and language must allow them to be able to hear the speech of others and to hear themselves for self-monitoring of their own speech. The procedure attempts to account for factors unique to infants and young children in the areas of audiometric assessment, electroacoustic selection, fitting and verification. A major feature of the procedure is the ability to use very limited data (a threshold at one frequency only) and through computer software that stores and calculates a wide range of information on infant and young childrens' ears, to calculate: (1) the desired sensation levels (DSLs) for amplified speech; (2) target real-ear aided response (REAR) and real-ear saturation response (RESR) values; and (3) target aided sound-field thresholds (Seewald, 1994). The basis of the procedure is to select hearing aid frequency/gain characteristics that place as much of the long-term speech spectrum as possible into the amplified range. Threshold data is converted to SPL (or measured preferably initially via insert earphones in SPL) and compared to the long-term speech spectrum stored in the computer. The computer program then calculates the amount of gain required to place the speech spectrum at the desired sensation levels for amplified speech. Predicted levels of amplified speech are used to select the desired real-ear SSPL values because UCL data is seldom obtainable in children.

After an instrument (BTE, ITE, ITC) and its coupling have been selected that meets the calculated requirements, the aided performance is verified using real-ear measurements, although functional gain measurements can also be used.

Because the procedure obtains all measures within the ear canal, the client is used as his/her own reference, regardless of age. Measurements are obtained, therefore, as in-situ gain as opposed to insertion gain. This permits real-ear to coupler differences (RECD) that allow for an accountability of the individual's ear and earmold acoustics. Additionally, because the acoustic difference between the real ear and the coupler have been defined, electroacoustic response shaping can be performed in the highly controlled acoustic conditions of the hearing aid test box with a very accurate prediction of how the hearing aid will perform on the individual

(Seewald, 1994). More recently, the DSL method has been proposed for adults as well, and also for evaluating linear and nonlinear hearing aid fitting in adults (Audioscan™, 1995).

Threshold-Based Procedures to Optimize Speech Recognition Based on the Articulation Index

The Articulation Index (AI) is a number ranging from 0.00 to 1.00, and represents that part of the total speech signal *available* to a listener from that presented. Calculation of the AI is made by dividing the frequency range into equal intelligibility bands, with each band's contribution determined by the dynamic range of speech that is available to the listener in that band. Each band's contribution may be reduced by external masking noise, filtering in the transmission path that attenuates part of the speech spectrum, or by reducing the level of speech so that parts of the speech spectrum are below threshold. It is the latter that has drawn the attention of the AI for use in hearing aid performance evaluations. In reality, these procedures are used as much or more for hearing aid verification purposes than for hearing aid electroacoustic performance prescription. The degree of difficulty in their use varies widely by procedure.

As used with hearing aids, these approaches use the audiogram and a formula to develop an optimum amplification curve. The bases for these methods are founded on calculations of the Articulation Index (AI) developed by French and Steinberg (1947), Fletcher (1952), or Kryter (1962), and on data obtained from the Harvard Report (Davis et al., 1947). The AI does not use loudness-based criteria. The goal is to provide amplification to allow the range of speech to be ***audible*** at each test frequency. It is assumed that achieving this goal will result in maximum speech recognition.

The earliest reported use of the AI was by Collard (1930). However, the most common use of the AI was developed by French and Steinberg (1947) to *predict,* rather than *measure,* the intelligibility of speech. AI theory holds that audible speech energy within a frequency band determines the intelligibility of the band. Therefore, the importance content of speech is directly related to the intensity of the signal at critical frequency bands. A number of 0.00 means that no speech sounds are audible, whereas a number of 1.00 indicates that all speech sounds are audible. In addition to the work by French and Steinberg (1947), others have proposed variations of the AI for various reasons. Beranek (1947) described a slightly less complicated version that changed the band contributions, altered the long-term average levels in each band, used male speakers only, and eliminated pauses between words in determining the speech level. Kryter's modification (1962) was to include corrections for upward and downward spread-of-masking, allowance for when the speech levels in a band exceed the listener's loudness discomfort levels, provided weights for calculating the AI from octave and one-third octave band analysis, and fused linear intensity weighting.

In addition to its ability to explain and predict the impact of hearing loss on speech intelligibility in quiet and in noise, the AI is also a sufficiently powerful tool for fitting hearing aids and for predicting the patient's aided ability to understand monosyllabic words and sentences in those same environmental conditions.

Fletcher (1952)

This modification uses the audiogram and a formula to develop an optimum amplification curve. Considering both conductive and sensorineural components of the hearing loss, the process involves complex calculations based on the Articulation Index, and is taken from data developed in the Harvard Report (Davis et al., 1947). He used "proficiency factors" to take into consideration the reduced speech discrimination abilities of listeners with sensorineural hearing loss. The formula and explanation are (Lybarger, 1978):

$$\mathbf{R = (response) = Bc + rBn}$$

Bc = conductive component of hearing loss in dB
Bn = sensorineural component of hearing loss in dB
r = a factor between 0.2 and 0.4

For sensorineural losses, R = rBn = 0.3 Bn.
For conductive losses a mirror image of the audiogram was called for and resulted in a downward sloping curve for a rising audiogram.

ANSI Standard S3.5-1969

The standard method for calculating the AI is ANSI Standard S3.5-1969 and is based on work by Kryter. It was developed to optimize telecommunications systems and contains useful tables showing the equal contribution to speech intelligibility of twenty individual frequency bands (Table 5).

Useful Hearing Aid Modifications

An objective method to evaluate the social hearing handicap (or benefit of amplification) would be to calculate the average hearing at a reference frequency within each of the 10 frequency bands. However, this is impractical and time consuming. Because of this, a number of proposals have been suggested for applying the

Table 5. Twenty frequency bands of equal contribution to speech intelligiblity (ANSI S3.5-1969).

Band No.	Frequency limits (Hz)	Mid-Frequency (Hz)
1	200-330	270
2	330-430	380
3	430-560	490
4	560-700	630
5	700-840	770
6	840-1000	920
7	1000-1150	1070
8	1150-1310	1230
9	1310-1480	1400
10	1480-1660	1570
11	1660-1830	1740
12	1830-2020	1920
13	2020-2240	2130
14	2240-2500	2370
15	2500-2820	2660
16	2820-3200	3000
17	3200-3650	3400
18	3650-4250	3950
19	4250-5050	4650
20	5050-6100	5600

principles of the Articulation Index, but in simpler forms (Briskey, Greenbaum, and Sinclair, 1966; Humes, 1986; Pavlovic, 1987, 1991; and Mueller and Killion, 1990) to the hearing aid selection and evaluation process. Methods differ primarily in the number of bands, the weightings assigned to each band, and the type of speech stimuli. Other hearing aid procedures that use AI principles, at least in part, include the DSL (1988) and the AIMax (Humes, 1986).

The AI is attractive in hearing aid outcomes measurements because (1) it provides a clear visual illustration of the effects of thresholds on the speech spectrum by a given hearing aid, (2) it allows for a comparison of different hearing aids with each other with respect to speech intelligibility without the need for speech testing, (3) it provides a possible method to adjust the hearing aid to maximize the AI, and (4) if the signal is heard it can contribute—or, if the signal is not heard, it can't contribute. It can be used in the hearing aid selection process with other indexes of user satisfaction. Also, a high score does not suggest a "best" hearing aid.

Mueller and Killion "Count the Dots" Procedure (1990)

Figure 15 provides an example of a simplified method for calculation of the AI. The dots (100) are distributed unevenly throughout the 30-dB speech dynamic range on the audiogram, when speech is presented at 70 dB SPL, or roughly 50 dB HTL. The greatest concentration of dots is in the higher frequencies and represents the significance of the frequency-dependent components of speech. Each dot contributes equally to speech discrimination. To calculate the AI, the number of dots that exceed threshold are counted and divided by 100. An AI of 0.5 means that 50% of the acoustic information that contributes to speech intelligibility is available to the person for use when speech is at normal conversational levels. If the threshold falls on top of any dot, it is still counted if half or more falls below the threshold. Other "count the dot" approaches have been proposed that vary somewhat from the procedure described here (Humes, 1991; Pavlovic, 1991). With these procedures, when the AI is used to determine the amount of speech cue information that is *available* to the listener, the term *Audibility Index* rather than *Articulation Index* is recommended to be used (Killion, Mueller, Pavlovic, and Humes, 1993).

Articulation Index Basics

Figures 16 through 22 illustrate AI basics (adapted from Pavlovic, 1988). The speech spectrum (overall intensity change of 30 dB) must be identified to use the AI, recognizing that it can change under everyday circumstances.

In interpreting the results of AI calculations, care should be taken. For example, (1) the threshold of discomfort is not taken into consideration, (2) the *speech spectrum* is shifted into a more audible range, and not that the *thresholds* have been changed, (3) an AI of 1.0 does not mean the auditory system is functioning normally, and (4) the application to nonlinear circuits is not clear. Still, there is a relationship that exists between the AI and speech intelligibility (Table 6).

Threshold-Based Procedure Using the Subject as the Reference

The "Benefit" Method (Sound-Field Method) of Fitting Hearing Aids (1992). This is a computerized method based on using the individual as his/her own standard to fit hearing aids, rather than referencing an average value based on pure-tone audiometry, as do pure-tone based fitting formulae. This procedure was developed at the Karolinska Hospital Clinical Department of Audiology, Stockholm, Sweden (Svärd, 1992; and Ahlner, 1994).

The Benefit Method recognizes that people understand poorer in noise, and that it is not possible to predict word recognition

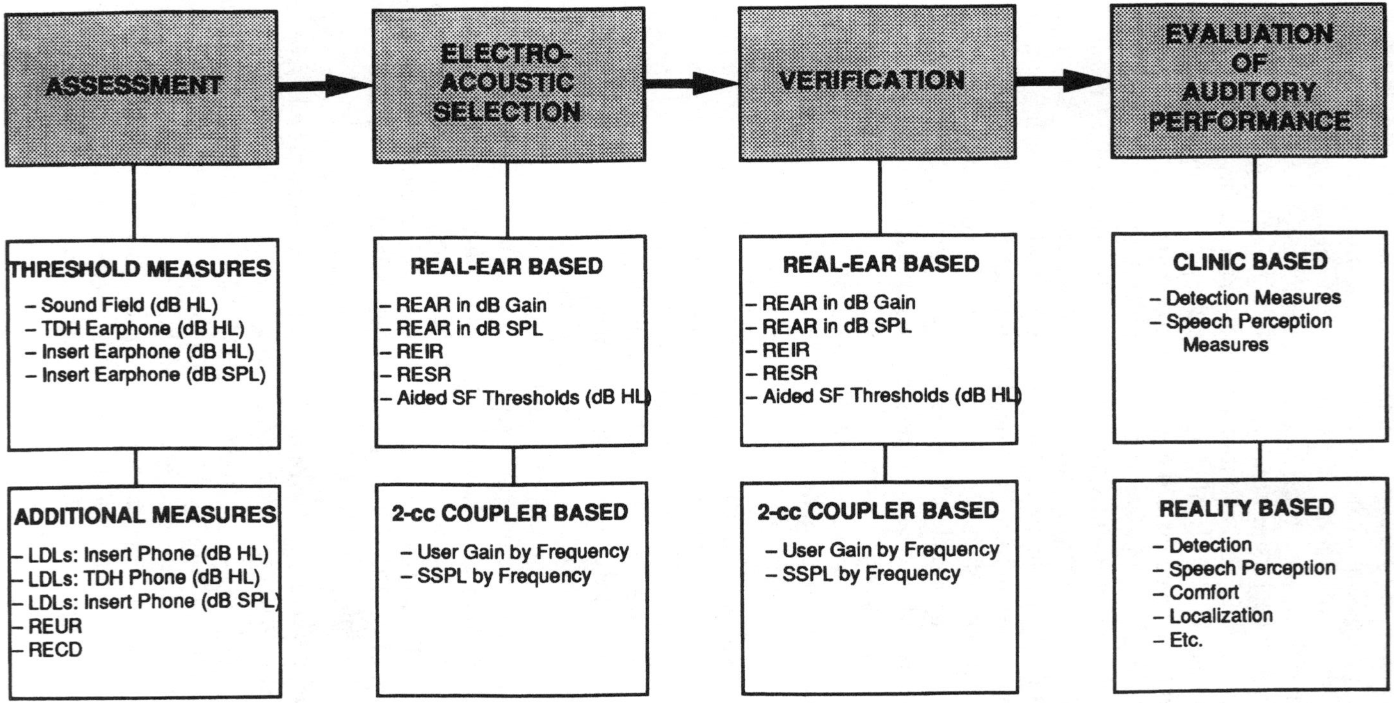

Fig. 15. The general structure and options (inputs and outputs) comprising the DSL method for hearing aid fitting in infants and children. (After Seewald, R. C. (1995), The desired sensation level (DSL) method for hearing aid fitting in infants and children, Phonak Focus, News/Ideas/High Technology/Acoustics, Nr. 20).

(a)	FREQUENCY (Hz)					
	250	500	1000	2000	4000	6000
Threshold (dB HL)	55	60	65	70	75	75
MAP (dB SPL)	73	73	75	85	90	93
DSLs (dB)	14	19	21	20	15	8
Amplified LTASS (dB SPL)	87	92	96	105	105	101
REAR (dB Gain)	24	28	39	54	63	59
RESR (dB SPL)	106	115	117	122	122	120
REIR (dB Gain)	23	26	37	42	48	52
Aided Thresholds (dB HL)	32	34	28	28	27	23

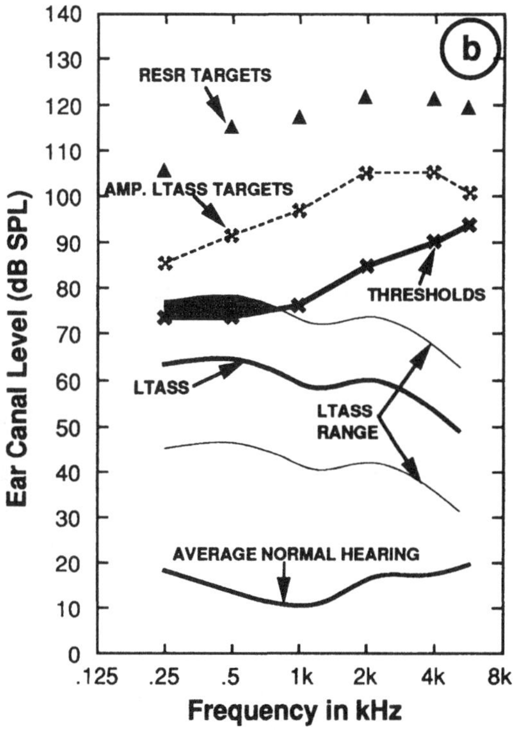

Fig. 16. Real-ear electroacoustic selection results derived for a loss using the DSL method, and by entering the threshold values only into the computer program. The seven calculations in (a) are made. Unaided information recorded in SPL (ear canal level) on a DSL SPL-O-GRAM (b). Thresholds are shown, along with average normal hearing sensitivity, the long-term average speech spectrum (LTASS), the associated LTASS range of approximately 30 dB, the amplified LTASS targets (DSLs), and the RESR targets. The shaded area in the unamplified speech spectrum area is all that is audible to this hearing loss. These values are calculated and plotted by the computer program, based on pure-tone thresholds. The theoretical end result of a hearing aid fitting for this loss would amplify the speech spectrum to levels above the thresholds, and not exceed the RESR targets. (After Seewald, R. C., (1995), The desired sensation level (DSL) method for hearing aid fitting in infants and children, Phonak Focus, News/Ideas/High Technology/Acoustics Nr. 20).

Count The Dots AI

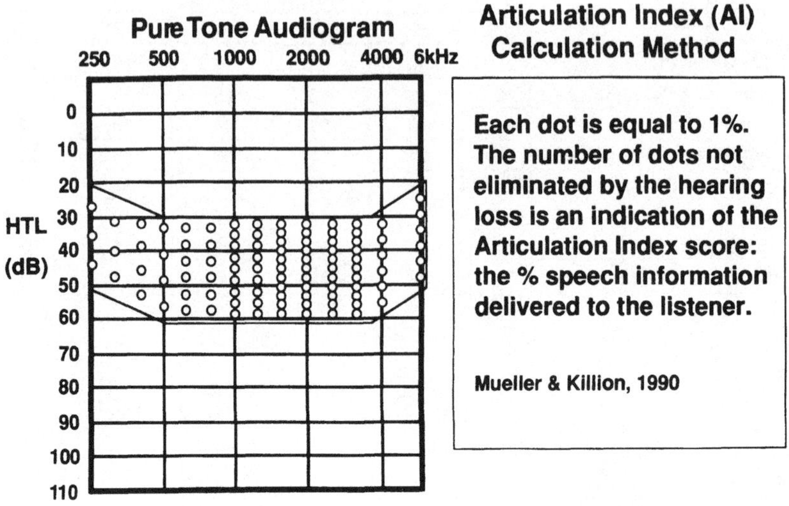

Fig. 17. "Count the Dots" Articulation Index calculation method. An explanation of its use is provided in the box. (Adapted from Mueller, H. G., and Killion, M. An easy method for calculating the articulation index. Hearing Journal, 1990:43:14–17.)

Articulation Index Basics

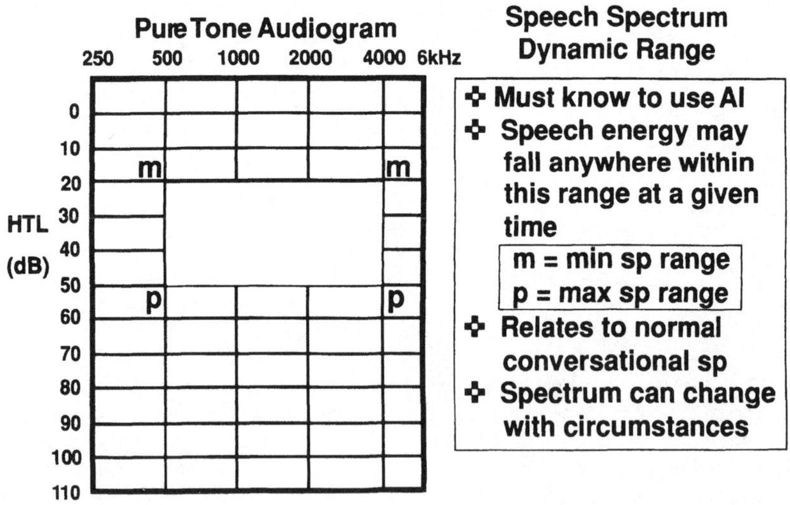

Fig. 18. Figures 18 through 24 are an attempt to explain the basics of the Articulation Index (AI) as modified for use for hearing aid evaluation. Note that other approaches will be somewhat different, but can be understood also, by referring to these series of Figures. This figure identifies the range and frequency distribution of the important speech spectrum dynamic range. (This series of Figures is adapted from Pavlovic, C. V. AI predictions of speech intelligibility in hearing aid selection, Asha, 1988:30;63–65.)

Hearing Loss and Dynamic Range

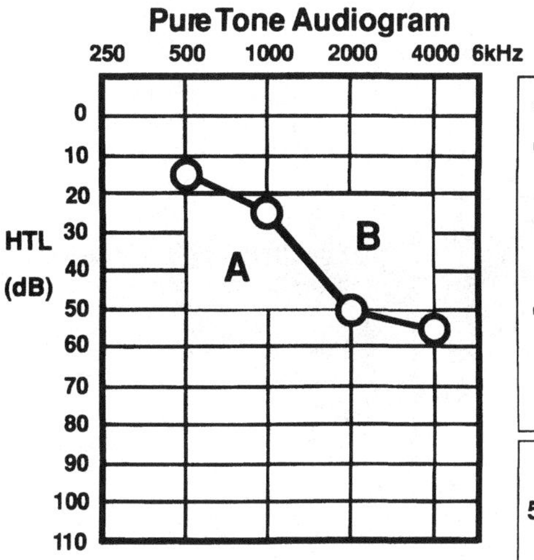

HL and Speech Dynamic Range

- HF Loss
- A = The part of the speech dynamic range that contributes to speech intelligibility
- B = Area lost due to the hearing loss. Does not contribute to speech intelligibility

Available DR in dB

500	1000	2000	4000 Hz
30	25	0	0

Fig. 19. Defining the available dynamic range (DR) in dB by comparing the audiogram to the speech spectrum dynamic range.

AI Calculation

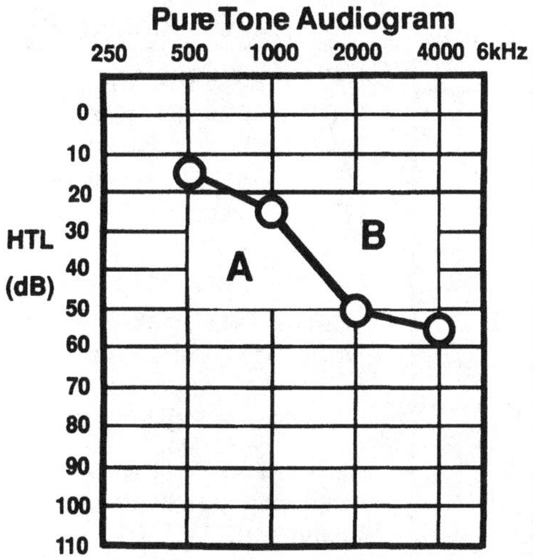

AI Calculation

- Add number of dB for the DR available at .5, 1, 2, and 4kHz
- Divide results by 120

Example

Freq.	DR (dB)
500	30
1000	25
2000	0
4000	0
	55

55/120 = 0.46
Speech information delivered to listener is 46%.

Fig. 20. Calculation of the AI by using the available DR information in dB. The total is divided by 120 (arrived at because four frequencies, each having a range of 30 dB, is 120). The unaided AI is 0.46, meaning that 46% of the speech information is being delivered to the listener.

Hearing Aid Improvement

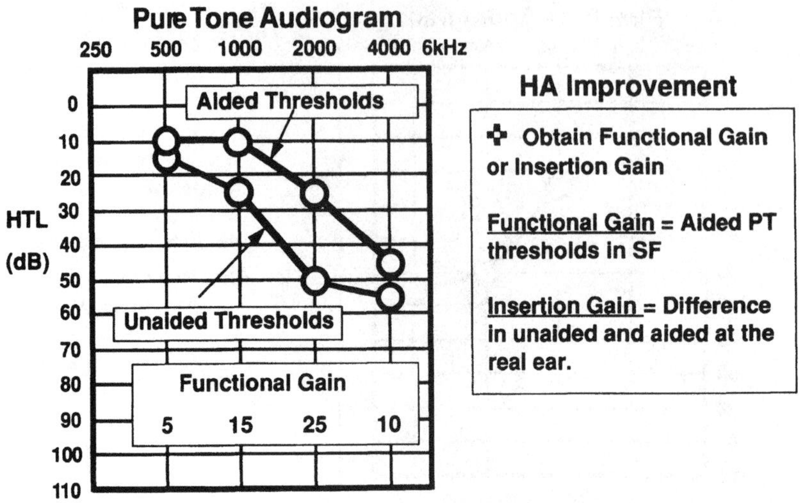

Fig. 21. Plotting of hearing aid improvement, whether by functional gain or insertion gain. The block at the bottom lists the functional gain improvements for the frequencies considered.

FG or IG Effect on Speech Spectra

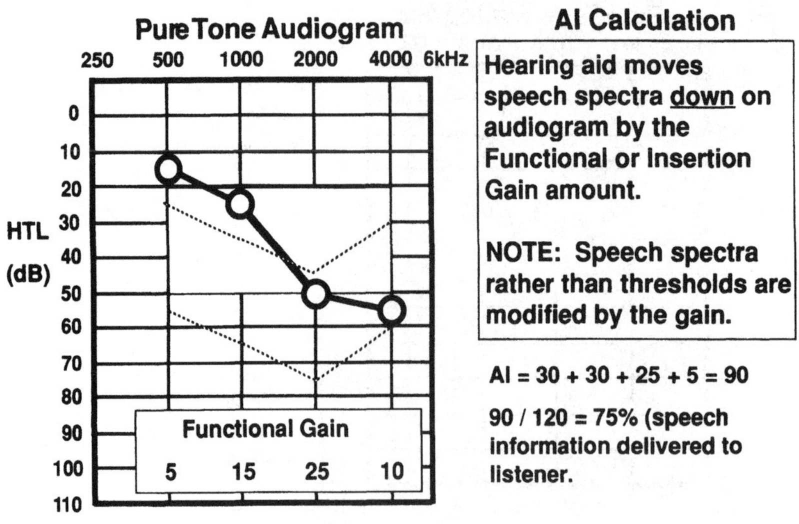

Fig. 22. The functional gain or insertion gain effect on the speech spectra. The effect is that the speech spectra, rather than thresholds, are modified by the gain. The speech spectra is moved *down* on the audiogram by the functional or insertion gain amount.

Table 6. Comparison of Articulation Index and speech intelligibility.

Articulation Index	Speech Intelligibility
1.00	100%
0.80	99%
0.60	98%
0.40	93%
0.20	50%
0.10	18%
0.05	8%

AI	% Sentence Understood	Speech Intelligibility
0.40–1.00	95–100	Excellent
0.20–0.40	80–95	Acceptable
0.10–0.20	30–80	Poor
0.00–0.10	0–30	None

scores in noise from those in quiet (word recognition scores are generally obtained in quiet because measuring these in noise is too time consuming and measurements have not been sufficiently reproducible). Still, because understanding in noise is critical, the Benefit Method takes this into consideration.

The test environment, instrumentation, and test procedure are as follows: The patient is surrounded by four loudspeakers creating a homogeneous noise field that simulates the difficult listening situation of the patient. The desired signal is presented by a separate loudspeaker located at a 45° angle to the patient (Figure 23). Test equipment is computerized, using damped wavetrain signals and PB (phonetically balanced) words as test stimuli, and includes components to measure the acoustics in the user's environment to use as the standard against which to test the benefit of amplification.

The test consists of four steps.

Step 1. Test word recognition in noise (no hearing aid) to assess the hearing problem. PB words are presented by the signal loudspeaker at 75 dB SPL (S/N + 10 dB). The purpose of this test is to assess the patient's everyday listening problem. This also provides some indication as to prognosis with amplification where several individuals are speaking at the same time.

Step 2. Perform an ***unaided*** threshold test using a controlled tone stimuli (damped wavetrain ad modum Victoreen, 1963)

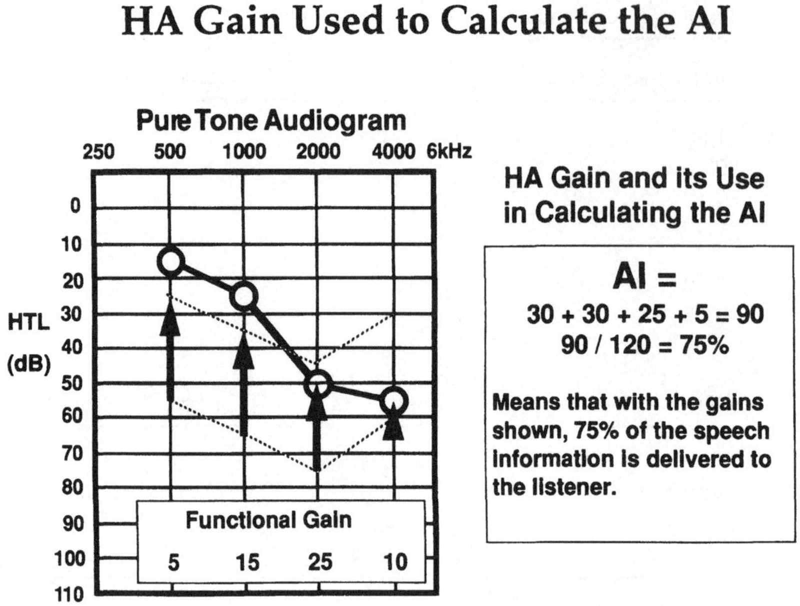

Fig. 23. This illustrates a calculated AI, but now with hearing aid use. The functional gain improvements from Figure 19 move the speech spectra down to the functional gain values obtained. The new DR values for the frequencies being evaluated are now 30, 30, 25, and 5 dB for the frequencies of 500, 1000, 2000, and 4000 Hz respectively. The aided AI is now 0.75, or indicating that 75% of the speech information is delivered to the listener as compared to the unaided AI of 46% in Figure 18.

attached to a Békésy audiometer, in speech-shaped noise. This provides more frequency specific information than speech audiometry. Threshold is assessed at 1000, 2000, 3000, and 4000 Hz in speech noise, unaided. The detection threshold is compared with the "normal" threshold from a reference group. The difference between the two thresholds (the patient's and the reference groups') is the minimum gain necessary to detect signals of a "normal" speech level (Figure 24). The test results, calculated by computer, show which sounds the hearing impaired individual must have amplified by the hearing aid.

Step 3. Perform an ***aided*** threshold test using the damped wave-train signal in speech noise. The hearing aid is set to the minimum gain necessary and the procedure of Step 2 is repeated. This shows to what extent the ear can make use of the amplification provided by the hearing aid. After normal threshold has been obtained (this may require some hearing aid adjustment), 10 dB reserve gain is recommended. This step identifies the optimum gain.

AI to Compare Hearing Aids

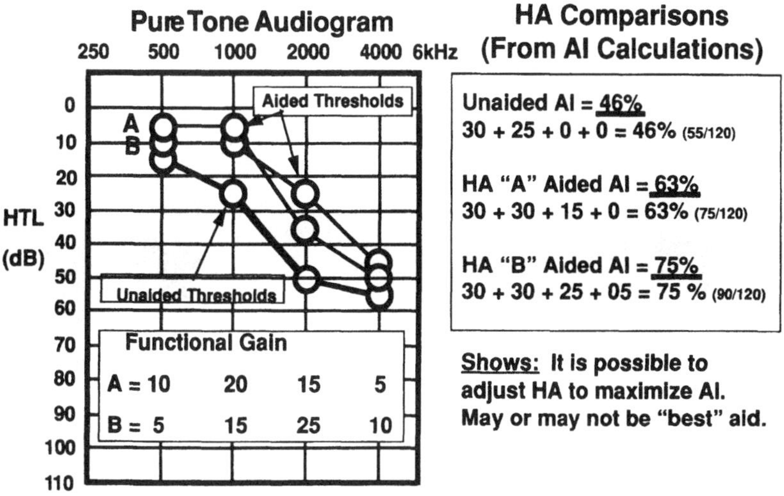

Fig. 24. This illustrates how the AI can be used to compare different hearing aids. As explained, this also shows that hearing aids can be adjusted to maximize the AI. Even if maximized, there is no evidence to suggest that the higher AI will provide the "best" hearing aid. What it does mean is that more speech information is available for the patient to use.

Step 4. Perform an aided word recognition score in speech noise with the aid that provides the best signal detection threshold. The difference between the results of Steps 1 and 4 is a measure of the benefit of the chosen hearing aid. The word recognition score shows the extent to which the patient's hearing aid can improve speech perception in noisy environments. This verifies the potential benefit of the prescribed hearing aid and its settings.

SUMMARY OF THRESHOLD-BASED PRESCRIPTIVE PROCEDURES

Threshold-based formulae, even when adjusted for volume control, do not provide equal target insertion gains, and may have differences as large as 20 dB at certain frequencies (Figure 25). In spite of this, what they have allowed for, is target frequency/gain selection, clinical verification of those target insertion gains, and the practice of frequency/gain modifications based on the verification results. Skinner et. al. (1982) suggest that even rather small changes in the overall gain, bandwidth, and frequency response in hearing aids produce results with varying degrees of effectiveness.

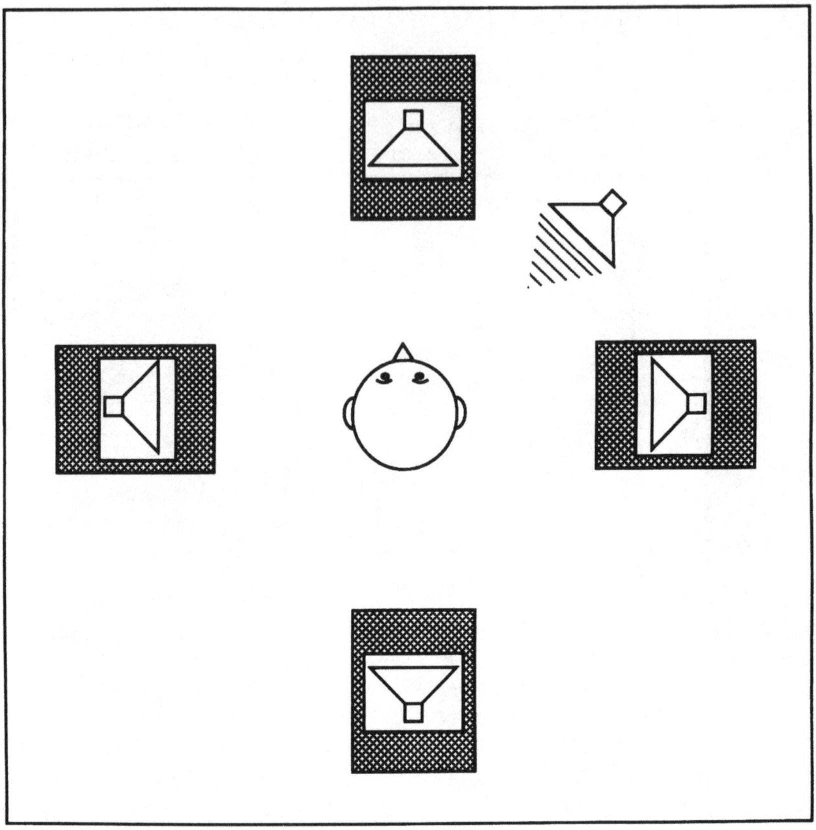

Fig. 25. Loudspeaker and room arrangement used for the "Benefit" method of hearing aid selection. Noise is presented through four loudspeakers, creating a difficult listening situation. The desired signal is presented by the separate loudspeaker at 1 meter distance and 45° to the patient. (Adapted from Svärd, I. and Spens, K. E., paper presented at the XXI International Conference on Audiology in Morioka, August 31–Sept. 4, 1992.)

And, although threshold-based formulae applied to linear circuitry hearing aids are the most frequently-used selection procedures today, advances in signal processing techniques and more complex hearing aid circuitry are expected to require new predictive approaches for the future.

PRESCRIPTIVE PROCEDURES BASED ON SUPRATHRESHOLD MEASURES OF LOUDNESS JUDGMENTS

The primary difference noted by advocates of suprathreshold-based procedures and threshold-based procedures involves the relationship between the two measures. Threshold-based advocates support the contention that knowledge of an individual's threshold will allow an accurate estimation of the MCL for that person. Suprathreshold-based advocates believe that the relationship between threshold and suprathreshold loudness measures such as MCL (most comfortable loudness), ULCL (upper limit of comfortable loudness), and LDL (loudness discomfort level) is **not** strong enough to permit accurate estimation of these loudness measures for individuals based on threshold data (Humes and Halling, 1994; Kamm, Dirks, and Mickey, 1978; Cox and Bisset, 1982). As a result, procedures are advocated that rely heavily on assessment of MCL to obtain gain at different frequencies, and in some cases, rely on audibility of the speech spectrum to set gain requirements. Regardless of whether MCL or some higher level measure at which sound becomes uncomfortably loud is used, both approaches attempt to place the spectrum of normal conversational speech at the MCL or preferred listening range of the patient. The belief is that amplification must be comfortable to listen to, or it will not be accepted by the patient.

Suprathreshold-based prescriptive procedures have achieved less popularity than threshold-based procedures primarily because: (a) the former are *believed* to take about twice as long, (b) manufacturers of hearing aids, especially custom-made devices, primarily request only pure-tone threshold data, (c) it is more difficult to obtain loudness judgments from children or patients having diminished intellectual capacity, and (d) test-retest variability is greater for MCL than for threshold (Humes and Halling, 1994). In spite of these shortcomings, Humes and Halling (1994) present compelling arguments in support of extended fuse of suprathreshold-based procedures. First, because the rationales for both suprathreshold and threshold methods are identical (amplify speech to MCL), an understanding of one will enhance our understanding of the other. Second, the hearing aid fitting process is undergoing radical changes related to (a) the emergence of programmable instruments, and (b) the use of real-ear probe microphone systems to validate fitting targets. If a goal is to provide amplification of speech at MCL, this can then be confirmed. Third, current threshold-based procedures were developed for hearing aids having linear amplifiers, but, many of the new non-linear amplifiers that allow gain and compression to be adjusted so that both soft and loud speech falls within the dynamic range, require verification that uses speech spectra at a number of overall levels (suprathreshold levels).

DSL METHOD? YES.

Direct MCL Judgments

These approaches either mirror the MCL curve or subtract from it the level of normal conversational speech to identify the gain required. The objective is for the hearing impaired to be fitted with gain characteristics that allow for amplifying speech to MCL. Watson and Knudsen (1940) and Kee (1972) were early proponents, recognizing that the practice of mirroring the pure-tone thresholds could easily result in exceeding the comfort level in the high frequencies.

Watson and Knudsen (1940). This was a first description for determining the response curve of a hearing aid. The procedure is designed to amplify speech to MCL. The curve is plotted as a mirror image of an equal loudness contour (Figure 26). A loudness match across octave frequencies is obtained to MCL at 1000 Hz.

Kee MCL Approach (1972). The procedure as outlined by Kee (1972) was to convert the pure-tone threshold in SPL so that it could be related more specifically to the hearing aid performance. All measurements are made under earphones. The critical elements of this procedure are as follows:

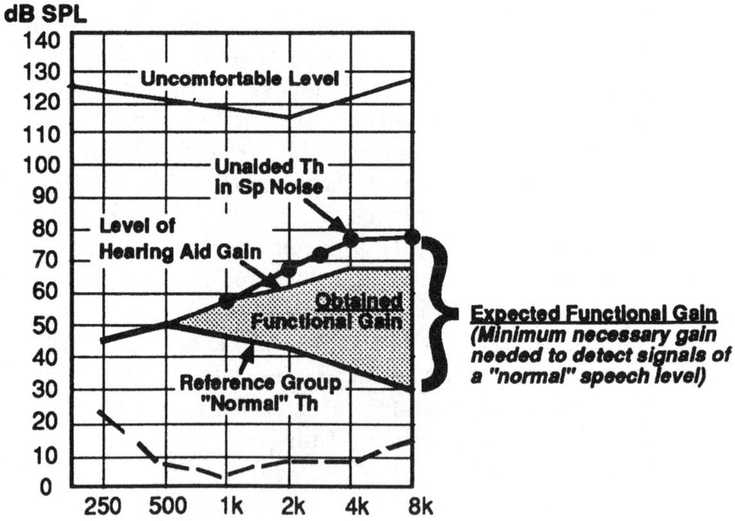

Fig. 26. Graphical representation showing the use of the "Benefit" method and the minimum necessary gain needed by the patient to obtain a "normal" threshold in noise. See text for explanation. (Adapted from Svärd, I. and Ahlner, B. H. The "benefit method" in the fitting of hearing aids. Bulletin of the American Authority Society, 1994;19:10–11,16.)

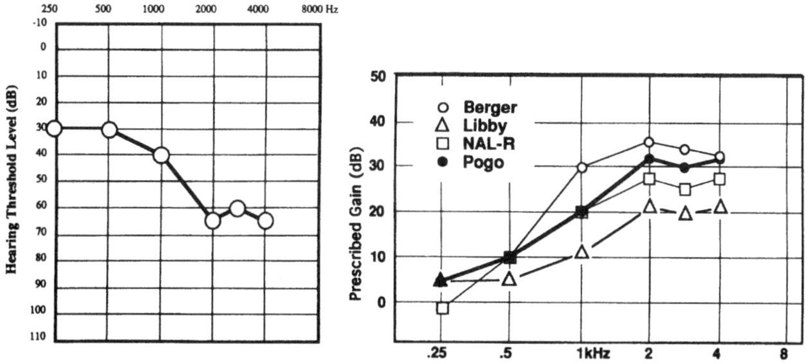

Fig. 27. Audiogram of a moderate hearing loss subjected to four different hearing aid fitting formulae, and the differences in prescribed insertion gains. (Adapted from McCandless, G. A. In Valente, M. (Editor) Strategies for Selecting and Verifying Hearing Aid Fittings. New York: Thieme Medical Publishers, Inc., 1994, p. 15.)

1. Measure hearing threshold levels and plot them using the numbers on the right side of the graph (Figure 27). By relating these to the numbers on the left side of the graph, it is possible to see easily how much sound pressure is required at each frequency for the ear to detect the test tone.
2. Three comfort levels are then determined at 500, 1000, 2000, and 3000 Hz, using pulsed pure tones. These are: too loud, comfortable, and too soft. (Too loud: a little too loud to be comfortable; too low to be comfortable—usually about 5 dB below the comfortable level; and comfortable—usually about 5 dB lower than too loud and 5 dB above too low). Collectively, these provide a range of comfortable listening levels that allow for defining the MCL more exactly. These data are plotted relative to the numbers on the left side of the chart, and should follow the curved lines when plotted for the frequency tested.
3. The gain required is the difference between the MCL and 65 dB at each frequency.

Shapiro MCL Approach (1975; 1976). Shapiro reported that a line bisecting a patient's pure-tone threshold and LDL occurred at about the MCL for the frequencies of 2000 and 4000 Hz. However, at the lower frequencies the MCL occurred at higher levels than the mid point. As a result of this, he recommended the following direct MCL procedure, even though the bases for it was formed from information obtained from bisection data:

1. MCL and LDL were determined for pulsed narrow band noise in octave frequencies from 250 through 4000 Hz, including

3000 Hz. MCL was defined as the level 5 dB below; the lowest intensity level described as being "too loud" 2 of 3 times. Using these data, he determined the ear with the largest dynamic range (DR) and highest LDL and used these to determine the aidable ear.

2. He subtracted 60 dB (customary input SPL for measuring hearing aid gain) from the MCLs at 1000, 2000, 3000, and 4000 Hz, using the resultant difference to determine the hearing aid gain required. At 500 Hz gain was determined by subtracting 10 dB, and at 250 15 dB was subtracted from the gain prescribed at 1000 Hz, assuming that less gain is required at the lower frequencies.
3. He then added 10 dB reserve gain at each frequency.

CID MCL Approach (1982, 1988). The Central Institute for the Deaf (CID) approach reported by Skinner, et. al., (1982) advocates amplifying the long-term average speech level (root mean square overall level of 65 dB SPL), to MCL. To use the procedure, it is first necessary to understand the "perceived speech spectrum" that amplification is intended to reach.

The assumption is made that average conversational speech should be amplified close to the listener's MCL. Because a single contour used to represent MCL is somewhat arbitrary, a graphical representation of the speech range and of average speech levels is shown in Figure 28 and plotted in SPL. This shows the shaded speech range (energy varies over approximately a 30 dB range from about 50 to 70 dB SPL), and average speech levels. At the lower end of the speech range, only about 1% of speech energy is not present (1st percentile), and the upper end of the range represents the 90th percentile (90% of speech energy should be detected. The curve identified as "average speech levels" indicates the 50th percentile, or the level at which 50 percent of the speech energy falls below and above. The use of MCL in specific frequency regions has been chosen as the criterion for estimating the level(s) at which speech cues will provide maximum discrimination ability. This is believed to reflect the listener's loudness growth.

The procedure is rather complicated and requires small computer capability. A complete presentation is beyond the scope of this Chapter and readers are referred to the original articles. Still, the following partial description is provided to allow readers some of the basic philosophy. Although this procedure utilizes both threshold and suprathreshold measurements, it is considered an MCL-based approach. Basic steps in the procedure, as summarized from Skinner, et. al. (1982) are as follows:

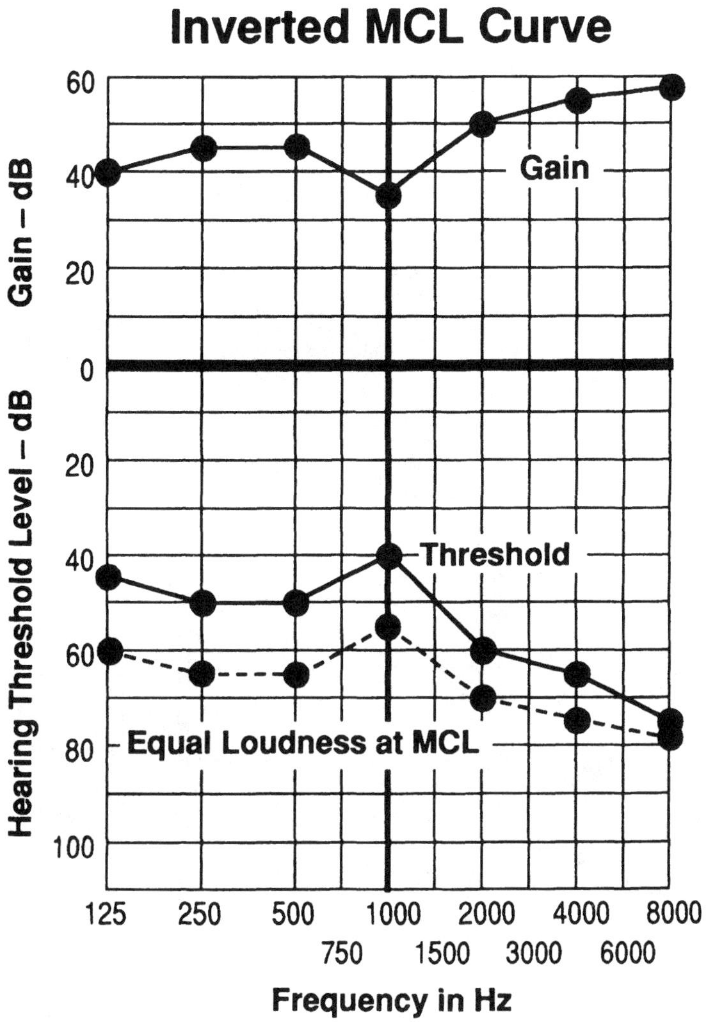

Fig. 28. Watson and Knudsen method for hearing aid response selection based on direct MCL judgments. The gain or response curve is a mirror image of an equal loudness contour at MCL.

1. The listener's auditory area is determined. Earphone delivered pulsed pure-tone threshold, MCL and LDL are obtained for audiometric frequencies from 250 to 6000 Hz, and later adjusted to reflect the condition in which a person listens to speech in everyday life (an unobstructed sound field environment).
2. The desired functional gain is then determined. A sample patient's auditory area (Figure 29) is shown in relation to the

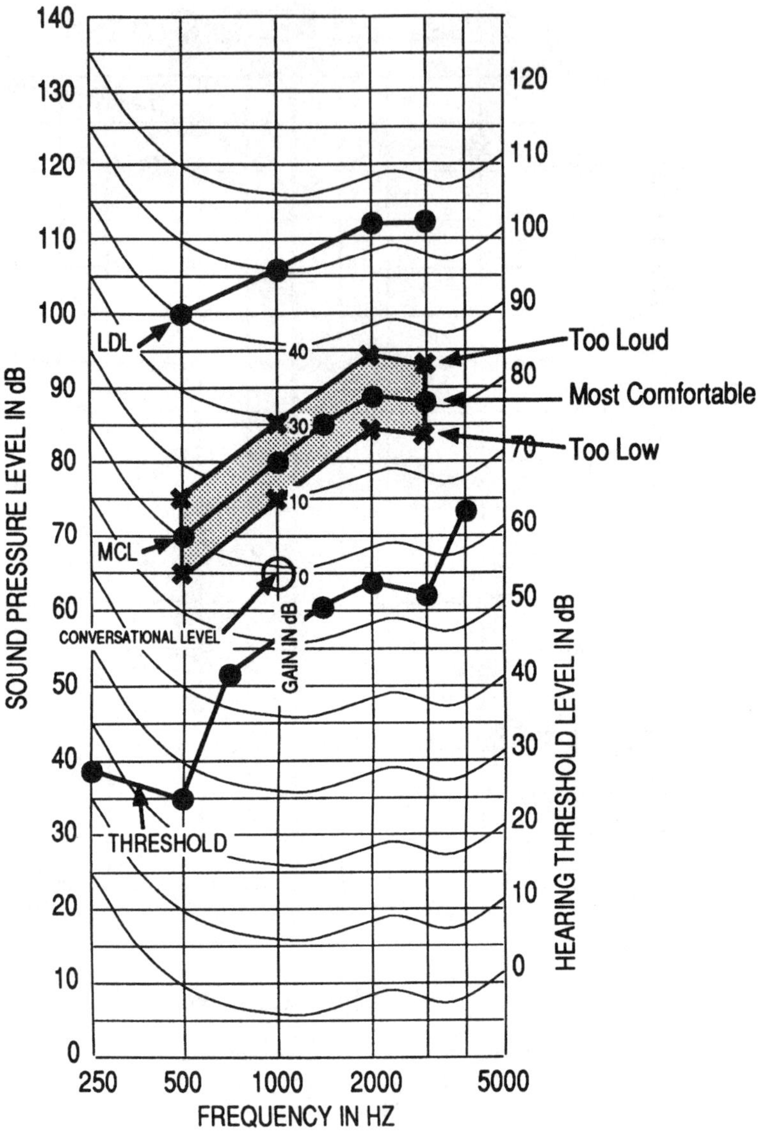

Fig. 29. Estimated hearing aid gain for various frequencies using direct MCL judgments (after Kee, 1992).

contour of average speech levels (unaided speech) described in Figure 28, but shown plotted in HTL in the sound field, rather than in SPL. Note that the unaided speech contour is above threshold (heard) only at 250 Hz, and is far below the MCL range. To amplify speech in the region of the MCL range, the functional gain denoted by the numbers on the vertical lines on the right-hand panel are required. The differences of approximation to MCL (dotted line) are an attempt to establish *loudness* relations similar to those received by normal hearing listeners. At 250 Hz amplification is reduced to a level that brings the speech spectrum to a midpoint between threshold and MCL in an attempt to reduce amplified low-frequency background noise. Subsequent modifications (Skinner, 1988) have called for amplification adjustments such that the only frequency to follow the initial amplification prescription to MCL is 500 Hz. The modified procedure advocates amplifying speech to halfway between threshold and MCL for 250 and 6000 Hz; 500 Hz to MCL; 1000 AND 2000 Hz to 90% of the range between threshold and MCL; and 2000 and 4000 Hz to 80% of the range between threshold and MCL. Conversions of thresholds obtained under earphones to sound-field thresholds are made as required.

3. Desired functional gain and actual functional gain are then compared. A hearing aid is chosen that, when coupled with an appropriate earmold, will provide approximately the desired functional gain and SSPL90. The listener adjusts the gain to running speech presented at 65 dB SPL so that maximum clarity and comfort is achieved. At this setting, the actual functional gain is recorded and then plotted against the desired functional gain (Figure 30A). Figure 30B shows the actual functional gain and desired functional gain differences, and Figure 30C shows the amount by which the listener's aid does not provide the desired functional gain.
4. Because the listener's auditory area (as measured on the head) is intended to be expressed in reference to the output of the hearing aid in a 2-cc coupler, an unobstructed-field to hearing-aid-microphone transfer function is obtained. This provides the difference between the level at the microphone in the hearing aid test box and that at the microphone port of the aid when worn on the head. This value is added to the patient's unaided thresholds, MCLs and LDLs.
5. Because the *actual* coupler gain of the hearing aid was measured with tubing on an artificial ear, to relate this measurement to the *desired* coupler gain, the difference between the two is added to the coupler gain to obtain the desired coupler gain.
6. The SSPL90 selection goal is to limit this level to just below the patient's LDL contour. The accuracy with which this can

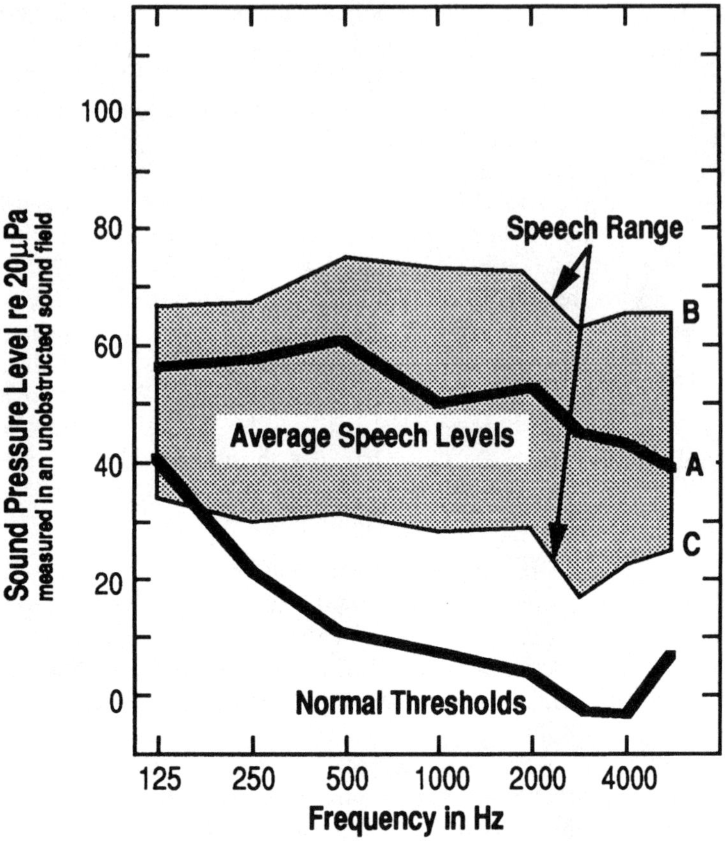

Fig. 30. Speech range (shaded area) and average speech levels (50th percentile) plotted in SPL, relative to normal hearing thresholds. This shows the approximately 30 dB range of normal speech energy, and also the level at which 50 percent of the speech energy falls below and above. This understanding forms an important basis for understanding the CID MCL approach to hearing aid fitting. (Adapted from Skinner, M. W., Pascoe, D. P., Miller, J. D., and Popelka, G. R.) Measurements to determine the optimal placement of speech energy within the listener's auditory area: a basis for selecting amplification characteristics. In Studebaker, G. A., and Bess, F. H. (editors) The Vanderbilt Hearing-Aid Report, Upper Darby: 1982 Monographs in Contemporary Audiology, p. 162, 1982).

be met can be determined by expressing the patient's LDL with reference to the output of the hearing aid. Subtract the functional gain from the unaided threshold, MCL and LDL values. These new values represent the "aided" levels at the microphone of the hearing aid. (This value can also be expressed in terms of the unobstructed field calibration. See original text).

The following criteria are used for selecting the desired SSPL90: (a) If the LDL is 18 dB or greater above the average MCL range at a given frequency, select 15 dB above MCL as the SSPL90. This allows linear amplification of the upper 15 dB of the 30 dB speech energy range, and still limits higher levels that may cause fatigue. (b) When there is insufficient range between MCL and LDL to allow this level of SSPL90, a clinical compromize can be made. Usually limit the output to 3 dB below LDL, regardless of the range. To do this, adjust the hearing aid in the test box so that the frequency with the SSPL90 closest to LDL is 3 dB below it at the output in the 2-cc coupler. A test to determine whether the SSPL90 is adjusted properly is to present narrow- and broad-bands of noise at intense levels that are likely to occur fairly often in everyday life (80–90 dB SPL). If the patient reports these to be loud, but acceptable, the SSPL90 is appropriately adjusted. If too loud, reduce the SSPL90. If the sounds become distorted before becoming too loud, the SSPL90 could be raised, or compression amplification considered.

Indirect MCL Judgments Based on Pure Tone Thresholds

Seiler (1971). This approach was one of the first formulae that considered the notable difference between hearing results obtained in a free field situation and those obtained when the ear is covered by an earphone or when an earmold is placed in the ear (Seiler, 1971). The resultant formula considered MCL, the ear resonance, the contribution of different frequencies to speech recognition, and the amount of gain required by the hearing aid. The formula assumed MCL values based on pure-tone levels (believing pure-tone MCL too difficult to obtain). The calculation for gain by frequency follows:

$$\mathbf{Gain = (TH_{HL} + MCL_{c} + ER_{dB}) \times Discrim_{\%} + 1/2(Gain)}$$

Where:

TH_{HL} = Threshold in HL (measured at frequencies of .5, 1, 2, 3 and 4 kHz)

MCL_{c} = Calculated MCL by adding 15 dB to each pure-tone threshold

ER_{dB} = Ear resonance values for those frequencies Weiner and Ross (1946)

$Discrim_{\%}$ = Weighted speech discrimination contributions for those frequencies (Fowler and Sabine, 1947). Weighting for speech discrimination contribution is

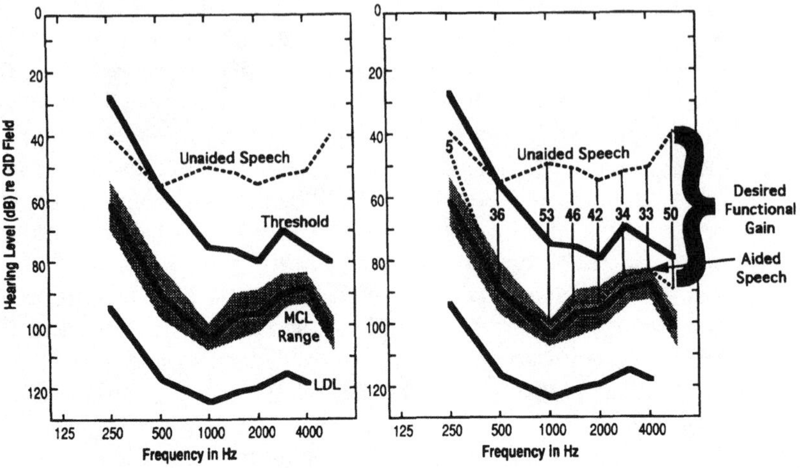

Fig. 31. CID MCL method to determination of desired functional gain. The left panel shows a listener's auditory area in HTL. Only at 250 Hz is the unaided speech contour heard. To amplify speech in the region of the MCL range, the functional gain denoted by the numbers on the vertical lines on the right-hand panel are required. See text for additional explanation. (Adapted from Skinner, M. W., Pascoe, D. P., Miller, J. D., and Popelka, G. R. Measurements to determine the optimal placement of speech energy within the listener's auditory area: a basis for selecting amplification characteristics. In Studebaker, G. A., and Bess, F. H. (editors) The Vanderbilt Hearing-Aid Report, Upper Darby: 1982 Monographs in Contemporary Audiology, p. 162, 1982).

512 Hz = 15%; 1024 Hz = 25%; 2048 Hz = 30%; 2896 Hz = 25%; and 4096 Hz = 5%, for a total of 100%.

Gain = HL thresholds at .5, 1, 2, 3, and 4 kHz with 15 dB added to arrive at a generalized MCL value for each frequency. These values are summed, and multiplied by 10% to provide a gain figure. This is then multiplied by .5 (the one-half gain rule) to arrive at the ½ gain figure (Figure 31) used in the formula.

Total conductive hearing losses required slight modifications in circuitry. Testing of the fitting included the use of cold running speech in quiet and noise (varying levels of the latter), checking VC reserve when the aid is used at MCL, and word recognition testing at MCL. These tests were to help determine if possible modifications should be made in the earmold, receiver, tubing, etc.

Indirect MCL Methods Based on the Dynamic Range (Bisection Approaches)

These techniques use audiometric threshold data in a suprathreshold prediction manner to relate the aided expectations to most comfortable loudness (MCL in SPL). Examples of the bisection approaches are provided by Balbi (1935), Wallenfels (1967), Bragg (1977), and by Cox (1983, 1985, and 1988). While vacations in the approaches exist, the basic attempt is to obtain an MCL response curve by bisecting the differences between the threshold of hearing and the threshold of discomfort, minus the input level for speech. Bisection techniques make the assumption that optimal hearing is close to MCL. However, bisection is not always the exact midpoint between the thresholds of sensitivity and discomfort. For example, in Figure 33, adapted from Wallenfels (1967), bisection is determined by the midpoints of a line drawn between the thresholds at 1000 Hz and 4000 Hz and extended to the lower limits of the response range. Other approaches use even different criteria.

Balbi (1935). This approach, patented in 1935, measured both threshold and LDL in SPL and then bisected them, making the assumption that this bisection would approximate the MCL and provide the shape of the amplification curve. Gain was determined as the dB SPL required to reach MCL at each frequency.

Wallenfels Bisection Approach (1967). The bisection procedure as suggested by Wallenfels (1967) is outlined as follows (Figure 32):

1. Obtain the pure-tone audiogram. Convert these data to SPL and plot them on a sound pressure graph.
2. Obtain the UCL using narrow bands of noise (or other stimuli). Convert these thresholds to SPL and plot them on the graph. The intent was to stay closer to the threshold curve if the dynamic range was narrow.
3. Plot the optimum listening level. Locate the midpoint between the threshold of sensitivity and the threshold of discomfort at 1000 Hz and also at 4000 Hz. Draw a line which bisects these two points and which extends below 1000 Hz. If the audiogram indicates a steep slope, the drawn line continues downward below 1000 Hz with that slope. However, if the slope between 1000 and 4000 Hz is less than 8 dB per octave, the recommended curve should have a slope below 1000 Hz between 8 and 10 dB per octave.
4. Subtract 65 dB from the optimum hearing levels at the various frequencies to determine the gain at each frequency. An

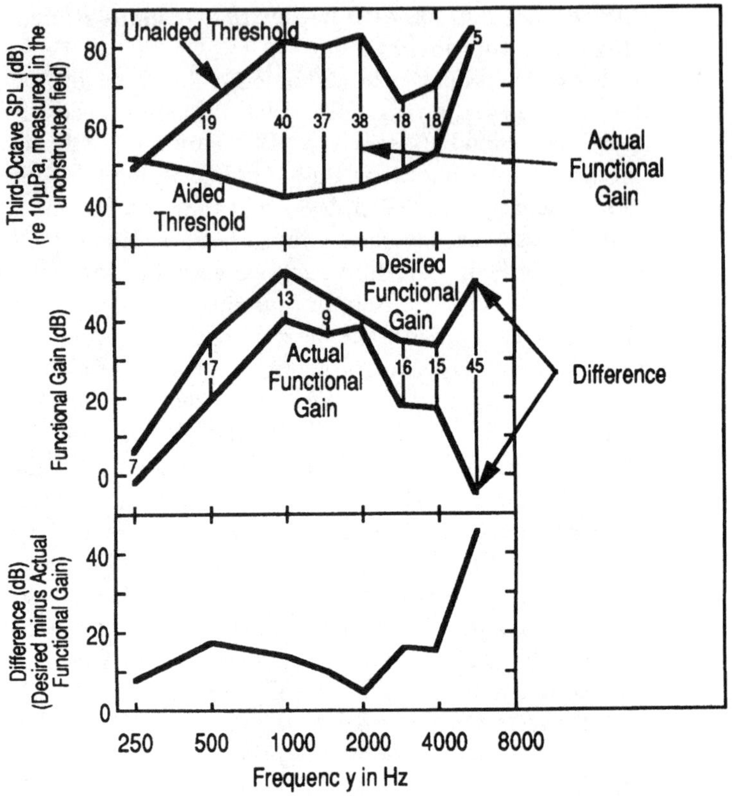

Fig. 32. CID MCL procedure comparing the actual functional gain (top panel), the desired functional gain compared to the actual functional gain (center panel), and the amount by which the patient's aid does not provide the desired functional gain (lower panel). (Adapted from Skinner, M. W., Pascoe, D. P., Miller, J. D., and Popelka, G. R. Measurements to determine the optimal placement of speech energy within the listener's auditory area: a basis for selecting amplification characteristics. In Studebaker, G. A., and Bess, F. H. (editors) The Vanderbilt Hearing-Aid Report, Upper Darby: 1982 Monographs in Contemporary Audiology, p. 162, 1982).

assumption is made that normal conversational speech is 65 dB at all frequencies. (In fact, this is not true, and accommodations can be made to more accurately reflect the actual inputs of speech at the different frequencies.)

Wallenfels assumed that the optimal hearing level was comparable to the patient's MCL. This was determined by taking hearing aids, as worn, and measuring their performance. He found that the optimum (predicted) level and the actual (measured) listening level were the same when patients were satisfied with their hearing aids, and were not the same when they were not satisfied with their aids.

Bragg (1977). This procedure defines a desired listening level (DLL) as being between "too-soft-to-hear" and "too-loud-to-bear." This is determined to be the amplification target, using a speech shaped 70 dB overall input signal. When applied to accompanying "hearing aid selector" charts, this overall level represents 60, 61, 58, 54, and 46 dB SPLs at octave frequencies from 250 through 4000 Hz. The listener's dynamic range is bisected, and the target gain is established as halfway between threshold and LDL from 1000 to 8000 Hz, and one-third between threshold and LDL at 250 and 500 Hz. If LDL is not obtainable, the stapedius reflex level is substituted. Two hearing aid selection charts allow for plotting of threshold and LDL (or stapedius reflex) data; one that allows for plotting in HTL and the other in SPL, with see-through overlays that allow easy comparison between the two reference levels. The goals of the selection procedure are to select or adjust hearing aids that best meet these criteria:

a. An SSPL90 from 250 through 4000 Hz that approaches at each frequency, but does not exceed the LDL.
b. Gain at each frequency should be sufficient to raise average speech to the DDL, plus a reasonable reserve. Between 5–15 dB reserve gain is added depending on the type of aid and conductive involvement (one-fourth the conductive loss). These reserve gain figures can be added to each frequency when selecting the hearing aid, or by setting the hearing aid volume control 5 to 15 dB below maximum when adjusting the aid.

MSUv3 (1983, 1985, 1988). This procedure, developed and modified by Cox (1983, 1985, 1988) at Memphis State University (MSU) over a number of years, bisects the listener's dynamic range and establishes the ***target gain*** to where the speech spectrum (a 70 dB SPL raised voice level) is amplified halfway between threshold and the measured or calculated ULCL (upper limit of comfortable loudness). Having evolved through versions 1.0 and 2.0, version 3.0 added a provision that prevents the target level for amplified speech at any frequency from being higher than ULCL-15 dB. This generally affects high-frequency gain and was added to manage the narrowed listening range (less than 30 dB) between SPHL and ULCL that occurs with such losses. A second provision allows the prescriptive procedure to be used based on threshold measures only, if needed. The procedure prescribes gain and SSPL90 for OTE (over-the-ear) and ITE (in-the-ear) hearing aids.

The procedure calls for obtaining hearing thresholds at several frequencies in SPL (HLSP) and loudness perception measurements of the upper limit of comfortable loudness (ULCL—also in SPL) for ⅓-octave noise bands or warble tones. The program has been designed to prescribe hearing aid gain and SSPL90 based on: (a) sound-field thresholds only, (b) earphone thresholds, (c) sound-field thresholds and ULCLs, or (d) any of the previous, singly or in combination with each other. Instrument selection is best done by computer, although hand calculations or a table look-up method can be used (Table 7), with the values used in the equations in Table 8. The prescription can include: (a) coupler gain at use volume control setting, (b) SSPL90, (c) aided sound-field threshold targets, and (d) insertion gain at each tested frequency. The prescription provides use gain, and not full-on gain values. Cox recommends full-on gain to be 10–15 dB greater than use gain at each frequency.

SSPL90 is prescribed at a level estimated to be high enough to avoid significant clipping of the speech signal under all likely listening conditions (12 dB added to the ULCL to account for speech peaks), and when adjusted to the highest level likely to be chosen by the listener. Because this prescriptive procedure does not specifically measure the listener's tolerance for amplified sound (it is predicted based on the measured or calculated ULCL, which is lower than the LDL), tolerance to loud, amplified sounds should be discussed with the client in follow-up interviews and adjusted accordingly.

ULCLs can be predicted from SPHL data rather than measured directly. Table 9 gives the equations for estimation of ULCL (dB SPL) from SPHL (dB SPL) for supra-aural or insert earphones. The equations can be used also for ⅓-octave band and warble tone stimuli. The error estimate for this prediction is on the order of 7–8 dB, and therefore, will often involve some inaccuracy, but has the advantage of being useful with clients who are unable to perform loudness judgments tasks. Cox (1988) also states that the highest level likely to be chosen by a listener for amplified speech is somewhat lower than the contour of ULCLs determined with NB noise or warble tone stimuli. Therefore, this level is now estimated at ULCL-5 dB plus some other correction factors. The reader is referred to Cox (1988) for a more complete explanation.

SUMMARY OF BISECTION TECHNIQUES

Bisection techniques that attempt to place amplified speech at a midpoint between threshold and some upper limit of the dynamic

Table 7. MSUv3 equations to calculate hearing instrument prescription.

EQUATIONS TO CALCULATE HEARING INSTRUMENT PRESCRIPTION (MSUv3)

(numbers in parentheses refer to columns in Table 8)

Gain for OTE Instrument

(a) Supra-aural earphone pretest:
Gain(HA − 1) = 1/2ULCL + 1/2SPHL − (1) − (2) + (5) + (6)*
or
Gain(HA − 1) = ULCL − 15 − (1) − (2) + (5) + (6)**

(b) Insert earphone pretest:
Gain(HA − 2) = 1/2ULCL + 1/2SPHL − (1) − (2)*
or
Gain(HA − 2) = ULCL − 15 − (1) − (2)**

*Gain option 1
**Gain option 2

Use gain option giving lower (smaller) value

Gain for ITE Instrument
Gain = [OTE gain(HA − 1)] − (3)

SSPL90 for OTE Instrument

(a) Supra-aural earphone pretest:
SSPL90 = ULCL − 5 + (4) + (5) + (6)

(b) Insert earphone pretest:
SSPL90 = ULCL − 5 + (4)

SSPL90 for ITE Instrument
SSPL90 = ULCL − 5 + (4) + (5) + (6)

Aided Sound Field Threshold (ASFT) Goals (ITE and OTE)
ASFT goal = (1) − 1/2ULCL + 1/2SPHL (for gain option 1)
or
ASFT goal = (1) + 15 − ULCL + SPHL (for gain option 2)

Estimation of Unaided Sound Field Threshold (USFT) from SPHL

(a) Supra-aural earphone pretest:
USFT = SPHL + (5) + (7)

(b) Insert earphone pretest:
USFT = SPHL + (6) + (7)

Insertion Gain (IG)
IG = USFT − ASFT goal

Estimation of SPHL from USFT

(a) Supra-aural earphone:
SPHL = USFT − (7) − (5)

(b) Insert earphone:
SPHL = USFT − (7) + (6)

Table 8. Values (dB) used in the equations of Table 7.

Freq. (kHz)	(1) Speech Spectrum	(2) OTE Head Baffle	(3) ITE re. OTE Input	(4) 1% Peak re. Long Term RMS	(5) Eardrum re. 6cc Coupler	(6) 2cc Coupler re. Eardrum	(7) FF re. Eardrum
0.25	60.0	0.5	1.0	17	−7.8	−4.0	−1.3
0.5	62.0	1.0	1.0	20	1.6	−4.0	−1.8
0.8	56.5	0.75	1.5	22	2.4	−4.0	−3.0
1.0	55.0	0.0	1.0	23	2.8	−5.0	−2.5
1.6	52.0	1.0	1.0	24	4.0	−7.5	−6.5
2.5	48.0	2.0	4.5	25	7.1	−9.5	−16.5
4.0	46.0	3.0	6.0	28	5.1	−12.0	−14.0
6.3	45.5	0.0	3.0	28	3.0	−14.0	−6.5

Table 9. Regression equations for estimation of ULCL (dB SPL) from SPHL (dB SPL) for supra-aural or insert earphone

ULCL (250)	= .37 (SPHL) + 85
ULCL (500)	= .25 (SPHL) + 83
ULCL (800)	= .45 (SPHL) + 73
ULCL (1000)	= .44 (SPHL) + 71
ULCL (1600)	= .41 (SPHL) + 69
ULCL (2500)	= .37 (SPHL) + 69
ULCL (4000)	= .39 (SPHL) + 68
ULCL (6300)	= .39 (SPHL) + 68

range may be flawed because although they might visually bisect the dynamic range, they may not bisect the dynamic range in loudness perception. This is understood with the recognition that loudness grows more rapidly at lower sensation levels than at higher sensation levels for both normal and impaired ears. Additionally, bisection procedures tend to under amplify high frequency losses (in the high frequencies). This problem arises when the assumption is made that the speech level at all frequencies is 65 dB (or 70 dB) SPL. Measurements show that long-term average speech spectra of high frequencies have much less energy (35 to 45 dB) than low frequencies (65 dB).

MCL SUMMARY

Differences in prescriptions among seven direct and indirect MCL methods compared by Humes and Halling (1994) show that the differences are generally greater for a rising with frequency sensorineural impairment and for the milder degrees of impairment across all audiometric configurations. The greatest differences among methods in their recommendations appear in average overall gain and low-frequency slope with little difference observed in high-frequency slope. From this comparison, these authors concluded that there are no data to clearly support the superiority of one MCL prescriptive method over another in terms of the frequency of successful fittings or the magnitude of success achieved in individual cases. They suggest that it may well be that both MCL and threshold methods have appropriate places in the hearing aid fitting process. It has been suggested (Humes and Hackett, 1990), for example, that it might be desirable initially to adjust a hearing aid for the wearer to maximize listening comfort (i.e., near MCL) or sound quality. Then it may be necessary to adjust the frequency-gain response of the instrument gradually to match more closely the response designed to maximize speech recognition.

COMFORTABLE LOUDNESS PRESCRIPTION PROCEDURES BASED ON A RANGE OF COMFORTABLE LOUDNESS

This category includes procedures that identify a **range** of comfortable loudness and use this in a variety of ways as a goal for hearing aid amplification.

Otometry (1963). This hearing aid selection procedure is based on the principle of determining a range of comfortable loudness, and of providing aided performance to return the hearing to a given equal loudness contour at 72 dB SPL. This procedure is the precursor and provides the foundation upon which loudness scaling hearing aid selection procedures are based. If the measured ear deviates from the normal flat 72 dB most comfortable loudness pressure curve (MCLP) by more than 6 dB, the ear should be considered for prosthetic correction.

The concept of fitting to loudness judgments, termed otometry (a "physical" science rather than a "behavioral" science), was developed by Victoreen in 1963. Otometry is based on the realization that 2-cc coupler data (used to measure standard hearing aid performance characteristics) is not related to real ear performance, nor to the audiogram in HTL, and hence, approaches all measurement procedures in sound pressure (including threshold and all loudness judgment data). Otometry attempts to return to the scientific method of expression, measurement, and numerical notation, and to move away from the behavioral approach that had found its way into audiometric measurement, but seemingly was not appropriate for hearing aid selection. Otometry is an attempt to determine how much hearing function is "left," not how much has been "lost," as does audiometry. The stimulus used for measurements is a damped wavetrain signal. A damped wavetrain signal was selected because it can be scientifically explained, is truly measurable, makes it feasible to obtain free-field measurements under practical conditions due to a reduction in standing wave or reflection problems, and yet takes the place of speech. The signal is considered as a pure-tone burst having a constant number of cycles regardless of the frequency of the signal. The signal was made to decay rapidly or fade out, much like speech, instead of coming to an abrupt end.

The principles of otometry do not in themselves tell how to prescribe a hearing instrument. They do, however, explain how an ear functions with a hearing instrument (Victoreen, 1973). As such, the procedure may function best when measuring the "outcome" of the fitting. Still, when performed in conjunction with a measured laboratory standard hearing instrument fitted with a custom-made earmold, a prescription for a hearing instrument for a given ear may be obtained using a substitution method (Melen, 1978; Hartenstein, 1978). As a predictor of the amplification required, otometry tends to suggest heavily high-frequency hearing aid characteristics. Therefore, it may lend itself better to post-fitting evaluation. However, if used as a prescriptive procedure for hearing aid amplification, Figure 35a through 33f illustrates the graphing and relationships of the measures required:

1. Measure the unaided free-field most comfortable loudness pressures (MCLP); identified also as the central loudness-pressure locus (CLPL) for each ear separately (other ear occluded, if necessary). The patient is seated at a distance of 28 inches at zero degree axis with the free-field speaker which presents the signals. MCLP is defined as the bracketed midpoint of loudness sensation between "loud" and "soft." Logically, this may be thought of as the most comfortable loudness pressure (although not defined subjectively by the listener.) The listener is asked to point to a card that has the words printed on it, "Loud," or "Soft." (Most individuals have a "comfortable" loudness range of about ±4 dB). The data are plotted on an Otometric chart in SPL from 250 to 6000 Hz (Figure 33c). If the measured ear departs from the normal flat 72 dB MCLP curve significantly (usually more than 6 dB), it is possible to consider the ear for prosthetic correction.
2. Measure the aided free-field "MCLP" for each ear separately (Figure 35c), with the other ear occluded, if necessary. A laboratory test aid (a normal hearing aid whose parameters can be modified as necessary by the manufacturer to fulfill the prescriptive measurements), with actual earmold coupling, is placed on the ear and the gain control of the hearing aid is adjusted (referenced) to MCLP for a 72 dB damped wavetrain signal at 1000 Hz (35d). Following this, signals at other frequencies are presented and plotted also for their most comfortable range and most comfortable loudness (35d), but with the volume control maintained at the referenced setting. (Measurements made with damped wavetrain signals have shown that normals and aided pathological ears respond at loudness

Seiler Formula Calculations (1971)

Frequency in Hz	500	1000	2000	3000	4000
Threshold (example)	45	45	60	70	80
+MCL	15	15	15	15	15
+ER dB	6	8	13	19	16
Sub Total	66	68	88	104	111
X Discrim. %	.15	.25	.30	.25	.05
Sub Total	9.90	17.00	26.40	26.00	5.55
+1/2 Gain	18.75	18.75	18.75	18.75	18.75
Response	**28.65**	**35.75**	**45.15**	**44.75**	**24.30**

MCL Th + 15 dB	
500 Hz	60
1000 Hz	60
2000 Hz	75
3000 Hz	85
4000 Hz	95
Total	375
X10%	
Gain	37.5
1/2 Gain	**18.75**

Fig. 33. Seiler indirect MCL hearing aid gain selection formula based on pure-tone thresholds. The formula considered, MCL, the ear resonance, the contribution of different frequencies to speech recognition, and the amount of gain required by the hearing aid. See text for explanation. (Adapted from Seiler, J. A. A formula for fitting hearing aids, The Hearing Dealer, March 1971, p. 19).

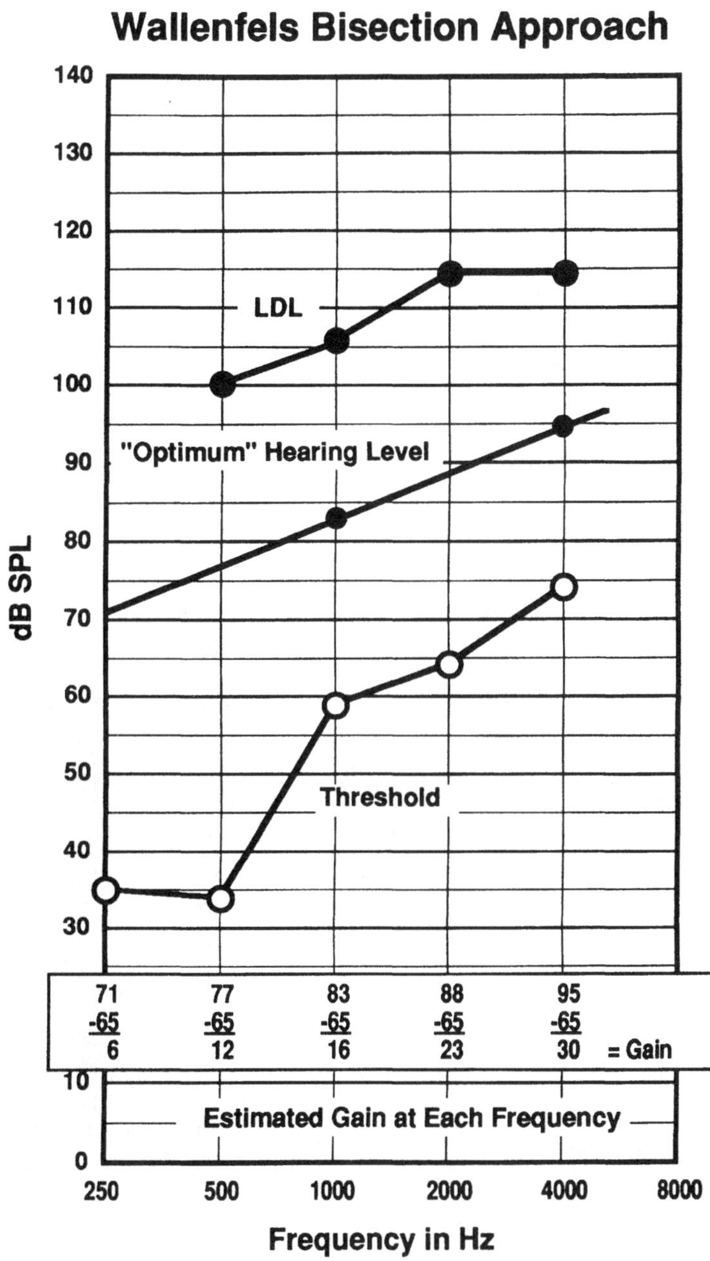

Fig. 34. Wallenfels bisection approach to determine the estimated hearing aid gain. The pure-tone audiogram is plotted in SPL, along with the LDL. The optimal listening level is plotted as a line that bisects the thresholds of discomfort (LDL) and sensitivity at 1000 and 4000 Hz, with 65 dB subtracted to determine the gain at each frequency. (Adapted from Wallenfels, H. G., *Hearing Aids on Prescription,* Charles C. Thomas, Springfield, IL, 1967).

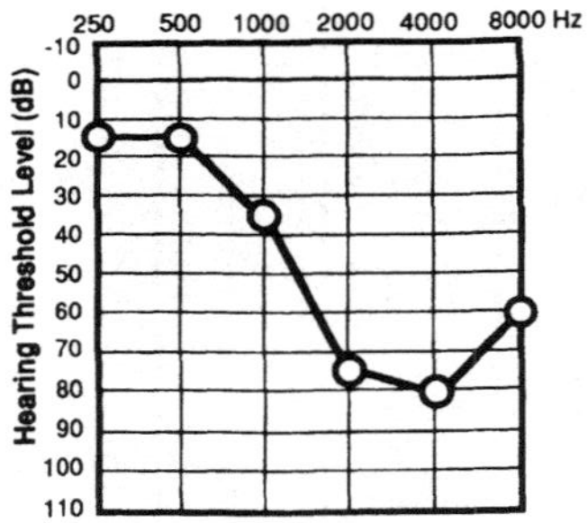

A

PRESCRIPTION TABULATION (DIRECT SUBSTITUTION METHOD)

Frequency	.25	.5	.75	1	1.5	2	2.5	3	4 kHz
Aided MCLP	78	76	74	72	72	72	72	74	76
MCLP Objective	96	84	78	72	72	72	72	72	72
Difference	-18	-8	-4	0	0	0	0	+2	+4
Test Instrument Gain in dB	—	22	35	43	47	55	57	59	52
Test Instrument Gain Values + difference = prescription (rx)	—	14	31	43	47	55	57	61	56

B

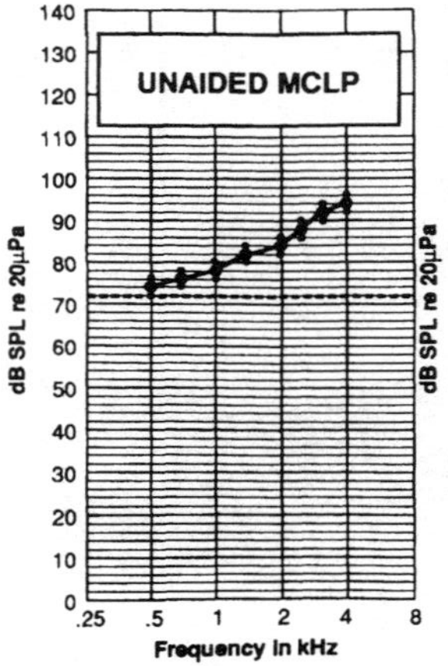

C

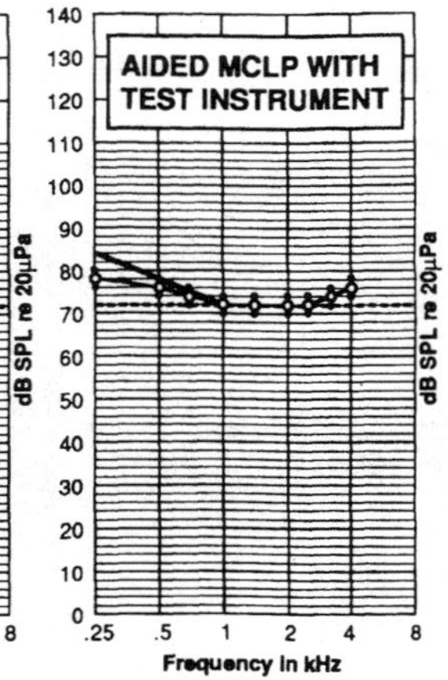

D

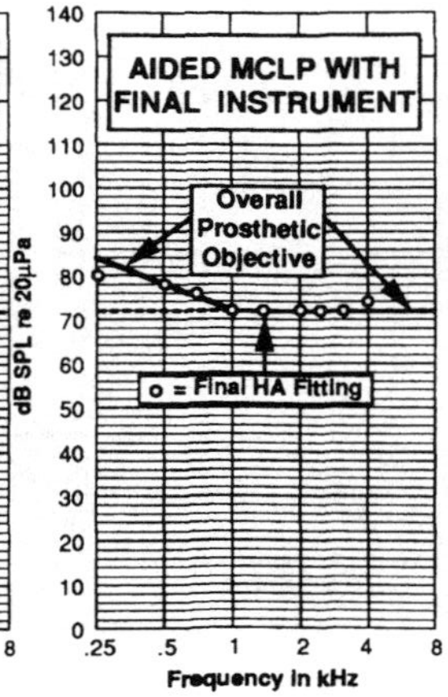

E

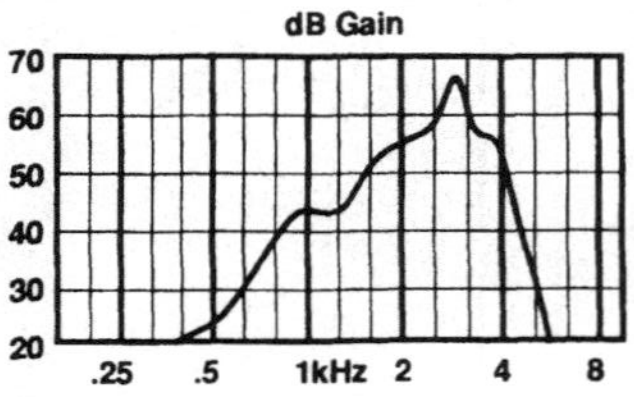

F

levels that are essentially at the same MCL). The "difference" between the SPL output required with the damped wavetrain signal to reach this level and 72 dB is recorded (35b, line 3).

The goal is to provide hearing aid gain and response to the defective ear so that it will duplicate the behavior of the "normal" ear. This level is at a comfortable loudness of 72 dB SPL for all frequencies (for a damped wavetrain signal) and is shown by the dashed line (Figure 35e). It is at this sound pressure level that the sensation of loudness is essentially independent of frequency for an average normal ear. This sound pressure level is said to coincide also with independently measured MCLs. It is also the approximate center of the loudness range of sound pressures. An arbitrary modification is made to adjust for the low frequencies and the potential upward spread of masking, relative predominance of low-frequency sounds in the environment, and relative lesser importance of low-frequency sounds for speech intelligibility. The modification as applied, is shown in Figure 35e by the solid line identified as "overall prosthetic objective," and is "rolled off" at a rate of 3 dB/octave for each 10 dB of in-use gain at 1000 Hz. For the loss in this example, the roll off is +6 dB at 500 Hz, and +12 dB at 250 Hz.

3. Once the previous measurements have been recorded, a prescription (or preselection) can be tabulated by a direct substitution method. This is obtained by taking aided measured values on the laboratory aid at the "in-use" gain setting (Figure 35f) and determining the difference between these gains

Fig. 35. (facing page) Graphing and the relationships involved in Otometry as described by Victoreen (1963), using a direct substitution method. For the audiogram identified in 33a, the unaided most comfortable loudness pressures (MCLP) are identified and plotted in SPL (33c), using a damped wavetrain signal. Normal unaided ear MCLP values are at 72 dB across the frequency spectrum (dashed line). MCLPs are then obtained from a "laboratory aid" (33d) after the gain control is adjusted to a comfortable level matching a 72 dB damped wavetrain signal input at 1000 Hz. This is identified as the "in-use" gain setting. Other frequencies are then matched in loudness to this level and their SPL values recorded. The actual differences in gain required to reach these levels at different frequencies are identified as the "difference" in 33b. To obtain these values, the "laboratory aid" is measured into a 2-cc coupler with the volume control as its reference setting. The "in-use" gain at 1000 Hz is the SPL output measured in the hearing aid at 1000 Hz minus the input signal. The "in-use" gain for this patient is 44 dB at 1000 Hz. The prescription (or preselection) can be tabulated by a direct substitution method. This is obtained by taking aided measured values on the laboratory hearing aid (33f) at the "in-use" gain setting and recording the differences between these gains and the difference values required to reach the prosthetic objective. These deviations from the prosthetic objective in measured MCLP are appropriately added or subtracted from the 2-cc coupler frequency response of the instrument, and a prescription is written (bottom line of 33b). The hearing aid prescriptive gain is the test instrument gain values plus the difference. See text for additional explanation.

and those difference values required to reach the prosthetic objective. These deviations from the prosthetic objective in measured MCLP are appropriately added or subtracted from the 2-cc coupler frequency response of the instrument, and a prescription is written (bottom line of 35b). The hearing aid prescriptive gain is the test instrument gain values plus the difference.

4. The aided MCLP values of the final (actual hearing aid from the manufacturer) hearing aid are compared with the MCLP objectives (solid line), and the differences recorded (Figure 35e). The final aided MCL, (using the damped wavetrain signal) is to be within ±2 dB of the predicted curve.
5. The aided tolerance of each ear separately is measured, with the other ear occluded. If a TD is reached before the limits of the equipment, the input sound pressure plus the gain of the aid may be used to specify the maximum tolerable pressure at that frequency.
6. Perform aided binaural "MCLP" to show if stereophonic perception has been achieved.

Essentially all hearing aid selection techniques based on loudness growth, have utilized certain concepts from Otometry.

Pascoe (1978). A hearing aid selection procedure considered simple and economical in time was proposed by Pascoe (1978) that was based on the acceptance of certain premises; namely:

1. That the frequency response of a hearing aid must be known or defined in terms of functional gain,
2. That although many changes in frequency response may be insignificant, those that reestablish the proper balance between the low-and high-frequency components of speech (two-humped configuration in the aided perceived speech spectrum) result in improved speech reception,
3. That wider bandwidth is correlated positively with improved discrimination: both ends of the spectrum must be retained to produce a pleasant, normal-sounding signal,
4. That amplification must be adjusted to variations in the dynamic hearing range; including compression, when needed, and
5. That hearing aids can be manufactured that meet these needs.

The suggested hearing aid selection procedure was explained as follows:

1. Define the dynamic range of loudness using pulsed third-octave bands of noise, monaurally at zero-degree incidence in the

sound-field, in SPL. Plug and muff the non-test ear. The listener selects from a five-point scale as follows: 1) Very soft; 2) Soft, but clear; 3) Just right; 4) A little loud, but OK; and 5) Too loud, uncomfortable. The trains of three or four pulses are given at various levels, and somewhat randomly; either ascending or descending sequences. The listener assigns a scale value following each pulse train. Earphones can be used (with appropriate corrections made to convert to sound-field levels) if the listener's hearing range precludes the use of sound-field signals. Suggested corrections from earphone SPL to sound-field SPL require the values below be subtracted from the earphone SPL values:

Frequency:	**250**	**500**	**1000**	**1500**	**2000**	**3000**	**4000**	**6000**	**Hz**
Phone-SF	−3	0	0	−2	−6	−12	−13	−9	dB

Obtaining three statements for each of five signal levels of eight noise bands will provide the basic information needed to select a hearing aid. As a minimum, exploration at the frequency bands around 500, 1000 and 2000 Hz should be defined fully.

2. Define the "desired signal levels." Input levels are to be defined that are expected to be reasonable facsimilies of the speech spectrum at or near normal conversational levels. Considering an overall input speech level of 65 dB SPL and a 20 dB range for speech, the following input levels are stipulated and are thought to approximate the 20% to 80% levels of speech as reported by Dunn and White (1940):

Frequency:	**250**	**500**	**1000**	**1500**	**2000**	**3000**	**4000**	**6000**	**Hz**
Maximum:	68	71	60	61	62	55	54	50	dB SPL
Mean:	58	61	50	51	52	45	44	40	(Third octave
Minimum:	48	51	40	41	42	35	34	30	band levels)

3. Derive the functional gain or functional frequency response of the hearing aid needed to amplify the above input levels to a listener's MCL.

4. Ensure that the minimum input levels reach the listener's thresholds but that the maximum input levels do not produce discomfort. If not, consider compression amplification to meet these needs.

5. Saturation output levels should be just below the discomfort levels previously described. If not feasible, consider compression amplification.

6. Use a "test aid" to describe the hearing aid characteristics in terms of coupler gain and/or frequency response. This "test

aid" should have characteristics that approximate the projected coupler requirements, aid type, and earmold coupling. Aided thresholds are obtained at each noise band. Again, if the unaided ear is believed to be participating, plug and muff that ear. Functional gain (aided thresholds subtracted from unaided thresholds) is calculated for each frequency band. The functional gains so defined are then compared to the hearing aid 2-cc coupler gains and functional vs. coupler corrections are calculated.

7. Specify the entire set of hearing aid characteristics in terms used by both the dispenser and manufacturer. This includes: style, ear fitted, gain and output characteristics, inherent noise level (below threshold), need for and type of compression or other form of output limiting.
8. Test the fitting with Step 6, using the "desired signal levels" of Step 2. Decisions must then be made as to whether departures from the required characteristics are significant or not, and whether further adjustments are necessary. These adjustments can be made electronically or acoustically. Although acceptable variances are difficult to specify, the fundamental goal is to have the sensations produced by the peaks of the high- and low-bands of speech to be within the most comfortable zone, while the frequencies of 1000 to 1500 Hz should be heard and described as "softer."

The results of this procedure can be translated into hearing levels and displayed on an audiogram, or they can be displayed in terms of SPL (Figure 36). This format is considered to be easily explainable and understood by the patient.

Loudness Growth in Octave Bands (1989) This test (identified as the LGOB test; an acronym for Loudness Growth in Octave Bands), introduced for use by a hearing aid from the ReSound Company was an extension of a vast body of scientific literature on the measurement of loudness sensation (Pluvinage and Benson, 1988). The test measures the growth of loudness as a function of frequency, with the dynamic range of an individual's hearing impairment readily calculated from the data. One-half octave bands of noise are presented and the patient is asked to make loudness judgments based on the following seven categories: 0) Cannot Hear, 1) Very Soft-VS, 2) Soft-S, 3) Comfortable-C, 4) Loud-L, 5) Very Loud-VL, and 6) Too Loud-TL.

The noise bands are presented at each of the octave frequency midpoints from 250 to 4000 Hz. The loudness growth is plotted for each frequency band using intensity versus loudness sensation,

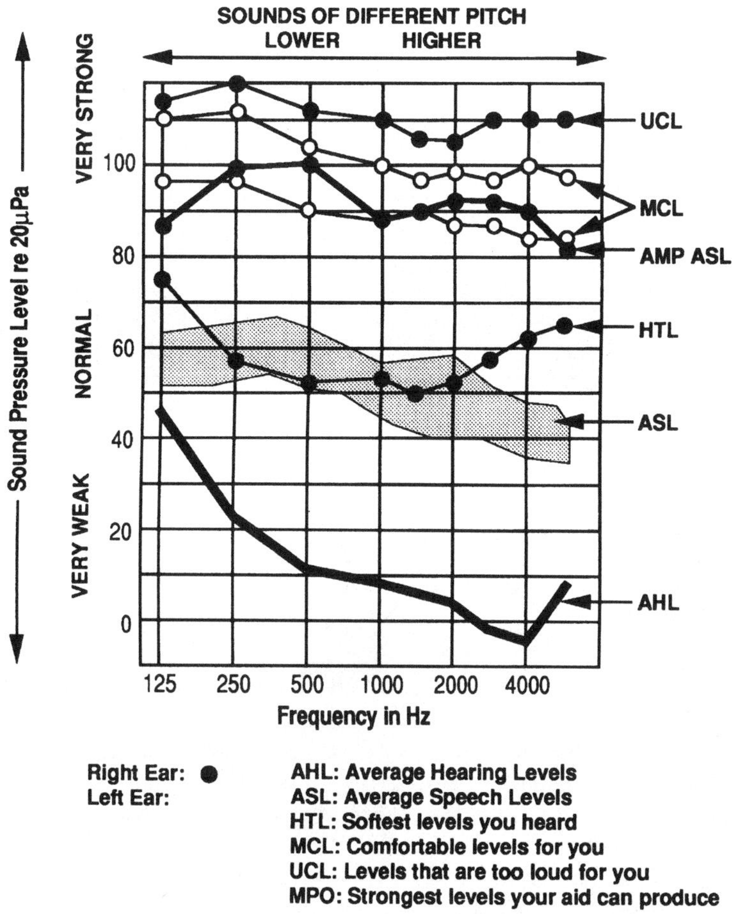

Fig. 36. Display of Pascoe hearing aid selection procedure and patient explanation information shown in SPL. The fundamental goal is to have the aided performance fall within the most comfortable zone of average speech levels.

and the equal loudness contours are then displayed. Presentations of noise levels and frequency bands are randomized and automatically given by a programmed computer, with the patient operating a hand-held selector from which the comfort level is selected (Figure 37) for each presentation sequence. Each presentation sequence consists of groups of three half-second bursts separated by half-second intervals of silence. During each stimulus presentation, all seven keys are lit up, prompting the patient to make a selection. Following a selection the light indicators are turned off, except for the selected key, which lights up for an extra second. The data obtained is used to determine the sound processing

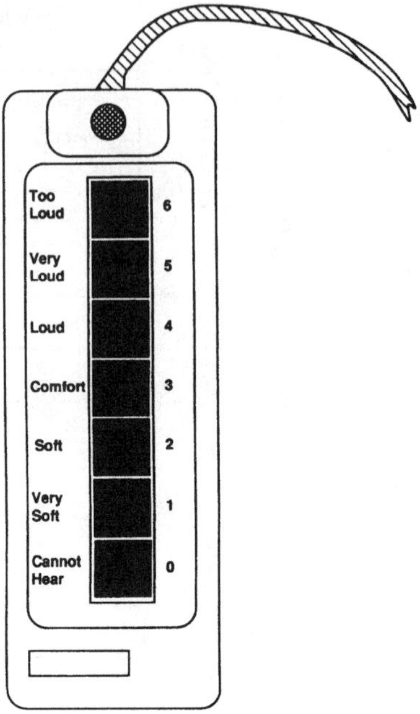

Fig. 37. Illustration of the Personal Selector used by ReSound to determine the patient's complete dynamic range, using the Loudness Growth in Octave Band (LGOB) procedure. See text for explanation.

required to fit an individual's dynamic range of hearing according to a proprietary fitting algorithm.

The actual test is divided into two sections. The first section collects data to determine the limits of the dynamic range. The intent is to evoke the VS and VL responses to avoid presentation of inaudible or uncomfortable stimuli during the second part of the test. In the second section of the test the data are averaged to compensate for changes in the patient's loudness criteria, avoiding those sounds exceeding the VS and VL levels. Based on the patient's dynamic range, intensity steps are presented from 6 dB for a normal dynamic range to 2 dB for a very narrow dynamic range. Figure 38 illustrates a comparison between a normal and abnormal loudness growth curve (the latter showing the spread and average) for a single frequency. Figure 39 shows equal loudness contours for each of the octave bands for a patient having a high-frequency hearing loss.

The LGOB test provides a method to obtain required diagnostic information of a patient's suprathreshold hearing profile. The degree of recruitment (abnormal loudness growth increase) can be quantified easily to distinguish between conductive, sensorineural, and mixed hearing impairments. From a hearing aid fitting perspective, the loudness growth patterns suggest sound processing options to best compensate a particular loss.

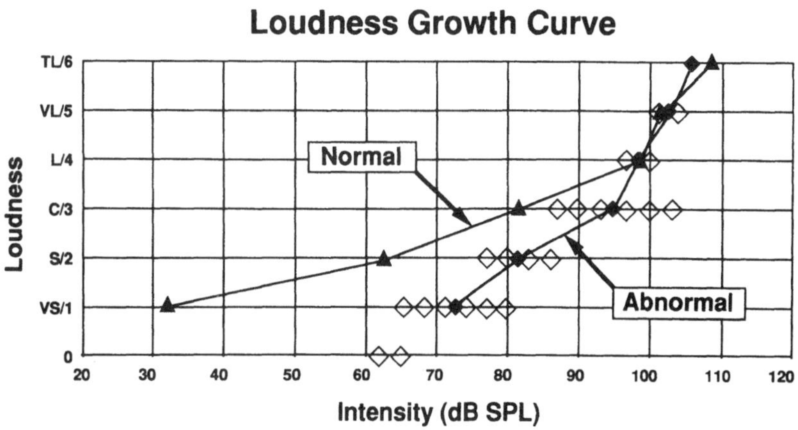

Fig. 38. A comparison between a normal and abnormal (rapid) loudness growth curve. The clear diamonds indicate the individual responses and the solid diamonds represent to the average intensity level for all presentations eliciting the same loudness selection. The loudness growth curve is obtained by connecting the solid diamonds. (After Pluvinage, Hearing Instruments, 39:3, 1989).

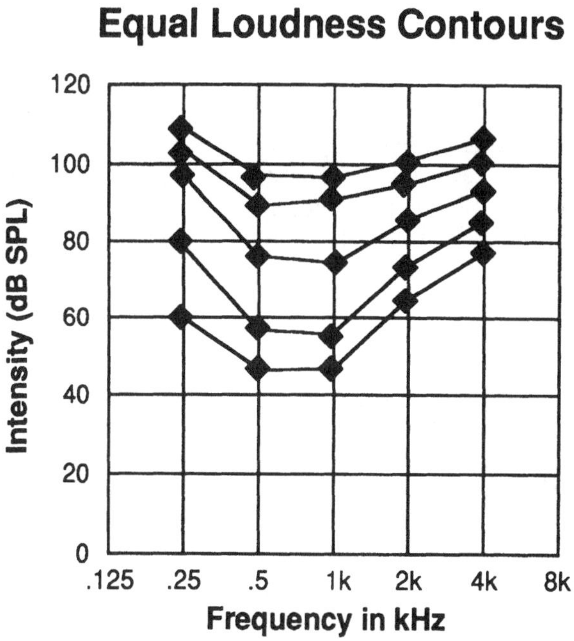

Fig. 39. Equal loudness contours for a patient having a high-frequency hearing loss. The patient's high-frequency hearing loss shows a decrease in the dynamic range (spacing between the curves) for the higher frequencies.

IHAFF (Independent Hearing Aid Fitting Forum, 1994). This group developed a protocol to respond to challenges presented by programmable and nonlinear technology. The protocol involves three components: (1) prefitting data collection of hearing thresholds, but with an emphasis on suprathreshold loudness-based measures, (2) amplification selection software, and (3) fitting and verification of benefit. The goal of the fitting procedure is to restore normal loudness appreciation of amplified speech cues that are audible for soft inputs, comfortable for normal speech levels, yet not uncomfortable or distorted for intense sounds.

The prefitting data collection (Phase I) involves obtaining pure-tone thresholds from 250 to 8000 Hz, and pulsed warble tones or narrow bands of noise loudness judgments (for seven levels ranging from very soft to uncomfortable) at a minimum of two frequencies, and then converting these to SPL (HA-1, 2-cc coupler measures). A median taken from four ascents for each loudness judgment is used (Figure 40). Insert earphone measurements are recommended to provide a common reference point to hearing aid measurements (and especially when the insertion depth is carefully matched between the earphone and the hearing aid earpiece). Loudness contour information is used to calculate the appropriate amplifier characteristics necessary to restore normal loudness perception. Loudness judgment testing can be administered manually or via computer, with a practice run from very soft to loud, followed by three ascending data collection runs for each judgment level presentation. The median value for each category is used to calculate the individual's loudness contour. The assumption is made that if a hearing aid restores the normal loudness perception sensations over a wide bandwidth, the patient will have a good opportunity to achieve maximum speech recognition ability. Also, an index of communicative handicap is obtained to assess the individual patient's needs and expectations from amplification, and to establish a baseline for comparison to aided conditions. For this latter phase, the protocol recommends the Abbreviated Profile of Hearing Aid Benefit, described later in this Chapter (APHAB, Cox and Alexander, 1994).

The hearing aid selection (Phase II) involves having casual, normal, and loud vocal effort speech levels targeted to fit appropriately within the individual's seven categories of loudness. The results of the loudness perception test are entered. Input/output curves derived from loudness perception data define the gain, slope, and output of the desired hearing aid. The loudness perceptions are used to determine the dynamic targets for various levels

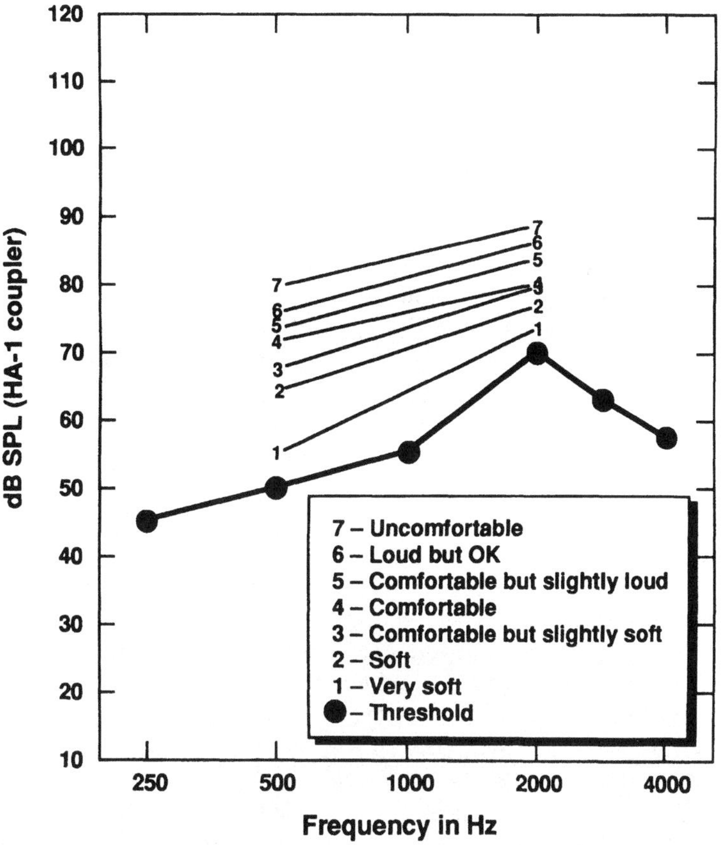

Fig. 40. Threshold audiogram with contour loudness judgments at 500 and 2000 Hz. (After Van Vliet (1995), Hearing Instruments, p. 30, March). Instructions for the loudness test: "The purpose of this test is to find your judgments of the loudness of different sounds. You will hear sounds that increase and decrease in volume. You must make a judgment about how loud the sounds are. Pretend you are listening to the radio at that volume. How loud would it be? After each sound, tell me which of these categories best describes the loudness. Keep in mind that an uncomfortably loud sound is louder than you would ever choose on your radio no matter what mood you are in."

of speech. The hearing aid microphone pickup location, loudness summation and other factors are considered in the equation. The program displays two input/output graphs at frequencies chosen by the dispenser, showing target values for the three speech input levels. The dispenser enters gain, compression ratio, compression threshold, and limiting levels of known circuits, and then matches the resultant calculated input/output curves for a match with the target values. While this process can be performed manually, it is best left to computer application. A computer program to assist in this selection process is termed VIOLA (Visualization of Input/Output Locator Algorithm). VIOLA helps make the determination as to what circuit parameters will achieve the amplification goals; what input/output function will maintain the relationship between the narrow bands of acoustic energy (used for loudness judgments) and wider band speech inputs. Figure 41 is a graphic of the VIOLA input/output display.

The fitting and validation (Phase III) can involve 2-cc coupler measures, aided sound field measures, and probe microphone assessment. A follow-up validation using APHAB is recommended. The 2-cc coupler measurements allow the instrument to be preset to meet the specifications as prescribed in Phase II. Special attention involves setting the correct SSPL90 and to ensure distortion measures lower than 10% at 90 dB SPL input. Aided measures of speech and sound are recommended as follows: conversational speech (65 dB SPL) is to be perceived at a loudness rating of 3, 4, or 5; low level sounds should fall in the 20–30 dB HL range; and high level speech (85 dB SPL) should be perceived at a loudness rating of 6. Probe microphone measures of real ear aided response (REAR) should show no excessive irregularities (peaks), and that the bandwidth is as wide as practical for the user. A real ear saturation response (RESR) to a swept warble-tone or smoothed pure-tone stimulus at 90 dB SPL is obtained to verify that a loudness discomfort rating of 7 is not reached at any frequency.

The IHAFF protocol is considered to be an ongoing process, and may be somewhat different than at the time of this writing.

FIG6 (1995) This computer-based fitting approach has been designed to fit non-linear hearing aids that have wide dynamic range compression (WDRC). The procedure is based on average loudness data that relates equal-loudness and threshold curves based on data from several published studies (Killion, 1995; Gitles and Tillman Niquette, 1995).

Patient audiometric thresholds are entered into the computer program and fitting curves are automatically calculated for low-level sounds (40 dB SPL), moderate level sounds (65 dB SPL), and high level sounds (95 dB SPL). Three target gain and frequency response curves were chosen because available knowledge of loudness growth data indicates that patients with sensorineural hearing loss typically require less gain for intense sounds than for weak sounds. Therefore, a single target gain is thought to represent a compromise between adequate gain for weak sounds, but too much gain for loud sounds. Although loudness tests would be ideal, they are not always possible or practical to obtain. FIG6 is based on the

Patient	Left 1	Left 2	Left 3	Right 1	Right 2	Right 3
Gaion at 40 dB	1			40		
Comp Threshold	82o			82o		
CR begin	10			10		
CR end	10			10		
Max Output	95			95		

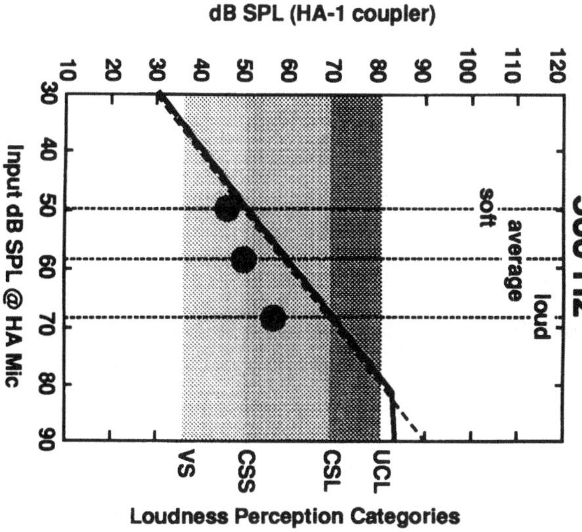

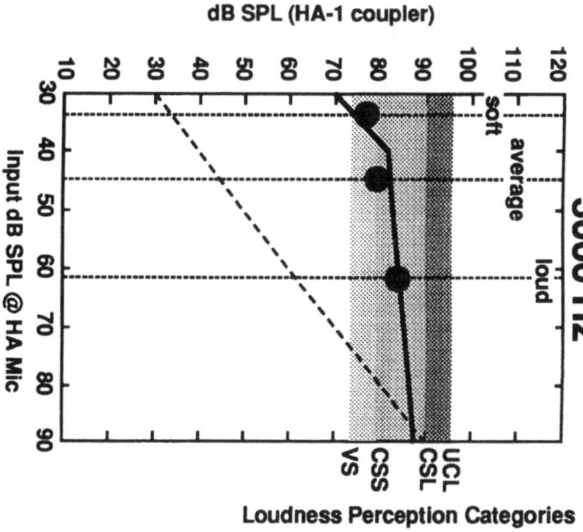

Fig. 41 This shows the hearing loss and loudness judgments for an individual with a mild hearing loss at 500 Hz, and a severe loss at 3000 Hz. The calculated "targets" (●) for the 500 Hz band are at less than unity gain, so no gain was selected for 500 Hz. A linear response up to a knee of 82 dB was selected for the 3000 Hz band. The output compression hearing aid selected has a 10:1 compression ratio and is limited at 95 dB SSPL90 output. (Modified from IHAFF, A comprehensive hearing aid fitting protocol, progress report, April, 1994).

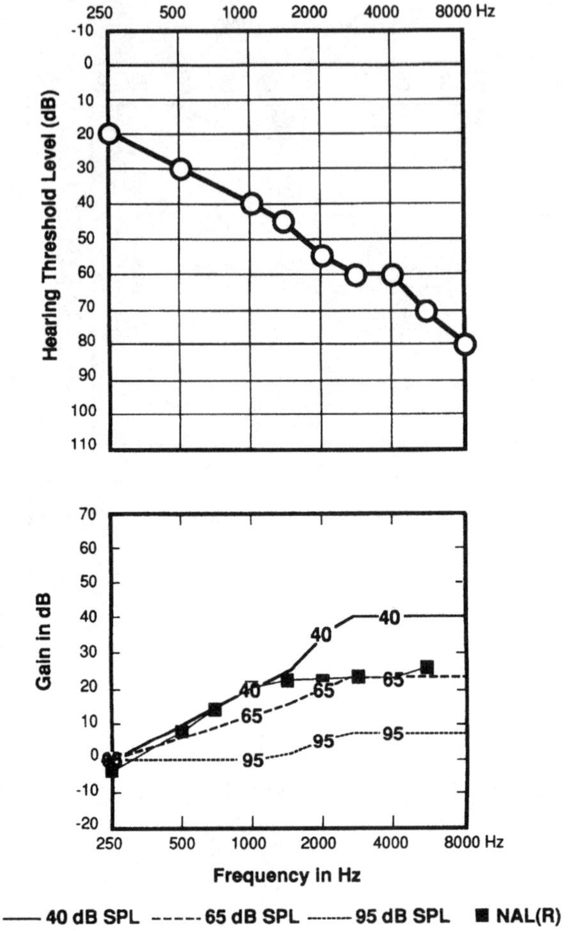

Fig. 42. FIG6 target gain curves for WDRC hearing aids with level-dependent frequency response, as compared with the NAL-R target curves, for the audiogram at the top. (Adapted from Gitles and Tillman Niquette, 1995, The Hearing Review, Nov/Dec, p. 30).

belief that targets based on average loudness growth data provide good first approximations of need. The use of FIG6 and WDRC is recommended for individuals having hearing losses between 20 and 70 dB HL, although individuals having more severe losses and reduced word recognition scores have been fitted successfully. FIG6 target gain curves for WDRC hearing aids having level-dependent frequency response are illustrated in Figure 42.

The program also calculates insertion gain targets (REIG) and 2-cc coupler response targets for BTE, ITE, ITC and CIC hearing instruments. These 2-cc coupler targets are used in combination with the manufacturer's published matrices.

SUMMARY OF PRESCRIPTIVE HEARING AID SELECTION APPROACHES

Hearing aid prescriptive formulae attempt to provide the dispenser with target gains, in general, or at specific frequencies. Considered advantages of a fitting formula include: (1) a level of objectivity is introduced into the evaluation process, (2) it is a first approximation of need—puts you in the right ball park, (3) provides a means for verifying the hearing aid fitting target in a sound-field or in a quiet room by measuring functional gain from the unaided to the aided condition, (4) it helps determine what modifications are needed to more closely approximate targets, and (5) it provides a means to discuss objective data with the patient.

These attempts at an "objective" method to determine amplified hearing aid performance have not, however, been without their distracters. It is well-known that the target gains based on pure-tone thresholds: (1) are influenced by the developers' beliefs in the significance of different frequency bands to intelligibility, (2) that they have been developed for hearing aids with linear amplification, and (3) that they have been developed based on 2-cc coupler measurements. Additionally, most prescriptive formulae have not taken into considerations the differences in hearing aid style or gain requirements for varying degrees of hearing impairment and some do not consider the UCL and subsequent SSPL90 requirements for the instrument. That almost all formulae have been derived from data obtained from sensorineural losses, occluding earmolds, and do not account for loudness growth changes further complicates fitting formulae.

In consideration of these issues, hearing aid fitting formulae are now being considered as a "first approximation of need" (Libby, 1989) in the selection process, rather than as providing the final target. That hearing aid formulae are based on average data seems to degrade their usefulness when applied to a given individual. Additionally, when measuring threshold, the practice of testing in 5 dB increments (± 5 dB variability) and the effects of ambient noise, suggest that formulae based on threshold data would be expected to have at least the same variability. On the other hand, threshold data may be the only information available upon which to base gain and frequency response projections. The greatest concern, however, is that of being able to substantiate that meeting a target provides even *appropriate* amplification. Meeting the "target" is also compounded by the inability of the electronics of the instrument to meet the requested target values, even with programmable systems. With the introduction and widespread utilization of new hearing aid options (such as nonlinear dynamic-range compression, multi-band, etc.), fitting formulae will need to be modified, as already explained with the IHAFF, FIG6, and revisions of the DSL.

An inherent limitation of most prescriptive approaches (threshold or suprathreshold) is that they were developed to predict the average gain required when the input to the hearing aid is **average** conversational speech presented in a quiet, nonreverberant environment at a distance of approximately three feet (or one meter). When input signal levels are less than this average conversational level, the amount of gain prescribed results in underamplification. Likewise, when the input signal levels are greater than this average conversational level, overamplification occurs. Unfortunately, prescriptive procedures do not generally take distance and input level changes into consideration.

Considerations that eventually lead to a given formula being used by the dispenser depend upon: (1) ease of use, (2) familiarity with the procedure, and most influential today (3) the procedure suggested and used by the manufacturers for their own circuit selection with custom-molded hearing instruments. To date, studies have not demonstrated a user advantage of threshold-based procedures over suprathreshold-based procedures, or vice versa. Also, the fact that it has been difficult to show that any single prescriptive procedures provides clearly superior speech intelligibility and speech quality makes it difficult to support a specific formulae (Sullivan, Levitt, Hwang, and Hennessey, 1988).

SSPL90 SELECTION

Some of the hearing aid selection approaches discussed previously, and some of those that follow, address the issue of SSPL90, or selecting the maximum output for the hearing aid. Many do not. However, because SSPL90 selection is considered to be a very important component of the hearing aid selection process, the author has taken the liberty to address the topic at this part of the chapter as a separate issue. Specifically, discussion presented will have a direct bearing on the usefulness and methods used to make this selection.

It is accepted that selecting an inappropriate SSPL90 can lead to outright rejection, inconsistent use, discouragement, or unsatisfactory use of the hearing aid. If the SSPL90 selected is too high and exceeds the patient's LDL, the fitting is considered to be inappropriate. (In this Chapter TD-Threshold of Discomfort; LDL-Loudness Discomfort Level; and UCL-Uncomfortable Loudness Level will be used synonymously). If the SSPL90 selected is too low distortions and a reduced amplified dynamic range will occur. It is suggested that the optimal SSPL90 setting is slightly below the LDL, but as high as possible to prevent limiting the amplified dynamic range (Mueller and Bright, 1994). These authors provide an excellent presentation on the selection and verification of maximum output and the reader is referred to it.

SSPL90 Prediction From Pure-Tone Thresholds

These procedures attempt to **predict** the LDL (rather than measure it) from pure-tone thresholds. These procedure are especially helpful when it is not possible to obtain LDL levels (non-verbal individuals, language problems, inability to respond, etc.). It is important to understand, however, that there is a nonlinear relationship between hearing levels and the LDL (McCandless and Miller, 1972; Kamm et. al., 1978), and that individual variability is rather large (in the order of 20 dB across frequencies). Figure 43, adapted from Kamm et al (1978) shows the relationship between hearing levels and LDL for pure tones at 500 and 2000 Hz, and for spondee words. Up to a 40–50 dB hearing level the average LDLs for individuals having a cochlear loss are very similar to normal hearing individuals. What is not shown is the large individual variability of 20 dB or more across frequencies. It is partly for these reasons that many believe that the LDL should be measured directly, when possible. Two methods for predicting SSPL90 requirements from pure tones have been discussed previously in this Chapter (MSUv3 and the DSL methods).

SSPL90 Selection From LDLs Using Other Types of Stimuli

Direct measurements of LDL have been made using a variety of stimuli. These have included, in addition to pure tones: (1) narrow bands of noise, (2) speech; in the forms of continuous discourse, sentences, spondees, nonsense syllables, filtered speech, etc., and (3) warble tones. Speech is often suggested as an appropriate stimulus because it represents what the patient listens to, and because it is often thought to provide information about loudness summation. On the other hand, those stimuli that provide frequency-specific information allow for comparisons to the SSPL90 curve selected.

A number of studies have compared LDLs obtained using various stimuli (Dirks and Kamm, 1976; Hawkins, 1980; Beattie and Boyd, 1986; Bentler and Pavlovic, 1989; Bentler, 1993; Filion and

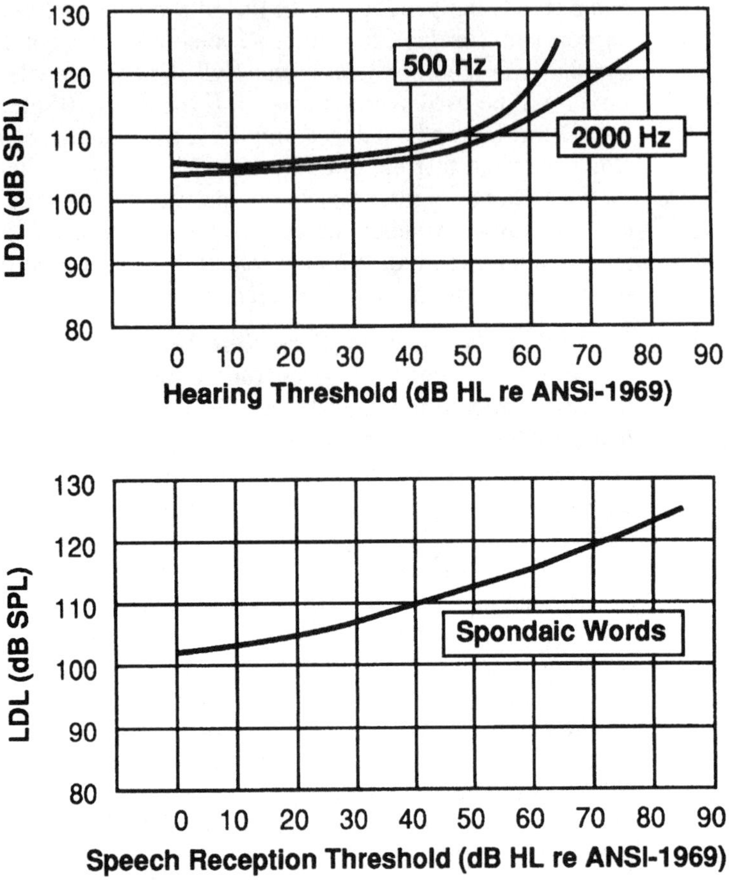

Fig. 43. Nonlinear function between a patient's hearing loss and the LDL for pure tones (top graph) and for spondees (bottom graph). (Adapted from Kamm, Dirks, and Mickey, 1978, JSHR, 21;688–691).

Margolis, 1992). The consistency is reasonably good between the LDLs obtained with the various stimuli, but as the signal type narrowed, the LDLs were somewhat higher in the low frequencies (differences up to about 10 dB between pure tones and wide band signals—Hawkins, 1980). Dirks and Kamm (1976) found no significant differences in LDLs between spondees and pure tones for a group of hearing impaired individuals, whereas Bentler and Pavlovic (1989) found a difference between normal and hearing-impaired individuals to pure tones and multitone (speech-like) stimuli, with multitone LDLs lower. Bentler (1993) further identified LDL inconsistencies to different kinds of environmental stimuli and annoyance judgments. Filion and Margolis (1992) reported that intensities exceeding the clinical LDL were seldom judged to be uncomfortable in the real world. When using six common formulae to prescribe the SSPL90, differences as great as 8 dB were found, but that differences as great as 25 dB were noted when the same individual was tested with each of the formulae (Hawkins, et. al., 1992).

Collectively, these studies seem to suggest that perhaps it might be desirable to use a variety of stimuli in measuring the LDL when using this measure for SSPL 90 selection. However, in general, using any of the afore-mentioned stimuli should give reasonably good clinical LDL measurements, with the understanding that verification, and possibly modification of the hearing aid's SSPL90 is a requisite part of the post-selection process.

Issues and Test Protocol for SSPL90 Selection

- What is best: actual measurement or prediction of LDL for SSPL90 selection? Whenever possible, measure LDL directly rather than predicting it from pure-tone data.
- What instructions should be given to identify the LDL? Beattie, et al., (1980) found that the LDL varied as a function of the type of instructions given. Suggested instructions (Hawkins, 1984) are as follows:

  > We need to do a test to determine where to set the amplifier on your hearing aid. We want to set it such that sounds do not become uncomfortably loud. You will hear some sounds, and after each one I want you to tell me which of the loudness categories on this sheet (Figure ?) best describes the sound to you. So after each sound tell me if it was "Comfortable," "Comfortable, But Slightly Loud," "Loud, But OK," or Uncomfortably Loud," etc. I will be zeroing in on the uncomfortably loud category because that is where we want the hearing aid to stop and not get any louder. So after each sound, tell me which category best describes the sound to you (p. 28).

- LDL Determination. Most current LDL measurements are obtained with tester-controlled procedures. A recommended approach is to employ a modified Hughson-Westlake technique (Carhart and Jerger, 1959), essentially the same as used for threshold determination. Using this technique, LDL is obtained in an ascending approach as follows:

  If using pure tones, test at .5, 1, 1.5, 2, and 3kHz.

  Alternately, if a single channel instrument is to be fitted, and knowledge of the peak SSPL90 is known, it may be sufficient to test at that frequency only (Mueller and Bright, 1994).

LEVELS OF LOUDNESS

Painfully Loud
Extremely Uncomfortable
Uncomfortably Loud
Loud, But O.K.
Comfortable, But Slightly Loud
Comfortable
Comfortable, But Slightly Soft
Soft
Very Soft

Fig. 44. Loudness categories descriptions for LDL measurements. (From Hawkins, 1984, Selection of a critical electroacoustic characteristic: SSPL90. Hearing Instruments, 35;28–32).

- Starting at MCL, increase the intensity in 5 dB increments until the listener indicates the sound is "Uncomfortably Loud."
- Drop the presentation level 10 dB and increase again in 5 dB increments until the listener indicates the sound is "Uncomfortably Loud."
- LDL is identified as the highest level indicated on two of three ascends. This may be defined better as the point midway between "Loud, But OK" and the "Uncomfortably Loud" categories. These categories are separated usually by only 4 to 6 dB.
- If measured in HTL, convert the LDL to 2-cc coupler SPL values. This is required to directly compare this value to the manufacturers' hearing aid specification of SSPL90.
- Select the hearing aid SSPL90 from the derived 20cc coupler values.
  - For pure tones the conversion values from Table 10 can be used.
  - If speech was used as the stimulus, add 20 dB to the HTL value to derive the SPL equivalent.
  - If insert earphones were used there is no need for the use of average correction factors, because precise corrections can be made. Place the insert receiver in the 2-cc coupler and measure the audiometer output at the dial setting obtained for LDL. If, for example, the dial reading on the audiometer was 80 dB and the measured 2-cc coupler reading was 85 dB, the conversion for this example

Table 10. Conversion Values from dB HL to dB SPL in a 2-cc Coupler

Frequency (Hz)	TDH-39	TDH-49 and 50
250	20.7	21.7
500	9.9	11.9
750	7.3	7.8
1000	5.5	6.0
1500	2.5	3.5
2000	5.2	7.2
3000	5.7	5.2
4000	−0.5	0.5
6000	−0.2	−2.2

(From Hawkins, D., 1992, Corrections and transformations relevant to hearing aid selection, in Mueller, Hawkins, and Northern (Eds), *Probe Microphone Measurements: Hearing Aid Selection and Assessment,* San Diego: Singular Publishing, pp. 251–268).

would be +5 dB. This calibration procedure need only be undertaken initially for the audiometer and insert earphone combination, and not for each patient. This procedure may be even more appropriate for children because the residual volume between the tip of the earpiece and the eardrum is smaller than in adults, resulting in a greater 2-cc to real ear output by as much as 15 dB or more (Feigin, et. al., 1989).

- If the LDL is 115 dB SPL, select a hearing aid whose SSPL90 is no greater than 115 dB SPL.

Issues and Test Protocol for SSPL90 Verification

This procedure follows the suggestions by Mueller and Bright (1994), who believe that verification is simplified if: (1) careful measurements are taken during the selection procedure, and/or (2) the hearing aid has an output control that has a wide range of adjustment. The procedure suggested uses both behavioral testing and probe-microphone measurements.

- Instructions. The same as for SSPL90 selection
- Patient position. In front of the loudspeaker (1 meter). Calibrate the sound delivery system to determine the dial setting that corresponds to a 90 dB SPL output for each frequency.
- Set the VC 5 dB above the use gain or prescriptive target gain if a new user (to account for potential higher use gain in some listening situations).

- Present pure tones at 90 dB SPL for the various frequencies. Use the LDL determination procedure described in the previous section. If the SSPL90 is set correctly the patient will respond to "Loud, But OK." If too loud, adjust the output control (or any other means to reduce the output—i.e., compression knee or compression ratio) of the hearing aid accordingly.
- If probe-microphone equipment is available, confirm the above results with an RESR (real ear saturation response) measurement. The RESR should correspond with the target RESR.
- The final test is to expose the patient to loud sounds that are similar to those expected to be encountered in the real world. At no point should the patient comment that any of the sounds are uncomfortably loud.

If using pure tones, test at .5, 1, 1.5, 2, and 3kHz.

Potential Correction Factors

- Exposure Effect. It has been reported that some individuals may show an increase in LDL of 6 to 8 dB following repeated LDL measurement sessions (Morgan and Dirks, 1974). As a result, it may be necessary to add an additional 3 dB to account for this variable (Hawkins, 1984; Cox, 1981; Libby, 1985).
- Hearing aids that provide very low distortion may be able to use a slightly higher SSPL90 than recommended by this procedure (Fortune, Preves, and Woodfuff, 1991).
- Binaural hearing aid fittings are treated as two separate monaural fittings (Mueller and Bright, 1994). Loudness discomfort does not seem to have a summation effect.

COMPARATIVE HEARING AID SELECTION APPROACHES

Traditional (Carhart; Classical; Sound Field Comparisons) Hearing Aid Evaluation

Best known as the Carhart, or Classical Procedure, this technique emphasizes word recognition performance in comparing a variety of preselected hearing aids. Based on sound-field comparisons of hearing aids, these approaches sought the hearing aids which would provide the: (1) greatest improvement in SRT, (2) best word recognition score in quiet, (3) widest dynamic range, and (4) satisfactory discrimination in the highest level of noise.

As reported by Carhart (1946), the procedure was developed to be used by hearing impaired veterans of World War II in the United States. The Army Rehabilitation Program goals were: (1) to find a hearing aid that would have optimal efficiency in everyday situations, (2) to provide an understanding of hearing aids, establish habits of efficient use, and initiate auditory training, and (3) to instill a full psychological acceptance of hearing aids.

Following otologic and audiologic evaluation, decisions about the type of aid and ear(s) to fit were made. A number of promising hearing aids were selected for trial use and evaluation. The clinic procedure, both before and during the selection process consisted of:

- Pure-tone air-, bone-conduction, and speech thresholds and word recognition (called speech discrimination) scores
- A confirming audiometric retest
- With each aid, aided gain for speech, and tolerance thresholds
- Word recognition tests in quiet and performance testing in noise
- Subjective evaluation of quality and acceptability

The procedure involved a subjective preselection of hearing aids that the evaluator thought might meet the needs of the patient. These instruments' performances (usually with similar electroacoustic characteristics) were then *compared* to each other using speech stimuli. The instrument that provided the best improvement in aided SRT and the highest word recognition score, was considered to be optimal, and was recommended.

The Classical hearing aid evaluation procedure was as follows:

Unaided:

- Pure-tone air-conduction, bone-conduction, speech discrimination, and SRT (both ears, under earphones: discrimination at 24, 25, 30, or 40 dB SL)
- Unaided sound-field SRT
- Unaided sound-field speech discrimination (in quiet) at 24, 25, 30, or 40 dB SL
- Unaided sound-field speech discrimination (in noise) at 24, 25, 30, or 40 dB SL, and at a +10 S/N ratio
- Unaided tolerance level for speech

The Hearing Aid(s) Were Placed on the Ears and:

- Speech presented at 40 dB re unaided SF SRT. Patient adjusted aid to a comfort level

At That Comfort Level, and Measured in a Sound Field:

- Aided SRT
- Aided speech discrimination (in quiet) at 24, 25, 30, or 40 dB SL

- Aided speech discrimination (in noise) at 24, 25, 30, or 40 dB SL, and at a +10 S/N ratio
- Aided tolerance

At Full Volume, and Measured in a Sound Field:

- Aided SRT
- Aided speech discrimination (in quiet) at 24, 25, 30, or 40 dB SL
- Aided speech discrimination (in noise) at 24, 25, 30, or 40 dB SL, and at a +10 S/N ratio
- Aided tolerance

Many variations of the original Carhart procedure have been undertaken, with most intended to shorten the evaluation time required or to improve the reliability of the procedure. Word recognition lists were shortened to 25 (from 50), and even some to 10 word lists (the latter of questionable value). Other modifications involved changing the words themselves to make the task more difficult or to provide words having high-frequency emphasis. A major difficulty with word recognition testing existed because unaided testing was generally presented at a comfortable loudness level to achieve "PB max," the best word recognition score for the individual. Aided testing, unfortunately, was measured also at a comfortable level to achieve "PB max." It was difficult, therefore, to tell a patient that " . . . without the hearing aid (but at a comfortable level that represented an aided condition) your ability to understand is 80% (example), and now with the hearing aids (again at a comfortable loudness level—often the same sensation level) your ability to understand is 80%." Many patients must have walked away wondering what good the hearing aids were doing or what kind of sham was being perpetrated! To circumvent this unacceptable approach, unaided word recognition was sometimes performed at a level of 50 dB HTL, (close to 65 dB SPL) regardless of the hearing thresholds, to approximate normal conversational speech levels. This provided a more realistic example of how the patient understood under normal unaided conditions, and how this then compared to their performance under aided conditions. In this way the advantages of having sound amplified by the hearing aid could be demonstrated.

The evaluation called for the use of "stock" hearing aids in the evaluation process. The dispenser selected a number of instruments from among the "best" of that stock and made aided comparisons, most often using "stock" earmolds as well. Once the "most adequate" of the preselected hearing aids was determined, a hearing aid was fitted that replicated the performance of the aid that performed best in the evaluation. Today this procedure is considered to be too subjective and time consuming.

Master Hearing Aid/Programmable Hearing Aid

What appears to be the original master hearing aid was patented by Hutchison in 1905. Early schematics and photographs of this and subsequent early units have been provided by Lybarger (1978), including those of Hincks in 1913, Tillyer is 1923, and of the Radioear "Selex-a-phone" patented in 1938.

The initial master hearing aid approach was based on the use of large external electronic devices to simulate or access various operating characteristics of hearing aids—to change the amplification characteristics via an external device rather than through changing the hearing aids to obtain those same characteristics. The intent of a "master hearing aid" is to identify patient-specific information by measurement or comparison of electroacoustical changes to which the patient can respond.

Master hearing aids have evolved to the point that today many of the programmable hearing aids have truly become "master hearing aids." Master hearing aids have progressed through at least three specific stages, with the last being programmable hearing aids as we know them today. These units continue to be used by some dispensers. The following descriptions recognize the evolution in these devices.

Master Hearing Aid: Initial Applications—Stage 1

As practical, operational devices, master hearing aids were first presented by Lybarger (1938). In the 40 years that followed, almost all manufacturers produced a master hearing aid that allowed dispensers to select the hearing aid characteristics for their particular line of hearing aids. These characteristics were expressed in sound pressure and consequently, the master hearing aid was often referred to as a pressure measuring instrument, SPL audiometer, supra-threshold testing device, or a hearing aid simulator. The use of master hearing aids often followed a comparative-prescriptive approach to hearing aid selection. Early master hearing aids featured the ability to change the frequency response, gain, output, binaural versus monaural, and other expectations for the hearing aid(s) to be selected (Figure 45). Most master hearing aids were combined with an audiometer and shared the HTL dial. These usually showed three sets of numbers: an outer row in HTL, a middle row in SPL (for speech), and an inner row in acoustic gain for MCL. Master hearing aids allow for binaural amplification estimates of the patient's performance, and often provide other useful

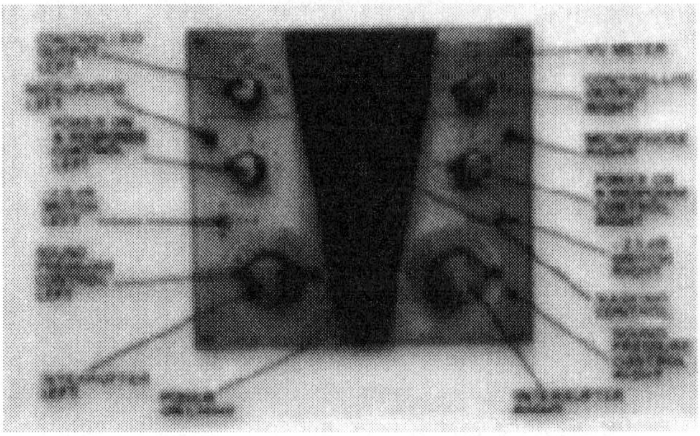

Fig. 45. Master hearing aid that used earphones to deliver the "modified" signal to the ear. The microphone was mounted in the center of the master hearing aid.

performance characteristics related to AGC-type function. The master hearing aid concept has been time efficient by allowing for rapid choices between different amplification characteristics. Additionally, the results can often be generalized to different brands of hearing aids, and the patient is exposed to a wider variety of frequency response configurations and output levels than with many other type selection applications.

The value of the master hearing aid was the ability to simulate a wide range of different hearing aid characteristics. In spite of these options, a legitimate criticism of these first master hearing aids was that although the hearing aid characteristics could be modified, the patient was listening through audiometric earphones rather than through hearing aid receivers, wider band microphones were used in the master device than what the hearing aid produced, and earmold coupling was unaccounted for. Therefore, the final fitting was rather different from the characteristics suggested by the master hearing aid.

Still, to explain how master hearing aids are used, the following explanation is offered:

Gain. An estimate of gain is obtained by determining the SPL required to provide adequate loudness of speech (MCL) for the patient. Usually, subtracting 60 to 70 dB, representing an average input speech level (depending upon the manufacturer and their fitting philosophy) from the middle row of numbers in SPL for speech, will give a gross estimate of the gain required. For example, an MCL of 90 dB HL is 110 dB SPL for speech. Subtracting 70 dB results in a 40 dB gain to reach MCL for the dial reading in

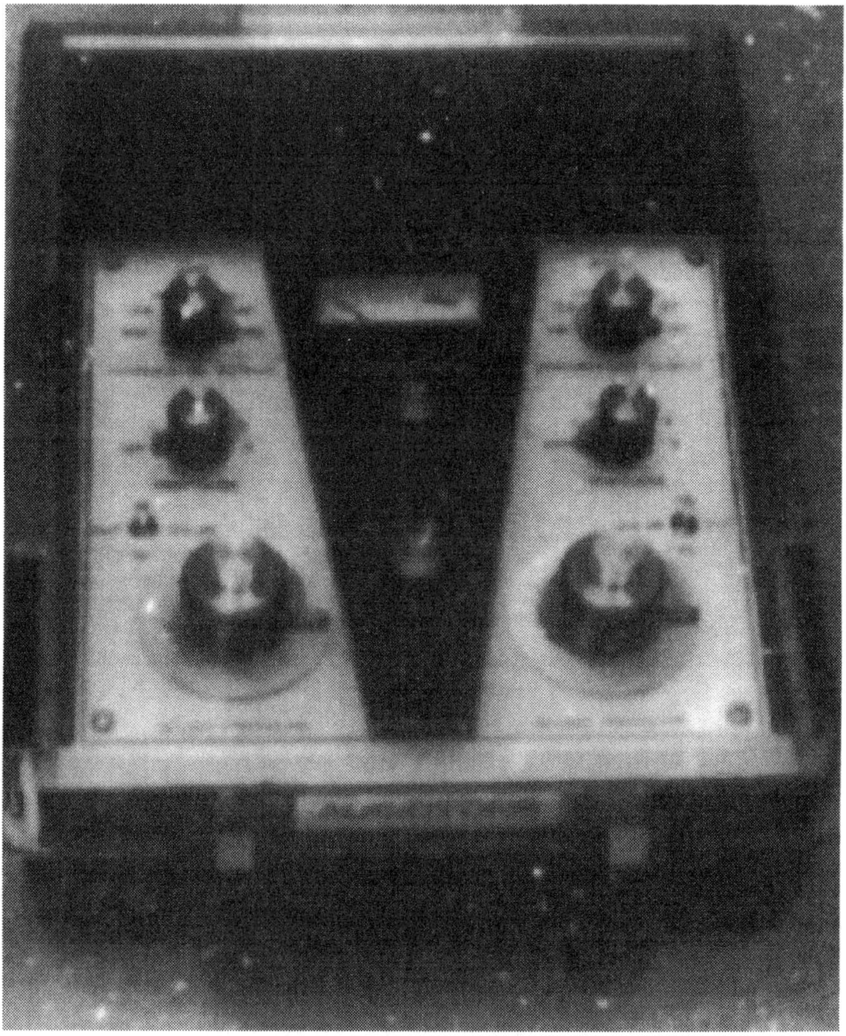

Fig. 46. Most master hearing aids were combined with an audiometer and shared the HTL dial. These usually showed three sets of numbers: an outer row in HTL, a middle row in SPL (for speech), and an inner row in acoustic gain for MCL. This latter number was determined by subtracting anywhere from 60 to 70 dB (depending upon the manufacturer and their fitting philosophy) from the SPL row.

Figure 46. The complete approach requires finding a combination of gain and response (or slope) that produces the best speech discrimination results. The gain levels change with the use of binaural versus monaural (less gain for binaural) and the frequency response slope (higher gain numbers as the response takes on more high-frequency emphasis to compensate for the loss of low-frequency energy).

SSPL90. The SSPL90 requirements are obtained by measuring the Threshold of Discomfort (TD), Loudness Discomfort Level (LDL), or Uncomfortable Level (UCL) for speech in SPL. Generally, the hearing aid selected should not have a SSPL90 that exceeds the obtained TD. As often used, TD is obtained while using both ears and achieving a balanced response (identified as directly in the center of the head or equally loud in both ears). If this is not done, the final fitting can result in the signal lateralizing to the ear where the aid has the higher output. (A 6 dB or greater difference will result in the signal lateralizing to the ear in which the aid has the higher output—Stenger effect). If balanced, even different outputs will sum into a single hearing experience. Differences at MCL are not as critical because the volume control of the hearing aid will allow the patient to balance the aids following the fitting.

Frequency Response. To help select the most appropriate frequency response, master hearing aids provide frequency response alternatives, from among which the most appropriate is selected. The hearing aid fitted eventually was expected to possess approximately the same frequency response (slope, gain per octave, rise per octave, pitch) that provided the clearest, most distinct, or intelligible speech. The frequency response characteristic interacted with the gain in that as the frequency response changes, corresponding adjustments in gain must be made to maintain speech at a comfortable and intelligible level.

Master Hearing Aid: Stage 2

To correct the inaccuracies to the final fitting as identified in Stage 1 Master Hearing Aids, the audiometric earphones and master hearing aid microphones were replaced with hearing aids (Figure 47). Additionally, this procedure allowed for the actual earmold coupling to be used. In other words, testing was performed under more "actual" conditions. The procedure was much improved, but the fact that not all hearing aids had the same microphones and receivers as did the master hearing aid units, continued to limit their accuracy. Additionally, the number of response slopes available in the master hearing aid was fairly limited (usually from four to six). This began to limit their use, especially when the number of hearing aids and their circuits began to proliferate with the growth of hearing aid types, styles, and circuits available from a given manufacturer. Additionally, programmable hearing aids have now substituted for many master hearing aids by offering true, in-situ circuit selection.

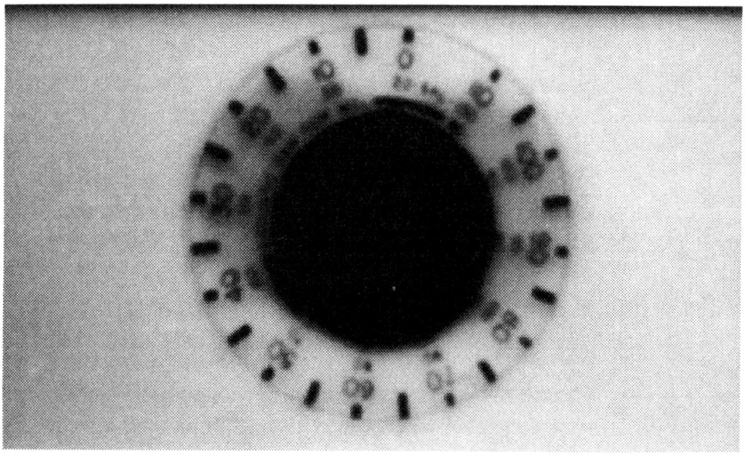

Fig. 47. Master HA that used ear level units containing hearing aid microphones and receivers so that the speech signal would be picked up by the hearing aid microphone, modified, and then delivered directly to the ear through a hearing aid receiver within the head level unit. The patient was fitted with the actual hearing aid coupling that was to be used for the final fit.

Master Hearing Aid: Stage 3 (Programmable Hearing Aids)

"True" master hearing aids exist today through programmable hearing aids and their associated external programmers. Even though their use is of fairly recent origin, the initial commercial use of such devices was presented as early as 1977 (Lawrence, Halladay, an Blackledge, 1977). Today's devices allow the dispenser and patient to work together to access a multitude (literally hundreds) of realistic hearing aid performance characteristics using the actual hearing aid the person will wear, including the exact ear coupling. These provide for the first time, true, in-situ circuit selection. A practical difficulty of having such a large number of electroacoustic options involves finding a correct starting point, and perhaps even more difficult, knowing when to conclude the fitting modifications, especially when combinations of options can reach into the thousands!

Programmable hearing aids consist of two primary components: (1) a hearing aid that has some type of memory module chip, and (2) an external microprocessor (computer) to access those memory locations or features within the chip. The memory module replaces the conventional trimmer potentiometer functions in the hearing aid and provides more varied and precise control. This control is sometimes referred to as an "electronic screwdriver." Programmable hearing aids are also known by names such as digitally programmable hearing aids and analog hearing aids with digital control. Once the desired electroacoustic performance is obtained, its characteristics are set and maintained within the hearing aid. Figure 48, illustrates the various components/functions available in today's programmable hearing aids (Staab, and Lybarger, 1994).

Some programmable hearing aids are simple and extremely portable (Figure 49) while others are much more complex (Figure 50). Still others are so large as not to be considered portable.

Programmable hearing aid electroacoustic performance selection occurs in a variety of ways. Three common methods used to select hearing aid performance are:

1. The application of one of any number of fitting formulae to pure-tone thresholds and use of that data to project a target gain/frequency response. Some form of real-ear or functional gain measurement is used to verify how closely the target was met. Adjustments can then be made through the external microprocessor. Most are prescriptive procedures based on pure-tone thresholds. Many times dispensers provide the basic audiometric threshold information to the manufacturer who, in turn, programs the instruments. This approach may still require fine adjustments on the part of the dispenser, who will then need a programming unit in the office. This latter requirement can prove costly to a dispensing facility, especially if a number of different manufacturers' hearing aid products are used. This could require purchasing a different programmer for each line of hearing instruments.
2. Other programmable hearing aids allow a comparison approach—" . . . do you prefer this sound or this sound?" This is a form of paired-comparison; storing different settings and allowing a rapid switching between them to determine patient preferences.
3. Still other programmable hearing aids base the hearing aid selection on suprathreshold data, such as MCL or a range of comfortable loudness.

In practice, programmable hearing aids most generally involve some kind of comparative listening, regardless of how the electroacoustics were selected. It is for this reason they have been included in this section on Comparative Hearing Aid Selection Approaches. Fitting strategies for programmable hearing aids take on a somewhat different aspect because these instruments often allow for alternate settings that provide a variety of electroacoustic responses at the command of the user. Setting hearing aids for

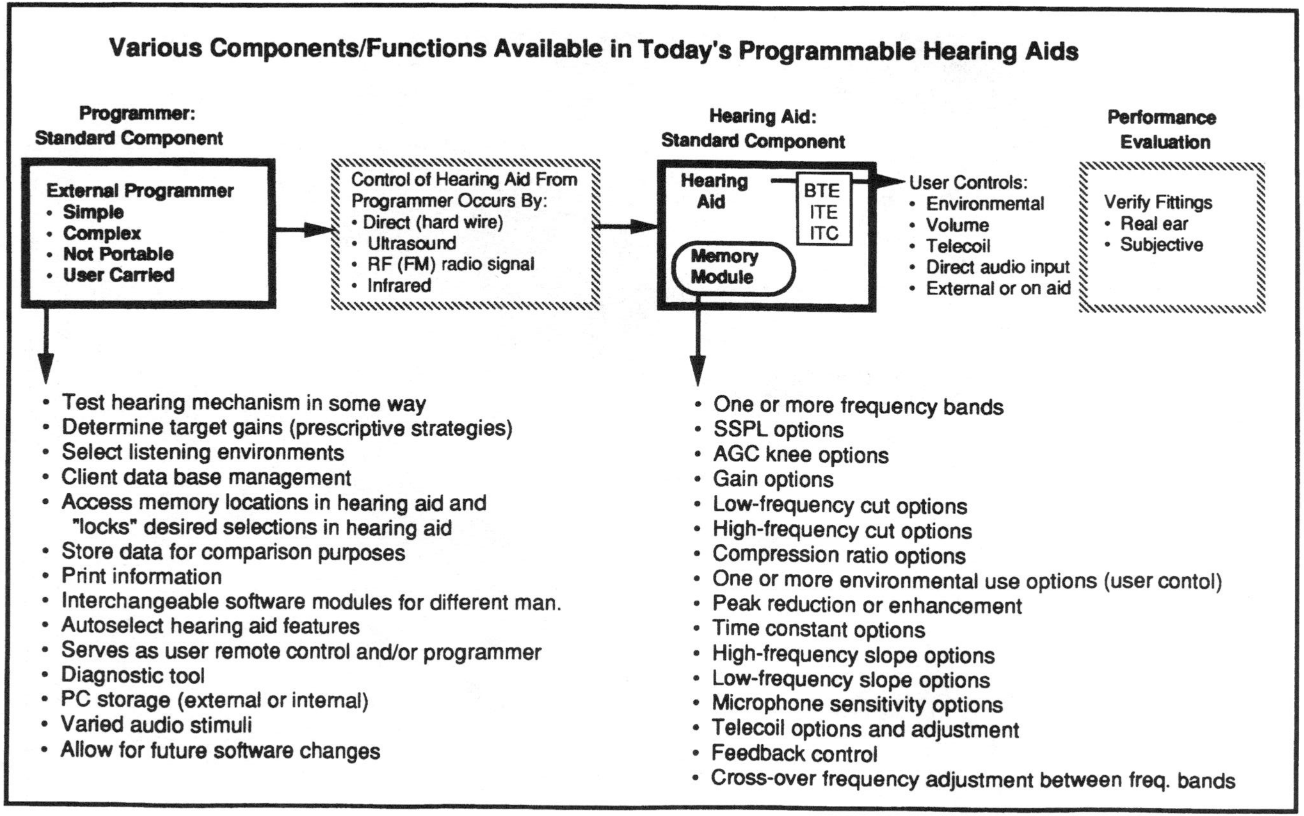

Fig. 48. Various components/functions available in today's programmable hearing aids. (With permission from Staab and Lybarger, 1994, Characteristics and use of hearing aids, in Katz (Ed) Handbook of Clinical Audiology, Fourth Edition, Williams & Wilkins: Baltimore, 1994).

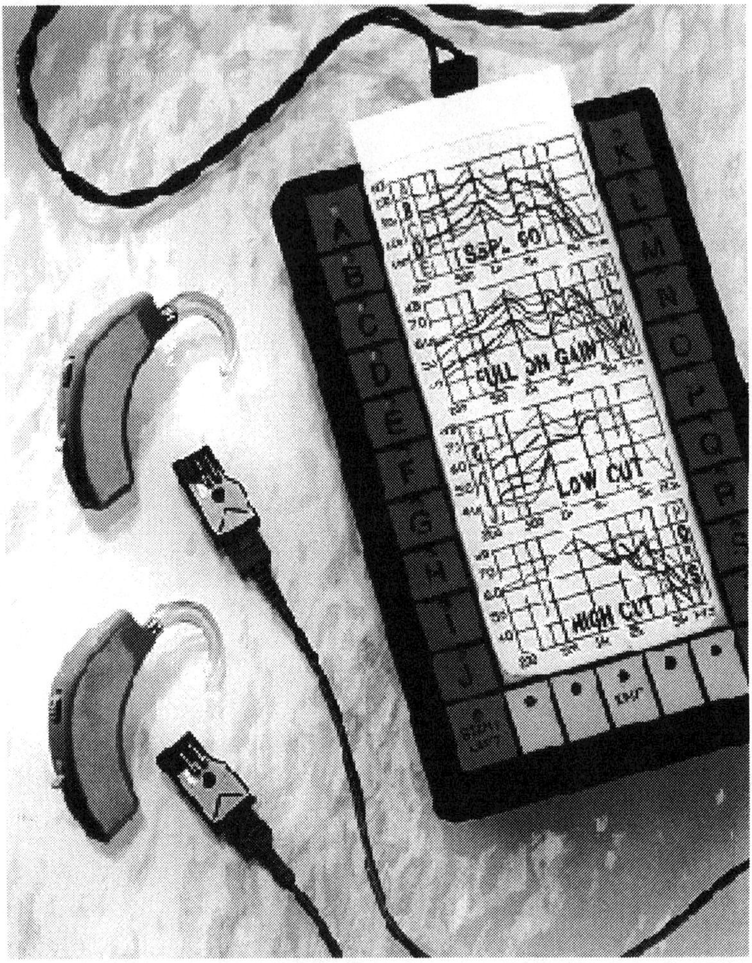

Fig. 49. Small and simple-to-use and understand programmable hearing instrument. It features options of SSPL90, full-on gain, low-cut, high-cut, and AGC or PC function. (With permission, Audiotone).

alternate electroacoustic responses do not follow the rules necessarily for prescription fitting.

Remote-controlled devices, to be used by the hearing aid wearer, are options with many programmable hearing aids. These allow the user to select pre-set electroacoustic characteristics for different environments, or to allow for gain adjustment without having to manipulate the instrument at the head level with the hand—thus avoiding annoying feedback or calling attention to the fact that a hearing aid is being worn. Some remote control units also allow the dispenser to program the hearing instrument.

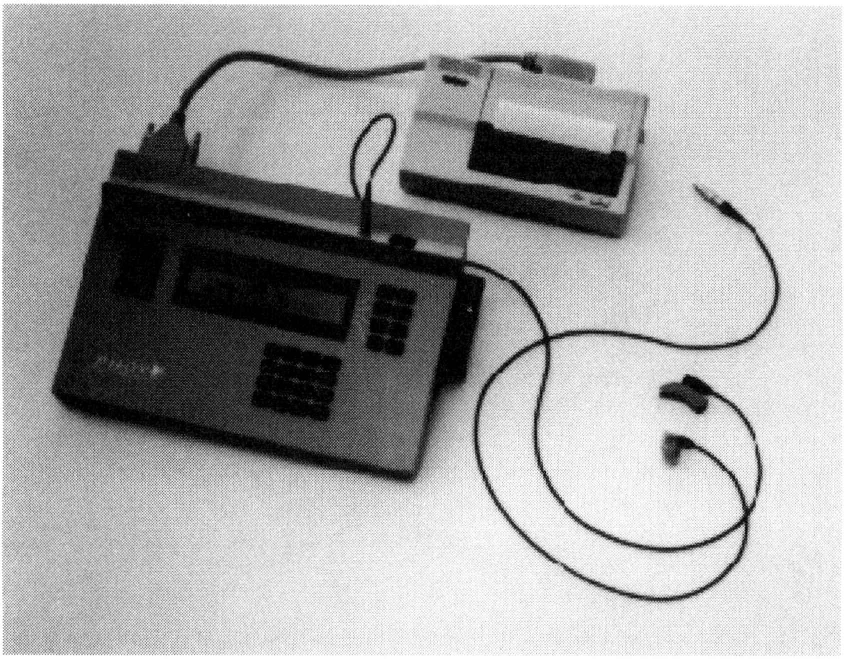

Fig. 50. Portable, but more complex digitally-programmable hearing aid system. (With permission, Maico/Bernafon).

An added feature of some of the more complex programming microprocessors is the ability to store patient data and electroacoustic information in a database management system for later use.

Programmable Multi-Channel (PMC) System. In an attempt to relieve dispensers from having to purchase a number of different programming devices, a group of manufacturers collaborated on a "universal" programmer called the Programmable Multi-Channel (PMC). The PMC allows for the adjustment of hearing aid parameters from different manufacturers, but all from one programming device. The PMC uses different software modules developed by each of the manufacturers that can be loaded into the programmer. Therefore, the extent to which any of the manufacturers' hearing aids can be programmed depends upon how extensive the manufacturers' product line of programmable instruments is. The PMC system is shown in Figure 51.

Paired Comparison Methods

These approaches emphasize the patient's judgement of "best" aided hearing. The patient is given a number of different output configurations in a given listening environment. The patient then selects from these various configurations what he/she judges as

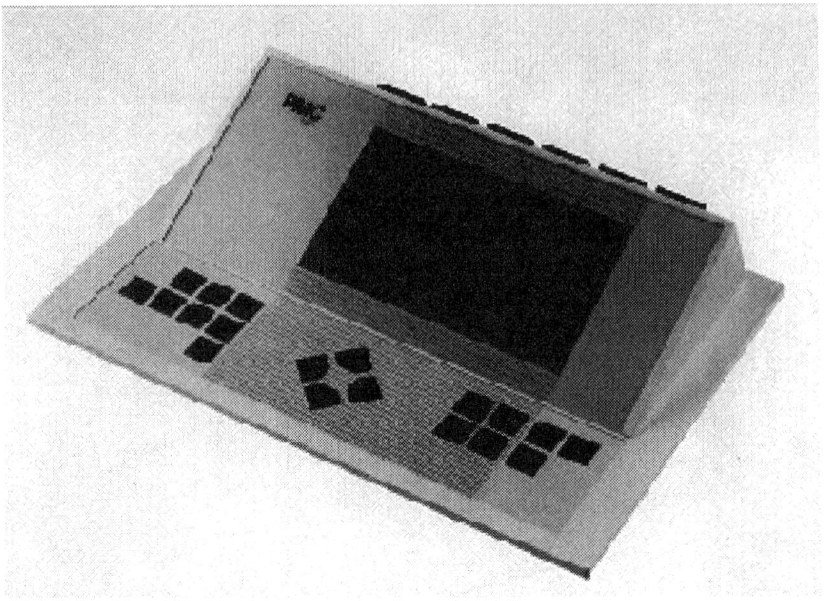

Fig. 51. The Programmable Multi Channel (PMC) is a universal programmer capable of programming hearing instruments from several different manufacturers. It uses an easy, menu-driven system. An easy-to-read display provides full information on the electro-acoustic parameters of the instrument to be programmed. Plug-in modules at the rear of the PMC are used by different manufacturers for their products.

best. There is no specific application of a fitting formula. Paired comparison approaches have considered value in that the patient participates in the decision-making process by determining "by comparison," which performance is best. Potential limitations of using this approach is that "best" may not be good in another environment, and the switching between configurations must be rapid to be meaningful. Figure 52 illustrates a simplical 5X5 matrix of different frequency response offerings used in such a procedure. The patient is presented alternately with the performance from two adjacent blocks and asked which is best. That block is then matched with another block's characteristics adjacent to it, and the patient is asked which is better. This continues until such time that the most appropriate amplification characteristic is selected.

INTEGRATED HEARING AID SELECTION PROCEDURES

Noah

A group of hearing aid manufacturers agreed, early in 1993, to establish a joint development group called the Hearing Instrument

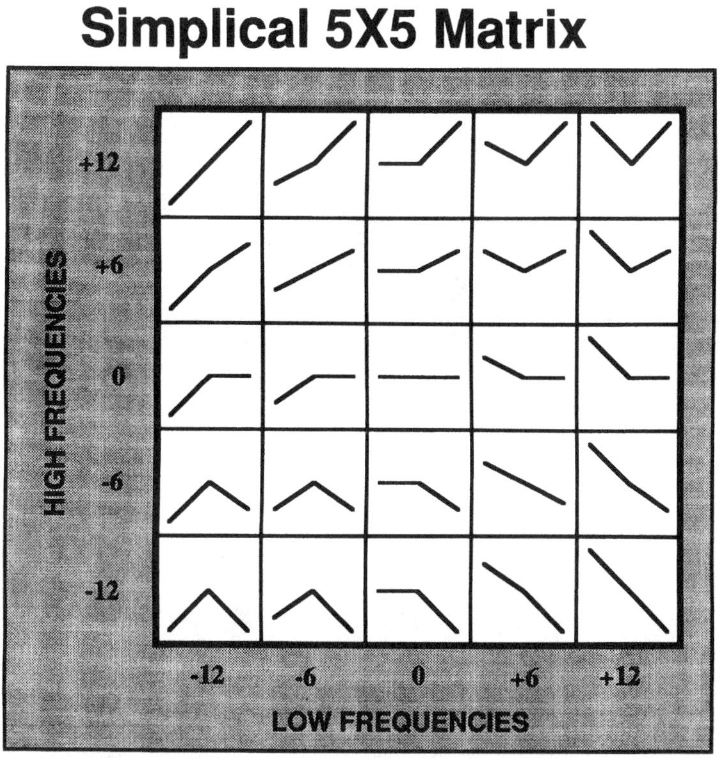

Fig. 52. Simplical 5X5 matrix that could be used in a paired-comparison approach to hearing aid selection. The numbers refer to filter changes with 1000 Hz as the center or pivot frequency.

Manufacturers' Software Association (HIMSA). Their mission was to: (1) design a standard for integrated hearing care software, and (2) develop an industry-wide software standard for fitting programmable hearing aids. The NOAH software system, introduced in 1994, is the result of this cooperative effort.

Essentially, the NOAH software system is a common platform that allows one office computer to link information (Figure 53) from:

- Programmable and non-programmable hearing aid fitting programs from different manufacturers
- Test equipment (NOAH compatible audiometers and real-ear test equipment)
- Office management software (i.e., Hearing Centers Network "PC/MacHear", Software and Systems "HearWare", and

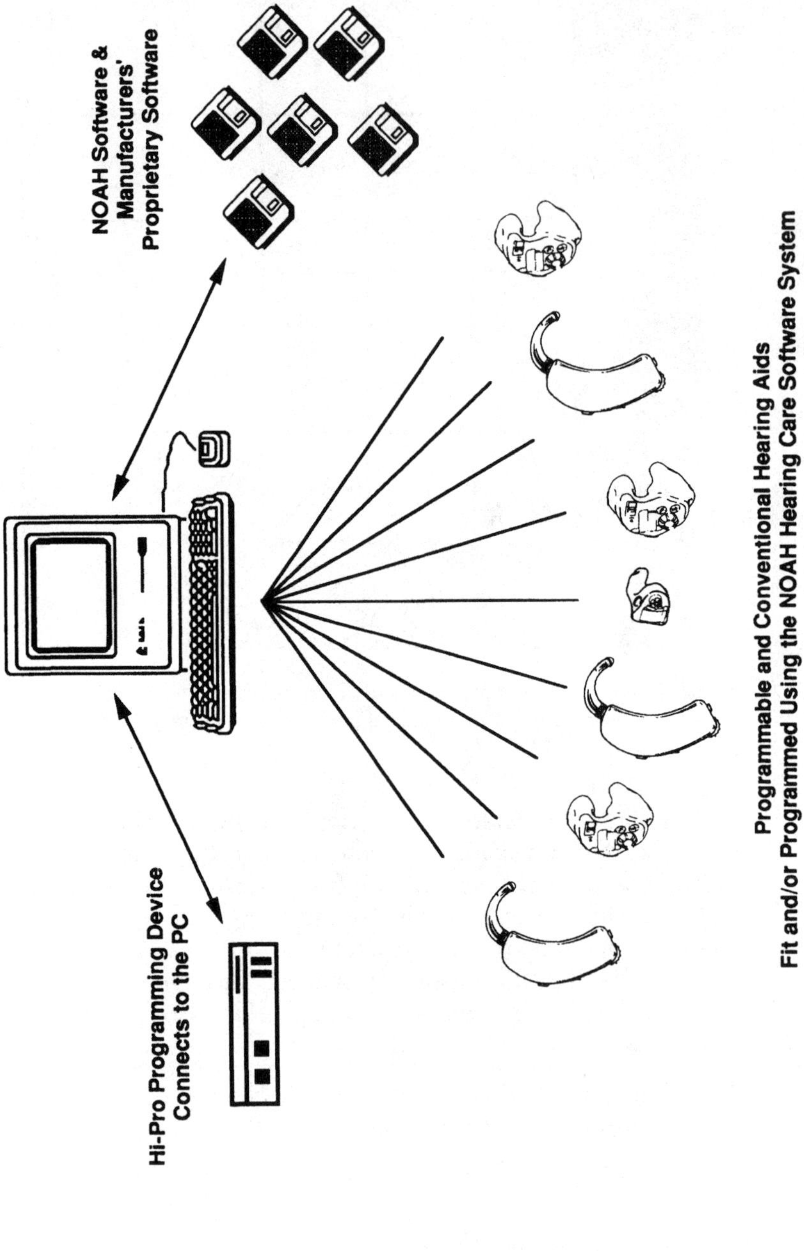

Fig. 53. NOAH hearing care system.

HIMSA America System Overview

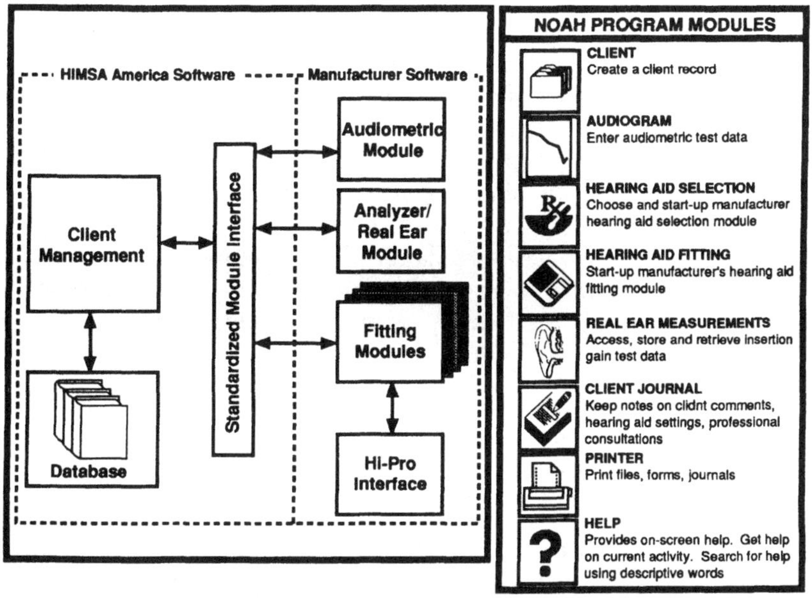

Fig. 54. HIMSA America system overview. The left side shows the NOAH hearing care system overview and identifies HIMSA software as opposed to that required by the manufacturer. The right side shows the NOAH applications managed by the dispenser in his/her office.

Starkey "Pro-Hear" support the NOAH software system at the time of this writing).

As a pictorial-icon-driven system, a NOAH session can consist of seven steps (or fewer, as desired), with the application program modules identified in Figure 54. A Help Module is provided to facilitate on-screen help.

The module activities are identified as follows (Jelonek, 1994):

1. ***Patient Module.*** Patient information is entered into the data base.

2. ***Audiometric Test Data.*** This is entered manually or transferred directly from an audiometer connected to the computer.

3. ***Hearing Aid Selection Module.*** This contains the proprietary software of those hearing aid manufacturers who are NOAH licensees. Each manufacturer's software provides product information, fitting recommendations, and fitting guidelines. This provides for computer-assisted fitting of conventional hearing aids.

4. ***Programming Module.*** This allows for computer-based programming of programmable hearing aids, but only from NOAH licensed subscribers. It takes the proprietary fitting software from the different manufacturers, all using different technologies, and makes them available in one software package. A cord supplied by the manufacturer couples the programmable hearing aid to the programming device (NOAH recommends and supports the HI-PRO interface programmer), which in turn is coupled by cable to the computer. NOAH creates a standardized program for fitting virtually all programmable hearing instruments. It is compatible with a wide range of hearing technologies, and with each licensed manufacturer's fitting module.
5. ***Real Ear Module.*** If real ear equipment has been connected to the computer and linked to NOAH's software platform, real ear data can be transferred and used in the hearing aid selection, fitting, or verification process.
6. ***Journal Module***. This allows the dispenser to add notes on fittings, troubleshooting activities, patient feedback, and professional consultations.
7. ***Printer Module.*** This allows for the printing of files, forms, or journals.

The NOAH system is intended for patient interaction by providing graphs and data on the screen that allow for informing and educating patients about their hearing, hearing aids, and the hearing aid purchase options. Not only does NOAH store and retrieve data within a given software module, it also transfers data from one software module to another, automatically. Because NOAH is modular it can be customized to the needs of the individual dispenser. It can be limited to one office or can be used to create an extensive hearing care network across multiple offices in different locations. At any time dispensers can add additional hearing aid fitting systems, integrate office management software, or connect test equipment, as long as it is NOAH licensed.

CONNEXX

CONNEXX is a programmable fitting program initiated by Siemens Hearing Instruments (1995), but used by other manufacturers as well. It uses the power of a personal computer to give the dispenser additional precision when fitting advanced technology programmable hearing instruments.

CONNEXX operates within the Microsoft® Windows® environment. It has an intuitive graphic interface allowing its learning and utilization to be easy. This system uses the HI-Pro hardware interface to program instruments and is compatible with NOAH as well.

This is a powerful consultation tool that demonstrates a hearing loss to a patient, and explains how the selection of the appropriate hearing aid can impact the end result of the fitting. The system is suggested especially for multi-band, multi-memory, compression hearing aids, that ordinarily take much guesswork and time. Changes in compression kneepoint and compression ratio can be made manually or automatically, and the results can be seen immediately on the screen.

The CONNEXX system is used in the following way:

- Enter the patient's audiogram, or download the audiogram from any compatible audiometer.
- Select from an internal list of popular prescriptive fitting methods.
- Select the manufacturer's advanced technology programmable hearing aid and allow the system to automatically select a "first fit." This taps the power of the computer to perform hundreds of thousands of calculations within seconds to optimize the set-up of the hearing aid. If the computer has CD-ROM and speakers, sound samples can be played and the instrument fine tuned. If the "first fit" approach is not preferred, the dispenser performs his/her own selections using a multitude of menus and features.
- On-line help is available.
- Results are available via an on-screen display.
- Multiple popular listening environments are available for use when fitting multiple-memory hearing aids.
- The software provides a full view of the range of adjustments for all controls on the computer screen.

OARS

OARS is an acronym for Open Audiometric Reporting Standard, which is a *proposal* for a simple, inexpensive, open cross-platform method for computerized products in the hearing health industry to communicate with each other to the degree necessary (Qualitone and dbc-Mifco, 1985). The intent is to allow hearing aid fitting systems to obtain information from an audiometer directly (eliminating the necessity for hand entry of the audiometric results). The proposal is to identify a method for being able to read, access, and modify data in a universal table language translator mode (graphs, and not just data). It is also intended to send graphical information to an office management system (OMS) for inclusion in a report.

NONCONVENTIONAL APPROACHES

Use Of Acoustic Impedance Measures in Hearing Aid Fitting

Completely different from the hearing aid selection procedures mentioned so far is the use of electroacoustic impedance measures to select certain parameters of the hearing aid, especially for those who are non-verbal or uncooperative.

McCandless and Miller (1972) first suggested its use in attempting to limit the output of a hearing aid for those individuals who were non-verbal. They attempted to relate acoustic reflex thresholds (ART) to loudness discomfort level (LDL). They found these to be about equal at about 95–100 dB SPL for both normal and cochlear losses when testing at specific frequencies. However, when using speech as a stimulus, they reported LDLs at 95 dB SPL and the ARTs at 89 dB SPL. They suggested that for hearing losses greater than 75 to 80 dB HL, that the ART and LDL were elevated 5 to 10 dB. Their recommendation for cochlear losses up to 75 dB HL was to set the SSPL90 for hearing aids at about 100 dB SPL, or at the point at which sound first becomes uncomfortable. Other studies have documented also the close relationship between LDL and the ART and the application of these to hearing aid fittings. Horning (1975) and Rainville (1976) recommended using average ARTs at 500, 1000 and 2000 Hz to specify the saturation output of hearing aids, whereas Snow and McCandless (1976) recommended that the saturation output on hearing aids be set to conversational speech or noise such that constant middle ear muscle contraction would not occur. Homes and Woodford (11) reported LDLs at a *lower* intensity than the ART for the majority of children having severe to profound hearing losses.

On the other hand, a number of studies have identified the ART much closer to the MCL than to the LDL (Rappaport and Tait, 1976; Berger; 1976; and Denenberg and Altshuler, 1976). Keith (1976) identified the ART for speech to be related to MCL for speech and the pure tone ART related to the LDL for speech. However, Preves and Orton (1978) found the ART to always be above the MCL and that the LDL was consistently higher than ART for all stimuli used (pure tones, speech spectrum noise). In both situations the individual variability was considerable. They concluded that the ART is an unreliable indicator of either MCL or UCL, and the large variability is felt to be due to variations in stimulus type and presentation format.

Tonisson (1975) used impedance measures to determine real ear gain by measuring the difference between the aided and unaided reflex thresholds. McCandless (1975) used impedance measures to adjust the gain of hearing aids. This was accomplished with the hearing aid on the head and turned on, the reflex was measured in the opposite ear (with speech input at 65 dB SPL). The gain of the aid was set to a point just below where the acoustic reflex occurred.

Attempts have also been made to use impedance measures to determine the most appropriate aided frequency response by measuring the acoustic reflex in the unaided ear and then comparing the acoustic reflex for different hearing aids (Snow and McCandless, 1976).

Synthetic Sentences

Reported by Jerger and Hayes (1976), this procedure follows the underlying philosophy that the hearing aid evaluation is not an end in itself, but is part of the total rehabilitation procedure. The method uses synthetic sentences and speech competition in varying "message-to-competition ratios" (MCR).

The goals of this technique are: (1) to determine the most suitable hearing aid arrangement, (2) to define differences among hearing aids in real life listening conditions, (3) to provide information on realistic expectations of aid use for patient counseling, and (4) to make accountable rehabilitative recommendations to patients.

The basic test set-up is diagrammed in Figure 55. The sentences are delivered at 60 dB SPL, while the competing message intensity is varied. The message-to-competition ratio varies from +20 to −20 dB. Results are obtained in the unaided, aided, and again unaided conditions. The patient's unaided and aided scores at each MCR are plotted graphically in relation to the performance of normal listeners in the same condition. (An example of a synthetic sentence is "women view men with green paper should.")

Use of ABR

The use of auditory brainstem response (ABR), or Brainstem Auditory Evoked Response (BAER) has been suggested as a technique in the prescription of hearing aids (Mokotoff and Krebs, 1976; Clark-Cox and Metz, 1980), especially for obtaining information about performance in young children where behavioral techniques may be of limited value. The intent is to use objective data upon which decisions regarding the choice of frequency response, gain setting, or a particular hearing aid can be made.

The results of ABR, displayed as seven scalp-positive waves that occur within the first 10 milliseconds following transient (short) acoustic stimuli (clicks and/or tone bursts covering a frequency range from approximately 1000 to 5000 Hz), are shown in

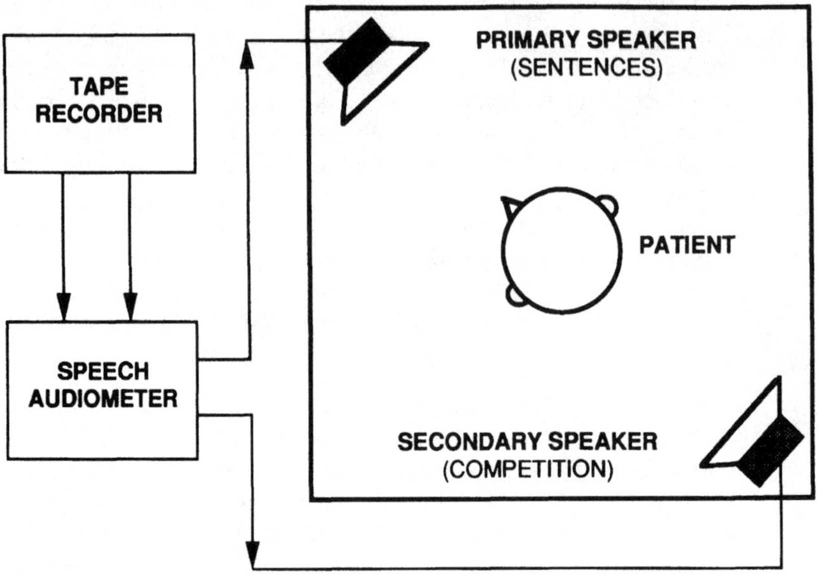

Fig. 55. Basic test set-up for hearing aid selection using synthetic sentences. Unaided and aided sentence scores are recorded at message-to-competition ratios from +20 to −20 dB (after Jerger and Hayes, 1976).

Figure 56. (Most efforts to use the ABR in hearing aid evaluations have involved click-evoked responses.) The seven waves are designated by Roman numerals with wave V typically being considered the most stable to be used in ABR testing. The figure shows a typical ABR trace for clicks under earphones and in a sound field.

To evaluate hearing aid performance, the hearing aid is fitted to the ear(s) with ABR data in sound field (or earphone suspended above the hearing aid microphone) obtained. Various methods have been used to select amplification characteristics of hearing aids:

A. The latency of wave V is noted in micro-seconds for all stimuli, with the intensity level of the stimuli being reduced in 10 dB steps. The hearing aids preselected for testing are then ranked, with the hearing aid producing the shortest latency ranked number one. Additionally, a hearing aid or hearing aid setting that produces an ABR at the lowest intensity level could be ranked number one (Clark-Cox and Metz (1980). By evaluating several aids with different response characteristics, information could be obtained that would indicate which aid produced the "best" ABR results. They reported that the hearing aid response that resulted in the shortest Wave V latency also provided the best speech intelligibility score.

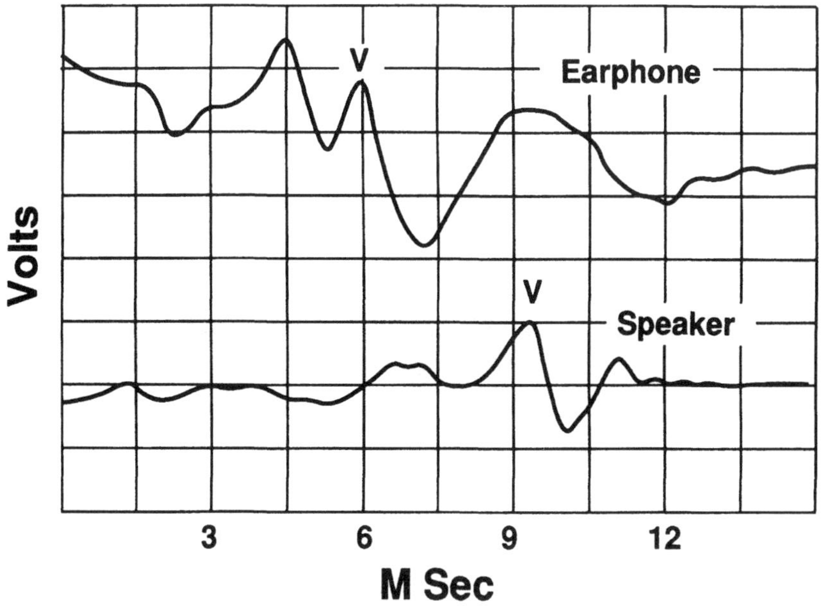

Fig. 56. Typical auditory brainstem evoked traces for clicks obtained from the same subject with earphones and free-field speaker at about the same intensity level for the clicks. The objective, scalp-positive waves which result from the presentation of these stimuli have been suggested for use with infants and young children to assist in the selection of hearing aids (Clark Cox and Metz, 1980).

B. The gain of a hearing aid is adjusted until a recognizable waveform is evident. Benefit is identified in terms of the difference between the aided and unaided ABR thresholds (Kileny, 1982; Mahoney, 1985).

C. The hearing aid's gain, output, and compression characteristics are adjusted until aided ABR latencies closely approximate normal latency values (Hecox, 1983).

Clark-Cox and Metz (1980) also suggest that the results from ABR are more accurate with some hearing loss configurations than others (i.e., fairly clear-cut results from precipitous configurations, but poorer results from sloping configurations). However, the complexity of the procedural problems inherent with ABR are cause for concern. For example, the abrupt click stimuli can produce ringing in the hearing aid (Seitz and Kisiel, 1990), or the use of tone bursts with longer duration, can create even greater artifacts (Kileny, 1982). Compression hearing aid circuits may respond too slowly to be reflected in the ABRs to click stimuli (Gorga, et. al., 1987).

The implications of studies with ABR suggest that it could be used with infants and young children to select hearing aid(s), but serious questions remain about the effectiveness of ABR to provide an accurate picture of the hearing aid's performance. Weber (1994) states that because of the procedural problems involved and with concerns about the validity of the technique, ABR is receiving very limited clinical use at this time for hearing aid selection/benefit.

HEARING AID VERIFICATION PROCEDURES

The qualification of a person's aided hearing performance is one of the most challenging problems confronting the hearing aid selection and fitting process. What follows later are approaches that have historical and current value. But first, an understanding of fundamental concepts in the verification of the hearing aid selected is warranted.

Functional Gain and Insertion Gain

Fundamental concepts in the verification of the hearing aid selection are those of functional (use) gain and insertion gain. Functional gain is a psychoacoustic or behavioral measurement whereas insertion gain is an electroacoustic term, both identified at the level of comfortable listening.

Functional gain is defined as the dB difference between unaided and aided thresholds, generally measured in a sound-field environment when using warble-tone stimuli at different frequencies, for speech, or narrow bands of noise.

Insertion gain is the dB difference between the sound pressure measured at or near the tympanic membrane location, with and without the hearing aid in place. Insertion gain is a method used to show the prescribed "target" for a particular hearing loss.

Figure 57 illustrates how functional gain and insertion gain are plotted.

These measures are used as follows in the hearing aid selection and evaluation process (Figure 58): (a) they first identify the prefitting calculations of desired gain (target functional gain or target insertion gain), and (b) they then allow for verification of how close those target gains were approximated while wearing the hearing aids (measured functional gain or measured insertion gain). Measured functional or insertion gain is also often referred to as real ear gain (this differentiates the measurement from 2-cc coupler measurements). For clinical purposes, functional and insertion gains are considered to be essentially similar (McCandless, 1982).

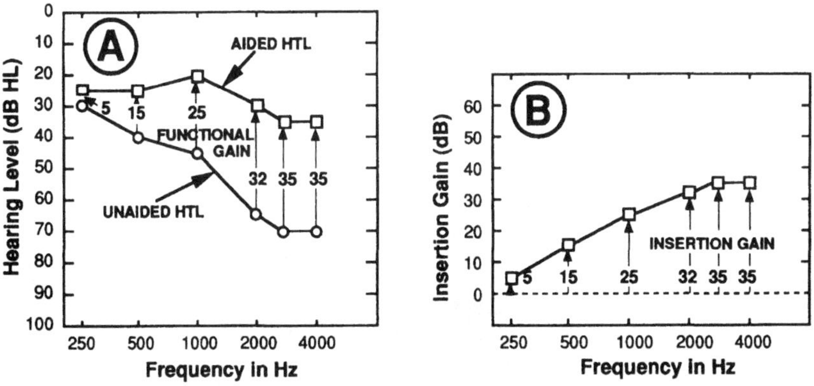

Fig. 57. The relationship between functional gain (A) and insertion gain (B) and how each is measured and plotted. (After McCandless, 1994, Overview and rationale of threshold-based hearing aid selection procedures, in Valente (Ed) Strategies for Selecting and Verifying Hearing Aid Fittings, Thieme Medical Publishers, Inc., New York, p. 7.)

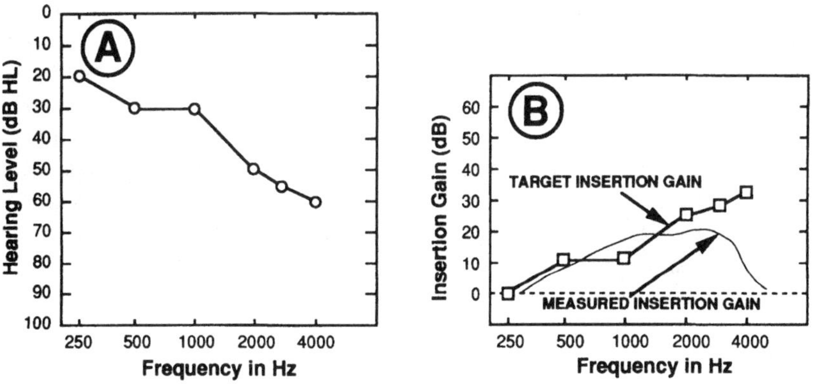

Fig. 58. Audiogram (A) and target insertion gain calculated from the prescriptive formula (POGO) (B). The measured insertion gain (B) shows too much gain in the mid-frequencies and insufficient gain in the high frequencies. (After McCandless, 1994, Overview and rationale of threshold-based hearing aid selection procedures, in Valente (Ed) Strategies for Selecting and Verifying Hearing Aid Fittings, Thieme Medical Publishers, Inc., New York, p. 7.)

Speech Audiometry

A number of hearing aid verification procedures have employed speech stimuli for verification (aided) measures. The Carhart procedure (1946) and modifications of it are notable examples, among others. Some of these verification procedures included aided (functional gain) versus unaided measures of Speech Reception Threshold sensitivity and word recognition scores. The emphasis on word recognition scores, however, has been widely criticized since a report by Shore, et. al. (1960). Specifically, concerns evolved around the unreliability and/or validity of speech stimuli, with its wide array of uncontrollable variables, as a reliable predictor of hearing aid performance. It was these concerns, in large part, that served to foster the movement toward predictive procedures based on pure-tone thresholds and/or other stimuli.

Pure Tones Presented in a Sound Field (Psychoacoustic Aided Hearing Measurements)

Goldberg (1986). This evaluation procedure (and to a lesser extent selection procedure) does not require language or the ability to recognize test words. The procedure is based on plotting results to steady-state sinusoidal signals presented in a calibrated, pure-tone sound field. All measurements are referenced to SPL and to normal hearing equal loudness contours (Goldberg, 1986). The basic principle recognizes and plots the "three most important" areas of hearing: (1) threshold of hearing, (2) preferred listening level (PLL), and (3) the UCLL—uncomfortable listening level. The final aided hearing measurements should meet or closely approach these three basic frequency contours. Moderate deviations to any of these three listening levels can result in a significant reduction in the usability of the selected aid, according to Goldberg. The procedure is intended to obtain measurements of the psychoacoustic contribution of the hearing aid, and can be referenced back to normal hearing equal loudness contour curves. Figure 59 shows the audiometric chart illustrating the important features of normal hearing, including the normal range of threshold sensitivity, the PLL for average normal listeners, and the UCLL. The lines for average best hearing and for UCLL are derived from normal equal loudness contour curves for minimum audible field (MAF) and the 110 dB phon, both corrected for a 90° presentation. The range of normal hearing sensitivity is plotted as being 25 dB. A concern of most dispensers relates to the use of pure tones through speakers (sound field), and the possibility of standing waves and interfering reflections from the furniture or reflecting walls on the room. To overcome this, a concentrated sound field is utilized, with a distance of nine inches from the speaker projections to the ear. This allows for up to two inches of patient head movement when centered between the speakers with a maximum error of 2 dB.

Related features include intensity level measurements in 2.5 dB increments. Testing is also recommended in speech noise, room noise, and street noise. The examiner should be able to mix these noises with selected tones to determine the degree of difficulty in

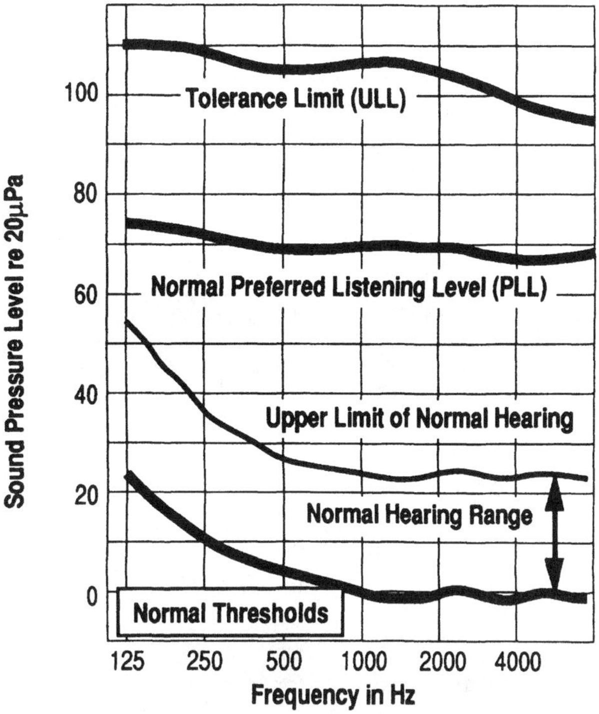

Fig. 59. Detailed 90° sound field audiometric chart showing the important features of normal hearing, including the normal range of threshold sensitivity, the preferred listening level for average normals and the uncomfortable listening level. The range of normal hearing sensitivity is shown as 25 dB.

noise. This procedure provides an estimation of use value in difficult listening situations.

The final aided hearing measurements, with the aid worn at the PLL, should meet or closely approach the three basic frequency contours at their designated intensity levels. Figure 60 shows the unaided and aided pure-tone sound-field audiogram. Four frequencies only are used (.25, .5, 1, and 3 kHz). An acceptable aided PLL is considered to be within ±4 dB from the recommended normal 70 dB equal loudness contour curve. (In many respects the procedure is similar to that of otometry). For aided hearing at PLL a flat frequency response is quite acceptable (all frequencies are loudness balanced against a reference 1000 Hz pure tone—essentially the average speech level of 69 dB SPL at one meter). In this example, the aided response exceeds the acceptable variability, and would require reduction. For both the unaided and aided UCLL, speech

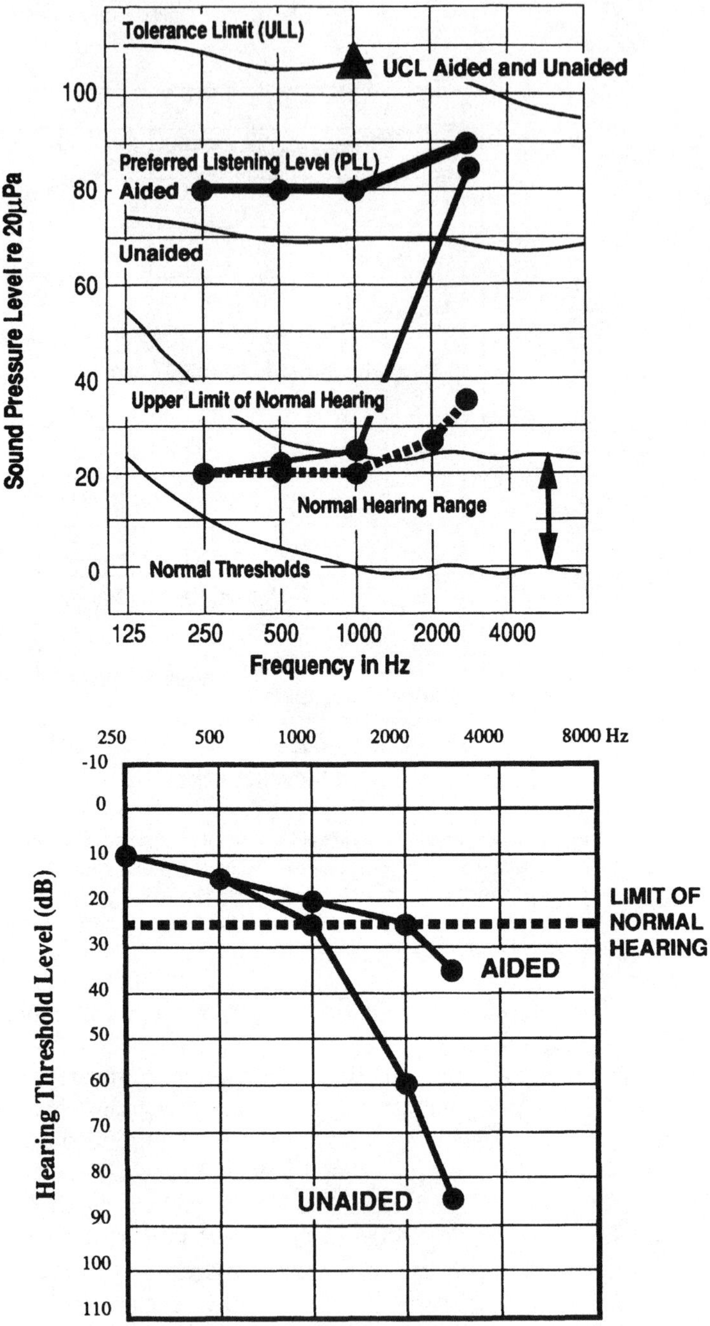

Fig. 60. Unaided and aided pure-tone sound field audiograms for the hearing loss shown in the lower graph. The final aided measurements, with the aid worn at the PLL, should closely approach the three basic curves at their designated intensity levels. An acceptable aided PLL is considered to be within ±4 dB from the recommended normal 70 dB equal loudness contour curve. This fitting shows that the aided response exceeds the acceptable variability and would require reduction.

noise (which should register the lowest unacceptable response, and because of its accuracy, ease of use, and repeatability) is used. Plotting these data in HTL can also be applied, using correction factors based on work by Shaw (1974) and Killion (1978), which are in Goldberg's report.

Probe-Microphone Measurements

A scientifically based method to assist in the selection, evaluation, and fitting of hearing aids has taken on an entirely new meaning with the advancements in microprocessor-based probe-microphone real-ear technology. Systems using this technology measure the amount by which a hearing aid changes the SPL in the external ear canal relative to the unaided condition. This approach allows the hearing aid and its associated coupling performance to be measured rapidly and objectively (voluntary response by the patient not required), near the tympanic membrane, while the hearing aids are being worn (*in situ*). As such, probe-microphone testing allows for verification of fitting formulae, helps determine if the hearing aids meet the patient's acoustic needs, and accurately displays what is occurring at the eardrum.

Although initial probe-microphone measurements within the external auditory canal were reported as early as 1946 by Wiener and Ross, it was not until 1981 that Harford presented a pragmatic approach to the use of probe-microphone measurements for hearing aid selection/benefit. A number of different systems are now available for probe-microphone measurements. (An excellent review of the use of probe-microphone measurements for hearing aid selection and assessment is provided by Mueller, Hawkins, and Northern, 1992.)

What is not fully understood, is that ***probe-microphone measurements are not a method of fitting hearing aids per se, but provide a method for evaluating whether prescriptive gain targets have actually been achieved when the hearing aids are worn. They do not determine or develop a fitting philosophy.*** For the most part, probe-microphone measurements are used to support prescriptive fitting approaches, if those prescriptive approaches are based on frequency specific gain, but can provide additional fitting information as well. Unfortunately, and as used primarily today, matching a prescriptive target gain does not assure that a successful fitting has been achieved, or even that speech has been made audible (Mueller, 1992).

Basic Concept

In real-ear probe-microphone measurements, (1) the natural resonance of the ear is measured near the tympanic membrane via a

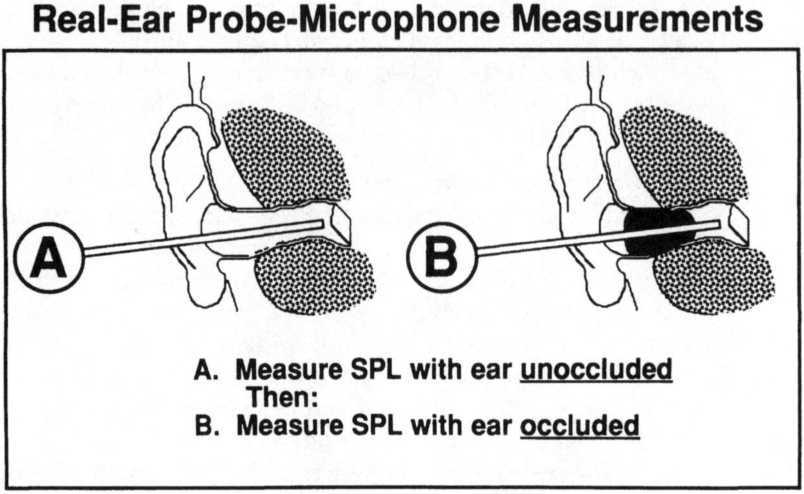

Fig. 61. Concept of real-ear probe-microphone measurements. In (A) the natural resonance of the ear is measured near the tympanic membrane by a probe microphone with the canal unoccluded, and then the measurements of amplification from the hearing aid can be measured with the ear canal occluded (B).

probe microphone with the canal open (unoccluded), and then (2) measurements of amplification are made with the hearing aid and its associated coupling (occluded) with the probe microphone in the same position (Figure 61). A variety of measurements that comprise the hearing aid selection and fitting procedures have been identified and follow later.

Probe-Microphone Systems

A number of different probe-microphone systems exist. Use of these instruments, regardless of manufacturer, involves two basic phases: (1) pre-measurement procedures to prepare the equipment and the patient, and (2) the real-ear measurement tests as listed in the previous paragraphs. A detailed explanation of probe-microphone systems can be found in Mueller, Hawkins, and Northern, 1992.

Phase 1. It is first necessary to conduct a series of pre-measurement procedures to prepare both the equipment and the patient. These are explained briefly as follows, realizing that these steps are handled somewhat differently by the various systems and, therefore, their operating manuals should be consulted:

A. *Equalization.* The purpose of this process is to control the sound-field signal so that its amplitude is at the same level across the frequency range.

B. *Probe Calibration.* The purpose of this procedure is to render the probe tube that will be placed in the ear canal ineffective—to make it essentially "acoustically invisible." The intent is to record measurements as if the microphone were located near the tympanic membrane. This step, and a close proximity of the probe tip to the tympanic membrane, is critical to the accuracy of real-ear measurements, especially at the high frequencies. A generalized insertion depth method is to place a ring marker on the probe 28 mm from the tip, and then place the ring marker at the tragal notch (for an adult). This is then the depth to which the probe should be inserted for all subsequent measurements. The probe calibration correction factor will automatically be applied by the instrumentation to all measurements.

C. *Patient Positioning.* The distance and angle to the loudspeaker must be taken into consideration. Distances from 0.5 to 1 meter are generally recommended. Facing angles from 0° to 45° are commonly used.

D. *Otoscopic Examination.* This is necessary prior to testing to determine at least if debris or excessive cerumen will interfere with the probe placement or potentially plug the probe.

Phase 2. Following real-ear set-up procedures, a series of measurements are made that help validate the hearing aid fitting process targets.

Real-Ear Unaided Response (REUR). This is usually the first of the measurements obtained and represents primarily the resonance characteristics of the open ear canal, but also the diffraction effects of the head, pinna and concha (Figure 62). An input level of 60 dB SPL is usually appropriate. The average adult REUR demonstrates a primary peak around 2700 Hz of about 17 dB, and a secondary peak of about 12–14 dB in the 4000 to 5000 Hz region.

The REUR has been used in at least three ways for hearing aid validation and selection: (1) it is most commonly used as a reference value to help calculate the hearing aid insertion gain: the insertion gain being used to validate prescriptive gain formulae targets, (2) the REUR has also been used when ordering custom-molded hearing aids to help determine the most appropriate 2-cc coupler response, and (3) to select a hearing aid real-ear frequency response that follows the same pattern as the REUR. The latter approach is not consistent with selective amplification prescriptive approaches and requires substantiation.

Real-Ear Occluded Response (REOR). This is the response of the ear canal and concha with the hearing aid in place but turned

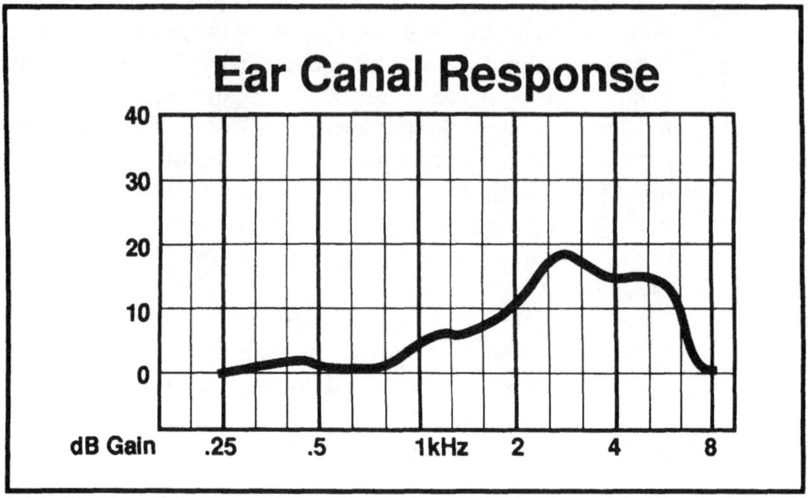

Fig. 62. REUR (Real-Ear Unaided Response). Ear canal response that represents primarily the resonance characteristics of the open ear canal, but also the diffraction effects of the head, pinna, and concha.

off, and with a 60 dB SPL input. This provides an estimate of the *insertion loss* created by placing a hearing aid or earmold in the ear (Figure 63). This measurement is not ordinarily obtained, but when recorded, REOR can provide some indications about the effect of venting of the coupling being used, or if feedback is being caused by the coupling.

Real-Ear Aided Response (REAR). This is normally measured immediately following the REUR and represents the aided ear measurement. It can be expressed in dB SPL or in dB SPL relative to the input. This includes the total response of the hearing aid system, including the REUR, and has been referred to in the past as the *in situ response,* or *in situ gain.* This measurement is similar of those obtained to 2-cc measurements; the exception being that the patient's own ear is used as the "load" rather than the 2-cc coupler.

REAR is used most commonly today to calculate *insertion gain,* and in some test equipment may not even be displayed. Still, REAR could be used to visualize other aspects of hearing aid performance (i.e., directional microphone performance, troubleshooting user complaints relating to feedback or unpleasant sound quality, or other types of signal processing applications). The relationships between REAR, REUR, and REOR are illustrated in Figure 63, left panel.

Real-Ear Saturation Response (RESR). This represents the aided ear with the hearing aid at saturation (rather than at use gain

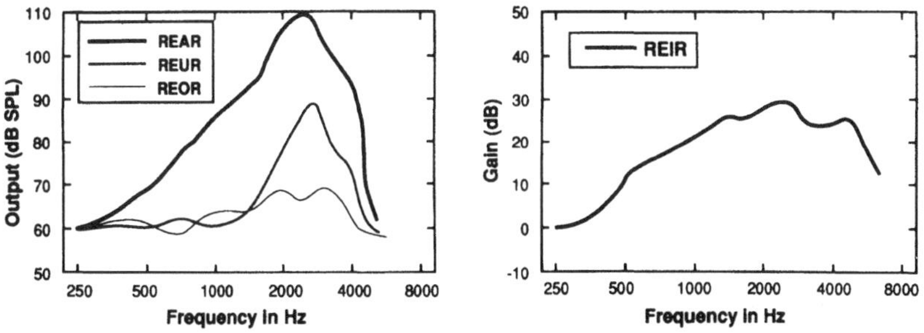

Fig. 63. Left panel: Illustration of the real ear unocluded response (REUR), the real ear occluded response (REOR), and the real ear aided response (REAR). The right panel shows the resulting real ear insertion response (REIR) for the measurements shown in the left panel. (Modified from Mueller, H. G., 1992, Terminology and procedures, in Mueller, Hawkins, and Northern (eds), Probe Microphone Measurements: Hearing Aid Selection and Assessment, Singular Publishing Group, Inc.: San Diego, p. 62).

as is the REAR) and is considered the real-ear counterpart to the SSPL90 measurement obtained on a 2-cc coupler. The use of this measurement seems to be especially important for the selection of hearing aid saturation outputs for those who are not able to provide qualified subjective judgments of loudness discomfort levels (young children and/or non responsive patients).

Real-Ear Insertion Response (REIR). This calculation is the REAR minus the REUR in dB (Figure 63), and represents the functional gain provided by the hearing aid worn. When identified at a specific frequency, it is referred to as the Real-Ear Insertion Gain (REIG). It is the amount of gain delivered when wearing a hearing aid that was not present before the hearing aid fitting. (REUR must be subtracted because it was present prior to the hearing aid fitting.)

REIR, as an electroacoustic measurement, approximates the behavioral measurement of functional gain (Dillon and Murray, 1987). As a result, REIG, especially, can be used to replace functional gain in formulae developed prior to the use of probe-microphone measurements. The importance of insertion response (gain) is that it agrees much more closely with subjective measures of hearing aid performance than do traditional coupler measurements.

REIR is used primarily to verify desired frequency specific target gains suggested by various fitting formulae. In fact, the measurement of REIR without a target becomes rather meaningless. Additionally, almost all probe-microphone test equipment can calculate and display prescriptive target insertion gains if puretone thresholds are entered. The target gains and REIR are often used during patient counseling to identify the success of the fitting.

Care must be taken, however, because it is rare for the target gains to be achieved at all frequencies.

***Real-Ear Coupler Difference* (*RECD*).** This is the difference in dB between the output of a hearing aid measured in the real ear versus that measured in a 2-cc coupler at the same settings. As suggested by Punch, et. al. (1990), this value combines the use of probe-microphone measurements with a prescriptive formula to arrive at a desired 2-cc coupler gain as an *individual* personal correction factor. This is different than correcting the 2-cc coupler response to derive the desired real-ear response. Because it includes the REUR for a particular person and then correcting for differences in the frequency responses in the 2-cc coupler versus that in the patient's ear, individualized target coupler gain can be specified as measured in a 2-cc coupler. This calculation would appear to allow for hearing aid selection, when used with prescriptive fitting approaches, to more closely approximate these prescriptive targets than are currently achieved by using average correction values.

Hearing aid success depends on having a goal. Real ear measurements are used to validate and verify the specific advantage provided by the HAs under evaluation. In general, the reliability of probe-microphone measures is relatively good, with some discrepancy at higher frequencies.

Just Able to Follow Speech

This procedure involves presenting continuous discourse at normal conversational speech levels from 0° azimuth, and some type of continuous competing noise from 180°. The noise is increased (ascending procedure) in level from the rear in 5 dB increments (2.5 dB increments would be better), until the patient can no longer follow the conversation from the front. This noise level is recorded. Alternate hearing aids, coupling, or modifications are made to the instrument and the test repeated with each alteration. The hearing aid combination that provides the highest noise level before speech can no longer be followed, is often considered the instrument of choice.

Estimation of Insertion Gain From 2-cc Coupler Measurements

Correction factors have been used to estimate insertion gain frequency response on real ears (or on KEMAR: Knowles Electronics Manikin for Acoustical Research) from 2-cc coupler frequency response data (Burkhard, 1978; Lybarger, 1978; Killion and Monser, 1980, Longwell and Johnson, 1980; Frye, 1982, McCandless and Lyregaard, 1983). This allows an approximation of the corrections needed and allows them to be applied to any hearing aid measured according to ANSI S3.22-1987.

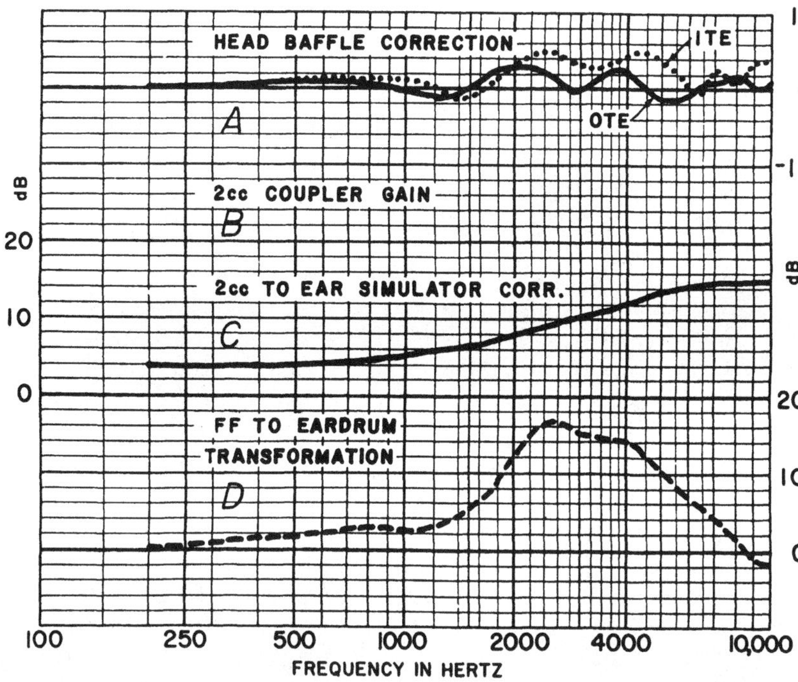

Fig. 64. Information used to estimate insertion gain from 2-cc coupler data (Lybarger, 1985).

Correction values can be practical if the following precautions are taken (Staab and Lybarger, 1994):

1. The correction used must be for the type of aid used, taking into account the microphone pickup location.
2. The physical, acoustic connection from the aid to the reference plane of the coupler or ear simulator must be identical acoustically with the user's tubing and earmold.
3. Corrections are applicable to closed coupler and occluded earmold conditions on a 2-cc coupler. (Estimates of venting effects can be applied after the estimated insertion gain is determined.)
4. Corrections are average. Large individual variations may exist.

Additionally, Lybarger (1985) has identified the combination of components involved in estimating insertion gain from coupler data (Figure 64). These include:

1. Head baffle.
2. 2-cc coupler response

3. 2-cc coupler-to-eardrum correction, and
4. Free field-to-eardrum transformation

Table 11 provides estimated 2-cc coupler to insertion gain corrections for various types of hearing aids by various investigators.

SELF-ASSESSMENT SCALES OF HEARING AID BENEFIT

Self-assessment scales have also been used to verify hearing aid performance. Although a number of self-assessment scales of hearing handicap have been developed, only a handful have been evaluated relative to their use for hearing aid benefit. When hearing aid benefit has been evaluated, the general purpose has been to determine if a reduction in hearing handicap is reported by the patient pre- and post-amplification. Self-assessment scales that have been evaluated for hearing aid benefit include the Hearing Handicap Scale (HHS) by Tannahill (1979); the Hearing Performance Inventory (HPI) by Dempsey (1986); the Hearing Handicap Inventory for the Elderly (HHIE) by Newman and Weinstein (1988); the Profile of Hearing Aid Performance (PHAP) by Cox and Gilmore (1990); the Abbreviated Profile of Hearing Aid Benefit (APHAB) by Cox and Alexander (1994), and the NAL Client Oriented Scale of Improvement (COSI), developed and investigated by the National Acoustic Laboratories (NAL) and distributed by Oticon (1996).

In the U.S. the APHAB is used fairly extensively and has had significant research conducted on it as a self-assessment tool for evaluating hearing aid benefit. As such, it is duplicated in Appendix A of this Chapter. The fact that other self-assessment scales are not reprinted does not mean that they are not preferred—only that a single example is used here to help explain the format and use of self-assessment scales.

SUMMARY OF HEARING AID SELECTION METHODS

Each hearing aid selection method has had some success. It is incumbent on the dispenser to decide the advantages and limitations of any system. Successful use of any procedure depends on more than just the electroacoustical end result. It also involves effective patient management, necessary counseling to allow the patient to understand and accept the hearing aids, verification procedures, and an understanding that the initial patient response may not prevail over time.

Table 11. Estimated 2-cc Coupler to Insertion Gain Corrections[a]

Frequency	BTE[b] (CALC)	ITE-1[c] (CALC)	ITE-2[d] L&T ('86)	ITE-3[e] B&B ('87)	ITC[f] (CALC)
200	**3.8**	**3.6**	4.8	2.5	**3.6**
300	**3.4**	**3.2**	3.5	2.4	**3.7**
400	**3.7**	**3.7**	3.3	2.2	**3.6**
500	**3.6**	**4.0**	2.7	2.0	**2.3**
600	**3.3**	**4.1**	2.2	1.5	**2.2**
700	**2.8**	**3.8**	1.9	1.5	**3.2**
800	**2.5**	**3.7**	2.0	1.6	**2.3**
900	**2.5**	**3.8**	2.8	2.2	**3.4**
1000	**2.7**	**4.2**	2.8	1.6	**5.1**
1200	**2.5**	**3.7**	2.6	2.3	**0.8**
1400	**1.4**	**1.1**	3.2	2.7	**−0.8**
1600	**2.2**	**0.7**	3.4	2.0	**−1.0**
1800	**1.5**	**0.4**	1.8	0.8	**−2.3**
2000	**−0.5**	**−0.6**	1.5	−1.2	**−2.4**
2200	**−2.8**	**−1.8**	0.6	−2.7	**−2.2**
2400	**−4.7**	**−2.4**	−1.8	−4.6	**−2.6**
2600	**−5.8**	**−2.4**	−3.7	−5.7	**−2.3**
2800	**−5.8**	**−2.1**	−3.4	−5.6	**−1.7**
3000	**−5.0**	**−1.6**	−1.2	−4.3	**−1.8**
3200	**−3.5**	**−1.0**	−0.9	−2.6	**−2.4**
3400	**−1.7**	**−0.4**	2.4	−1.0	**−2.2**
3600	**−0.5**	**0.5**	3.5	0.5	**−1.0**
3800	**0.3**	**1.3**	4.5	1.8	**−0.3**
4000	**0.5**	**2.5**	6.7	2.8	**0.6**
4500	**0.3**	**5.2**	10.0	5.1	**5.1**
5000	**1.8**	**6.9**	8.6	6.7	**6.1**
5500	**4.0**	**7.7**	10.2	10.3	**7.8**
6000	**6.5**	**7.6**	12.6	11.6	**7.3**
6500	**9.6**	**8.5**	15.3	14.8	**8.9**
7000	**11.5**	**13.3**	18.2	19.7	**11.0**
7500			16.7	17.2	
8000	**15.1**	**14.1**	15.2	16.8	
9000	**15.7**	**19.5**			
10000	**17.4**	**20.6**			

[a] Add values to 2-cc curves to obtain estimated insertion gain
[b] BTE = Calculated correction (Lybarger, 1985; Lybarger and Teder, 1986)
[c] ITE − 1 = Calculated correction (Lybarger, 1985; Lybarger and Teder, 1986)
[d] ITE − 2 = S3-48 Round Robin. One aid, six labs, on KEMAR (Lybarger and Teder, 1986)
[e] ITE − 3 = Ten different ITEs on KEMAR (Burnett and Beck, 1987)
[f] ITC = Calculated (Lybarger, 1985; Lybarger and Teder, 1986)

ELECTROACOUSTIC CHARACTERISTICS

An understanding of the electroacoustic characteristics of a hearing aid is important to the hearing aid specialist. The measurement of these characteristics, however, can be quite variable between measurement sites and individuals. Still, good use can be made of these measured characteristics, as long as the methods of measurement and what is measured are understood.

Unfortunately, some hearing aid dispensers measure hearing aid performance in the hard-walled 2cc couplers specified by various "Standards" and attempt to apply these data directly to the fitting of a hearing aid. This is not what the Standards* were developed to do. Rather, they were all developed to assist in the *comparison of hearing aid performance from one facility to another and one aid to another.* (A more extensive explanation of technical standards relating to measurement instrumentation and approaches can be found in Chapter 43, Katz Handbook of Clinical Audiology, by Staab and Lybarger, 1994).

HEARING AID COUPLERS

Hearing aid couplers are also known as "artificial ears." This is a standard device needed to couple the hearing aid to the measurement microphone. When used for bone-conduction devices it is known as an "artificial mastoid."

In the measurement system the hearing aid must be measured into a "load resistance." The load resistance was speculated to be approximately 2-cc and an artificial ear was developed around this volume. Theoretically, this is approximately the same volume of air in an occluded ear canal between the tip of an earmold inserted into an ear and the tympanic membrane (Figure 65).

Figure 66 illustrates FOUR popular methods for coupling hearing aids to an artificial ear for measurement purposes—all into a 2cc volume coupler. Figure 66A and 66B show the HA-1 type coupler. This HA-1 coupler is adapted to test earphones using plastic tubing, such as in behind-the-ear or eyeglass hearing aids (66A), and actual earmolds (66B—i.e., in-the-ear hearing aids), etc. The test results should state the nature, dimensions, and material of the

*The term "standard" implies consensus and approval and that they have regulatory power. However, it is important to realize that U.S. "Standards" as identified herein do not mandate anything, but that they are recommendations that may be followed on a voluntary basis. It is only when they are adopted by a regulatory agency that their measurements become required rather than voluntary (i.e. FDA). (Preves, 1996).

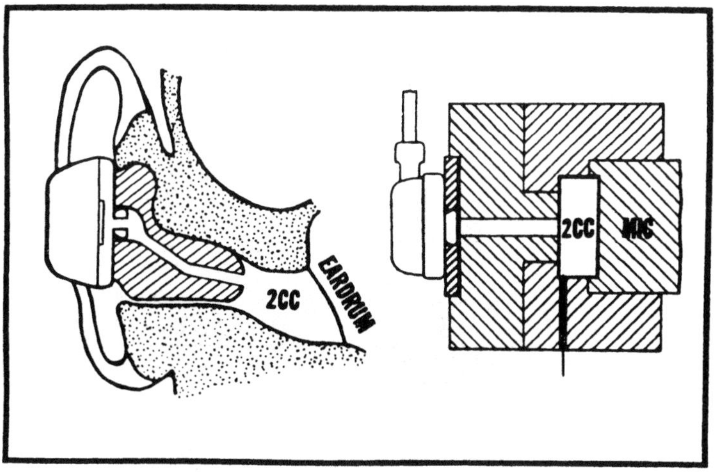

Fig. 65. A conventional type receiver on the ear and on a 2-cc coupler to show how the latter simulates an actual ear. (With permission, Staab, W. J. 1978, *Hearing Aid Handbook,* Blue Ridge Summit, PA, p. 166).

components forming the acoustic tube. The HA-2 coupler is shown in 66C and 66D and is used with earphones provided with a nub (66C—as in body-worn hearing aids), or for earphone coupler with entrance through a tube (66D). Figure 66E is a special form of the HA-1 coupler and is intended for testing the module portion of a modular ITE hearing aid and/or nonbattery (insert) type receivers. It uses a rigid or flexible sealing construction, and unless otherwise specified, has a tube diameter of 1.93 mm and a length of 10 mm. The proposed HA-4 coupler (66F) is a variation of the HA-2 coupler and is intended for BTE or eyeglass testing. It has a sound path bore through the earmold from the end of the earhook of a BTE aid, or from the end of the sound outlet on the eyeglass aid. A uniform diameter of 1.93 mm and a length of 43 mm is assumed.

The hearing aid specialist should understand that hearing aid measurements using different coupler volumes and connections will result in different performance measurements, but they can still function well for standards or comparison purposes. For example, even though the 2cc coupler volume was developed prior to World War II, it was recognized that measurements obtained with it were only approximations of what would happen in the real ear. Therefore, a variety of couplers have been developed, with most having smaller volumes than 2-cc. The reason for this is that real ear probe microphone measurements indicate that 2-cc

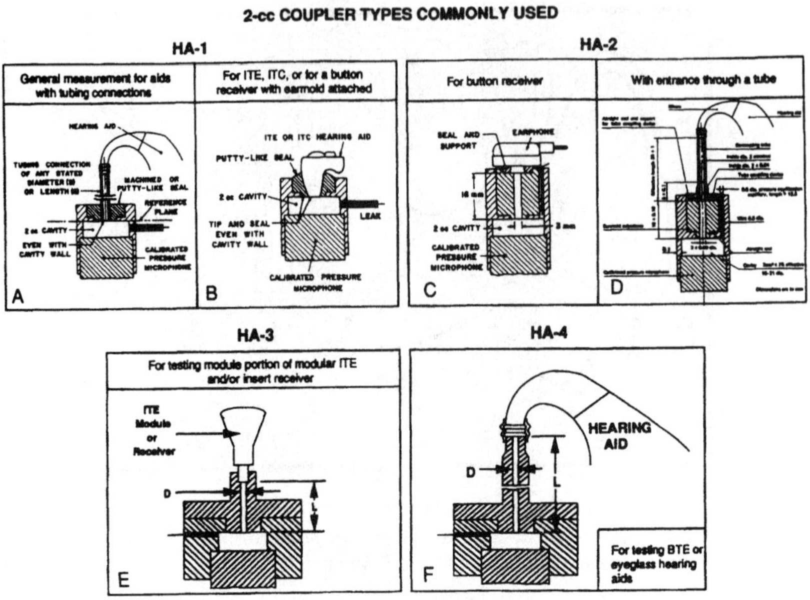

Fig. 66. 2-cc couplers commonly used in hearing aid measurement. (A) and (B) are the most generalized forms used. The relatively large opening in the sound entrance face allows almost any tubing, earmold, ITE, or ITC aid to be mounted on the coupler with a suitable formable material. (C), for use with a button receiver, and (D) having a dual diameter entrance tube that has a serious disadvantage in that it does not replicate general earmold manufacturing practice. (E) and (F), recent coupler designations for ITE modules and/or insert receivers and for BTE or eyeglass hearing aids, respectively. (With permission from Staab, W., and Lybarger, S, 1994, Characteristics and use of hearing aids, in Katz, J., Ed. *Handbook of Clinical Audiology, Fourth Edition.* Baltimore: Williams & Wilkins, p. 705).

volume is too large and, therefore, does not provide as good an indication of real ear performance as could be available.

As a result, the 2-cc coupler, while considered the "workhorse" coupler for hearing aid measurements, has some limitations; the greatest of which is the fact that the SPL in average actual ears is generally higher over the frequency band than measured in a 2-cc coupler. This indicates that the volume of the coupler is larger than optimum. What this means is that the 2-cc responses differ from real ear probe tube microphone measurements. Still, the 2-cc coupler has performed well for the purpose for which it was designed: the comparison of hearing aids. The response curves obtained with the 2-cc coupler are absolutely reproducible, making the coupler invaluable for inspection control. The coupler is also simple and robust in design—desirable features of any standard device. Because it is standardized through the world it will continue to be used for many years.

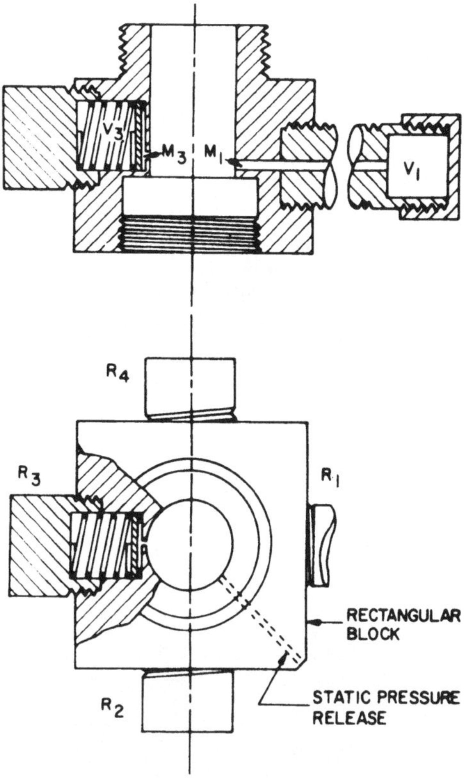

Fig. 67. Diagram of a Zwislocki type four-branch ear simulator. There are four resonant side branches tuned to produce a standardized acoustical input impedance similar to that of typical human ears. (Courtesy of Knowles Electronics, Inc., Itasca, IL).

ALTERNATE COUPLERS

In spite of the fact that the 2cc coupler will continue to be used for many years, alternate couplers have, and will continue, the be developed. What makes it difficult to decide on any coupler is to select one which would be typical for all ears. Unfortunately, the acoustic impedance of the ear canal in which a hearing aid receiver must work is substantially different for various types of pathological conditions. However, since most losses fitted with amplification are sensorineural, the use of "normal" acoustic impedance parameters seem most desirable for standardization.

The most commonly used alternate is the Zwislocki Coupler. Described in 1970 by Zwislocki, this coupler has four acoustical networks having an acoustical impedance that more accurately matches the impedance of the average normal ear (Figure 67). This coupler has a cavity volume of 1.2-cc. Adapters have been designed to simulate HA-1 and HA-2 type connections.

A comparison of output sound pressure differences obtained from a 2cc versus a Zwislocki coupler are show in Figure 68. The

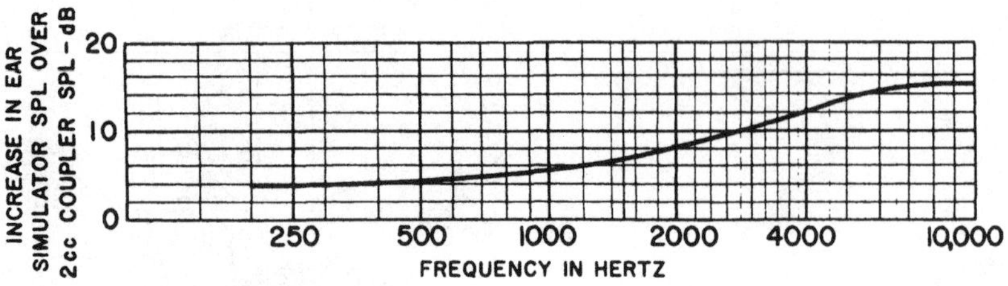

Fig. 68. Curve showing approximate relationship of the SPL in an ear simulator to that in a 2-cc coupler. (With permission from Staab, W., and Lybarger, S., 1994, Characteristics and use of hearing aids, in Katz, J., Ed. *Handbook of Clinical Audiology, Fourth Edition.* Baltimore: Williams & Wilkins, p. 707).

difference is about 4 dB before 800 Hz, and as high as about 14 dB at 5000 Hz.

BODY EFFECTS ON HEARING AID PERFORMANCE

Body effects should be considered by the hearing aid dispenser when hearing aid measurements are made. While more difficult to control, consideration should be made of: (1) body diffraction and clothing effects, (2) the accounting for and use of the head, pinna, concha diffraction, and resonances, and (3) the mounting of the hearing aid to the head.

Two potential solutions appeared to be: (1) standardize an artificial head and torso, and (2) adopt standard correction or equalizing curves applied to free field measurements. KEMAR (Knowles Electronics Manikin for Acoustic Research—Burkhard and Sachs, 1975) is an attempt at the first potential solution (Figure 69).

With KEMAR the influence of head and body diffraction can be included in hearing aid measurements. KEMAR is an imitation of the upper part of the human body. The design of the ear canal and eardrum simulator, made to match the acoustic data of the real ear, is based on use of the Zwislocki coupler. Consequently, all KEMAR measurements are made using a Zwislocki coupler—although a Zwislocki coupler can be used for hearing aid measurements without KEMAR.

DESCRIPTIVE PERFORMANCE OF THE HEARING AID

The performance characteristics of a hearing aid (how an input signal is changed as it is taken from acoustic to electric to acoustic)

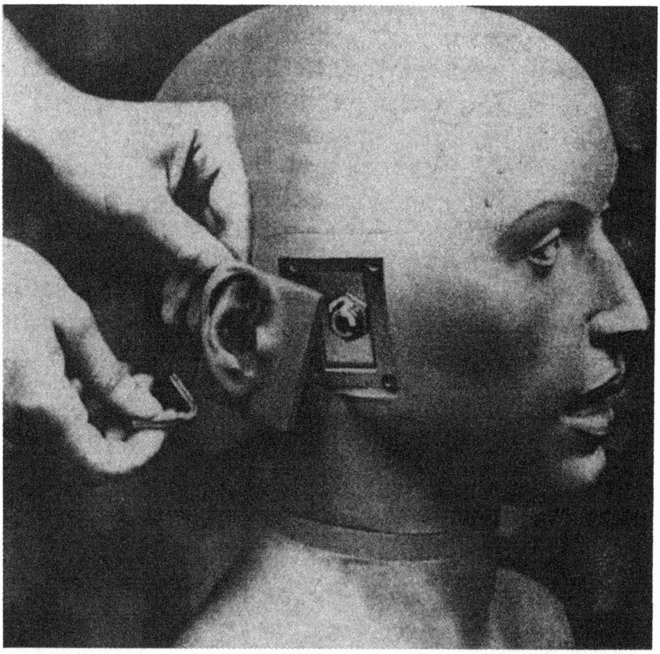

Fig. 69. KEMAR, showing removable ear with part of Zwislocki coupler showing. KEMAR consists of a standardized artificial head and torso to provide an indication of body effects on hearing aid performance.

are known as the electroacoustic characteristics. The main characteristics are described according to the following basic formula:

INPUT + GAIN = OUTPUT

INPUT

While not a performance characteristic, no measurements can be obtained without an input stimulus. Input is the sound source to the microphone and is measured in SPL.

ACOUSTIC GAIN

Acoustic gain is the amount (in dB) that the SPL in the amplifier exceeds the SPL received by the microphone.

60 + ? = 110
Gain = 50 since gain equals output minus input

ACOUSTIC OUTPUT

Acoustic output is the sum (in dB) of SPL at the microphone plus gain.

60 + 50 = ?
Output = 110 since output equals input plus gain

SATURATION

Saturation is also known as overload, maximum power output (MPO), and saturation sound pressure level (SSPL). Saturation is the maximum SPL the hearing aid can produce with a given gain and frequency—regardless of the input level. In the following example, the saturation of this hearing aid is reached at an input level of 80 dB input. Note that no further changes in the output level occurred beyond this level, even though the input continued to increase. The saturation level had been reached at an output level of 130 dB.

INPUT	+	GAIN	=	OUTPUT
30	+	50	=	80
40	+	50	=	90
50	+	50	=	100
60	+	50	=	110
70	+	50	=	120
80	+	50	=	130
90	+	50	=	130
100	+	50	=	130

FREQUENCY RESPONSE

A hearing aid does not amplify all frequencies equally. The resultant curve or configuration depends on the combined responses of the microphone, amplifier, and receiver. A hearing aid frequency response curve shows relative gain as a function of (1) constant input, and (2) frequency. This will be described in more detail later in this section.

DISTORTION

Distortion is the failure of the system to reproduce the received acoustic waveform with exactness. Distortion is by definition, any signal component or characteristic present at the output which was not present at the input. Various types of distortion include: nonlinear, frequency, phase, transient, and noise.

SIGNAL/NOISE RATIO

Signal/Noise ratio is the difference in dB between the signal and noise in a system. It is used to determine the inherent noise level of a hearing aid.

HEARING AID STANDARDS

Historically, methods have existed to measure and express hearing aid performance for an accurate comparison of aids. These have consisted of Measurement Standards versus Performance Standards.

Hearing aid standards have as their secretariat the Acoustical Society of America (ASA). They accredit the following American National Standards Institute (ANSI) Committees: S1–Acoustics; S2–Mechanical Shock and Vibration; S3–Bioacoustics; and S12–Noise. Hearing aid standards fall under the scope of the S3–Bioacoustics committee. This committee provides standards, specifications, methods of measurement and test, and terminology in the fields of mechanical shock and physiological acoustics, including aspects of general acoustics, shock, and vibration that pertain to biological safety, tolerance, and comfort. A number of their issues relate to hearing aids. These are: S3–48, Hearing Aids; S3–80, Probe Tube Measurement of Hearing Aid Performance; S3–37, Coupler Calibration of Earphones; and S3–81, Assistive Listening Devices. Most of what follows is related to work developed by the S3–48 working group (Preves, 1996).

The original Measurement Standards consisted of the ANSI (American National Standards Institute) S3.3-1960 "Methods for Measurement of Electroacoustical Characteristics of Hearing Aids" in the United States. This standard was based on one of the first hearing aid measurement standards developed, ASA Z24.14-1953, titled American Standard Method for Measurement of Characteristics of Hearing Aids (Lybarger, 1994). The S3.3 standard has been reaffirmed repeatedly, first in 1971, and last in 1990. Note that the S3.3 standard preceeded the ANSI S3.22, which was requested specifically by the FDA in 1976. However, the latter did not replace S3.3. Therefore, any approach to standards must also consider what went prior to the change, and be included, when not specifically eliminated or replaced. Internationally, and having somewhat similar features, was the IEC Electrotechnical

Commission) Recommendation 126-1961. The ANSI S3.22 and IEC 126 documents dealt with specific measurement techniques and procedures that should be followed when making electroacoustic measurements.

The original Performance Standards for committing the measured data to paper were the USA Standard Method of Expressing Hearing Aid Performance (1971), and the Hearing Aid Industry Conference Standard Method of Expressing Hearing Aid Performance (1974). The purpose of these Performance Standards was to arrive at an expression of hearing aid performance using a single number—such as for gain, output, frequency range, and several related matters.

ANSI S3.22-1976 (REVISIONS 1982, 1987)

This Standard, first approved by the Acoustical Society of America (ASA) and then later by the American National Standards Institute (ANSI), both in 1976, combined the earlier Measurement Standards and Performance Standards into one document. In addition, it (1) suggested changes in measuring techniques, and (2) recommended tolerances—the first time in a standard. This Standard now titled the "American National Standards of Hearing Aid Characteristics ANSI S3.22-1987 (ASA 7-1987)" is also used by the Food and Drug Administration (FDA) of the United States to express its technical data values for hearing aid labeling.

The ANSI S3.22-1987 is being updated and is expected to be adopted as ANSI S3.22-1996. Some of the changes being incorporated into this revision consist of: (1) a simulated telephone sensitivity rating, (2) simulated room loop ration (optional), (3) input-output curve and attack/release times at active frequencies (optional), (4) modified attack time rest, (5) same reference test position for AGC and linear aids, (6) output noise as a function of frequency (optional), and (7) quiescent and peak battery current ratings (optional)—(Cole, 1995). It appears also that because a 90 dB input SPL may not cause saturation, and also to attempt to be more consistent with IEC 118 series of standards, the term Saturation Sound Pressure Level for 90 dB input SPL and its abbreviation SSPL90 will be replaced with Output Sound Pressure Level with a 90 dB input SPL and OSPL90, respectively (ANSI S3.22-199x draft, 1995).

With the exception of a change in input level used to measure harmonic distortion at 1600 Hz (65 dB instead of 70 dB SPL), the 1982 revision of the S3.22 standard consisted primarily of editorial changes. Other standards of related significance, but not dis-

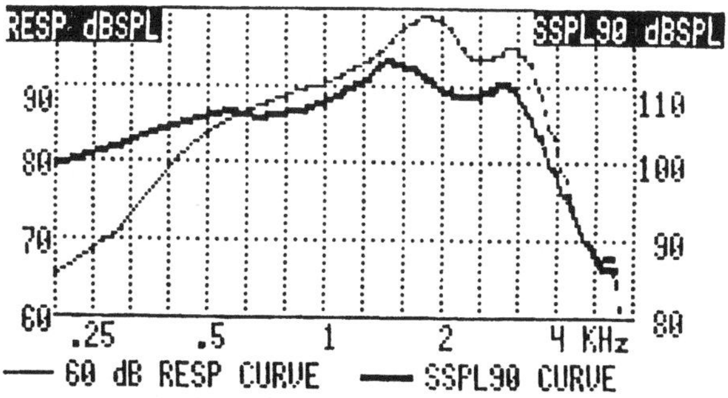

MAX SSPL90: 113.3 dB AT: 1500 Hz HF AVG: 110.1 dB	RESP LIMIT: 73.5 dB F1= 330 Hz F2=4500 Hz	
HF AVG FULL ON GAIN: AT 60 dB IN 37.3 dB RESPONSE CURVE GAIN: 33.5 dB REFERENCE TEST GAIN: 33.1 dB	THD FREQ SRC 1.0 % 500 Hz 70 dB 1.8 % 800 Hz 70 dB 0.9 % 1600 Hz 65 dB EQ INP NOISE: 22.6 dB BAT (1.3 V) 0.93 mA	ANSI S3.22-1987 LINEAR TYPE AID F.O.G. AT 60 dB

Fig. 70. Automatic ANSI print-out for a linear hearing aid. (With permission from Staab, W., and Lybarger, S., 1994, Characteristics and use of hearing aids, in Katz, J., Ed. *Handbook of Clinical Audiology, Fourth Edition.* Baltimore: Williams & Wilkins, p. 712).

cussed in this Chapter include: Occluded Ear Simulator (ANSI Standard S3.25–1979); Manikin Measurements (ANSI Standard S3.35–1985); and Noise Test Standard (S3.42–1992).

FDA required labeling for hearing aids is responsible for the data provided by hearing aid manufacturers for each hearing aid. Figure 70 provides a representative sample of what is required, followed by a line-by-line explanation of the data provided, how the data was obtained, and what the required tolerance is for that measurement. Other hearing aids would have their performance expressed by different values.

SSPL90 Curve Run at 90 dB SPL Input

General Explanation. The input signal used to develop the maximum output on the graph was developed with 90 dB SPL input. Since this is not an actual performance measurement, it has no other interpretations or tolerances.

SPPL90 = 113.3 dB SPL @ 1500 Hz

General Explanation. This figure refers to the peak saturation output of the hearing aid—or how strong the instrument is, and the frequency at which it occurs. In some cases, it might be desirable to select a hearing aid which has a saturation output no greater than a measured UCL.

Data Development. An output curve is to be developed over a range from 200 to 5000 Hz with an input of 90 dB and with the volume control of the aid set to the full-on setting.

INPUT + GAIN = OUTPUT
90 + FULL = OUTPUT CURVE

Tolerance. The peak output of 113.3 dB SPL at 1500 Hz is not to be exceeded for this particular hearing aid. Because of this, most manufacturers will produce hearing aids having values somewhat below this figure so as not to exceed this number.

HF AVE SSPL90 = 110.1 dB

General Explanation. This is the high-frequency average saturation sound pressure level taken from the output curve generated shown above. It is felt to provide a better overall estimate of the output of the hearing aid than the single figure shown in the example above.

This might provide a better indication of the saturation level at which to limit the hearing aid than the single peak value.

Data Development. The figure for this is derived from the SSPL90 curve. It is the average of 1000, 1600, and 2500 Hz.

1000 Hz = 108.0 dB
1600 Hz = 113.3 dB
2500 Hz = 109.0 dB
TOTAL = 330.3 dB

HF-AVE SSPL90 = 330.3/3 = 110.1 dB

Tolerance. Tolerance for HF-average SSPL90 is plus or minus 4 dB.

RTP (RTS; RTG) 5 33.1

General Explanation. This Reference Test Setting is used to adjust the hearing aid gain for the measurements of: (1) frequency response, (2) harmonic distortion, (3) equivalent input noise level, and (4) battery current. This level was chosen because this gain (1) is close to the typical "use" setting of the hearing aid, especially for high gain aids, (2) measures distortion closer to the maximum output of the aid, and (3) is more representative than a full-on setting. It was felt that the gain control for certain tests should be related to the saturation output capacity of the aid. This is the setting of the hearing aid volume control so that the average of the earphone coupler sound pressure levels at 1000, 1600, and 2500 Hz, with a pure tone input sound pressure level of 60 dB, is 17 dB (plus or minus 1 dB) less than HF-average SSPL90.

RTS = HF-Avg SSPL90–17 dB (and also minus the 60 dB input level).

Data Development. With an input of 60 dB, the gain of the hearing aid is varied so that the output of the hearing aid is the HF-avg SSPL90 minus 17 dB. If the aid does not have enough gain to achieve this, the volume control is to be set to the full-on setting.

INPUT + GAIN = OUTPUT
60 + VARY = HF-AVE SSPL90 MINUS 17 dB

Tolerance. There is no measurement tolerance for this value. This setting is important in that it is this value to which the volume control of the hearing aid is adjusted for measurements of frequency response, harmonic distortion, equivalent input noise level, and battery current.

HF-AVE FULL ON GAIN = 37.3 dB @ 60 dB IN

General Explanation. Potentially, gain can be measured at three settings; full-on gain, reference test gain control setting, or at 50 dB input for AGC hearing aids. In this measurement, the figure is the high frequency average of 1000, 1600, and 2500 Hz taken from the full-on gain curve. It is a measure of the general amplification of the aid.

Data Development. The average is obtained from an output curve obtained with an input of 60 dB and the volume control set to the full-on setting. In Addition to the HF-avg full-on gain, the maximum full-on peak gain can be expressed. The frequency should be stated. There is no tolerance figure for this peak gain value.

INPUT + GAIN = OUTPUT
60 + FULL-ON = OUTPUT

Tolerance. A hearing aid should be within plus or minus 5 dB of its stated HF-avg. full-on gain value. Remember to subtract the input level of 60 dB to obtain the gain figure.

1000 Hz	= 93.1 dB
1600 Hz	= 101.1 dB
2500 Hz	= 97.1 dB
TOTAL	= 291.0/3 = 97.0 dB
HF-AVE	= 97.3 − 60 dB input = 37.3 dB
FULL-ON GAIN	= 99.0 dB − 60 = 39.0 dB

In 1987 S3.22 was revised to accommodate those hearing aids with extreme high-pass or extreme low-pass frequency responses. This revision allowed the hearing aid manufacturer to select "special purpose frequencies" with which to form a special purpose average (SPA) full-on gain and a SPA SSPL90 that more closely represented the passband of the hearing aid. The Standard defines a "special purpose" hearing aid as one whose full-on gain at *any one* of the three test frequencies (1000, 1600, or 2500 Hz) is more than 15 dB below the maximum (peak) full-on gain *at any frequency.*

Response Limit: 73.5 dB (F1 = 300 Hz; F2-4500 Hz)

General Explanation. The frequency response curve describes the performance of the hearing aid over a range from 200 to 5000 Hz. The lower frequency limit is defined by F1 and the upper frequency limit is defined by F2. Together, they define the frequency range of the hearing aid.

Data Development. The frequency response curve is obtained by using an input of 60 dB, setting the volume control of the aid to the Reference Test Position, and recording the frequency response curve over a range from 200 to 5000 Hz. To determine the frequency range, 20 dB is subtracted from the average of 1000, 1600, and 2500 Hz. A horizontal line is drawn on the graph at that average value. F1 is the lower point at which the horizontal line crosses the response curve and F2 is the upper crossing of the two.

INPUT + GAIN = OUTPUT
60 + RTGS = OUTPUT

Tolerance. The frequency response curve is divided into two bands for tolerance compliance. The low band is 1.25 F1 to 2000 Hz. The high band is from 2000 Hz to 4000 Hz or 0.8 F2 (whichever is lower). The allowable tolerance in the low band is plus or minus 4 dB, and in the high band plus or minus 6 dB. A template can be moved vertically any amount. Horizontally, it can be moved to plus or minus 10% in frequency. Both bands must lie within the template tolerances.

Total Harmonic Distortion

General Explanation. Harmonic distortion results when new frequencies are generated by the hearing aid output as a result of nonlinearity. The lower the number, the lower the distortion.

Data Development. Harmonic distortion measurements are obtained with an input of 70 dB for 500 and 800 Hz and 65 dB input for 1600 Hz. The volume control is set to the reference test position. The total harmonic distortion in the coupler output for frequencies of 500, 800, and 1600 Hz are recorded. In the event the response curve rises 12 dB or more between any distortion test frequency and its second harmonic, the distortion test at that test frequency may be omitted since it will not be accurate. When this occurs, the frequency and distortion will be bracketed or omitted.

INPUT + GAIN = OUTPUT
70 70 65 + RTGS = INPUT
500, 800, 1600

Tolerance. The tolerance for harmonic distortion is a "not to exceed figure." Whatever the manufacturer lists as a distortion figure at any of the three test frequencies should not be exceeded.

EQ Input Noise Level 22.6 dB SPL

General Explanation. This is a figure of how much noise the hearing aid has. The lower the dB SPL the lower the noise. EQ stands for *equivalent.*

Data Development. The hearing aid is first tested with an input level, and then without an input level, and the difference between these two outputs is a measure of the internal noise of an aid. The formula for computing this figure is $L_n = L_2 - (L_{avg} - 60)$dB. L_2 is no input and the L_{avg} is the average output of 1000, 1600, and 2500 Hz. In the above example, $L_2 = 97.3$ and $L_{avg} = 37.3$.

INPUT + GAIN = OUTPUT
60 + RTGS = OUTPUT

Then

INPUT + GAIN = OUTPUT
0 + RTGS = OUTPUT

Tolerance. The Ln or equivalent noise level for the hearing aid should not exceed the value specified.

BATTERY I = 0.93 mA @ 1000 Hz, 65 dB IN

General Explanation. Battery current drain provides an indication of the expected battery life for a given hearing aid.

Data Development. The battery current is measured with a 1000 Hz input signal at 65 dB SPL and the gain control of the hearing aid set to the Reference Test Position.

INPUT + GAIN = OUTPUT
65 + RTP = OUTPUT
1000 HZ

The actual current drain is calculated from the following formula:

$$\text{HRS} = \frac{\text{MILLIAMPERE HRS (mAH)}}{\text{CURRENT DRAIN (I mA)}}$$

For example, a 76 size cell may have a capacity of 190 mAH. If the current drain is 1.5 mA, the life expectancy of that cell is approximately 125 hours. Of course, this is all dependent upon the type of aid and the environmental conditions.

Tolerance. The current drain should not exceed the value recorded by the manufacturer for a given hearing aid.

BATTERY V = 1.3 V

General Explanation. This is a description of the battery voltage used in the measurement of the hearing aid in question. There is no tolerance requirement for the battery.

SSPL90 CURVE

This is the darker curve shown in Figure 70 and provides a graphic display of the saturation output of the hearing aid. This was explained earlier.

Full-On Gain Curve

This curve is most often referred to by the manufacturer as an indication of the performance of a hearing aid. It is convenient to run during production because the volume control is set to the full-on gain position. How this curve was developed was explained earlier.

Frequency Response Curve Run with the VC in the Reference Test Position

This curve is less frequently seen in the data provided by the manufacturer for each hearing aid because of the time involved in proper setting of the volume control to achieve the reference test position setting. However, it is usually recorded in the User's Instructional Booklet provided with each hearing aid. The explanation for this curve was given earlier.

Induction Coil Sensitivity

General Description. This data is ordinarily obtained from the specification sheets which accompanies each hearing aid. It is a measure of the strength of the telecoil of the hearing aid (if the hearing aid incorporates this feature).

Data Development. The output of the hearing aid is obtained with the volume control set to the full-on position and with the hearing aid placed in an alternating magnetic field having a frequency response of 1000 Hz and a magnetic field strength of 10 mA/m (milliampere per meter).

INPUT + GAIN = OUTPUT
MAG FIELD + FULL = OUTPUT
10 mA/m
1000 Hz

Tolerance. An example of induction coil sensitivity might be 100 dB @ 1000 Hz. The tolerance for this measurement is plus or minus 6 dB at the frequency specified.

AGC Hearing Aids

Certain measurements pertain to AGC hearing aids only. The two primary differences include: (1) All gain results are obtained with an input of 50 dB rather than 60 dB (although a current draft suggests that both AGC and linear aids use a 60 dB input level with the gain set to the RGP). (2) The procedures are "attempts" to measure the dynamics of the AGC (automatic gain control) hearing aids.

Input-Output Characteristics

General Explanation. This is a graph which shows how the hearing aid performed with different inputs (Figure 71).

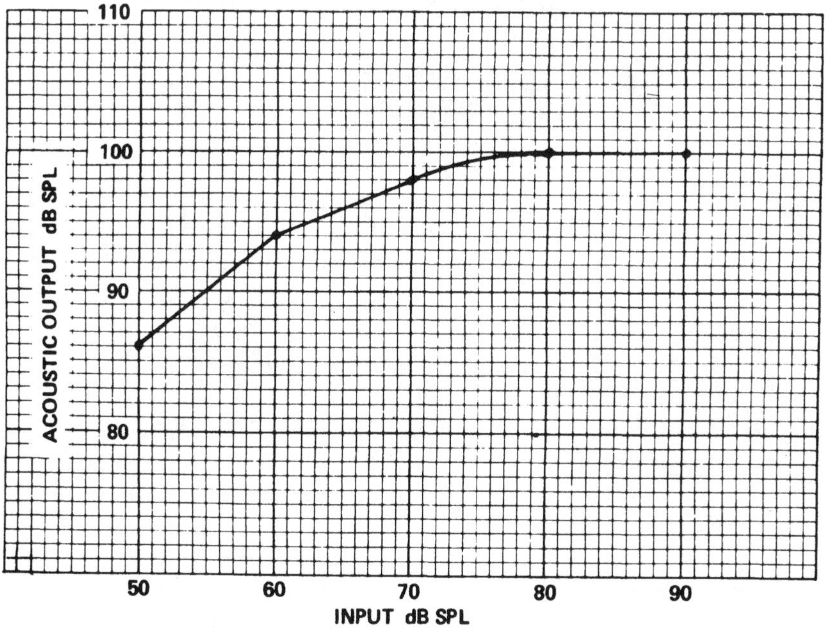

Fig. 71. Input/output characteristic of an AGC hearing aid, showing how the output is effected with changes in the input level.

Data Development. This graph shows the output at 2000 Hz for input sound pressure levels from 50 to 90 dB in 10 dB steps.

INPUT + GAIN = OUTPUT
50, 60, 70, 80, 90 + FULL = OUTPUT
2000 Hz

Tolerance. With the measured and specified curves matched at 70 dB input level, the measured curve at 50 and 90 dB input levels shall have an output of plus or minus 4 dB from the specified curve.

Dynamic AGC Characteristics

General Explanation. This measurement is an attempt to show how well the hearing aid can follow the dynamic characteristics of the input signal. In other words, how rapidly does the AGC system function, both going into compression for loud sounds (attack time), and in going out of compression when soft sounds are being picked up by the hearing aid microphone (release time).

Data Development. The performance of the aid is measured with an input signal which jumps back and forth between 55 and 80 dB (to simulate soft and loud input signals) at 1000 Hz and with the volume control of the aid set to the full-on position. The aid is to be measured in its maximum compression (greatest amount of compression).

INPUT + GAIN = OUTPUT
55 & 80 + FULL = OUTPUT
2000 Hz

A measure of the time constants (attack and release times) of the hearing aid are recorded. The attack time is the time between the abrupt increase from 55 to 80 dB and the point where the level has stabilized to within 2 dB of the steady state value for the 80 dB input SPL. The release time is the interval between the abrupt drop from 80 to 55 dB and the point where the signal has stabilized to within 2 dB of the steady state value for the 55 dB input SPL (Figure 72). Future considerations are to modify this from 2 to 3 dB for the attack time and from 2 to 4 dB for the release time. This recommendation is being made to accommodate newer hearing aids having variable time constants.

Tolerance. The tolerance allowed on attack and release times is plus or minus 5 msec (milliseconds) or plus or minus 50%, whichever is larger of the values specified for the model. Table 12, taken from Staab and Lybarger (1994) provides a complete sum-

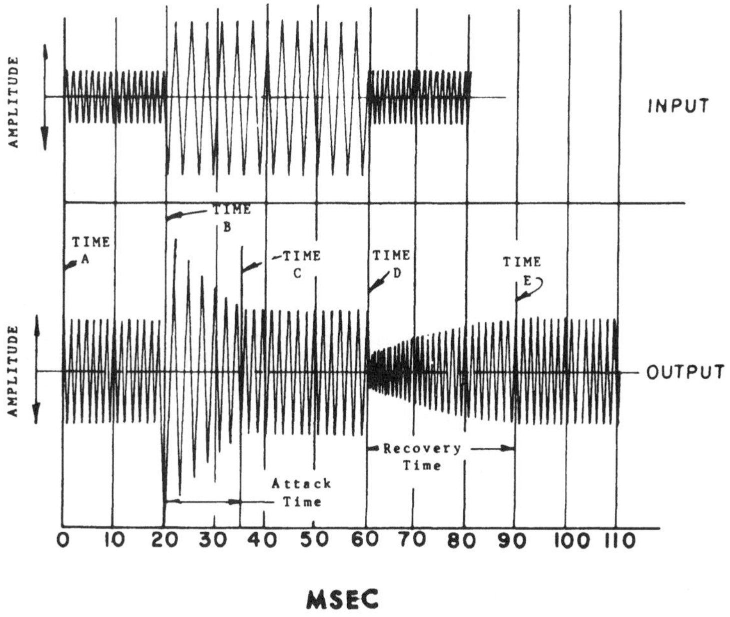

Fig. 72. Input signal (top) and aided (bottom) recording of a hearing aid showing the effects of attack and recovery times on the amplified signal.

mary of the ANSI S3.22-1987 (and revisions) that specify the hearing aid characteristics and their tolerances.

COHERENCE TESTING

The coherence function describes the cumulative effect of different forms of signal corruption by a hearing aid (Preves and Newton, 1989; Preves and Woodruff, 1990; Dyrlund, 1989; Bareham, 1990). It is a direct measure of the linearity of a hearing aid and represents, in a number from 0 to 1, what part of the output signal of a hearing aid is due only to the input signal over the frequency range of interest. The determination of the coherence function indicates how much of the output signal has been caused by the input signal and how much by circuit noise and distortion in the hearing aid. At this time coherence measurement is not a standard and is not widely available in hearing aid test equipment. However, measurement of the coherence function is utilized by the Veterans Administration as a part of their hearing aid selection process. Coherence function as a hearing aid measurement has

Table 12. ANSI 53.22-1987 (ASA-1987) Specification of Hearing Aid Characteristics Summary

Characteristic	Input SPL dB re 20 μPa	Frequency (Hz)	Gain Control Setting	Presentation	Tolerance Requirements
SSPL 90 Curve	90	Frequencies between 200 and 5000	Full on	Curve State maximum value dB	No more than 3dB above mfr. stated maximum value
HFA SSPL90	90	1000, 1600, 2500	Full on	Value (dB) (3-frequency average)	Mfr. specified value ±4 dB
HFA Full-On Gain or SPA Full-on Gain	60 or 50 (state which) 50 for AGC or where aid would overload	1000, 1600, 2500 or SPA frequencies	Full on	Value (dB) (3-frequency average)	Mfr. Specified value ±5 dB
Frequency Response	60 or 50	200–5000	Ref. Test Gain Control Pos. Set gain control back to give output SPL 17 dB less than average SSPL90, or full on for low gain and AGC aids		±4 dB in low band ±6 dB in high band
Frequency Range	60	200-5000 Line 20 dB below 3-freq. avg.	Reference Test Position	State f_1 (low limit) and f_2 (high limit)	For information only

Total Harmonic Distortion	70	500, 800, 1600	Reference Test Position	Number (%)	No more than 3% above mfr. specified value
Equivalent Input Noise Level, L_n	60	1000, 1600, 2500 (Avg. to get L_{av})	Reference Test Position	Number (dB) $L_n = L_2 - (L_{av} - 60)$	No more than 3 dB above mfr. specified value
Battery Current	65	1000	Reference Test Position	Value (mA)	No more than 20% above mfr. specified value
Telephone Pickup (Induction Coil)	10 mA/m rms magnetic field	1000	Full on	Greatest value (dB)	Within ±6 dB of mfr. specified value
Input-Output Curves (AGC only)	50 to 90 in 10 dB steps	2000	Full on	Curve Input = abscissa Curve Output = ordinate	Match specified and measured curves at 70 dB input, then to be within ±5 dB of specified value
Attack and Release Times (AGC only)	Abruptly alternating between 55 and 80 dB	2000	Full on	Values (ms)	Mfr. specified values ±5 ms or ±50%, whichever is larger.

been recommended in the ANSI S3.42 standard, ensuring this standard a higher profile and greater use.

MEASURING CONDITIONS

Certain conditions are to be met when hearing aid measurements are taken. These include:

1. RMS (Root Mean Square) response.
2. 2cc coupler HA-1 or HA-2 with either rigid or flexible tubing.
3. Ambient conditions
    a. Temperature 23 plus or minus 5 degrees centigrade (73 plus or minus 9 degrees Fahrenheit).
    b. Relative humidity 0 to 80%
    c. Atmospheric pressure 760 plus or minus 35, minus 150 mm of Mercury.
4. Supply voltage (state type and voltage of battery).
5. Tube dimensions (for BTE and eyeglass aids).
    a. Length 2.5 cm. (0.984″) plus or minus 4%
    b. Internal diameter 0.193 cm (0.076″) plus or minus 2%
6. Earhook or filters (if used, must be on the aid when making measurements).

IEC VERSUS ANSI STANDARDS

The standards used in the U.S. are not the same as for all parts of the world. Shortly after the publication of ANSI S3.22-1976, the IEC (International Electrotechnical Commission) developed the 118 series of hearing aid measurement standards. Although these standards followed the general intent of the ANSI S3.22 standard, they did not follow the specific detail. The standard for the Measurement of Performance Characteristics of Hearing Aids for Quality Inspection for Delivery Purposes was 118-7 and uses the same 2-cc coupler as does the S3.22. However, IEC 118-0, which characterizes hearing aid standard Measurement of Electroacoustic Characteristics, uses the IEC 711 ear simulator. Another significant difference is that the IEC uses a single frequency to set the gain control to reference test position (rather than the 3-frequency average of S3.22), and uses a 15 dB gain control setback (rather than the 17 dB as used in S3.22). Table 13 (adapted from

Table 13. Comparison of Main Test Methods and Conditions Specified in ANSI S3.22-1987 to Those in IEC 118-7.

Subject	IEC	ANSI
RTGCP	Single frequency, 15 dB gain control setback	HFA (SPA), 17 dB gain control setback
Battery current	60 dB SPL input	65 dB SPL input
Input, full-on gain	50 dB SPL if OSPL90-SPL60 is <5 dB	50 dB SPL if OSPL90-SPL60 is <4 dB
Distortion	1 frequency	3 frequencies
Frequency range	No	Yes
Tolerances	No	Yes
AGC measurements	No	Yes
Directional mic.	No	Yes
Ambient condition		Small differences

RTGCP = reference test gain control position. Redrawn from Dyrlund, 1992.

Dyrlund, 1992) provides additional information on the differences between the tests in ANSI S3.22 and IEC 118-7.

SUMMARY

In selecting appropriate amplification systems, the hearing aid specialist must acquire knowledge of those conditions affecting normal hearing which necessitate amplification use. He/she must be aware of the individual's emotional and psychological needs as well as probable use of hearing aids. The dispenser must be aware of those techniques employed in the selection process as well as the limitations imposed by them. It is critical that one be aware of the accepted methods for measuring the acoustic performance of hearing aid devices to confirm their suitability for use by the hearing impaired person. Such emphases should have been apparent in this chapter.

REFERENCES

ALPINER, J. G. (1967). Aural rehabilitation and the aged patient. *Maico Audiological Library,* 4;9–12.

AMERICAN NATIONAL STANDARDS INSTITUTE. (1992). Testing Hearing Aids with a Broad-Band Noise Signal (ANSI S3-42-1992). New York: Acoustical Society of America.

American National Standard Method of Expressing Hearing Standard for the Specification of Hearing Aid Characteristics (ANSI S3.22-1982/ASA 7-1982), New York ANSI.

American National Standard Method of Expressing Hearing Aid Performance, S3.8-1967 (R-1971), *American National Standards Institute, New York.*

American National Standard for Measurement of Electroacoustical Characteristics of Hearing Aids, S3.3-1960, *American National Standards Institute, New York.*

American National Standard Specification of Hearing Aid Characteristics, (ANSI S3.22-199x, revision of ANSI S3.22-1987, 2nd draft—not approved by ANSI, August, 1995), New York.

Balbi, C. M. R. (1935). Adjusted sound amplification. U.S. Patent No. 2,003,875.

Bareham, J. (1990). Part 2: hearing instrument measurements using dual channel signal analysis. Hearing instruments, 41;32–33.

Beattie, R. C., and Boyd, R. L. (1986). Relationship between pure tone and speech loudness discomfort levels among hearing-impaired subjects. *Journal of Speech and Hearing Disorders,* 51;120–124.

Beattie, R. C., Svihovec, D. A., Carmen, R. E., et. al. (1980). Loudness discomfort level for speech: comparison of two instructional sets for saturation sound pressure level selection. *Ear and Hearing,* 1;197–205.

Bentler, R. (1993). Relationship of perceived quality dimensions to threshold of discomfort, abstract. *Audiology Today,* 5;40–41.

Bentler, R., and Pavlovic, C. (1989). Comparison of discomfort levels obtained with pure tones and multitone complexes. *Journal of the Acoustical Society of America,* 86;126–132.

Berger, K. W. (1976). Prescription of hearing aids: a rationale. *Journal of American Auditory Society,* 2;71–78.

Berger, K. W. (1976). The use of uncomfortable loudness level in hearing aid fitting. *Maico Audiological Library Series,* XV, 2.

Berger, K. W., and Millin, J. (1968). Hearing aids, in *Audiological Assessment,* Edited by D. Rose, Englewood Cliffs: *Prentice Hall,* 471–517.

Bragg, V. C. (1977). Toward a more objective hearing aid fitting procedure. *Hearing Instruments,* 28;9:6–9.

Brooks, D. N. (1972). The use and disuse of medresco hearing aids. *Sound, 4;80–85.*

Burkhard, M. D. (1978). Ed. Manikin Measurements. Itasca, IL: *Knowles Electronics.*

Burnett, E. D., and Beck, L. B. (1987). A correction for converting 2cm coupler responses to insertion responses for custom in-the-ear non-directional hearing aids. *Ear and Hearing, 8;5 Suppl:89S-94S.*

BURKHARD, M. D. and SACKS, R. M. (1975). Anthropometric manikin for acoustic research. Journal of the Acoustical Society of America, 58;214–222.

BYRNE, D., and TONISSON, W. (1976). Selecting the gain of hearing aids for persons with sensorineural hearing impairments. *Scandinavian Audiology,* 5;51–59.

CARHART, R. (1946). Selection of hearing aids. Archives of Otolaryngology, 44;1–18.

CARHART, R. and JERGER, J. (1959). Preferred method for clinical determination of pure tone thresholds. *Journal of Speech and Hearing Disorders, 24;330–345.*

CARSTAIRS, V. (1973). Utilization of hearing aids issued by the national health service. *British Journal of Audiology, 7;72–76.*

CLARKE COX, L., and METZ, D. A. (1980). ABER in the prescription of hearing aids, *Hearing Instruments,* 31;12–15,55.

COLE, W. A. (1995). Ten facts about hearing aid standards. Product brochure, Audioscan, Sept. 11.

CORNELISSE, L. E., SEEWALD, R. C., and JAMIESON, D. G. (1994). Wide-dynamic-range compression hearing aids: the DSL[i/o] approach. *The Hearing Journal, 47:10;23–26.*

COX, R. M. (1981). Using LDLs to establish hearing aid limiting levels. *Hearing Instruments, 5;16–20.*

COX, R. M. (1983). Using ULCL measures to find frequency/gain and SSPL90. *Hearing Instruments, 7;17–21, 39.*

COX, R. M. (1985). A structured approach to hearing aid selection. *Ear and Hearing, 6;5:226–239.*

COX, R. M. (1988). The MSU hearing instrument prescription procedure. *Hearing Instruments, 39;1:6,8,10.*

COX, R. M., and ALEXANDER, G. C. (1994). The abbreviated profile of hearing aid benefit (APHAB). In submission.

COX, R. M. and GILMORE, G. C. (1990). Development of the profile of hearing aid performance (PHAP). *Journal of Speech and Hearing Research, 33;343–357.*

CRANMER, K. (1983). Hearing aid dispensing—1983. Hearing Instruments, 34;5:99–12.

CRANMER-BRISKEY, K. (1994). 1994 hearing instruments dispenser survey results. *Hearing Instruments, 45;9:13–16.*

CURRAN, J. R. (1977). Formulas don't work. *Hearing Aid Journal. 31:10;78–81.*

DAVIS, H., STEVENS, S. S., NICHOLS JR., R. H., HUDGINS, C. V., MARQUIS, R. J., PETERSON, G. E., and ROSS, D. A. (1947). *Hearing Aids, An Experimental Study of Design Objectives, Harvard University Press, Cambridge.*

Dempsey, J. (1986). The hearing performance inventory as a tool in fitting hearing aids. Journal of the Academy of Rehabilitative Audiology, 19;116–125.

Denenberg, L., and Altschuler, M. (1976). The clinical relationship between acoustic reflexes and loudness perception. Journal of the American Audiological Society, 2;3:79–82.

Dillon, H., and Murray, N. (1987). Accuracy of twelve methods of estimating the real ear gain of hearing aids. Ear and Hearing, 8;2–11.

Dirks, D., and Kamm, C. (1976). Psychometric functions for loudness discomfort and most comfortable loudness level. Journal of Speech and Hearing Disorders, 19;613–627.

Dunn, H. K., and White, S. D. (1940). Statistical measurements on conversational speech. Journal of the Acoustical Society of America, 11;278–288.

Dyrlund, O. (1989). Characterization of non-linear distortion in hearing aids using coherence analysis, a pilot study. Scandinavian Audiology, 18;143–148.

FDA, Dept. HEW, Subchapter H, Medical Devices, Part 801. (1977). Hearing aid devices. Federal Register, 42;31:9286–9296.

Feigin, J., Kopun, J., Stelmachowicz, P., and Gorga, M. (1989). Probe-tube microphone measures of ear-canal sound pressure levels in infants and children. Ear and Hearing, 10;254–258.

Filion, P. R., and Margolis, R. H. (1992). Comparison of clinical and real-life judgments of loudness discomfort. Journal of the American Academy of Audiology, 3;193–199.

Fletcher, H. (1952). The perception of speech sounds by deafened persons. Journal of the Acoustical Society of America, 24;490–497.

Fortune, T., Preves, D., and Woodruff, B. (1991). Saturation-induced distortion and its effects on aided LDL. Hearing Instruments, 42;37–42.

Fowler, E. P., and Sabine, P. E. (1947). American Medical Association Council on Physical Medicine.

Frye, G. J. (1982). "In situ" and "etymotic" hearing aid testing. Hearing Instruments, 33;32–36.

Gitles, T. C., and Tillman Niquette, P. (1995). FIG6 in ten. The Hearing Review, Nov/Dec., 28, 30.

Goldberg, H. (1986). Psychoacoustic aided hearing measurements, Hearing Instruments, 37;6:17,19,51.

Gorga, M. P., Beauchaine, K. A., and Reiland, J. K. (1987). Comparison of onset and steady-state responses of hearing aids: implications for use of the auditory brainstem response in the selection of hearing aids. Journal of Speech and Hearing Research, 30;130–136.

HAIC Standards for Hearing Aids. (1974). Hearing Aid Conference, New York.

Harford, E. (1981). A new clinical technique for verification of hearing aid response. Archives of Otolaryngology, 107;463.

HARTENSTEIN, R. W. (1978). Clinical use of otometry in hearing aid dispensing. Department of Otolaryngology, The Hammond Clinic, Munster, Indiana.

HAWKINS, D. B. (1980). The effect of signal type on the loudness discomfort level. Ear and Hearing, 1;38–41.

HAWKINS, D. B. (1984). Selection of a critical electroacoustic characteristic: SSPL90. Hearing Instruments, 35;28–32.

HAWKINS, D., BALL, T., BEASLEY, H., et. al. (1992). A comparison of SSPL90 selection procedures. Journal of the American Academy of Audiology, 3;46–50.

HECOX, K. (1983). Role of auditory brainstem response in the selection of hearing aids. Ear and Hearing, 4;51–55.

HODGSON, W. R., and SKINNER, P. H. (1977). *Hearing Aid Assessment and use in Audiologic Habilitation,* The Williams and Wilkins Co., Baltimore, MD.

HORNING, J. (1975). TYMPANOMETRY AND HEARING AID SELECTION. HEARING AID JOURNAL, 28;6:8.

HUGHSON, W., and THOMPSON, E. (1944). Hearing aids. Archives of Otolaryngology, 39;245–249.

HUMES, L. E. and HACKETT, T. (1990). Comparison of frequency response and aided speech-recognition performance obtained for hearing aids selected by three different prescriptive methods. Journal of the American Academy of Audiology, 1;101–108.

HUMES, L. E., and HALLING, D. C. (1994). Overview, rationale, and comparison of suprathreshold-based gain prescriptive methods. In Valente (Ed) *Strategies for Selecting and Verifying Hearing Aid Fittings,* Thieme Medical Publishers, Inc., New York, pp. 19–37.

IHAFF (INDEPENDENT HEARING AID FITTING FORUM). (1994). A comprehensive hearing aid fitting protocol, progress report.

INTERNATIONAL ELECTROTECHNICAL COMMISSION (IEC) 126: IECE reference Coupler for the measurement of hearing aids coupled to the ear by means of ear inserts. (1961).

JERGER, J., and HAYES, D. (1976). Hearing aid evaluation. Archives of Otolaryngology, 102;214–225.

KAMM, C., DIRKS, D. D., and MICKEY, M. R. (1978). Effect of sensorineural hearing loss on loudness discomfort level and most comfortable loudness judgments. Journal of Speech and Hearing Research, 21;688–691.

KEE, W. R. (1972). Use of pure tone measurement in hearing aid fittings. Audecibel, Winter, 9–15.

KEITH, R. (1976). An acoustic reflex technique of establishing hearing aid settings. Paper presented at the American Speech and Hearing Association Convention, Houston, TX.

KILENY, P. R. (1982). Auditory brainstem responses as indicators of hearing aid performance. Annals of Otol., 91;61–64.

KILLION, M. C. (1978). Revised estimate of minimum audible pressure: where is the missing 6 dB? Journal of the Acoustical Society of America, 63;5:1501.

KILLION, M. C. (1995). Personal communication. FIG6 computer disc and handout.

KILLION, M. C., and MONSER, E. L. (1980). CORFIG: coupler response for flat insertion gain. In Stedebaker, G. A., and Hochberg, I. (Eds). *Acoustical Factors Affecting Hearing Aid Response.* Baltimore: University Part Press, 149–168.

KODICEK, J., and GARRAD, J. (1955). The hearing aid in use: a survey of 1459 patients. Journal of Laryngology and Otology, 69;807–820.

LAWRENCE, D. W., HALLADAY, H. E., and BLACKLEDGE, V. O. (1977). Part 1: listener performance as a criterion for setting frequency selective parameters of hearing instruments. Audiology & Hearing Education, Feb/March, 26, 28–29.

LIBBY, E. R. (1985). The LDL to SSPL90 conversion dilemma. Hearing Instruments, 36;15–16,68.

LONGWELL, T. F., and JOHNSON, J. H. (1980). Estimating hearing aid insertion gain from coupler gain. Hearing Instruments, 31;20–22, 30.

LYBARGER, S. (1994). Hearing aid related standards published by American Standards Association, United States of America Standards Institute and American National Standards Institute, Personal communication with David Preves.

LYBARGER, S. F. (1938). U.S. Patent No. 2, 112,569.

LYBARGER, S. F. (1957). Radioear basic fitting procedure (condensed form for clinical use), Radioear Corporation, Original written June 14, 1955, Revised July 10, 1957.

LYBARGER, S. F. (1957). Some factors that we consider important in hearing aid design. American Speech and Hearing Association Meeting, Cincinnati, OH, November.

LYBARGER, S. F. (1963). Simplified fitting system for hearing aids," *Radioear Specifications and Fitting Information Manual,* Oct., 1–8.

LYBARGER, S. F. (1944). U.S. patent Application SN543-278.

LYBARGER, S. F. (1978). Selective amplification—a review and evaluation. Journal of the American Audiology Society, 3;6:258–266.

LYBARGER, S. F. (1981). Modified unpublished definition of a hearing aid, provided for use by Audiotone, with permission by S. F. Lybarger. (The original definition is as follows: A hearing aid is an ultra-small electro-acoustic device that is always too large, that has to faithfully amplify speech a million times without bringing in any noise, that has to work without failure—in a flood of perspiration or a cloud of talcum powder, or both, that one usually puts off buying for ten years after he needs it because he doesn't want anyone to know he is hard of hearing but which he can't do without for thirty minutes when it needs serviced).

LYBARGER, S. F. (1985). Relationship between coupler measurements of hearing aids, as required by the Food and Drug Administration (FDA) labeling regulations and the performance of an aid under actual use conditions. American Auditory Society Carhart Memorial Lecture, Atlanta. Corti's Organ, 10, No. 3.

LYBARGER, S. F., and TEDER, H. (1986). 2 cc coupler curves to insertion gain curves. Hearing Instruments, 37;36–37,40.

MCCANDLESS, G. A. (1982). In-the-ear canal acoustic measures, in STUDEBAKER, G. A., BESS, F. H. (eds): *The Vanderbilt Hearing-Aid Report.* Upper Darby, PA: Monographs in Contemporary Audiology, 170–173.

MCCANDLESS, G. (1975). Special consideration in evaluating children and the aging for hearing aids. Proceedings of the Lexington Hearing Aid Conference, June.

MCCANDLESS, G. (1980). Real-ear measures of hearing aid function. Hearing Aid Journal, May, 8–9, 30.

MCCANDLESS, G. A., and LYREGAARD, P. E. (1983). Prescription of gain/output (POGO) for hearing aids. Hearing Instruments, 34;16–21.

MCCANDLESS, G. A., and MILLER, D. L. (1972). Loudness discomfort and hearing aids. Hearing Aid Journal, 25;8:7.

MARTIN, M. C., STEVENSON, P. W., and GROVER, B. C. (1978). Some aspects of auditory space, speech perception and the use of hearing aids. Scandinavian Audiology Supplement, 6;141–161.

MEDICAL RESEARCH COUNCIL SPECIAL REPORT NO. 261. (1947). Hearing aids and audiometers. *London: His Majesty's Stationery Office.*

MAHONEY, T. M. (1985). Auditory brainstem response hearing aid application. In JACOBSON, J. T., Ed. *The Auditory Brainstem Response.* San Diego, CA: College-Hill Press, 349–370.

MELEN, L. A. (1978). Application of otometric principles in binaural hearing aid fittings. Project 76-12 of the Guthrie Foundation for Medical Research, Sayre, PA.

MOKOTOFF, B., and KREBS, D. F. (1976). Brainstem auditory-evoked responses with amplification. Paper Presented at the 92nd meeting, Acoustical Society of America, Nov.

MORGAN, D. E. and DIRKS, D. D. (1974). Loudness discomfort level under earphone and in the free field: the effects of calibration methods. Journal of the Acoustical Society of America, 56;172–178.

MUELLER, H. G. (1992). Insertion gain measurements. In MUELLER, H. G., HAWKINS, D. B., and NORTHERN, J. L., Eds. *Probe Microphone Measurements: Hearing Aid Selection and Assessment.* San Diego, CA: Singular Publishing Group, Inc., 113–143.

MUELLER, H. G., and BRIGHT, K. E. (1994). *Selection and verification of maximum output.* In VALENTE, M. (Ed) Strategies for Selecting and Verifying Hearing Aid Fittings, Thieme Medical Publishers, Inc., New York, 38–63.

Mueller, H. G., Hawkins, D. B., and Northern, J. L. (1992). *Probe Microphone Measurements: Hearing Aid Selection and Assessment.* San Diego, CA: Singular Publishing Group, Inc.

Mueller, H. G., and Killion, M. (1990). An easy method for calculating the articulation index. Hearing Journal, 43:14–17.

Newman, C., and Weinstein, B. (1988). The hearing handicap inventory for the elderly as a measure of hearing aid benefit. Ear and Hearing, 9;81–85.

Oticon. (1996). About COSI (the NAL client oriented scale of improvement). Oticon publication distributed in March, 1996, Breckenridge, CO Otology and Auditory Conference.

Pascoe, D. (1975). Frequency responses of hearing aids and their effects on the speech perception of hearing-impaired subjects. Annals of Otology, Rhinology, and Laryngology. Vol. 84 (Supplement 23).

Pascoe, D. (1978). An approach to hearing aid selection. Hearing Instruments, 29;12–16, 36.

Pascoe, D. P. (1990). Clinical measurements of the auditory dynamic range and their relation to formulas for hearing aid gain, in *Presbyacousis and Other Age Related Aspects.* 14th Danavox Symposium, 129–147.

Pavlovic, C. V. (1987). Derivation of primary parameters and procedures for use in speech intelligibility predictions. J. Acoust. Soc. Amer., 82;2, August.

Pluvinage, V. (1989). Clinical measurement of loudness growth. Hearing Instruments, 39;3.

Pluvinage, V., and Benson, D. (1990). New dimensions in diagnostics and fitting. Hearing Instruments, 39;8:28-30.

Punch, J., Chi, C., and Patterson, J. (1990). A recommended protocol for prescription use of target gain rules. Hearing Instruments, 41;12-19.

Preves, D. A. (1996). Standardizing hearing aid measurement parameters and electroacoustic performance tests. In Valente, M. (Ed) *Hearing Aids: Standards, Options, and Limitations,* Thieme Medical Publishers, Inc.: New York, 1-71.

Preves, D. A., and Newton, J. R. (1989). The headroom problem and hearing aid performance. Hearing Journal, 42;21.

Preves, D. A., and Woodruff, B. D. (1990). Some methods of improving and assessing hearing aid headroom. Audecibel, 38;8–13.

Qualitone and dbc-Mifco. (1995). The open audiometric reporting standard (OARS).

Rainville, M. (1976). Impedance measurements in evaluation of hearing aid performance. Hearing Instruments, 27; 11:39.

Rappaport, B., and Tait, C. (1976). Acoustic reflex threshold measurement in hearing aid selection. Archives of Otolaryngology, March, 102;129–132.

Reddell, R. C. and Calvert, D. R. (1966). Selecting a hearing aid by interpreting audiologic data. Journal of Auditory Research, 6;445–452.

RESNICK, D., and BECKER, M. (1963). Hearing aid evaluation—a new approach. ASHA, 5;695–699.

RICE, J. (1966). Hearing aids. Journal of Laryngology and Otology, 80;583–600.

SEEWALD, R. C. (1994). Fitting children with the DSL method. The Hearing Journal, 47;9:10, 48–51.

SEEWALD, R. C. (1995). The desired sensation level (DSL) method for hearing aid fitting in infants and children. Phonak Focus, News/Ideas/High Technology/Acoustics, Nr. 20.

SEEWALD, R. C., ROSS, M., and SPIRO, M. K. (1985). Selecting amplification characteristics for young hearing-impaired children. Ear and Hearing, 6;48–53.

SEILER, J. A. (1971). A formula for fitting hearing aids. The Hearing Dealer, March, 18–19, 30.

SEITZ, M. R., and KISIEL, D. L. (1990). Hearing aid assessment and the auditory brainstem response. In Sandlin, R., Ed. *Handbook of Hearing Aid Amplification, Vol. II: Clinical Considerations and Fitting Practices.* Boston: College Hill Press, 203–223.

SHAPIRO, I., (1975). Prediction of most comfortable loudness levels in hearing aid evaluation. Journal of Speech and Hearing Disorders, 40;434–438.

SHAPIRO, I. (1976). Hearing aid fitting by prescription. Audiology, 15;163–173.

SHAW, E. A. G. (1974). Transformation of sound pressure level from free field to the eardrum in a horizontal plane, Journal of the Acoustical Society of America, 56;6:1848.

SHORE, I., BILGER, R., and HIRSH, I. (1960). Hearing aid evaluation: reliability of repeated measurements. Journal of Speech and Hearing Research, 25;152–170.

SIEMENS, PC CONNEXX. (1995). Product brochure 37 15070 10/95 A 0908 20k.

SILMAN, S., GELFAND S. A., SILVERMAN, C. A. (1984). Late-onset auditory deprivation: effects of monaural versus binaural hearing aids. Journal of the Acoustical Society of America, 76;1357–1362.

SKINNER, M. W., PASCOE, D. P., MILLER, J. D., and POPELKA, G. R. (1982). Measurements to determine the optimal placement of speech energy within the listener's auditory area: a basis for selecting amplification characteristics. In STUDEBAKER, G. A., and BESS, F. H. (editors) *The Vanderbilt Hearing-Aid Report,* Upper Darby: 1982 Monographs in Contemporary Audiology, 161–169.

SNOW, T., and MCCANDLESS, G. (1976). The use of impedance measures in hearing aid selection. Hearing Aid Journal, 29;3, 32.

STAAB, W. J. (1978). *Hearing Aid Handbook,* Tab Books, Blue Ridge Summit, PA.

STAAB, W. J., and LYBARGER, S. F. (1994). Characteristics and use of hearing aids, in KATZ, J., Ed. *Handbook of Clinical Audiology, Fourth Edition.* Baltimore: Williams & Wilkins, 657–722.

SULLIVAN, J. A., LEVITT, H., HWANG, J., and HENNESSEY, A. (1988). An experimental comparison of four hearing aid prescription methods. Ear and Hearing, 9;22–32.

SVÄRD, I. and AHLNER, B. H. (1994). The "benefit method" in the fitting of hearing aids. Bulletin of the American Auditory Society, 19;10–11, 16.

SVÄRD, I. and SPENS, K. E. (1992). Paper presented at the XXI International Conference on Audiology in Morioka, Japan, August 31–Sept. 4.

TONISSON, W. (1975). Measuring in-the-ear gain of hearing aids by the acoustic reflex method. Journal of Speech and Hearing Research, 18;17–30.

VICTOREEN, J. A. (1963). *Hearing Enhancement,* Springfield, IL, Charles C. Thomas.

VICTOREEN, J. A. (1973). *Basic Principles of Otometry,* Springfield, IL, Charles C. Thomas.

WALLENFELS, H. G. (1967). *Hearing Aids on Prescription.* Charles C. Thomas, Springfield, IL.

WATSON, N. A., and KNUDSEN, V. O. (1940). Selective amplification in hearing aids. Journal of the Acoustical Society of America, 11;406–419.

WEBER, B. A. (1994). Auditory brainstem response: threshold estimation and auditory screening. In KATZ, J., Ed. *Handbook of Clinical Audiology, Fourth Edition.* Baltimore: Williams & Wilkins, 375–386.

WIENER, F., and ROSS, D. (1946). The pressure distribution in the auditory canal and progressive sound field. Journal of the Acoustical Society of America, 18;401–408.

ZWISLOCKI, J. J. (1971). Ear-like coupler for calibration of earphones. Journal of the Acoustical Society of America, 50;110(A).

ZWISLOCKI, J. J. (1970). An acoustic coupler for earphone calibration. Report LSC-S-7. Laboratory of Sensory Communication, Syracuse, NY.

APPENDIX A

ABBREVIATED PROFILE OF HEARING AID BENEFIT

Name: ________________________ Today's Date: __/__/__ Date of Birth: __/__/__
Last *First*

Address: ____

Telephone: (home) ______________ (work) ______________ SSN: ______________

HEARING AID EXPERIENCE:	DAILY HEARING AID USE:	EMPLOYMENT:
__ Less than 6 weeks	__ Less than 1 hour per day	__ Full-time
__ 6 weeks to 11 months	__ 1 to 4 hours per day	__ Part-time
__ 1 to 10 years	__ 4 to 8 hours per day	__ Not employed outside the home, or retired
__ Over 10 years	__ 8 to 16 hours per day	

INSTRUCTIONS: Please circle the answers that come closest to your everyday experience. Notice that each choice includes a percentage. You can use this to help you decide on your answer. For example, if a statement is true about 75% of the time, circle "C" for that item. If you have not experienced the situation we describe, try to think of a similar situation that you have been in and respond for that situation. If you have no idea, leave that item blank.

A Always (99%)
B Almost Always (87%)
C Generally (75%)
D Half-the-time (50%)
E Occasionally (25%)
F Seldom (12%)
G Never (1%)

	Without My Hearing Aid	With My Hearing Aid
1. The sound of a fire engine siren close by is so loud that I need to cover my ears	A B C D E F G	A B C D E F G
2. When a speaker is addressing a small group, and everyone is listening quietly, I have to strain to understand	A B C D E F G	A B C D E F G
3. It's hard for me to understand what is being said at lectures or church services	A B C D E F G	A B C D E F G
4. When I am at the dinner table with several people, and am trying to have a conversation with one person, understanding speech is difficult	A B C D E F G	A B C D E F G
5. When I am in a theater watching a movie or play, and the people around me are whispering and rustling paper wrappers, I can still make out the dialogue	A B C D E F G	A B C D E F G
6. When I'm in a quiet conversation with my doctor in an examination room, it is hard to follow the conversation	A B C D E F G	A B C D E F G

A Always (99%)	E Occasionally (25%)
B Almost Always (87%)	F Seldom (12%)
C Generally (75%)	G Never (1%)
D Half-the-time (50%)	

	Without My Hearing Aid	With My Hearing Aid
7. When I am listening to the news on the car radio, and family members are talking, I have trouble hearing the news	A B C D E F G	A B C D E F G
8. The sounds of running water, such as a toilet or shower, are uncomfortably loud	A B C D E F G	A B C D E F G
9. When I am having a quiet conversation with a friend, I have difficulty understanding	A B C D E F G	A B C D E F G
10. I can understand conversations even when several people are talking	A B C D E F G	A B C D E F G
11. The sounds of construction work are uncomfortably loud	A B C D E F G	A B C D E F G
12. I have trouble understanding others when an air conditioner or fan is on	A B C D E F G	A B C D E F G
13. I have trouble understanding dialogue in a movie or at the theater	A B C D E F G	A B C D E F G
14. Traffic noises are too loud	A B C D E F G	A B C D E F G
15. When I am in a small office, interviewing or answering questions, I have difficulty following the conversation. . . .	A B C D E F G	A B C D E F G
16. I miss a lot of information when I'm listening to a lecture	A B C D E F G	A B C D E F G
17. I have to ask people to repeat themselves in one-on-one conversation in a quiet room	A B C D E F G	A B C D E F G
18. Unexpected sounds, like a smoke detector or alarm bell are uncomfortable	A B C D E F G	A B C D E F G
19. I can follow the words of a sermon when listening to a religious service	A B C D E F G	A B C D E F G
20. When I am in a crowded grocery store, talking with the cashier, I can follow the conversation	A B C D E F G	A B C D E F G
21. I can communicate with others when we are in a crowd	A B C D E F G	A B C D E F G
22. The sound of screeching tires is uncomfortably loud	A B C D E F G	A B C D E F G

A Always (99%)	E Occasionally (25%)
B Almost Always (87%)	F Seldom (12%)
C Generally (75%)	G Never (1%)
D Half-the-time (50%)	

	Without My Hearing Aid	With My Hearing Aid
23. I have difficulty hearing a conversation when I'm with one of my family at home	A B C D E F G	A B C D E F G
24. When I am talking with someone across a large empty room, I understand the words	A B C D E F G	A B C D E F G

FOR AUDIOLOGIST USE ONLY

HEARING AND FITTING:	HEARING AID TYPE:	HEARING AID:
___ Unilateral	___ CIC	Make ______________
___ Bilateral	___ ITC	Model ______________
___ Directional Mic	___ ITE	Ser. # ______________
___ Compression	___ BTE	Fitted ______________

Comments: ____

____

____

____

____

VII

PRINCIPLES OF SOUND FIELD AUDIOMETRY

ROBERT E SANDLIN, Ph.D.

INTRODUCTION

In any professional discipline, change is inevitable. Depending on the underlying motivation for change, it may be orderly or random. There have been significant changes over the past eight to ten years in how hearing aid performance is assessed. Most of these changes have been in objective clinical methods, suggested either by various fitting formulae, or in instrumental measurement, exemplified by real ear assessment.

Our task, here, is to discuss sound field audiometry. In its strict sense, sound field assessment is those procedures that use test signals presented through a loudspeaker system in a sound controlled environment rather than through headphones. In a larger sense, however, this chapter stresses subjective assessment in hearing aid selection and fitting. It is rather straight forward to suggest that only through subjective measurement can one obtain hard data on the processing capabilities of the auditory system. To fit hearing aid devices without some assessment of the patient's ability to utilized hearing aid amplification in communicative situations is untenable.

In hearing instrument dispensing, early attempts to reasonably conclude that a given hearing aid was appropriately fitted utilized some form of sound field testing. Patients were placed in a sound treated chamber and instructed to respond to one or more acoustic stimuli. By carefully selecting the stimulus, the dispenser was reasonably certain that differences between aided and unaided responses were strong indicators of probable success with the hearing aid. Whether the stimulus was a phonetically balanced word, pure tone, warble tone, narrow bands of noise, amplitude modulated signal, damped wave train, or a variety of other signals, the patient's response to these stimuli was the final arbiter in deciding the value of the amplification system under test. Even though hearing aid selection procedures differed from one facility to the other, clinicians generally assumed the instrument that performed best, by whatever criteria, was the instrument of choice.

Investigators have reported the utility of sound field testing. Yet, it has been demonstrated beyond reasonable doubt that the more recent introduction and utilization of probe tube microphone measurements yielded a stable, objective and repeatable assessment of hearing aid performance. A more definitive control over the response parameters of the hearing aid was possible through use of a probe microphone (see Chapter VIII by McCandless.)

There is a tendency among professional disciplines to embrace new, challenging and exciting procedures, which provides useful clinical information not available prior to the introduction of the technology. Unfortunately, there is also a tendency for some to discard older procedures that have provided very useful information. One would hope that objective measures of hearing aid performance will not replace, entirely, subjective measures of performance and patient acceptance.

Sound field and probe tube microphone measures yield distinctly different kinds of information. Sound field measures provide information about the patient's response to acoustic signal(s) processed by the auditory system. The patient judges whether the signal is present or absent, loud or soft, distorted or undistorted, intelligible or unintelligible. Probe microphone measurement provides objective information about the acoustic characteristics of the signal impinging on the eardrum.

This chapter does not pit one assessment protocol against another. It has not been demonstrated conclusively that one method of assessment is more valid than the other in determining the hearing aid of choice. There is ample evidence to suggest that each method provides specific information about the performance of the hearing aid under test. The reader may question why a portion of this chapter devoted to sound field assessment deals with objective measurement of hearing aid performance. The reason is rather straight forward: It is to demonstrate that objective and subjective measurements contribute to the determination of "optimal" amplification.

CHAPTER OBJECTIVES

This chapter reviews the advantages and limitations of sound field testing to determine hearing aid performance and its appropriateness for the hearing impaired patient. This chapter does not extol the virtues of one measurement system over another. Rather it suggests that the principles underlying sound field measurement can be of clinical value when used intelligently. It is not a *how-to* chapter, but one which stresses the utility of sound field testing in the fitting of hearing aid devices.

HISTORICAL PERSPECTIVE

In the late 1930's, the University of Wisconsin's Speech and Hearing Center introduced sound field assessment. The center was under the direction of Dr. Robert West. During and after World War II, it was common for speech and hearing centers to use sound field testing in rehabilitation practices for veterans with hearing loss due to their war experiences. The principle dictating the use of sound field assessment was to provide information about the patient's response to acoustic stimuli with and without a hearing aid. Although the validity of some sound field measurement was questioned, information gained contributed to the hearing aid selection process.

A number of authors have reported the application and value of some form of sound field assessment. The reader is referred to Carhart (1946), Ross and Duffy (1961) Duffy (1967), Victoreen (1973), Duffy (1978), Punch & Parker, (1978), Goldberg (1981), Zelnick (1982), Preves (1984), Walker, et. al. 1984), Gabrielson et al. (1988), Studebaker & Sherbecoe (1988), Walker (1981) Sandlin (1990), Cox & McDaniel (1992) and Farby & Shum (1994).

SUBJECTIVE ASSESSMENT IN HEARING AID FITTING

In this chapter, subjective assessment is defined as testing of the manner in which individuals perceive and process acoustic information. It involves the physical event (the sound) and the psychological events (perception and processing). It includes psychoacoustics, . . . *[the] branch of psychophysics which deals with the quantification of sensation and the measurement of the psychological correlates of the physical stimulus. Psychoacoustics thus embraces the study of the psychological response to acoustical stimulation* (Durrant & Lovrinic 1984, p. 214).

Subjective assessment implies more than the perception of sound. It involves judging the contribution of perceived sounds to the intelligibility of the intended message. It entails measuring sound quality. It means determining whether a complex, amplified acoustic signal, such as speech, is acceptable to a hearing aid user. It implies evaluating whether or not two or more acoustic signals can be discriminated when delivered to the ear at the same time. It signifies appraising whether or not the auditory system perceives loudness changes in a normal or abnormal manner. It is interesting to note that some type of subjective assessment has been used for a number of years by engineering laboratories to make some differentiation among sound transmission circuitry. (Munson, et. al., 1962 and McDermott, 1968).

Sound field assessment refers to responses to acoustic signals produced in a sound field. Many audiologists and hearing instrument dispensers use it in some form in making the final determination of successful hearing aid use. Their work falls into that behavioral category of subjective measurement knows as psychoacoustics; the study of human perception and response to acoustic events.

The following are some psychoacoustic measures used in assessing the human auditory system. Normally, they are presented in the aided and unaided condition in a sound field:

- *Preferred listening level.* The level at which the patient judges speech to be at its optimal level for attending to sustained discourse.
- *Uncomfortable listening level.* The level at which the patient judges speech or other acoustic signals to be uncomfortably loud. That is, any further increase in the acoustic signal might result in the rejection of amplification.
- *Word recognition ability:* The percent of words correctly identified when presented at an optimal listening level.
- *Binaural performance:* The contribution to the perception and discrimination of acoustic signals presented to both ears, as opposed to one ear only.
- *Word recognition in noise:* The discrimination of words in the presence of background noise at some specified signal-to-noise ratio (S/N R).

- *Dynamic range:* The subjective assessment of the level at which a given acoustic signal violates the uncomfortable listening level subtracted from the level at which the patient is barely able to detect the presence of that signal.
- *Rollover phenomenon:* That phenomenon occurring when, above a certain input intensity level, word recognition is degraded.
- *Central processing disorder:* A disorder in which the peripheral auditory system is functioning adequately, but other structures such as the brainstem, midbrain and the auditory cortex are incapable of normal processing of speech and other acoustic signals.
- *Speech reception threshold.* The presentation level at which the patient is able to correctly identify 50% of the bisyllablic words presented, as well as other speech stimuli.
- *Difference limen for frequency (pitch):* The point at which the patient can just detect differences between two signals of different frequency when presented at the same level.
- *Difference limen for intensity (loudness).* The point at which the patient can just detect differences between signals of different intensities.
- *Loudness growth:* The rate of perceived loudness growth as the intensity of the signal increases.
- *Magnitude estimation:* The subjective intelligibility rating of speech or speech-like material presented at specified output levels.
- *Pure tone threshold sensitivity:* The point at which the individual perceives the presence of a pure tone signal.

Not all of these tests are performed on all patients fitted with hearing instruments. However, the length of the list reflects the value and extent of psychoacoustic measures in the decision-making process. Most who select and fit hearing aids conclude that the patient is the final arbiter of perceived benefit. This is true regardless of the method(s) employed to determine the electroacoustic properties of the hearing aid.

OBJECTIVE MEASUREMENTS IN HEARING AID FITTING

Although this chapter deals with the contributions of sound field measurement, it is appropriate to present a brief overview of objective measurement.

Objective measures do not require a response from the patient during the hearing aid assessment, or more accurately, do not require some intentional or cognitive processing of the acoustic signal(s) to which the patient is asked to attend. The measurement of one's threshold response to a pure tone signal may be considered objective. The person either hears it or doesn't. In another sense, it is subjective. The patient decides whether or not the signal was heard. The same is true when the patient is asked whether a signal is too loud or too soft. It is an either-or response. Since the patient either does or does not correctly identify the word, some argument can be made that a word recognition score is also an objective assessment.

Among the methods used in objective assessment is real ear probe tube measurement. In real ear measurement, the examiner places a probe tube close to the tympanic membrane, presents a sound, and measures its acoustic characteristics. The examiner judges if the acoustic signal at the eardrum meets predetermined criteria. A number of acronyms have been proposed to reflect the contributions of real ear probe tube measurements. Among them are:

- REIG real ear insertion gain
- REIR real ear insertion response
- REAR real ear aided response
- REUR real ear unaided response
- REOR real ear occluded response
- RESR real ear saturation response

Each measurement provides information about the acoustic signal at the ear drum and the means to decide whether or not it meets predetermined criteria.

There have been a number of individual efforts over the past several decades to devise an effective and objective fitting formula. The result have resulted in a number of proposed fitting formulae, each of which differs from the other. Most suggests that the recommended target gains for selected frequencies are those best suited to meet the acoustic needs of the patient. The following list is not an exhaustive one, but serves to underscore the continuing search for some objective method of successfully fitting hearing aid devices:

1930—Balbi

1940—Watson & Knudsen

1944—Lybarger
1946—Carhart
1954—Davis
1966—Redell & Calvert
1972—Key
1973—Victoreen
1975—Pascoe
1976—Byrne & Tonnison
1976—Skinner
1977—Berger
1983—McCandless & Lyregaard
1985—Cox 1985
1986—Byrne & Dillon (NAL)
1986—Libby 1986.

Whenever possible, the intent of each fitting method is to make the speech spectrum audible to the hearing impaired person. Most of the approaches suggest the degree to which specific frequencies should be amplified to achieve audibility of the speech spectrum. Figure 1 shows the recommended insertion gain for three different fitting methods for a moderately sloping high frequency hearing loss. Note that the gain responses have been normalized at 1000 Hz. The three methods, Berger, Libby and Lybarger, do not produce the same recommended insertion gain values for the same target frequencies.

Although these differences exist, it does not mean that such methods can not be useful. It suggests the clinician should select that method which represents best the acoustic needs of the patient. Usually some clinical experimentation is needed before one can conclude if one fitting method is superior to another. All compromise the amplification needs for given listening environments. That is, fitting formulae specify the best output response for the quiet listening environment. None recommends the appropriate responses for listening in various types of environmental backgrounds such as crowd noise, traffic noise, industrial noise, etc.

Current fitting strategies to determine insertion gain requirements are based on sensorineural losses, occluding earmolds and linear hearing aid amplifiers. For the most part, linear aids do not change their acoustic gain response as the listening environment changes. A signal processing instrument or a multimemory hearing

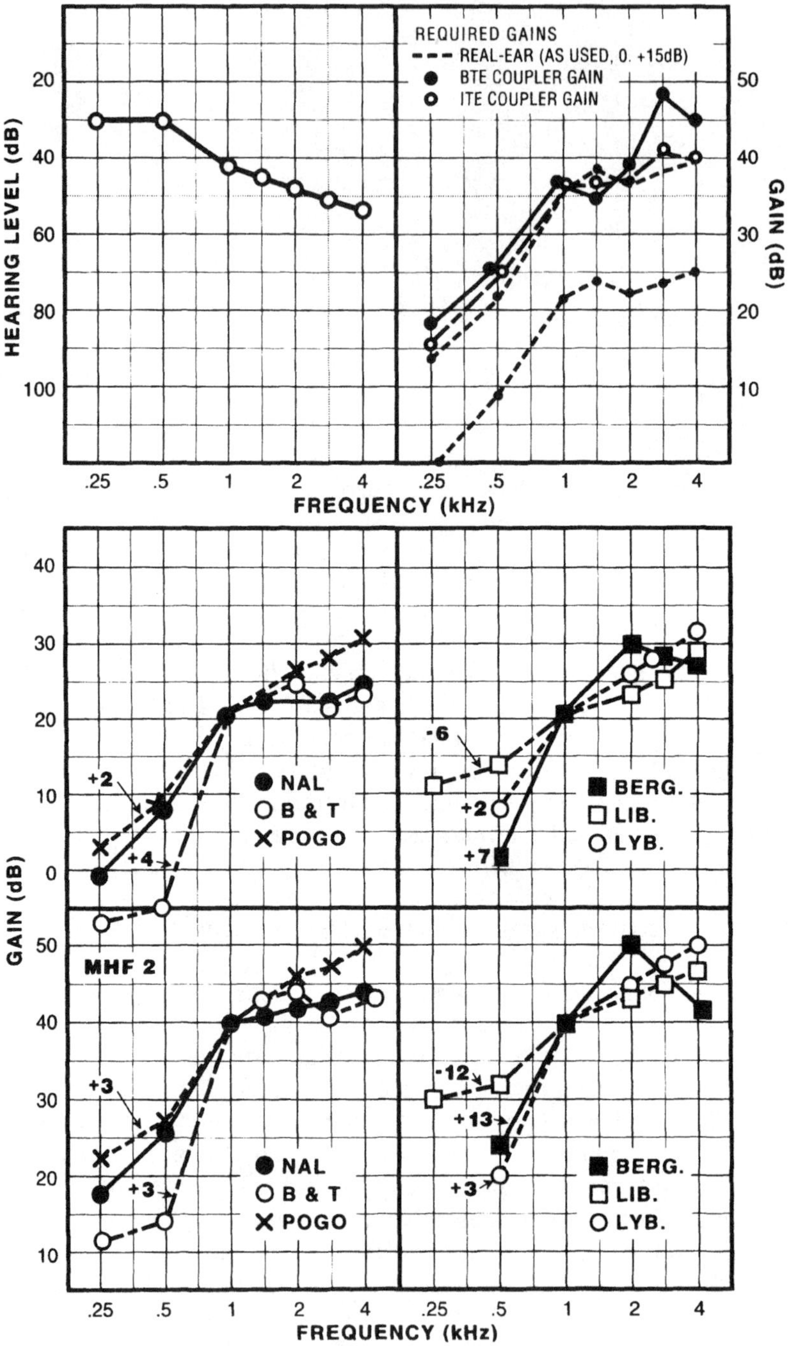

Fig. 1. Recommended insertion gain for a moderately sloping high frequency hearing impairment using three different fitting methods. Note that required target gain differs from one method to another.

aid may be best for meeting amplification needs as a function of listening environment. With the myriad of programmable hearing aids available, the dispenser is faced with the task of deciding that electroacoustic response best for a given listening condition. The reader is referred to Valente's definitive work in this textbook (Chapter IX) for a review of programmable hearing aid instrumentation and their utility.

Regardless of the fitting method employed, real ear probe tube measurement is an effective tool in measuring insertion gain. It is a rapid and accurate measurement of insertion gain at target frequencies. It offers a positive confirmation of whether or not target gains have been achieved. For a definitive review of real ear measurement, the reader is referred to an excellent textbook by Mueller and his colleagues (1992).

Current methods prescribe what the insertion gain should be for a linear hearing device. They fail to accurately define hearing aid response when the input is increased or when non-linear hearing aids are used. There is no broad-based acceptance of selection and fitting guidelines for setting the electroacoustic parameters for instruments with compression or other automatic signal processing functions.

Fabry and Schum (1994) make the following comment regarding the utility of probe microphone assessment and the application of fitting formulae: "*. . . other problems hamper this approach, including (1) there are nearly a dozen published prescriptive threshold formulae, and none has been demonstrated to be clearly superior to all others, (2) it is difficult to quantify what is meant by an "adequate" match to target gain; (3) many prescriptive formulae do not include prescription of maximum hearing aid output levels; and (4) these methods do not suffice for many of the advanced circuits such as automatic signal processing (ASP) or programmable hearing aids that have low compression thresholds (i.e., 45–55 dB SPL) and variable compression ratios.*

A primary issue becomes the accuracy of a hearing aid fitting model that uses only pure-tone thresholds and probe tube measurements for prescription and assessment of hearing aid performance, respectively. This strategy disregards the preferences of the person who ultimately provides the final determinant of hearing aid effectiveness. (p. 136.)

The issue is not whether objective or subjective procedures can be clinically defended. The issue is whether the acoustic needs of the patients are met by the clinical method employed. Jerger (personal correspondence 1987) offers a reasonable summary of present needs by stating:

Although systems for the measurement of real ear gain of hearing aids represent a significant technologic advance over analogous closed coupler measurements in quantifying the frequency response of a hearing aid system, it is important to remember that successful fitting of a hearing aid involves much more than the determination of the optimal frequency response. The audiologist must answer the following questions:

1. *Is the use of any hearing aid appropriate?*
2. *What is the best arrangement and configuration of the hearing aid system (e.g., BTE, ITE, canal aid, monaural vs. binaural; CROS, BICROS, etc.)?*
3. *Does the patient perform adequately with the recommended aid in the sense of understanding speech in realistic environments?*
4. *Is there a better solution than a hearing aid (i.e., assistive listening device)?*

To answer those questions, a thoughtful and responsible audiologist must necessarily incorporate into the evaluative system measures that go far beyond the real ear frequency response. They will typically involve some measure of the patient's ability to understand real speech in a realistic environment. They may involve quality judgments, paired comparison, adaptive measures of signal-to-noise ratio, or more traditional speech audiometric measures. Whatever their nature, however, they will broaden the evaluative spectrum beyond the narrow confines of frequency responses.

THE SOUND TREATED CHAMBER

To achieve reliable and repeatable psychoacoustic measurements in a sound field, it is necessary to place the patient in an area where ambient noise levels are controlled. A *sound field* is enclosed by the walls, floor and ceiling of a sound room. The room's construction should prevent ambient sounds from interfering with the patient's ability to respond to acoustic stimuli presented by the examiner. To create an optimal test environment, the test chamber should be acoustically treated to reduce sound reverberation (standing waves) to a minimum. If the acoustic stimulus from a sound field speaker becomes highly reverberant, it may interfere with the patient's recognition and/or proper assessment of the test signal. To create acceptable test conditions, sound absorbing materials dampen sounds in the test chamber, reducing standing waves to a negligible amount. One must be aware, however, that in the "real world" some sound reverberation is present and constitutes part of a normal listening environment. Nevertheless, the task is one of constructing a test chamber in which standing waves do not distort or interfere with the patient's response to a given acoustic stimulus.

DIRECT AND REVERBERATING SOUND FIELDS

Sound fields are direct or reverberating. The direct sound field is one that is dominated by directly radiated sound. Sound generated at the source (the sound field speaker) radiates directly to the listener. The reverberant sound field is one dominated by the sound reflected by a number of surfaces. The extent to which this reverberating sound field can be controlled will determine the accuracy of all measurement obtained in that field. It is not necessary to create an anechoic chamber (one without any standing waves) to conduct the sound field tests required to fit and select hearing aids. A direct field is present throughout an anechoic test chamber. That is, there is no reflected sound which alters the sound level at the eardrum. An attempt to create a truly anechoic environment would be expensive and of questionable clinical value. Very few professionals have access to, need, or can afford, such a test facility.

The dispenser should be aware of the need to control sound levels within the test chamber. External, ambient sounds must not interfere with the patient's ability to properly assess test signals generated within the chamber. To attenuate outside sounds, the test chamber is constructed of materials that provide stiffness and mass. The degree to which external sounds are attenuated depends on the types and amount of material used in the construction of the sound room. Attenuation is also frequency specific. Low frequencies, having longer wave lengths, are more difficult to attenuate than higher frequencies having shorter wave lengths.

Noise levels in the test chamber might interfere with measuring organic thresholds (Macrae & Frazer 1980; Zemplenyi, Dirks, & Gilman, 1985). As mentioned previously, unless one can afford the expense of constructing something that approaches the characteristics of an anechoic chamber, the hearing health professional must accept some minimal error in threshold assessment, regardless of its magnitude. As long as the ambient noise in the sound chamber is at or below 45 dB(A), the effect on getting reliable measures of hearing aid performance is minimal.

Figure 2 shows the averaged hearing threshold sensitivity to selected pure tone stimuli in a sound room. The ambient noise level is 45 dB(A). All threshold measures are expressed in dB SPL. Measurements were made with the sound source at 90 degrees azimuth, with the sound field speaker placed approximately 9 inches from a Type 2 sound level meter positioned where the person's head would be during the test. A 45 dB(A) ambient level may interfere with audibility as the azimuth or distance from the speaker-to-ear is altered.

Still, most persons being tested in a sound field have a bilateral hearing impairment. For this patient population, a 45 dB(A) ambient noise level would seldom create a problem in obtaining reliable threshold measurements over a broad frequency range.

The presence of standing waves and the effect of head movement can effect test reliability. For example, obtaining reliable measures of unaided and aided thresholds for specific frequencies require adherence to sound field conditions permitting only minimal error. In general, when assessing the patient's sound discrimination or word recognition function, less strict control of sound field parameters would be acceptable.

This section is not intended to provide specific information about sound chamber construction and acoustic performance. It suggests, rather, the degree to which the sound chamber construc-

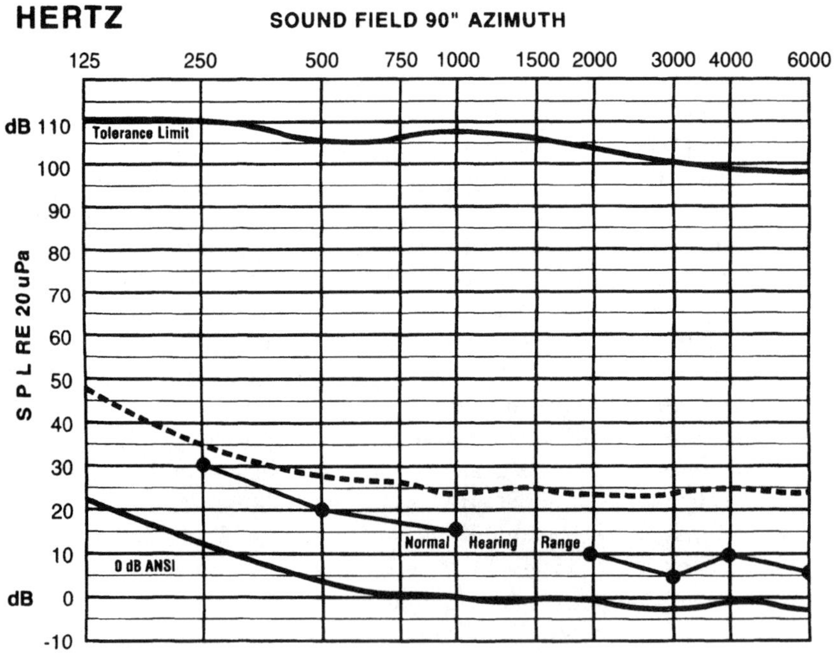

Fig. 2. Shown here is the averaged hearing threshold sensitivity to selected pure tone stimuli for six normal hearing individuals. The averaged ambient noise level is 45 dB (A) and the signal source is at 90 degrees. The solid and dashed lines indicate the range of thresholds for monaural presentation.

tion controls internally and externally generated sounds. For a more complete description, the reader is referred to the scholarly report of Walker (1988), who provides an extensive review of the technical considerations for sound field audiometry.

RATIONALE FOR PROPER PLACEMENT OF THE PATIENT IN THE SOUND ROOM

Accurate sound field measurement of an individual's response to acoustic stimuli is not without problems. Patients must be positioned so that the desired signal level at the ear is not greatly influenced by the sound room characteristics. The sound pressure of a given signal at the patient's ear should be constant and not influenced by standing waves. If control of the field can not be accomplished, signal intensity at the eardrum can vary greatly and lead to erroneous measurement. To achieve stability, the patient must be placed far enough from reflecting surfaces so that there is no disturbance from change in sound pressure (D'Antonio, 1986; Preves & Sullivan, 1987). The distance of the patient from the sound field speaker can influence the signal stability at the ear drum. Figure 3 (Vol. 1) shows signal intensity variability as a function of distance. As the distance from the sound source increases, the more pronounced is the signal level variability. Most authorities recommend that the patient be placed approximately one meter from the sound field speaker to reduce the influence of standing

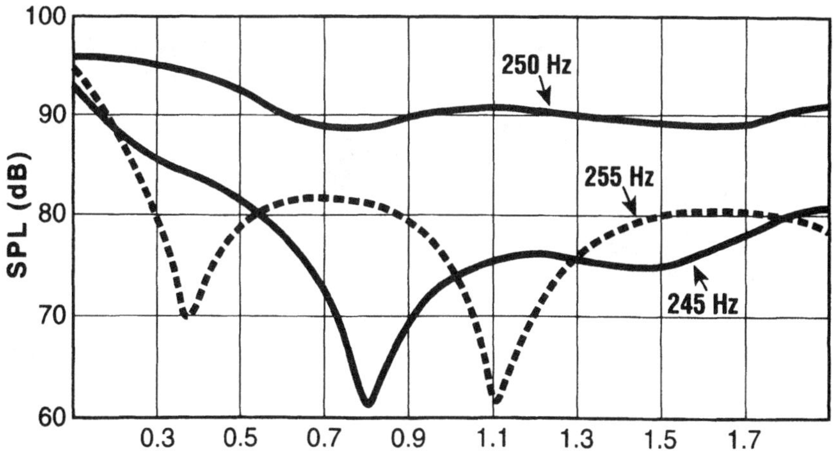

Fig. 3. Signal intensity variability in level for three pure tones, five Hz apart, as the distance increases from the sound source.

waves. The patient's head must be held as steady as possible. The patient's orientation to the sound field speakers is shown in Figure 4. They type of signal generated in the sound field will determine variations in sound pressure when the head is moved only slightly. In general, pure tones are not the most appropriate stimuli to use in a sound field assessment. Depending on the frequency of the pure tone, slight movements of the head may create significant changes in the signal intensity. Goldberg (1979), however, has suggested that pure tones can be used successfully if the sound source is only nine to twelve inches from the ear. Restricting the

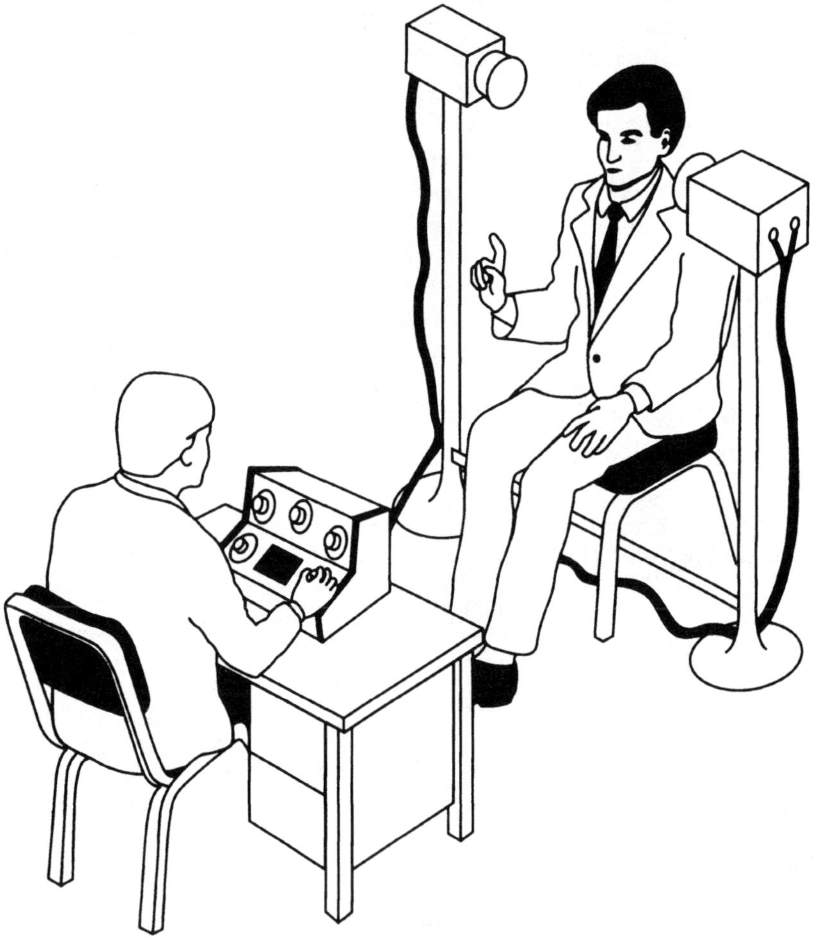

Fig. 4. Subject position in a sound chamber in obtaining pure tone threshold measurements. Note that the sound source is at 90 degrees azimuth and the speaker is about nine inches from the ear under test.

source-to-listener distance greatly reduces the deleterious effects of standing waves.

Woodward and Tecca (1985) suggest that; *If use of pure tones in a sound field yield reliable measures of auditory sensitivity, the application of these stimuli in assessment of functional gain for various modes of amplification may prove more accurate than alternative stimuli. When a hearing aid is introduced, the potential for client response to components of frequencies other than the normal test frequency or any alternative stimuli may be affected not only by the slope of an individual audiogram, but also by the frequency response of the hearing aid and the interaction of these two variables (p.22).* For example, if one uses a "warble tone" signal in assessing organic thresholds in a sound field, the frequency deviation and modulation rate constitute two parameters that must be controlled. Frequency deviation refers; *to that difference between an unmodulated carrier frequency and the lowest or the highest instantaneous frequency attained by the waveform during modulation.* (Lundeen 1988, p. 32). Modulation rate simply refers the rate that frequency change occurs.

Depending on what stimuli are to be presented, more than one sound field speaker may be necessary. For example, in assessing the patient's binaural response to acoustic signals, more than one sound field speaker is needed, in that one signal may come from one speaker and another from a different sound field speaker. In general, if only one sound field speaker is used, it is placed at 0 degrees azimuth when assessing aided and unaided monaural response. When assessing binaural response, two speakers are used and should be placed at 45 degrees azimuth, relative to the patient's head position in the sound field.

A number of complex signals have been suggested as suitable for sound field measurement. Commonly used complex signals are the frequency modulated (warble tone) signal, and narrow bands of noise. However, their spectral characteristics may vary, depending on the audiometer used. Other types of complex signals include amplitude modulated tones (Goldberg 1979) and damped wave-trains (Victoreen 1974). The rationale for the use of these signals is that they have acoustic energy centered around the nominal frequency. Figure 5 shows the response of a pure tone and two modulated tones (5 and 20% respectively) as a function of distance from the sound source. Note that there are significant differences among the sounds, with the 20% modulated tone having the least variability of the three.

Care must be exercised in selecting the slope of the filter skirts. If the skirts are not "steep" enough, then there is a possibility that

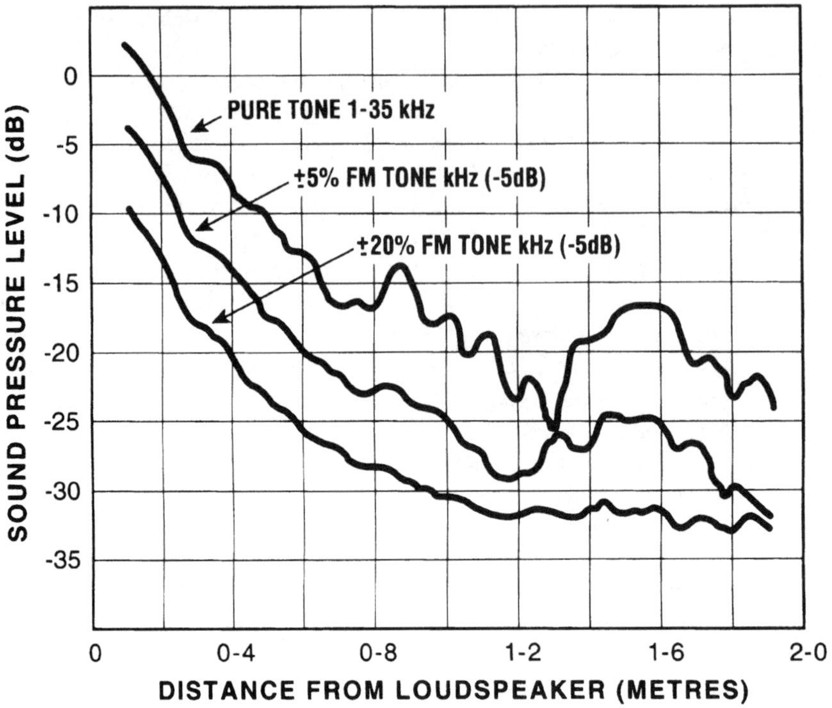

Fig. 5. The sound pressure levels generated by an unmodulated and two modulated tones with the same center frequency but different bandwidths, as a function of distance from the speaker. The overall levels of the tones have been arbitrarily separated by 5 dB.

one sacrifices frequency specificity. This is especially true for those patients having rapidly falling hearing loss. That is, the filter skirts should be steep enough to prevent loss of frequency specificity.

In selecting the appropriate test stimulus, hearing instrument dispensers should consider those suggestions offered by Dillon and Walker (1982).

- *It must be reasonably frequency specific because frequency specific information is needed for a satisfactory definition of the client's hearing status and amplification needs.*
- *The sound pressure level generated in the field must be stable over the whole region that the client's head could occupy, during testing.*
- *The sound pressure level generated at the client's ear must be stable for small shifts in frequency, such as may occur in an oscillator's output between calibrations.*

- *The results obtained in the sound field must be relatable to similar measurements made with pure tones under earphones. (page 153)*

Acoustic stimuli employed by the clinician must be those that contribute significantly to making a decision about the amplification needs of the patient and permit determining whether the desired psychoacoustic performance has been achieved.

THE USE OF SPEECH OR SPEECH-LIKE STIMULI IN A SOUND FIELD

Practitioners agree that the single most compelling reason for hearing aid use is to improve the individual's ability to understand conversational speech. There is considerable disagreement, nonetheless, regarding the speech stimulus of choice in the evaluation process. Regardless of the stimulus employed, improved speech discrimination is one of the desired goals.

The task is to determine the most appropriate speech stimulus to use when assessing the clinical contributions of a hearing aid. Early on, Carhart (1946) suggested that when word recognition scores differed by only 8%, the hearing aid yielding the better score was the instrument of choice. However, the use of monosyllabic, phonetically balanced words to define real differences among two or more hearing aids is fraught with error (Thornton & Rafin, 1978). The total number of monosyllabic words needed to consistently and reliably differentiate among hearing aids far exceeds the amount of time one can devote to the evaluation process. Additionally, Shore, Bilger and Hirsch (1960) established that word recognition tasks do not consistently differentiate among hearing aids. Schwartz and Walden (1983) demonstrated that word recognition scores for eight patients, extending over a five day period, varied as much as 30 percent.

Other than using monosyllabic words to assess word recognition scores between hearing aids, a number of other speech based or speech-like procedures have been recommended to determine hearing aid performance. Such test as the Nonsense Syllable Test (NST) developed by Levitt and Resnick (1978), the Synthetic Sentence Identification (SSI) offered by Speaks and Jerger (1965), and the Speech Perception in Noise devised by Kalikow, Stevens and Elliot (1977), have contributed to one's ability to determine the best hearing aid from a number of instruments evaluated.

There are other speech based procedures one can use in sound field testing to estimate the value of hearing aids. However, determining speech performance is only one of a host of clinical procedures to select and fit hearing instruments. These procedures will be covered in a subsequent section of this chapter.

It is possible for individuals to judge the intelligibility of a paragraph or selected sentences by the process of magnitude estimation (Purdy and Watson (1990). Magnitude estimation can be defined as the subjective task of assessing the intelligibility of selected discourse, or other speech samples, presented at a specified level. That is, the patient simply estimates the percent of understanding of a spoken passage. There is a close approximation between magnitude estimation and actual measures of intelligibility.

Magnitude estimation is useful in assessing the intelligibility of speech material in the presence of background noise or completing messages at specified signal to noise ratios. In a sound field, the hearing health professional can determine differences between aided and unaided performance for one or more hearing aids for which the same acoustic stimuli are presented. In this manner, the only variable affecting magnitude estimation is the electroacoustic response of the hearing aid(s). The reader is referred to the work of Cox and McDaniels (1989, 1992 & 1994) in their germinal studies of intelligibility rating of connected discourse and its application to hearing aid selection. The reader is referred, also, to the study by Studebaker & Sherbecoe (1988) for their pioneering work in the application of magnitude estimation measures.

Not only is magnitude estimation useful in assessing the intelligibility of connected discourse, it is also valuable in determining quality judgments, signal sharpness and clarity, and the comfort of connected speech. Each of these measures can be instrumental in helping the hearing health professional judge overall hearing aid performance.

Duffy (1987) makes a good argument for phoneme recognition testing. A phoneme may be defined as any speech sound associated with a family of sounds having identifying acoustic characteristics distinguishing it from any other phoneme. There are some forty four different phonemes in the English phonological system. The acoustic characteristics of a given phoneme must be audible and identifiable by the listener, if it is to be correctly perceived. Determining of phoneme recognition is possible, with or without hearing aid devices, demands some type of sound field, subjective assessment. Such sound field assessment determines the extent to which the patient is able to use amplification and the subsequent contributions of the hearing aid. Obviously, the extent to which a hearing aid device can reinstate the essential acoustic information contained in any phoneme, and the extent to which the auditory system is capable of processing this information, is critical to successful aural rehabilitation. Not only is such assessment valuable for monaurally function but binaural function as well.

DETERMINING THE MOST COMFORTABLE LISTENING LEVEL

Hearing impaired persons will adjust hearing aid gain to maintain a most comfortable listening level, the level at which a person listens to connected discourse for extended periods of time without adjusting the hearing aid volume or sensing the need for volume change to maintain comfort. The hearing loss type and magnitude, the signal processing capabilities of the hearing aid and the environment in which listening takes place help determine the preferred listening level.

To determine the most comfortable listening, the patient must make some judgment on the acceptable level for the hearing aid under test. Fitting formulae assume that if the hearing aid achieves recommended target gain, a most comfortable listening level results (Leijon, Eriksson-Mangold, & Berch-Karlsen, 1984). There are those who feel that current fitting methods utilizing a half-gain rule may not be valid in setting the hearing aid gain for mild hearing impairments. Other fitting protocols, such as that proposed by Libby (1986) recommend that the 1/3 gain is more appropriate for mild to moderate hearing losses. Further, various fitting methods do not accurately predict insertion gain requirements to achieve most comfortable listening for those with severe to profound hearing impairment. An impetus arose to modify the fitting criteria for the severe to profoundly deaf persons, based on the patient's psychological assessment of the gain required to achieve a comfortable level of listening. Subsequently, some fitting methods have been revised to more closely reflect the insertion gains needed to achieve acceptable levels (Libby, 1986, Schwartz, Lyregaard, & Lundh, and Byrne, Parkinson, & Newall 1991).

The patient determines the acceptability of the hearing aid relative to listening comfort. The dispenser can best confirm it in the sound field. Assuming that current fitting methods provide a first approximation of need, the task is to *fine tune* hearing aid performance to achieve patient acceptance. It is this fine tuning that requires a subjective response from the person being evaluated.

The clinician should know there is, or can be, a difference between the amplification needed to achieve a most comfortable listening level and that required to best understand the intended message. In an early study, Posner and Ventry found that . . . *subjects with sensorineural loss did not achieve PB max (maximum intelligibility of monosyllabic, phonetically balanced words. ed.) when listening at the most comfortable loudness (MCL). While the mean MCL for their subjects was 14.6 dB SL, PB, max did not occur until a mean SL of 37.2 dB* (Hodgson, 1977, p. 117)

Whether the issue is one of a most comfortable listening level, or a level to achieve maximum word recognition, such measures can only be accomplished through some type of psychoacoustic, sound field assessment. The dilemma is whether or not to set the response of the hearing aid to provide an acceptable comfort level or to gain the best discrimination function. A compromise may be to counsel the patient about the limitations and advantages of adjusting the volume level to meet comfort or intelligibility needs. For some patients, counseling can result in the acceptance of that response offering maximum understanding without violating the comfort level.

An unrelenting challenge for the hearing health professional is determining how to maintain a comfortable listening level when there is noise or a competing message in the background. Current fitting formulae do not provide for the best electroacoustic response when the patient is exposed to environmental conditions other than quiet. The reason for this is rather straight forward. Current fitting formula are based on the use of a linear hearing aid. Since linear systems do not change acoustic behavior as a function of ambient noise levels, it is of little consequence. As a result, the recommended hearing aid response is a deliberate compromise. The acoustic parameters of the hearing aid are set to yield a response that is "as adequate as possible" for listening conditions to which the person may be exposed on a frequently occurring basis.

However, with the number of non-linear hearing aids available today, comfortable listening levels may be more closely approximated for a number of listening environments. This is especially true for multi-memory, digitally controlled, programmable hearing aid systems. Such hearing instruments permit the manipulation of the electroacoustic response of two or more programs to provide an appropriate interface with specific background conditions. Even with multimemory hearing aids, the hearing health professional must determine what the response of the instrument should be for each of the available memories. Some hearing aid companies have attempted to assist the dispenser by providing fitting guidelines for multiprogrammable systems. Widex, for example, has developed a fitting guide for their multimemory hearing aids, which recommends the necessary changes in the output response to maintain comfortable listening level for a number of listening environments.

Regardless of the linear or non-linear characteristics of today's hearing aids, a most comfortable level as a function of listening environment can only be confirmed realistically in a sound field. Sound field assessment provides clinically useful information, relative to the patient's determination of his or her comfort level as the listening environment changes. Sound field measurement provides equally useful information of the effects of non-linear hearing aids on the determination of a most comfortable listening level.

DETERMINING THE LOUDNESS DISCOMFORT LEVEL

If this author were limited to a single measure for determining hearing aid acceptance, it would be the direct measurement of loudness discomfort. Any person involved in the selection, fitting and follow up care of hearing impaired patients can attest to the advantage of correctly determining this value. The error which many practitioners commit is that of providing an SSPL 90 function that unrealistically represents the maximum sound pressure the user is willing to accept. For too many years we may have assumed that a sensorineural hearing impairment required higher SSPL 90 values. However, subsequent studies have indicated that such may not be the case.

Objectively, some fitting formulae assume that loudness discomfort can be predicted from target frequency thresholds. As McCandless (1994) has stated: *Although the use of prescriptive procedures has become popular, no general agreement has been reached as to what measurements should be used to calculate the prescribed gain, (e.g., hearing thresholds, MCL or UCL). However, most dispensers and manufacturers currently use threshold-based procedures for calculation of the prescribed frequency-gain response since the pure-tone audiogram is easily obtained and always available* (p. 4).

McCandless is suggesting there may be other ways to obtain a more accurate assessment of functions such as loudness discomfort. Moreover, Mueller (1992) states: *One of the primary goals of the hearing aid fitting procedure is to assure that maximum output of the hearing aid is both comfortable and safe. While this can be accomplished with some degree of accuracy with adult patients without using probe-microphone measurements, by combining the RESR (Real Ear Saturation Response. . . . ed.) with aided LDLs*

(Loudness Discomfort Levels . . . ed.), more precise fitting of the hearing aid's output can be obtained (page 60). This statement suggests that combining objective measurement with subjective responses from the patient may contribute more useful information than any one single measurement.

Getting a reliable estimation of loudness discomfort by subjective methods in a sound field is not without difficulty. Most clinicians concede that the subjective assessment of loudness discomfort is, in part, a function of the instruction given. For example, if the instruction is that of asking the patient to determine when the sound level creates a sensation of tickle, pain or dizziness, it is unlikely that the result approximates a realistic SSPL 90. Conversely, if the instruction is that of asking the patient to determine when the sound is "just" becoming annoying, it may underestimate the SSPL90 required for optimal hearing aid performance. The most appropriate instruction, therefore, may be that of determining at what point the sound level is acceptable for brief periods of time without violating the discomfort level.

Problems encountered, if the patient is fitted with hearing aids providing excessive SPL 90, are twofold. In the first instance, the patient will adjust the volume control downward to guard against sudden exposure to overly loud sounds. When this happens, it may cause certain speech sounds (primarily the consonants) to be inaudible; thus creating a loss of speech cues needed to understand the intended message. However, when the patient turns the volume up to understand clearly the message, sudden loud sounds violate comfort levels. In the second instance, the patient may turn the hearing aid off during those moments of discomfort. Such activity may lead, ultimately, to the person's rejection of amplification.

FOLLOW-UP SOUND FIELD ASSESSMENT

There is general agreement that any fitting procedure, subjective or objective, is a "first approximation" of the appropriateness of the recommended hearing aid(s). There is often a need to change some of the acoustic response parameters of the hearing aid to achieve optimal performance. The need for change is based on the individual's experiences with hearing aid amplification. Experiences indicating a need for change in hearing aid performance, such as excessive SPL 90, minimal improvement in word recognition function, significantly reduced discrimination in the presence of noise, signal distortions produced by the hearing aid, are best assessed in a sound field.

For example, if the patient complains of poor aided word recognition ability, assessing change in performance following modification of hearing aid response, sound field testing will show the magnitude of those changes. It is possible to determine which phonemes are unintelligible and which are correctly identified. If the patient complains of poor performance in the presence of specific noise environments, sound field assessment following modification of frequency response indicates whether a positive change has been generated. If the patient feels that monaural performance is more acceptable than binaural performance, sound field assessment identifies the magnitude of difference in performance. If the patient complains that the hearing aid is too loud or too soft to be acceptable, subsequent sound field testing confirms whether electroacoustic changes in hearing aid performance has satisfied the complaint.

It should be self-evident that successful fitting of hearing aids must involve some form of the patient's assessment of value received. One of the problems faced by the hearing health professional is that of meeting the patient's acoustic needs without violating acceptance of amplification. Established acoustic performances to meet needs are not the same as the individual's acceptance of the recommended hearing aids. Experienced hearing instrument dispensers know that patients may reject the hearing aid(s), even though the electroacoustic response meets all reasonable criteria.

Among the advantages of sound field testing is that of using test results to counsel patients regarding what is needed and what is acceptable. If the patient is aware that improved performance is possible with the recommended hearing aid, strategies may be developed over time, which permit acceptance of the desired response. That is, the clinician can compare optimal acoustic performance with that which the patient is willing to accept and suggest that he/she is best served by adapting to the recommended hearing aid characteristics.

SOME THOUGHTS ABOUT THE ARTICULATION INDEX

The popularity of a simplified articulation index (AI) (Mueller and Killion (1990), Humes (1991), and Pavlovic (1991) is based on the ease with which a threshold audiogram can be obtained. Having measured organic thresholds for selected frequencies, one can count the dots (Mueller and Killion, 1990) that fall below the unaided thresholds and predict articulation function. Additional impetus was given to the use of some form of AI by the clinical report of Humes (1991) who found that there was a very positive correlation between the articulation function predicted by an AI procedure and actual sound recognition scores obtained by a nonsense syllable test. That is, if one can determined the extent to which the speech spectrum is made audible by hearing aid devices, a reasonable estimation of AI can be predicted.

When one reports word recognition scores for a group of individuals, the assumption is that an individual within that group will produce a score consistent with the average of the group. Although, the use of some AI may yield a reliable predictor of function and, thus, reflect accurately the articulation skills of the hearing impaired patient, such is not always the case. Again, such statements as this are not intended to indict the use of some AI, but rather to caution against the tendency to assume that the obtained AI accurately represents the patient's ability to perform.

There are a number of factors that may influence the patient's ability to understand the intended word message. For example, the ability of the auditory system to process information, even though the speech spectrum may be audible, may be highly compromised. Regardless of the type of amplification provided, the system simply can not correctly process enough information to correspond to the predicted function of an AI procedure. Such conditions consistent with central auditory processing disorders, which often accompany the aging process, influence one's ability to discriminate acoustic events. Various cochlear distortions may degrade the kinds of neural input to the processing system needed to correctly identify the intended message. Further, distortion products produced by the hearing aid, i.e., intermodulation distortion, harmonic distortion, internal noise, symmetrical and asymmetrical peak clipping, etc, may provided significant barriers to understanding the intended signal or message.

We had spoken earlier in this chapter about the value of "first approximation" of need provided by current hearing aid fitting formulae. Such may very well be true when discussing the application of a given AI procedure. It gives the hearing health professional some indication of improved word recognition function. No audiologist or hearing instrument dispenser is unaware of this possibility, yet the caution is still present not to accept as an absolute the predicted functions.

This rather extended preamble serves to suggest that sound field assessment of word recognition skills is still a viable clinical procedure. There is considerable concern about what kind of speech material should be used when testing the individual's ability. One realizes that such tests as the CID W22 word lists, or perhaps other recognized word lists and other measures of speech recognition performance, may fall short of yielding reliable scores. However, the value of such measures may, in some cases, be more clinically useful than predicted measures. Studebaker (1991) presents a provocative overview of the limitations of measures of intelligibility.

SOME THOUGHTS ABOUT DIGITALLY PROGRAMMABLE HEARING AIDS

No textbook dealing with hearing aid amplification would be complete without some comment on the utility of digitally programmable hearing aid systems. This chapter, however, will only review the need for subjective, sound field assessment relating to how one decides on the most appropriate hearing aid response for different listening environments. Not only what the output response is of the hearing aid, but whether some form of signal processing is indicated, compared to conventional hearing aid systems. There is no need to defend the advantages offered by programmable systems. In his chapter, Valente ably manages that task.

It is difficult to arrived at some absolute standard by which one sets the various acoustic parameters for specific listening conditions. This is so because one can not replicate all acoustic environments to which a hearing impaired individual may be exposed. It would seem appropriate to get information from the patient, relative to those listening environments to which he/she is exposed frequently. Having done so, one may then attempt to replicate in a sound field, as nearly as possible, the acoustic conditions of the environment. The extent to which a number of environments can be treated successfully, depends on whether the instrument is a single or multi-memory unit. If a multiple memory system, the task is that of gathering appropriate patient information to set the various acoustic responses for two or more listening conditions to best interface with need.

Based on the magnitude of the hearing impairment and the auditory processing capabilities, it may not be possible to meet all of patient's acoustic needs for all possible listening conditions. Sound field assessment offers the best method at this time to approximate optimal amplification needs to a specific background environment. This statement is not to indict those efforts to provide a cookbook, or recipe, for presetting the hearing aid to provide, but rather to state that such methods offer a first approximation of need. The "fine tuning" of the hearing aid response demands some patient input, preferably obtained in a sound field.

SUMMARY AND CONCLUSION

Sound field assessment is a useful tool in the selection, fitting, evaluation and verification process of hearing aid utilization. Sound field audiometry provides a method of assessing unaided and aided responses to specific acoustic stimuli in a controlled sound environment. By comparing aided to unaided responses, the dispenser can measure the contributions of the hearing aid under test.

The application of sound field assessment does not imply that other measurement protocols are of little value in the selection and fitting of hearing aids. The argument is not whether objective or subjective methods are best. The argument to be defended is that of utilizing the clinical contributions of each to assess superiority of those hearing instrument(s) evaluated.

It is a gross error in clinical judgment to deny the contributions made by objective measurements of hearing aid performance. Probe microphone measurement has been beneficial in determining the help offered by amplification. Further, to deny the objectivity of current fitting methods would be less than astute. Despite the lack of consensus about how much gain is required at what target frequencies, such fitting protocols do provide an approximation of need. Conversely, it would be equally absurd for one to reject the contributions of subjective, sound field assessment.

In the final analysis, an individual's response to acoustic stimuli in a controlled sound field is important in determining the appropriateness of the hearing aid device. In a broader sense, the audiologist and dispenser are advised to utilize measurement protocols, objective and subjective, which best contribute to the proper selection of hearing aid amplification. Doing so greatly enhances the person's ability to enjoy the acoustic world in which he or she lives. However, caution is advised in limiting one's clinical investigation to only objective measurement. By so doing, the patient is being eliminated as an active participant in the decision making process regarding hearing aid amplification.

A word of concern is given here to those who hesitate to use new or advanced methods to fit hearing aids. Unfortunately, there are those few hearing health professionals who select and fit hearing aid devices without adherence to or the understanding of any assessment method. Even though sound field audiometry is of significant value, they refuse to do even basic sound field measurements. They ask the patient, "How do you like it?" or "Does this sound better to you?" If the patient responds in the affirmative, the hearing aid fitting is a success. This type of "divine" evaluation should be abandoned.

This author's crystal ball is no clearer than others in predicting the future of those measurement criteria to be employed in determining the best hearing aid. Undoubtedly, such future requirements must measure, in part, the patient utilization and acceptance of hearing aid amplification and the extent to which word recognition and the use-value of other acoustic stimuli are enhanced.

GLOSSARY

Articulation Index A method of predicting intelligibility of speech or speech-like sounds based on pure tone threshold data.

Direct Sound Field A room, area or chamber in which the sound source (loudspeaker) radiates acoustic signals directly to the listener.

First Approximation The use of some objective or subjective method of assessing the probability of the appropriateness of a hearing instrument fitting.

Magnitude Estimation The subjective task of assessing the intelligibility of selected discourse, or other speech samples presented as specified levels.

Loudness Discomfort Level The level at which sounds at the ear are excessively loud and unacceptable to the listener.

Most Comfortable Level The level at which a person will listen to speech or other acoustic signals for extended periods of time, without rejecting them because of too little or too much sound level.

Objective Fitting Method A system by which audiometric data are used to determine the response characteristics of a hearing aid to interface with a given hearing impairment.

Phoneme Any speech sound associated with a family of sounds having identifying acoustic characteristics distinguishing it from any other phoneme.

Probe Microphone Measurement Objective assessment of the properties of an acoustic signal(s) at or near the eardrum of the person under test.

Professional One who adheres to ethical and legal standards of performance dictated by the group or organization to which he/she belongs.

Programmable Hearing Aid System A system which permits the dispenser to program the hearing instrument to some selected acoustic performance, or to reprogram the hearing aid should such be necessary. Programmable hearing aids may be single or multimemory systems.

Psychoacoustics The study of human perception and response to acoustic events.

Reverberating Sound Field A room, area or chamber in which the sounds are reflected by one or more surfaces.

Sound Field Any room or chamber in which acoustic signals originate from a loudspeaker system.

Sound Field Assessment Those procedures that use test signals presented through a loudspeaker system in a sound controlled environment rather than through headphones.

Subjective Assessment Measuring the patient's response to one or more simple or complex acoustic signals normally presented in a sound field.

REFERENCES

BYRNE, D., PARKINSON, A., & NEWALL, P. Modified hearing aid selection procedures for severe/profound hearing losses. In G. Studebaker, F. Bess & L. Beck (eds.), The Vanderbilt Report Hearing-aid Report II. (1991) pp 295–300. Parekton, MD: York Press.

CARHART, R. The selection of hearing aids. Archives of Otolaryngolgy, (1946) 44, 1–18.

COX, R. M. & MCDANIEL, D. M. Intelligibility rating of continuous discourse: Application to hearing aid selection. *J Acoust Soc Am.* (1992). 76:758–766.

COX, R. M. & ALEXANDER, G. C. Maturation of hearing aid benefit: Objective and subjective measurements. *Ear Hear* (1992)143:131–141.

COX, R. M. & MCDANIEL, D. M. Evaluation of the speech intelligibility rating (SIR) test for hearing aid comparisons. *J. Speech Hear Res.* (1992) 35:686–693.

DILLON, H. & WALKER, J. Comparison of stimuli used in sound field audiometric testing. *J. Acoust. Soc. Am.*, (1992) 71, 161–172.

DUFFY, J. K. Audio-visuals speech audiometry and a new audio-visual speech perception index. *Maico Audiological Library Services,* (1967) 5 (9), 1–3.

DUFFY, J. K. Sound field audiometry and hearing aid advisement. *Hearing Instruments* (1978) 29(2), 6–12.

DUFFY, J. K. Sound field audiometry and hearing aid selection. In E. Zelnick (ed.) Hearing Instrument: Selection and Evaluation. Livonia, Michigan. NIHIS. (1987) pp. 179–215.

DURRANT, J. D. & LOVRINIC, J. H. Bases of Hearing Science (Second Edition). Baltimore: Williams & Wilkins, (1981).

FABRY, D. A. & SCHUM,. D. J. The role of subjective measurement techniques in hearing aid fittings. In: M. Valente (ed). Strategies for

MUELLER, H. G., HAWKINS, D. & NORTHERN, J. Probe Microphone Measurements: Hearing aid selection and assessment. San Diego: Singular Publishing Group, Inc. (1992)

MUELLER, H. G. Terminology and procedures. In G. Mueller, D. Hawkins & J. Northern (Eds.) Probe microphone measurements: Hearing aid selection and assessment. San Diego, CA. Singular Press, Inc. (1992) pp. 41–66.

MUNSON, W. A. & KARLIN, J. E. Isoreference method of evaluating speech-transmission circuits. *J Acoust Soc Am.* (1962) 34: 762–774.

PAVLOVIC, C. Speech recognition and five articulation indexes. *Hearing Instruments,* (1991) 42, 20–24.

POSNER, J., & VENTRY, I. Relationships between comfortable loudness levels for speech and speech discrimination in sensorineural loss. *J. Speech Hear. Disord.* (1977) 42, 370–375.

PREVES, D. Principles of signal processing, In: R. E. Sandlin (ed). *Handbook of Hearing Aid Amplification, Vol. I.* (1990) (pp. 81–120) San Diego: College-Hill Press.

PUNCH, J. L. & PARKER, C. A. Pairwise listener preferences in hearing aid evaluation. *J. Speech Hear Res;* (1981) 24: 366–374.

PURDY, S. C. Reliability, sensitivity, and validity of magnitude estimation, paired comparisons, and category scaling. Unpublished doctoral dissertation, The University of Iowa, Iowa City. (1990)

ROSS, M. & DUFFY, J. Report on sound field audiometry. Paper presented at the American Speech and Hearing Convention, Chicago, IL. (1961)

SANDLIN, R. E. Clinical application of sound-field audiometry. In: R. E. Sandlin (ed). *Handbook of Hearing Aid Amplification, Vol. II.* (1990) pp. 257–278. San Diego: College-Hill Press.

SCHWARTZ, D., LYREGAARD, P. & LUNDH, P. Hearing aid selection for severe-to-profound hearing loss. *Hearing Journal,* (1988) 41, 13–17.

SHORE, I., BILGER, R. & HIRSH, I. Hearing aid evaluation: Reliability of repeated measurements. *J. Speech Hear. Disord.,* (1960) 25, 142–170.

SPEAKS, C., & JERGER, J. Method for measurement of speech identification. *J of Speech and Hear Res.* (1965) 8, 185–194.

STUDEBAKER, G. A. Measures of intelligibility and quality. In G. Studebaker, F. Bess, & L. Beck (Eds.), The Vanderbilt hearing-aid report II (1991), pp. 185–195. Parkton, MD: York Press.

STUDEBAKER, G. A., & SHERBECOE, R. L. Magnitude estimations of the intelligibility and quality of speech in noise. *Ear Hear.* (1988) 9:259–267.

THORTON, A. & RAFIN, M. Speech discrimination scores modeled as a binomial variable. *J. Speech Hear. Res.,* (1978) 21, 507–518.

VICTOREEN, J. Hearing Enhancement. Springfield, IL: Charles C. Thomas. (1973)

WALDEN, B. E., SCHWARTZ, D. M. & WILLIAMS, D. L. et al.: Test of the assumptions underlying comparative hearing aid evaluations *J. Speech Hear Dis* (1983) 48:264–273.

WALKER, G. DILLON H, & BYRNE. The use of loudness discomfort levels for selecting the maximum output of hearing aids. *Austr J. Audiol.* (1984) 6:23–32

WALKER, G. Technical Considerations for Sound Field Audiometry. In: R. E. Sandlin (ed). Handbook of Hearing Aid Amplification: Volume I. (1990) pp 147–164. San Diego: College-Hill Press

WOODWARD, C. M. & TECCA, J. E. The use of pure tone stimuli in a soundfield. *Hearing Journal,* (1985) 38: 21–27.

ZELNICK, E. Selecting frequency response. *Hearing Journal,* (1982) 35(3), 31

VIII

PROBE MICROPHONE MEASUREMENTS

GEARY A. MCCANDLESS, Ph.D.

INTRODUCTION

The purpose of any hearing aid fitting procedure is to restore, as best possible, the ability to hear sounds, especially those of speech. If applied correctly, it is assumed a hearing aid will permit normal speech and other environmental sounds to be heard as clearly as the hearing loss will permit at comfortable listening levels. In order to accomplish these goals, it is essential that hearing aids be provided with frequency response, gain, output, and other electroacoustic properties appropriate for each individual user. In order to reasonably guarantee that proper electroacoustic properties are provided, real-ear measures (REM's) are performed and are defined as those tests which reflect the electroacoustic or psychoacoustic characteristics being delivered to the unaided ear or while a specific aid is in place and turned on[1].

As will be discussed in this chapter, real-ear measures are typically used as part of the process of verification or validation of fit. It should be stressed that real-ear measures, which meet a previously calculated target or formula, do not necessarily guarantee user satisfaction. Real-ear data are useful but are not the only determinant of a successful hearing aid fitting. When electroacoustic measures of a hearing aid are to be used as part of a selection and fitting process, it is important they be obtained on the patient and not only in 2-cm^3 or other couplers, since hearing aid performance cannot be accurately predicted for an individual user based only on coupler data. When performing real-ear measurements it may be necessary to make adjustments to the hearing aid and earmold to make sure that electroacoustic goals have been met and that the aid is comfortable.

An important distinction must be made here between the various types of real-ear measures. Broadly speaking, functional gain (FG) is a real-ear measure derived by subtracting the aided from the unaided sound field threshold[2,3]. With functional gain, the hearing aid, the ear, nerve transmission pathways and perception of the individual are all factors contributing to this measure. As used in the context of this chapter, however, real-ear measures will refer to as insertion responses or probe microphone measures. It is defined as sound pressure measures taken within an individual's ear canal using a small probe tube with or without a hearing aid. By comparing insertion measures both with and without a hearing aid, it is possible to quantify the amount of gain and other characteristics produced by a specific hearing aid while actually being worn by the user. The amount of gain is particularly important in the verification of fit because it reflects the expected functional shift toward normal threshold or degree of elevation of speech and environmental sounds into the users audible area[1,4,5].

CHAPTER OBJECTIVES

It is the intent of this chapter to present a strong rationale for both new and experienced dispensers in utilizing real-ear measures as an integral part of the hearing aid fitting and verification process. It is expected that such use will result in objective measures with which to gauge user function and satisfaction.

Of considerable importance is the notion presented in the chapter that real-ear measures yield specific measures which can be used either to verify target gain, frequency response and output characteristics or when targets are not met these data show where specific modifications are required in the instrument.

A final objective is to present the required details of the actual real-ear testing process. These steps, along with those provided by the various manufacturers, should guide the dispenser through the real-ear verification process.

WHY REAL-EAR MEASURES

In current practice, desired electroacoustic characteristics of hearing aids are usually selected on the basis of some predetermined target gain or prescripted formula based on pure tone thresholds, most comfortable loudness levels or other psychoacoustic tests. These fitting formulae assume that if calculations of desired gain or other characteristics are met, the fitting will more likely result in user satisfaction by providing acceptable sound quality, clarity and will be more comfortable to the patient than if not used[6]. The use of speech recognition tests or subjective responses from patients for validation of fit, do not provide detailed frequency-specific data provided by real-ear measures. Further, speech tests cannot be used to insure that target gain goals have been met at specific frequencies. Real-ear measures, on the other hand, provide detailed profiles of gain, linear or compression characteristics, saturation levels and other measures which reflect target characteristics. With such objective sound pressure information available at the time of fitting, it is possible to insure that target criteria have been met[7]. These data can also be used at the time of fitting to all small adjustments of the aid to be made which meet clarity or comfort requirements of the user.

It should be remembered that the intent of real-ear measures is to assess gain, output or other electroacoustic characteristics using a specific hearing aid with given settings on a single patient. These measures reflect the sum of the interactions of the hearing aid, ear mold and acoustic characteristics of the users ear. Knowing how a specific fitting works together with the acoustics of an individual ear canal is essential in the fitting process since electroacoustic characteristics on group data or coupler measurements do not adequately predict what might be produced in an individuals' ear[1]. Another use of real or insertion responses is to document baseline data at the time of fitting a hearing aid. Over time, should hearing threshold or function of the hearing aid change, real-ear insertion records can be invaluable in determining the need for new instruments, or to appropriately change gain, output or other parameters.

There is a basic assumption that verification of fit using real-ear measures correlates with higher user satisfaction, however real-ear measures alone do not guarantee user success[8]. Prescribing gain, output or compression characteristics is of relatively little value, if subsequent tests are not administered at the time of fitting which insure specific targets and goals have been met. Merely asking the user how the hearing aids sound is insufficient in itself as the sole validating criteria for good fit. Figure 1 illustrates this point. Curve

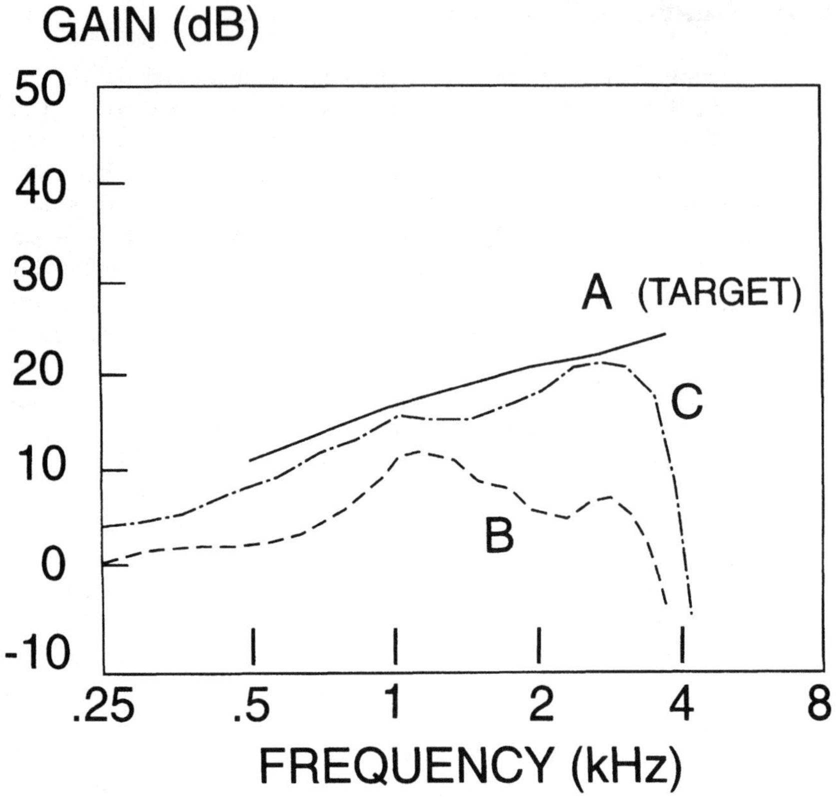

Fig. 1. Target response (A) and a real-ear hearing aid response not meeting target criteria, (B) judged to sound "very good" by the patient. Different hearing aid (C) meets target criteria and sounds subjectively "much better" than original hearing aid.

A shows the POGO target or desired insertion gain for an individual with a mild-to-moderate sensorineural hearing loss. Curve B is the real-ear insertion response (REIR) for the hearing aid as received from the manufacturer but does not conform to the target or desired gain in this case. In spite of this disparity, this first time user reported the aid sounded "great" and that it "seemed to help." By contrast, Curve C shows the real-ear responses from a second aid which more closely approximates the target curve. Not only does the real-ear gain curve conform more closely to the calculated target or ideal gain but the patient reported the second aid as sounding clearer and of much better general quality than the original hearing aid previously judged to be quite acceptable.

To summarize, specifying target or desired characteristics to the manufacturer is of little value unless real-ear measures are used at the time of fitting to insure target criteria have been met on an individual ear. Likewise, performing real-ear measures are of little value if the fitter has previously established no target criteria to be met.

Based on the above assumptions, implementation of either threshold-based or other prescriptive procedures require at least three steps including matrixes provided by the manufacturer:

1. A calculation of prescribed frequency gain characteristics based on audiometric, psychoacoustic or other data.
2. A conversion of desired or target gain into standardized hearing aid measurements which can be used to order or adjust a hearing instrument with specific characteristics.
3. Verification of fit using measures of functional or insertion gain, output or other electroacoustic characteristics[9].

It should be noted that while some of the newer hearing aids can be programmed to fit a wide-range of hearing loss, final selection of the electroacoustic characteristics is best done using an iterative process where gain, compression, output or other parameters are derived from the MCL or other measures directly from the hearing aid candidate. Whether using adaptive fitting techniques or threshold based prescriptive procedures, real-ear measures are still essential in the final verification process. Stated differently, real-ear measurements are useful whether the aid is a linear, peak-clipping type or a nonlinear hearing aid or whether it is programmable[10].

DEFINITIONS

As real-ear probe measurements evolved, procedures have been established and modified considerably in recent years. While there is yet no mandated standards by the American National Standards Institute (ANSI) for terminology or measurement techniques, many of the terms have gained popular use among dispensers and researchers and will be used here. Care must be taken to insure that all measurements be performed with identical stimuli and speaker location and with a patient's head in the same position.

As stated earlier, REMs are used primarily in the verification process of hearing aid fitting, but exactly what is being verified? First, REMs help describe the gain and potential benefit of a specific hearing aid. Second, REMs provide valuable information to the dispenser as to whether or not specific targets have been achieved. Third, REMs can be used to identify minor acoustic changes required to improve a subjects' perception of clarity or sound quality. Finally, REMs provide an excellent objective record of a hearing aids function and serves as a baseline for future fittings.

Although a number of specific REMs have evolved, most dispensers are interested primarily in the amount of gain or functional improvement between the aided and unaided condition. With this in mind, the difference in gain between a probe-measured response without a hearing aid then with a hearing aid yields the amount of improvement or gain provided by the instrument.

REAL-EAR UNAIDED RESPONSE (REUR)

The first of the real-ear procedures usually performed is the real-ear unaided response (REUR) and is defined as the sound pressure over a specified frequency range obtained when using a probe-tube microphone pick-up located at or near the tympanic membrane. The units used to express this response are either sound pressure level or gain relative to the stimulus level at the entrance of the ear canal. Individual REURs vary considerably as shown in Figure 2 showing real-ear unaided responses from three different adults. Note the resonant peak is characteristically seen just above 2000 Hz in most individuals[11].

The REUR serves as a reference or baseline for the calculation of insertion gain. The real-ear unaided response represents the gain in sound pressure from all the factors which might influence or modify sound including the pinna, head, torso and ear canal. The REUR must be measured with care and the insertion depth of the probe tube taken in the unaided condition must remain the same depth and position as when the hearing aid is in place.

REAL-EAR AIDED RESPONSE (REAR)

The Real-Ear Aided Response (REAR) is defined as the sound pressure level across frequencies measured in the ear canal at or near the tympanic membrane with the hearing aid in place and turned on, usually set to a comfortable setting level. The REAR is of vital importance because it represents the difference between the real-ear unaided response and the real-ear aided response and indicates the sum effects or gain produced by the hearing aid. Figure 3 illustrates the real-ear unaided response and aided response from a patient with a moderate sensorineural hearing loss.

REAL-EAR INSERTION RESPONSE (REIR)

The difference between the REUR and REAR is referred to as the real-ear insertion response (REIR) or real-ear insertion gain

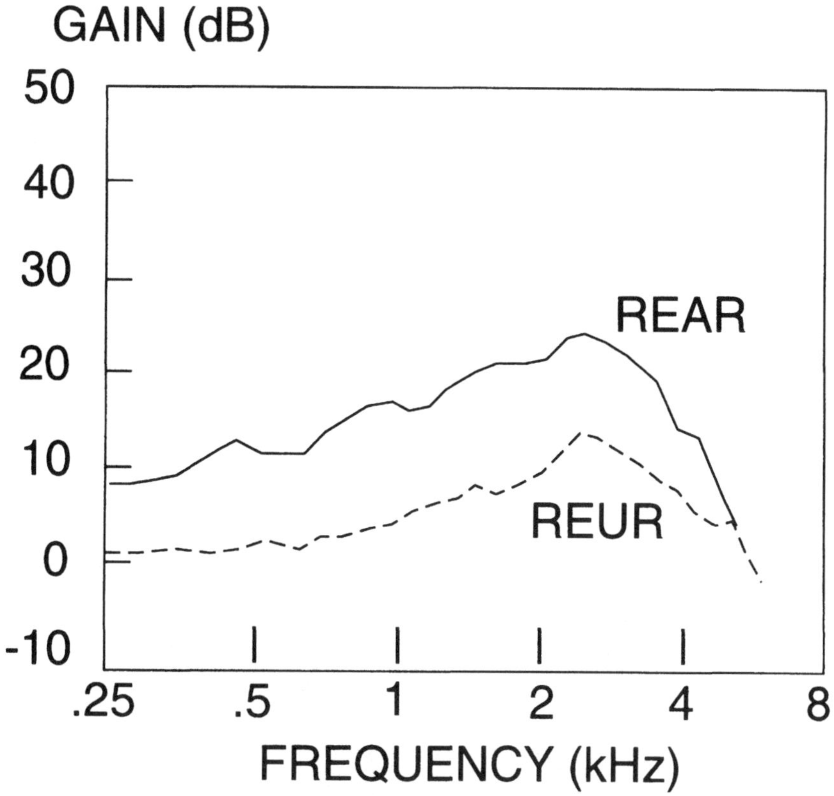

Fig. 2. Real-Ear Unaided Response from three different adults.

(REIG). This response curve reflects the amount of gain across frequency produced when a hearing aid is in place over the unaided condition. Figure 4 illustrates an example of the REIG across frequency derived from the difference between the REUR and REAR.

Whereas the REIR is the gain across a broad frequency range produced by the hearing aid, the term real-ear insertion gain (REIG) is defined as the amount of gain at specific frequencies or average of selected frequencies. For example, in Figure 4 note that the amount of insertion gain at 2000 Hz is about 15 dB.

Neither REIG or REIR across frequencies are direct measures of hearing. It must be remembered that they are physical measures of sound pressure. Functional gain can be generally inferred from insertion gain measures and if both are obtained with care, they result in nearly equivalent values[5,12,13]. Because functional and insertion gain values are typically very close, insertion gain measures are most often preferred for office use since they can be performed

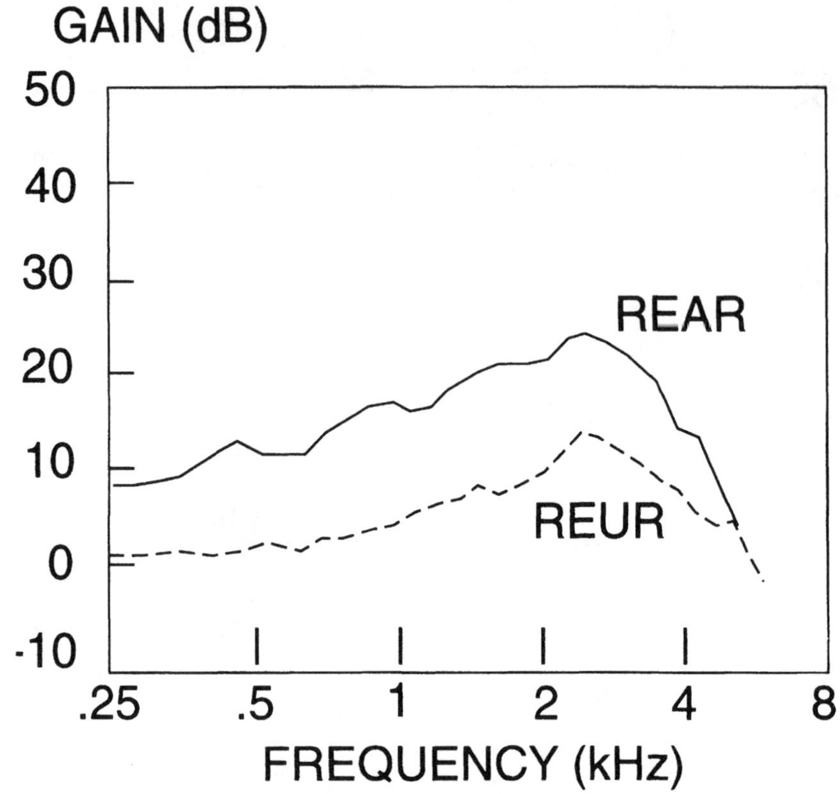

Fig. 3. REUR and REAR from a patient with a moderate 50 dB hearing loss.

in much less time than can aided and unaided sound field audiograms (functional gain). Also, REIR measures generally have less variability than do those of functional gain. Insertion gain measures have the added advantage of not requiring a sound room for administration and employ wide uses of stimuli such as pure tone, narrow bands of noise, speech weighted signals, etc.

OTHER REAL-EAR MEASURES

REAL-EAR OCCLUDED RESPONSE (REOR)

This response is a measure of the sound pressure across frequency obtained with a hearing aid in place but turned off. Stated differently, the REOR is an indication of the amount of attenuation caused by the insertion of an ear mold or hearing aid into the ear canal. This measure is not used routinely by all dispensers but can

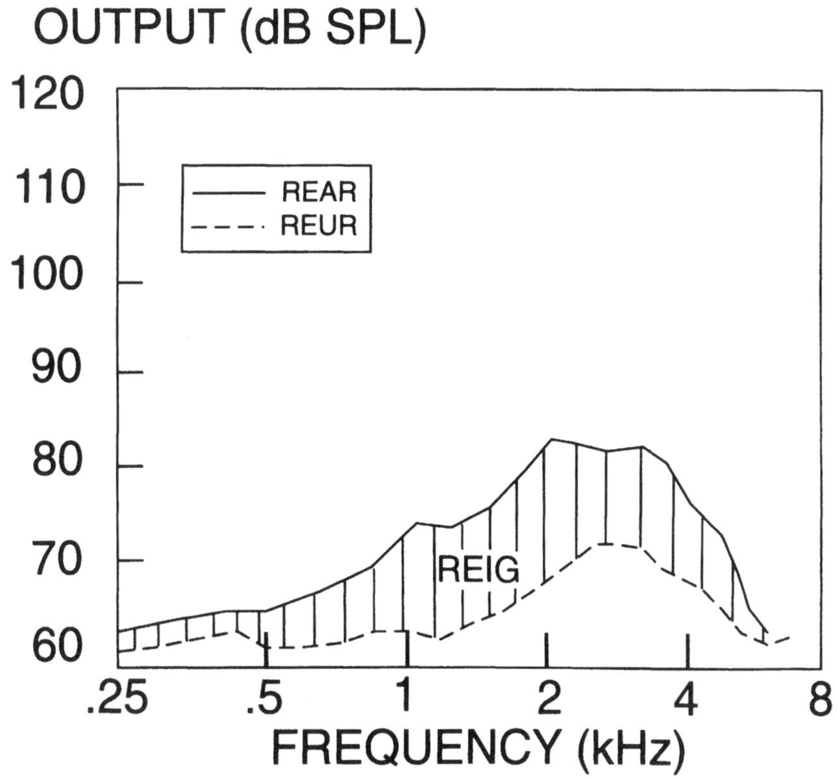

Fig. 4. REUR, REAR and REIG from a patient having a mild hearing loss.

be valuable in those cases where the insertion of the hearing aid produces an unusual occlusion affect or large insertion loss[15].

A a general rule, the deeper the hearing aid or earmold is inserted, the greater the occlusion effect. The REOR can be particularly useful when the interaction of the occlusion and canal affect the aided response in an unusual manner. Use of the REOR is not necessarily recommended for use on a routine basis but can be highly valuable in special cases where achieving smooth aided responses or adequate gain at specific frequencies are difficult to achieve.

REAL-EAR SATURATION RESPONSE (RESR)

The RESR is defined as an insertion gain measure obtained with the hearing aid in place and turned on and with the stimulus level sufficiently intense and hearing aid gain turned sufficiently high as to saturate the hearing aid. Since a fairly high intensity input signal is required to produce a saturation response, some dispensers are reluctant to perform this measure in the patient's ear. In most hearing aids, however, the maximum output of the aid should fall far below any damage risk criterion but may be subjectively very loud or annoying. If it is to be used, it is important to counsel the potential user that the stimulus will likely be loud but will not be harmful. An alternate procedure is to perform SSPL-90 measurements in a 2-cm^3 coupler. Except in rare instances, this will yield a useful approximation to real-ear measures with appropriate real-ear to coupler conversions[5,15,16,17].

INSTRUMENTATION

Probe microphone measurements near the tympanic membrance have been performed since the 1940's but only recently have commercial instruments become available which perform these tests quickly and automatically. Real-ear measures have been used for some time in Europe, but were not widely used in the United States until the mid-1980's[18]. At present, it is estimated that there are nearly twenty different computerized or self-contained real-ear systems sold in the Unties States. Some systems are computer based whereas others are dedicated systems. It should be remembered that these instruments are still evolving and will no doubt be improved considerably in the next few years. They all have some common functions in that they can measure real-ear unaided responses, real-ear occluded responses and real-ear aided responses. However, some have special calculations or display features not found in other instruments. Nearly all current devices are capable of displaying idealized target responses which can be used to visually compare target responses with those obtained from an individual as a base-line for verification of fit (Figure 5).

MEASUREMENT PROTOCOL

Probe tube measurements can be extremely valuable if performed with care and consistency. It should be recognized, however that such measurements cannot be performed on all patients. The primary reason real-ear measures cannot be used is when the earmold or hearing aid fits so tightly as to prevent placement or squeezing the soft probe tube between the mold or aid and the ear canal wall. Deeply inserted earmolds, or in the canal (CIC) hearing aids, also present a similar problem. In these cases the mold or aid extends so deeply into the ear canal that little room is left to accommodate

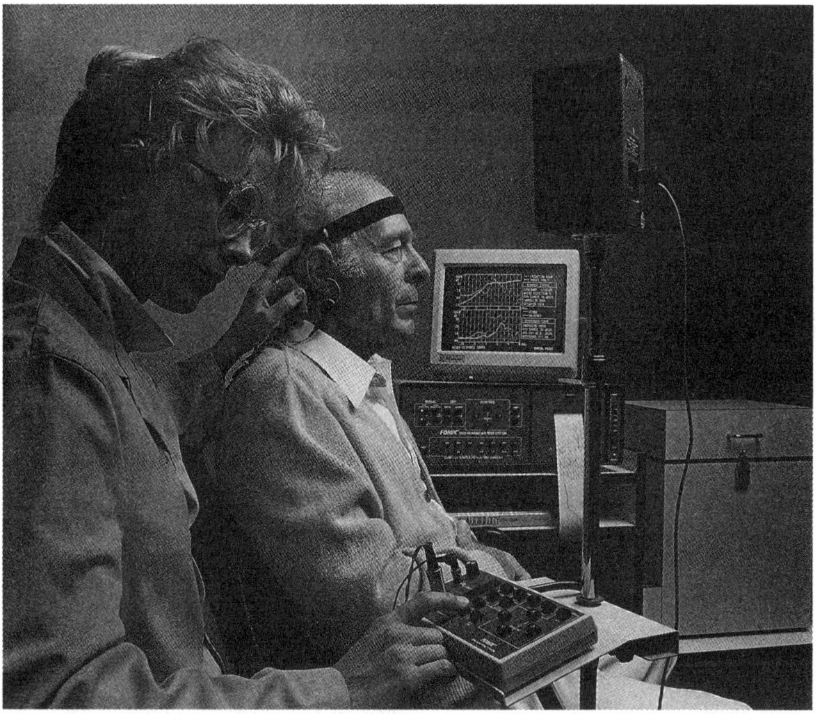

Fig. 5. Patient being tested for real-ear measures. (Courtesy Phonix Inc.)

the probe tube. Some manufacturers on request, will mold a small diameter hole into canal aids to allow probe tube measurements to be performed at the time of fitting where sufficient space permits. When testing is completed these holes are then sealed.

EQUALIZATION AND CALIBRATION

Signal calibration and equalization of any real-ear system is critical to the validity of probe-tube measures[19]. Calibration of the signal at a known distance from the loudspeaker insures that a standard intensity is produced at a specific distance from the loudspeaker. Calibration also insures that compensation is made for characteristic resonances of the probe tube. The purpose of equalization is to compensate for effects of distance, room acoustics and changes in the signal imposed primarily by the size and length of the probe tube. Equalization is defined as a procedure of controlling or shaping the stimulus signal at a specific location so as to insure the amplitude and spectrum remains at a stable level while testing. There are several methods of equalizing the test stimuli[14,20]. The modified pressure method is most commonly used wherein a reference microphone is placed near the hearing aid microphone (but not in the ear) and makes a series of automatic real-time corrections of the input signal to an appropriate shape and level. It is suggested that equalization be performed at least daily or whenever a response is suspect for any reason. Once equalized, subsequent measures should be valid unless the instruments are moved or the test environment changes.

Each manufacturer usually details the recommended calibration and equalization protocols for their respective probe tube systems. These procedures are usually performed with the probe microphone a specified distance from the loudspeaker off the head with no reflective surfaces nearby.

The most common factor affecting calibration or equalization is plugging of the probe-tube by cerumen and checks should be performed each time the probe tube is cleaned or changed. Calibration of stimulus intensity and equalization should be performed with the microphone located at the same azimuth and distance from the loudspeaker as will be used in actual testing. Most manufacturers recommend that the speaker be placed at 0 azimuth. The tests can be administered with the speaker at 45 degrees or other location but the resultant waveform will differ with varying locations[21,22].

TYPE AND LEVEL OF TEST SIGNAL

A variety of test signals can be used in securing real-ear measures, including pure tones, narrow bands, wide bands or bursts of speech-like noise. The signal used depends, in part, on those selected by the manufacturer and built into the real-ear instruments. Whereas ANSI standards specify types of stimuli and input levels to be used in coupler measurements, no such standards have yet been specified for real-ear measurements. The setting of an appropriate signal level is determined by the information desired by the dispenser. Uniform stimulus standards for all instruments will likely be integrated into all real-ear test instruments in the near future.

Selection of an appropriate signal depends to some degree on the purpose of a given test. For example, if you wish to determine how a hearing aid responds to discrete signals, then pure tone stimuli would likely be the signal of choice. If you wish to know how a hearing instrument handles multiple frequencies simultaneously the selection of a speech spectrum or other broad band noise would be more appropriate. Narrow bands or pure tones are currently the stimuli of choice when detailing the input-output characteristics of compression circuits.

For the present, two principles should be followed when selecting testing levels:

1. The level of the test signal should be at a level roughly comparable to sound levels encountered in normal hearing aid use. This level is typically at 50–70 dB SPL and is sufficiently high so that ambient background noise will not interfere with the test.
2. When measuring gain, the test level should be at a sufficiently low level so as not to drive the hearing aid under test into saturation nor cause undue discomfort to the patient. Where determination of saturation output is desired, or if compression function is measured, higher input levels may be needed. In this case, special care must be taken to insure that excessively loud sounds are not delivered to the patient.

INSERTION OF THE PROBE TUBE

Both the insertion technique and depth into the ear canal are critical factors in obtaining valid real-ear measures. To the beginning practitioner, inserting the probe tube into the ear canal causes considerable anxiety due to fear of physical injury or pain to the patient. If well designed tubing is provided by the meanufacturer and proper insertion is performed with reasonable care, there is little chance the tube itself will damage normal ears. There is much greater likelihood the tube insertion will cause only a tickling sensation or cough reflex and at worse, be slightly painful if the tympanic membrane is touched.

As a general principle, the closer the probe tip is placed to the tympanic membrane, the better the measurements[23]. Shallow insertion has greatest effect on the higher frequencies. A shallow insertion extending just beyond the tip of an earmold, for example, may cause a measurement error of 2–10 dB at frequencies above 1500 Hz. If insertion can be within 5 mm of the tympanic membrane, measurement error will typically be accurate within 2–3 dB up to 8000 Hz.

Some individuals insert the probe until the tympanic membrane in touched, then withdraw the tube about 5 mm. This technique is not recommended for general clinical use because of the discomfort and anxiety caused to the patient. A better and equally precise technique is to insert the tube to a standard depth for all adult subjects. Due to the rather small variance in canal length among adults (about 35 mm), the tube should be inserted 27 to 30 mm beyond the tragus. This can be easily accomplished by marking the tube at this length and slowly placing it into the ear canal to a point where the mark reaches the tragus base[24].

HEARING AID SETTINGS

Real-ear measures are performed primarily to determine the insertion response or gain at specific frequencies while the candidate is wearing a particular hearing aid at specific settings. It is important, therefore, that the hearing aid volume control be set at a level most likely to be used in real life situations. Setting the volume control at a comfortable level for real-ear testing should be done very carefully, either by the patient or dispenser. If the aid is set at too low a level it will underestimate the potential benefit of the aid and will not meet target criterion. If set too loud it will overestimate the target gain and in real life situations will subjectively be too loud.

TEST SEQUENCE

Although the testing sequence for real-ear measures is arbitrary and up to the discretion of the dispenser, performing certain procedures in a particular sequence improves the efficiency considerably.

1. *Equalize*
It is not mandatory that equalization be done prior to testing every patient but it is recommended when any change in stimulus type, test setting or replacement of the probe tube, that calibration and equalization be performed prior to real-ear measures on patients.

2. *Otoscopic Examination*
Careful otoscopy prior to testing is essential first to assure that no medical pathology is present and also to insure that excessive cerumen is not present which might alter the probe microphone measurements.

3. *Set Stimulus Parameters*
Real-ear insertion responses aided or unaided can be obtained using a variety of levels and stimulus types. It is important that the level selected by well above the background level of the room yet sufficiently low as not to produce saturation in the hearing aid. The level usually chosen is 60 dB SPL. The selection of pure tone versus broad band noise is also an important parameter since measuring by discrete pure tone stimuli may indicate different amounts of gain than when bursts of speech-like noise are used.

4. *Insertion of the Probe Tube*
As a general rule, the probe placement should be at a constant position across patients. It is also essential that the probe tip ex-

tend beyond the hearing aid or ear mold by at least 5 millimeters (mm). In order to reduce test variability in the higher frequencies, it is important that the probe tip be within 8–10 mm of the tympanic membrane. Some current instruments now have the capability of automatically measuring the distance of the probe tip from the tympanic membrane.

5. REUR

The REUR serves as the baseline which when subtracted from the aided response yields the real-ear insertion response and real-ear insertion gain. In most cases it is best to obtain this response before testing in the aided condition.

6. Placement of the hearing aid on the patient and adjust volume control.

7. REAR/REIG

Clinical instrumentation calculate and display the aided response automatically, however the fitter must determine and preset the volume control levels.

8. Optional Real-Ear Measures

REOR/RESR: The real-ear occluded response is rarely used by dispensers but can be valuable in cases where there may be unusual resonance characteristics caused by the pinna canal or canal size. The real-ear occluded response can also be valuable in trouble-shooting in those cases where it is difficult to achieve the target gain.

Real-Ear Coupler Difference: The real-ear coupler difference is defined as the difference in decibels as a function of frequency between outputs of a hearing aid measured in a real-ear versus a 2-cm^3 coupler[14]. This calculation is useful in reconciling some of the differences seen between a 2-cm^3 hard wall coupler and the real-ear measures of an individual patient whose acoustic characteristics differ considerably from that standard.

REAL-EAR MEASURES WITH NON-LINEAR AND PROGRAMMABLE HEARING AIDS

All real-ear measures are considered static in that they assess function at a single input level or series of discreet levels. Real ear measures will no doubt assume an increasingly important role in hearing aid fitting in the future as we become better able to assess the interactions of various sound processing strategies, differences in compression function and effects of multi-channel gain and compression ratios[10]. Also, special real-ear measures have potential value in assessing the gain and output characteristics of hearing aids using special speech processing or other circuitry. When complex or multiple signals are introduced to a hearing aid as found in real life situations, real ear measures may indicate how well a given instrument handles these multiple signals to enhance speech recognition without producing distortion and reducing the effects of unwanted ambient noise.

Still another promising application of real-ear measures is its inclusion as part of an iterative fitting process wherein the characteristics of programmable hearing aids are modified while worn by the patient. Specific electroacoustic characteristics can be modified in situ to achieve best comfort, speech recognition and sound quality. Real-ear measures are ideally suited to achieve these objectives.

SUMMARY

This chapter has attempted to define the various real ear measures and describe their use as part of the validation process in fitting hearing aids. Also included are some recommended protocols and testing sequences. This chapter also stresses the importance of establishing detailed, valid fitting objective having a strong rationale. Unless clear objectives are set, real-ear measures are of little value.

Real-ear measures play a valuable role in the validation segment of hearing aid fittings. The particular value of these measures is their objectivity, reliability and speed with which data can be acquired. There is growing evidence that if fitting objectives are chosen having a well supported rationale, hearing aid users will be better satisfied and speech will be more recognizable under a variety of environmental conditions. Environmental sounds will also be more comfortable and natural. Real-ear measures provide valuable objective data which reflect the gain, frequency response and output characteristics of a specific hearing aid on an individual ear. Using these measures, we no longer have to infer certain hearing aid characteristics from measures taken from coupler data.

GLOSSARY

Functional Gain difference in dB derived by subtracting the aided from the unaided sound field thresholds at specific frequencies across the audiometric frequency range.

Insertion Gain (IG) the difference in sound pressure levels at specific frequencies or an average of frequencies derived by subtracting the unaided from the aided levels. Insertion gain implies that measures are obtained using a probe-tube microphone placed at or near the tympanic membrane.

Real-Ear Aided Response (REAR) response curve expressed in SPL across frequency relative to a specific input level measured at or near the tympanic membrane with the hearing aid in place and turned on.

Real-Ear Insertion Response (REIR) difference in the response (curves) between the REUR and REAR.

Real-Ear Occluded Response (REOR) response curve expressed in SPL across frequency related to a specific input level measured at or near the tympanic membrane with the hearing aid in place and turned off.

Real-Ear Probe Tube Measures the measurement in sound pressure at or near the tympanic membrane using a small flexible probe-tube microphone. Measures may be with or without a hearing aid in place and turned on. The most frequently used measures are frequency response, gain, and maximum output.

Real-Ear Saturation Response (RESR) response expressed in SPL across frequency relative to a specific input level sufficient to produce saturation in the hearing aid (usually 90 dB SPL), measured at or near the tympanic membrane with the aid in place and turned to full volume.

Real-Ear Unaided Response (REUR) response curve expressed in SPL across frequency relative to a specific input level measured at or near the tympanic membrane in a unoccluded ear.

REFERENCES

1. Tecca, J. E. (1994). Use of real-ear measurements to verify hearing aid fit tings in Valente, M (ed) *Strategies for Selecting and Verifying Hearing Aid Fittings,* 88–107.

2. Hawkins, D. B., & Schum, D. J. (1984). Relationships among various measures of hearing aid gain. *Journal of Speech and Hearing Disorders,* 49, 94–97.

3. Dillon, H., & Murray, N. (1987). Accuracy of twelve methods for estimat ing the real ear gain of hearing aids. *Ear and Hearing,* 8(5, Suppl.), 60–67.

4. Hawkins, D. B. (1987). Clinical ear canal probe tube measurements. *Ear Hear,* 8:74–81.

5. Zemplenyi, J., Kirks, D., & Gilman, S. (1985). Probe-determined hearing-aid gain compared to functional and coupler gains. *Journal of Speech and Hearing Research,* 28:394–404.

6. Hawkins, D. B. (1992). Prescriptive approaches to selection of gain and frequency response, in Mueller G, et al (eds). *Probe Microphone Measurements,* 91–112.

7. Tecca, J. E. (1990). Clinical applications of real-ear probe tube measurement, in Sandlin RE (ed): *Handbook of Hearing Aid Amplification, Volume II, Clinical Considerations and Fitting Practices,* 225–255.

8. Mueller, G. H. (1992). Insertion gain measurements, in Mueller, G. H., Hawkins, D. B. & Northern, J. E.: *Probe Microphone Measurements,* 113–143.

9. McCandless, G. A., & Lyregaard, P. E. (1983). Presription of gain/output (POGO) for hearing aids. *Hearing Instruments,* 34(1), 16–21.

10. Mueller, G. H & Hawkins, D. B. (1992). Assessment of hearing arrangements, special circuitry, and features in Mueller, G. H., Hawkins, D. B. & Northern, J. L.: *Probe Microphone Measurements,* 201–225.

11. Shaw, E. (1974). Transformation of sound pressure from the free field to the eardrum in the horizontal plane. *Journal of the Acoustical Society of America,* 45, 1848–1861.

12. Mason, D., Popelka, G. R. (1986). Comparison of hearing-aid gain using functional, coupler, and probe-tube measurements. *Journal of Speech and Hearing Research,* 29:218–226.

13. Stelmachowicz, P. G. & Lewis, D. E. (1988). Some theoretical considerations concerning the relationship between functional gain and insertion gain. *Journal of Speech and Hearing Research,* 31:491–496.

14. Mueller, G. H. (1992). Terminology and procedures in Mueller, G. H., Hawkins, D. B. & Northern, J. L.: *Probe Microphone Measurements,* 41–66.

15. Hawkins, D. B. & Haskell, G. B (1982). A comparison of functional gain and 2 cc coupler gain. *Journal of Speech and Hearing Disorders,* 47:71–76.

16. Schum, D. J. (1986). Inter-subject variability effects on coupler to real ear correction curves. *Hearing Instruments,* 37(3):25–26.

17. Burnett, E. D., & Beck, L. B. (1987). A correction for converting 2 cm^3 coupler responses to insertion responses for custom in-the-ear nondirectional hearing aids. *Ear Hear,* 8:89–94.

18. Northern, J. L. (1992). Introduction to computerized probe-microphone real-ear measurements in hearing aid evaluation procedures in Mueller, G. H., Hawkins, D. B., & Northern, J. L.: *Probe Microphone Measurements,* 1–19.

19. Preves, D. A., & Sullivan, R. F. (1987). Methods of sound field equalization for real ear measurements with probe microphones. *Hearing Instruments,* 38(1):16–20.

20. Moskal, N. L. & Goldstein, D. P. (1992). Probe tube systems: Effects of equalization on real ear insertion and aided gain. *Ear Hear,* 13:46–54.

21. Killian, M. C. & Revit, L. J. (1987). Insertion gain repeatability versus loudspeaker location: You want me to put my loudspeaker W-H-E-R-E? *Ear Hear,* 8:68–73.

22. Ickes, M. A., Hawkins, D. B., & Cooper, W. A. (1991). Effect of reference microphone location and loudspeaker azimuth on probe tube microphone measurements. *Journal of the American Academy of Audiology,* 2:156–163.

23. Hawkins, D. B. & Mueller, G. H. (1992). Procedural considerations in Probe Microphone measurements in Mueller, G. H., Hawkins, D. B. & Northern, J. L.: *Probe Microphone Measurements,* p. 67–89.

24. Hawkins, D. B., Alvarez, E., & Houlihan, J. (1991). Reliability of three types of probe-tube microphone measurements. *Hearing Instruments,* 42:14–16.

IX

PROGRAMMABLE HEARING AID SYSTEMS

MICHAEL VALENTE, Ph.D., MAUREEN VALENTE, M.A., AND LISA G. POTTS, M.S.

INTRODUCTION

Programmable hearing aids have been available for approximately six years and at least seventeen manufacturers currently offer programmable hearing aids (Mueller, 1994). However, in 1993, programmable hearing aids accounted for only 3.19% of the total number of hearing aids dispensed in the United States and programmable hearing aids are not expected to exceed 7.5% of the market by 1995 (Hall and Roth, 1994).

Several reasons may account for dispensers' apparent reluctance to recommend programmable hearing aids for their patients. These reasons were outlined by Valente, Skinner, Valente, Potts, Jenison and Coticchia (1994), but a brief review may be helpful. First, there is the increased invoice cost of the hearing aids and the additional equipment necessary to program programmable hearing aids. Second, there is an avoidance by some to accept, or even try the new technologies or fitting strategies which are required to successfully fit programmable hearing aids. Third, and perhaps most important is an inescapable fact that most dispensers request that manufacturers select the electroacoustic characteristics of hearing aids they order for their patients. With programmable hearing aids, the decisions related to adjusting the various parameters are the exclusive responsibility of the dispenser. It may be that most dispensers are simply not adequately trained or prepared to make those decisions and avoidance is the safest alternative. Fourth is the feeling that there is a paucity of sufficient scientific evidence in peer-reviewed journals clearly supporting the advantages provided by programmable hearing aids. Finally, many third party payers do not reimburse as well for programmable hearing aids as they do for nonprogrammable hearing aids.

CHAPTER OBJECTIVES

This chapter will provide an overview of the potential advantages of programmable hearing aids for both the dispenser and patient. Hopefully, this information will be a catalyst for dispensers to pursue the advantages of programmable technology for themselves and for their patients.

WHY PROGRAMMABLE?

Most, if not all, programmable hearing aids are more expensive to the dispenser and patient than nonprogrammable hearing aids. The increased cost to the patient is the result of the additive effects of a) the increased invoice cost of programmable hearing aids to the dispenser; b) the cost of the programmer or personal computer (PC) required to program the hearing aids; c) the initial increased time required to dispense some programmable hearing aids; and d) the time-off necessary for dispensers to attend seminars to learn and integrate the numerous software and product updates from the manufacturer. Finally, some programmable hearing aids have warranties which are one to two years longer than the typical one year warranty delivered with most nonprogrammable hearing aids. All of these factors typically enter into determining an appropriate charge for the hearing aids and professional services associated with dispensing programmable hearing aids. The following question must be raised, "what are the advantages of programmable hearing aids to justify the increased cost to the dispenser and the patient?" Hopefully, the information contained within the following pages will provide some answers.

ADVANTAGES OF PROGRAMMABLE HEARING AIDS

The first section of this chapter will present the numerous advantages offered by programmable technology. First, there is the benefit of having the ability to ***immediately*** change the electroacoustic characteristics of the hearing aids in a ***wider*** variety of ways to compensate for changes in hearing loss. The advantage is that the patient does not have to purchase new hearing aids or wait for the hearing aids to be returned from the manufacturer because a new matrix needed to be ordered to correct for the change in hearing loss. Second, there are ***numerous adjustable parameters*** available with programmable hearing aids which are simply not available with nonprogrammable hearing aids. These include the ability to divide the frequency response into two or more frequency bands via a programmable ***crossover frequency (Cf)*** so that changes can be programmed into one frequency band independent of the adjacent frequency band. Other adjustable parameters available with programmable hearing aids which are not available with nonprogrammable hearing aids include the ability to program: ***compression ratio, compression kneepoint and compression release time; feedback notch filter, compensation at 3000 Hz; resonant peak control and the appropriate balance in gain between the low frequency and high frequency bands.*** In addition to the numerous parameters available, the advantage of programmable hearing aids extends to the greater range and precision in which the changes can be made using programmable technology.

Other advantages of programmable hearing aids include the ease in which changes can be incorporated into the hearing aids via a remote control, dedicated programmer or personal computer (PC); the presence of ***multiple memories*** within the same hearing aids and the use of ***paired comparisons*** to help the patient determine which combination of adjustable parameters provides the greatest user satisfaction. Finally, there is the issue of superior ***signal processing*** available in some programmable hearing aids which can lead to increased user satisfaction in a wider variety of listening environments.

A. COMPENSATION FOR CHANGES IN HEARING LEVEL

There are numerous hearing disorders which are known to result in changes in hearing thresholds (i.e., ***progressive or fluctuating hearing loss***). Examples include autosomal recessive hearing loss (high frequency, low and mid-frequency and early onset), autosomal dominant hearing loss, X-linked hearing loss, Usher's Syndrome, Alport's Syndrome, Pendred's Syndrome, Paget's Disease, Meniere's Disease, otosclerosis, strial dysplasia, meningitis, labryrinthitis, rubella, cytomegalovirus (CMV), syphilis, leukemia, ototoxicity, presbycusis, hypothyroidism and perilymphatic or round window fistula (Potts and Valente, 1995).

With nonprogrammable hearing aids, it is often necessary for the user to purchase new hearing aids if the hearing loss changes significantly from the time the hearing aids were originally purchased. With programmable hearing aids it is easy for the dispenser to re-connect the hearing aids to the ***remote control, dedicated programmer or PC*** and re-configure the electroacoustic characteristics of the hearing aids to compensate for the change in hearing loss.

In addition, changes in hearing loss will ultimately result in changes in the ***dynamic range*** (i.e., the residual hearing between hearing threshold and threshold of uncomfortable loudness). Usually, changes in the dynamic range are more likely to be restricted to the high frequency region. Several programmable hearing aids allow the dispenser to change the electroacoustic characteristics ***exclusively in the high frequency band*** by programming the ***crossover frequency (Cf)***, which will be discussed in greater detail in a later section. For example, ReSound (Trede, 1992; Pluvinage, 1994) and 3M hearing aids (Stypulkowski, Raskind and Hodgson, 1992; Stypulkowski, 1994) allow the dispenser to increase or decrease the width of the high frequency band by programming a lower or higher Cf. Fitting strategies to account for the reduced dynamic range may include ***reducing the output*** (3M and Maico Gamma), ***programming a more aggressive compression ratio*** (ReSound) or ***programming a lower compression kneepoint*** (3M) ***exclusively in the high frequency band*** where the dynamic range is narrower in comparison to the dynamic range within the low frequency band.

B. ADJUSTABLE PARAMETERS AVAILABLE IN PROGRAMMABLE HEARING AIDS

Table 1 summarizes fourteen adjustable parameters for the seventeen programmable hearing aids the authors have had the opportunity to dispense in the last five years. As can be seen in Table 1, not all of the fourteen parameters are available in all of the seventeen programmable hearing aids. In some cases, only three adjustable parameters are available, while in other programmable

Table 1. Summary of 14 adjustable parameters across 17 programmable hearing aids

	Adjustable Parameters													
Hearing Aids	1	2	3	4	5	6	7	8	9	10	11	12	13	14
AUDIOTONE	Y	Y	Y	Y	N	N	N	N	N	N	N	N	N	N
RESOUND	Y	N	Y	Y	N	N	N	N	N	N	Y[3]	Y	N	N
PHOX	Y	Y	Y	Y	Y	Y	Y	Y	Y	Y	N	N	N	N
STAR42	Y	Y	Y	Y	Y	Y	Y	Y	Y	Y	N	N	N	N
EUROSTAR	Y	Y	Y	Y	Y	Y	Y	Y	Y	Y	N	N	N	N
GAMMA	Y	Y	Y	Y	Y	Y	Y	Y	Y	Y	N	N	N	N
TRITON	Y[1]	N	N	N	Y[1]	N	N	N	N	N	N	Y[1]	N	N
INFINITI	Y	N	Y	Y	Y	N	N	N	N	N	N	N	N	N
TRILOGY I	Y	N	Y	Y[2]	N	N	N	N	N	N	N	N	N	N
TRILOGY II	Y	Y	Y	Y[2]	N	N	N	N	N	N	N	N	N	Y
RESOLUTION I	Y	Y	Y	Y	Y	N	N	N	N	N	N	N	Y	N
RESOLUTION II	Y	Y	Y	Y	Y	N	N	N	N	N	N	N	Y	Y
SIGMA	Y	Y	Y	Y	Y	N	N	N	N	N	N	N	Y	N
3M	Y[3]	Y[3]	Y	Y	Y[3]	N	N	N	N	N	N	Y	Y[3]	N
QUATTRO/DUO	N	Y	Y	Y	N	Y	N	N	N	N	N	N	N	N
LOGO	Y	Y	Y	Y	N	N	N	Y	N	N	N	N	N	N
PICS	Y	Y	Y	Y	N	Y	N	Y	N	N	N	N	N	N

1 = Gain
2 = Output
3 = Low cut
4 = High cut
5 = AGC threshold
6 = LF slope
7 = HF slope
8 = AGC type
9 = 3k peak
10 = High Frequency Emphasis
11 = Compression Ratio
12 = Crossover Frequency
13 = Release Time
14 = Feedback Notch Filter
[1] = In two or three bands
[2] = Resonant Peak Control
[3] = In two bands
Y = Yes
N = No

hearing aids as many as ten adjustable parameters are available. The first four parameters (***overall gain, low frequency cut, high frequency cut and overall output***) are available with many nonprogrammable hearing aids and will not be discussed in great detail in this chapter. However, as will be illustrated in a later section, even with these parameters, programmable hearing aids may still be advantageous in terms of the ***range of adjustability*** as well as the ***precision*** with which the adjustment can be made. At this point the authors will discuss the numerous adjustable parameters available on programmable hearing aids which are not typically available with most nonprogrammable hearing aids.

1. Low and high frequency slope

In addition to a ***low and high frequency cut,*** another method of shaping the low and high frequency response is the ability to adjust the ***slope,*** or steepness of the low and high frequency response. For example, the Maico PHOX (Wallace, 1992) uses switch capacitor filters to allow the dispenser to reduce low and high frequency gain by an additional 6, 12, or 18 dB, relative to the gain at 1000 Hz, by pressing the low or high frequency slope parameter on the PX8 programmer (Figure 1). Other programmable hearing aids which allow for adjustment of the low or high frequency slope are the Widex Quattro and Duo, Starkey Star42 and Eurostar, Maico Gamma (programming F1, F2, F3 and F4 to program filter settings between 300-4000 Hz for the low frequency slope and between 6000 and 875 Hz for the high frequency slope) and Phonak PiCs.

2. Crossover frequency

As can be seen in Table 1, most programmable hearing aids do not allow for programming a crossover frequency (Cf) and are referred to as ***single-band hearing aids*** (Maico PHOX and Gamma, Starkey Trilogy I (Curran, 1992), Audiotone 2000 (Rutledge, 1992), Siemens Infiniti (Burton 1992; 1994). Unitron Sigma, Widex Quattro, Duo and Logo (Sandlin, 1992; Westermann, 1994) and Phonak PiCs). The absence of a programmable Cf does not allow the dispenser to change the electroacoustic characteristics in one frequency region (***band or channel***) relative to another segment of the frequency region. That is, any change made to the hearing aids via the programmer effects the electroacoustic performance of the entire frequency response of the hearing aids.

As mentioned earlier, several programmable hearing aids allow the dispenser to divide the frequency response, which is typically between 200 to 6000 Hz, into two or three bands by programming the Cf. For example, in order to accurately fit ReSound hearing

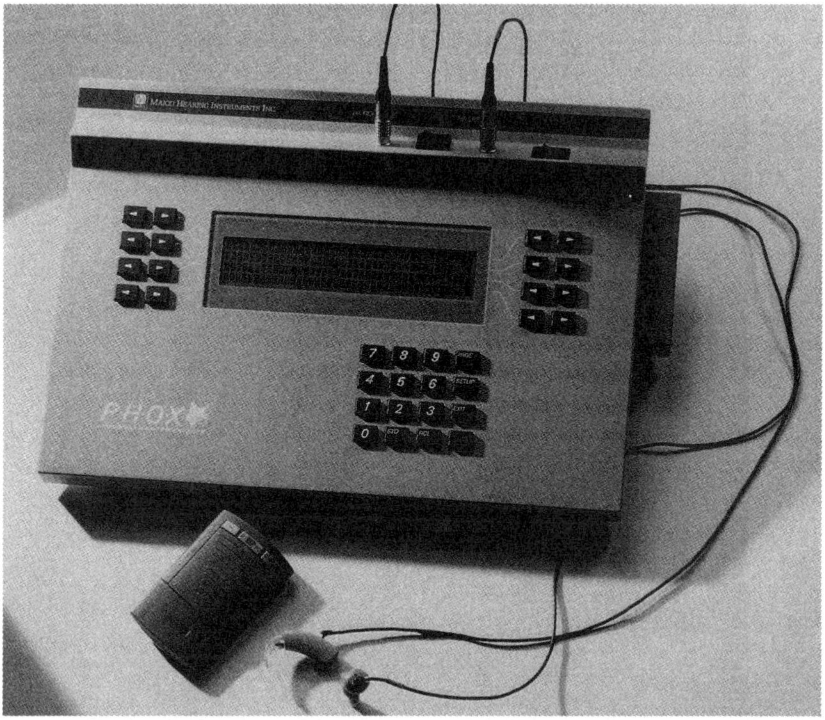

Fig. 1. Maico PX8 programmer with Gamma RD101 BTE and RD311 ITC hearing aids and remote control (Reproduced with permission from Maico Hearing Instruments Inc).

aids, the dispenser is encouraged to evaluate the patient's loudness growth by using the ***Loudness Growth in Octave Bands (LGOB)*** test generated when using the ReSound P^3 programmer, ER-3A insert earphones and personal selector (Figure 2). With this test, the listener presses a button on the personal selector which corresponds to his loudness perception of ½ octave bands of noise centered at 500, 1000, 2000 and 4000 Hz presented in groups of three ½ second bursts separated by ½ second intervals of silence (Allen, Hall and Jeng, 1990; Pluvinage and Benson, 1988; Pluvinage, 1994). The patient can press the button corresponding to ***"cannot hear" (0), "very soft" (#1), "soft" (#2), "comfortable" (#3), "loud" (#4), "very loud" (#5) and "too loud" (6).*** During a trial phase, the LGOB test initially measures the limits of the patient's dynamic range between very soft" and "very loud" so as not to present sounds which are inaudible or uncomfortable during the second phase of the LGOB test. This phase measures the loudness growth in 2 to 6 dB steps, depending upon the dynamic range of the ear in that particular frequency band. During the trial phase,

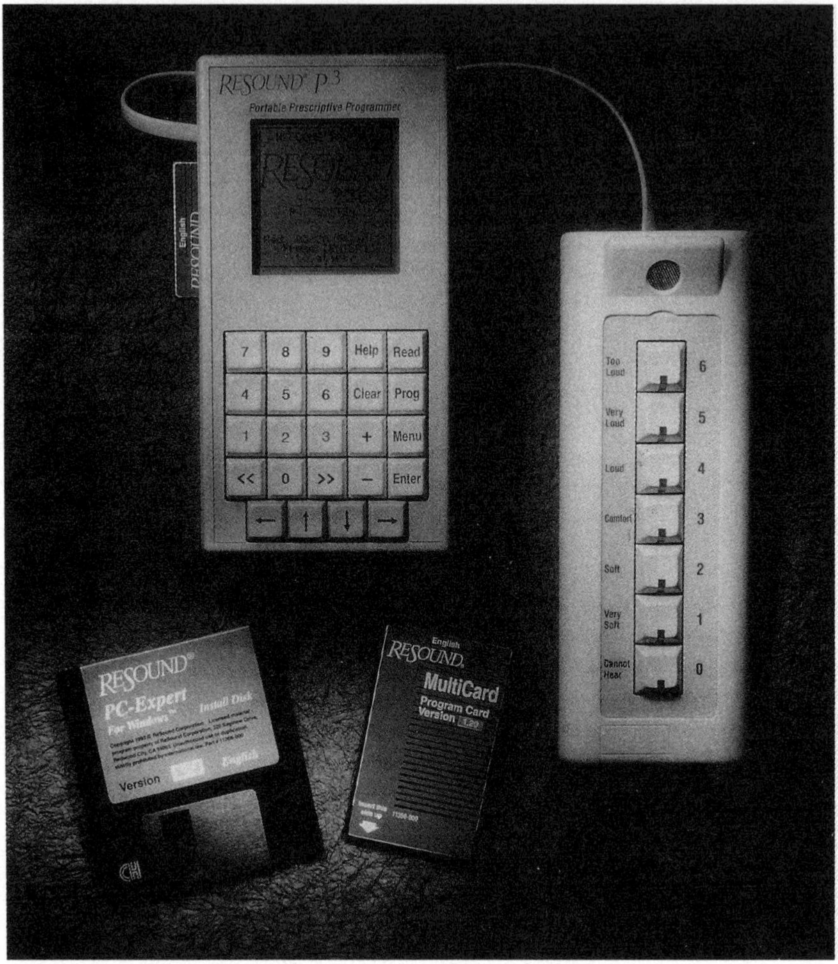

Fig. 2. ReSound P3 programmer, personal selector, PC-Expert software and programming card for the P3 (Reproduced with permission from ReSound Corporation).

frequency is held constant while intensity is presented in random order. However, during the second phase both frequency and intensity are presented in random order.

Figure 3 illustrates the results of the LGOB test for the four test frequencies. For each frequency, the printout reports the results for the LGOB test for normal listeners (***dashed line***) for the hearing impaired patient (***solid line***). The horizontal axis represents the input level (0-120 dB SPL measured in a HA-1 2cc coupler) and the vertical axis (1-5) represents loudness judgment from "very soft" to "very loud."

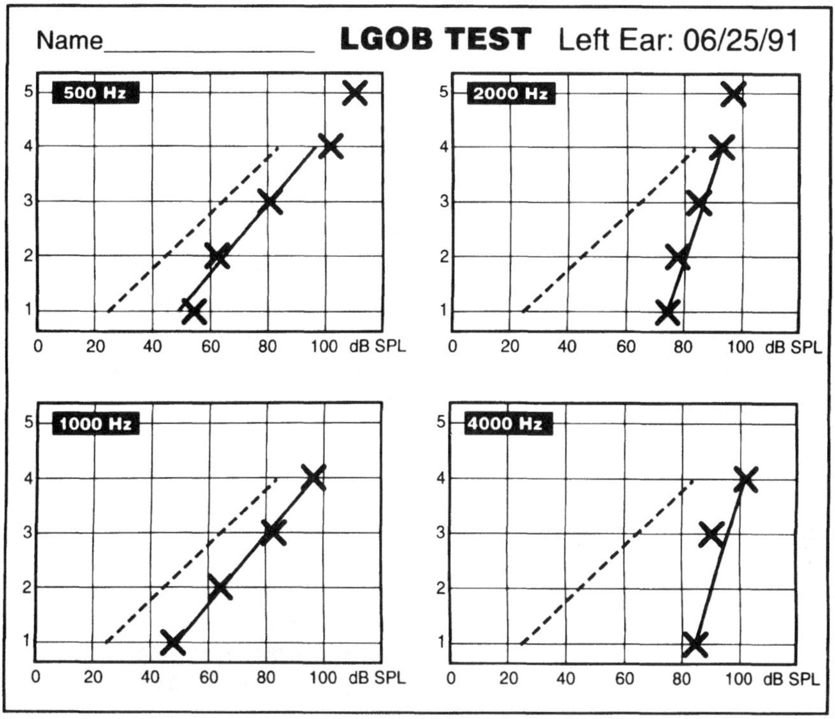

Fig. 3. Results of Loudness Growth in Octave Bands (LGOB) test for a patient (solid line) at 500, 1000, 2000 and 4000 Hz. The dashed line represents the results of the LGOB for listeners with normal hearing.

At 500 Hz, the solid line indicates that the patient has a 26 dB hearing loss because the solid line (at 50 dB) is shifted to the right along the horizontal axis by 26 dB of the dashed line (at 24 dB) for the loudness judgment of "very soft." In addition, the ***dynamic range for the normal ear*** is 60 dB wide (84 dB for "loud" - 24 dB for "very soft") and the ***slope*** of the line is a little less than 45°. However, the ***dynamic range for the patient*** has been reduced slightly to 46 dB (96 dB for "loud" - 50 dB for "very soft") and the ***slope*** has increased slightly to almost 50°. The presence of a ***narrower dynamic range*** (46 dB versus 60 dB) and a ***steeper slope*** indicates the need for a slight amount of compensation for the reduced dynamic range in the low band. In fact, this finding would require a compression ratio of approximately 1.3:1 at 500 Hz. For the interested reader, one method of determining the overall compression ratio is to divide the dynamic range of the normal ear by the dynamic range of the impaired ear. In this case it would be 60 dB/46 dB which would result in a compression ratio of 1.3:1. That is, for each 1.3 dB increase in input at the microphone of the hearing aid in the low band, there would be only a 1.0 dB increase in the output from the receiver. Another way to interpret the results of the LGOB is to realize that for the softer input levels (horizontal axis), greater gain is required because of the greater separation between the normal and patient LGOB curves. However, at higher input levels, slightly less gain is required because the separation between the normal and patient LGOB curve is diminished.

In contrast, observe the LGOB results at 4000 Hz in the lower right box. The solid line is shifted approximately 58 dB (84 dB-26 dB) re: the dashed line indicating a moderate-severe hearing loss at 4000 Hz. In addition, note that the patient required 84 dB to establish a loudness perception for "very soft" (#1) and 100 dB to establish a loudness perception for "loud" (#4). This results in a ***dynamic range*** of only 16 dB (100 dB - 84 dB) between "very soft" and "loud" and a ***slope*** of approximately 75°. On the other hand, the dynamic range between "very soft" and "loud" for the normal ear (dashed line) was 56 dB wide (82 dB for "loud" - 26 dB for "very soft"). This calculates into a compression ratio of approximately 3.5:1. That is, for each 3.5 dB increase in input at the microphone of the hearing aid in the ***high band,*** there would be only a 1.0 dB increase in the output from the receiver. Again, another way to interpret the LGOB results is to realize that for the softer input levels (horizontal axis), even greater gain is required at 4000 Hz (re: 500 Hz) because of the greater separation between the normal and patient LGOB curves. However, at higher input levels, significantly less gain is required because the separation between the normal and patient LGOB curve has nearly disappeared.

Thus, in looking at the LGOB curves in Figure 3 it becomes easier to understand that this patient requires a different method of compression in the low band (500-1000 Hz) because the LGOB results are nearly ***linear*** (or parallel to the normal LGOB results) which requires essentially equal gain for both soft (50 dB) and loud (80 dB) input levels. However, in the high band (2000-4000 Hz), ***nonlinear*** amplification is required due to the reduced dynamic range (i.e., steeper slope) requiring greater gain for soft input levels and significantly less gain for higher input levels. In this situation the dispenser might program a Cf of 1300 Hz to separate the frequency response into two bands to provide more linear amplification in the low band below 1300 Hz and nonlinear amplification in the high band above 1300 Hz. In addition, because of the greater hearing loss for softer input and less loss for louder input levels (re: normal), greater gain will be prescribed for soft input levels (50 dB) and less gain will be prescribed for high input levels (80 dB). This is especially true for the high frequency band.

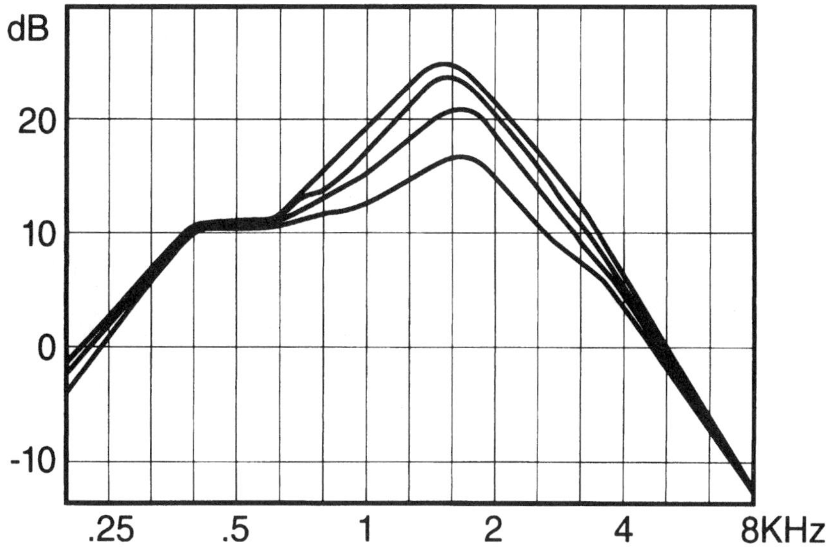

Fig. 4. Real Ear Insertion Response (REIR) at input levels of 50–80 dB in 10 dB increments for a ReSound ED3. The crossover frequency (Cf) was programmed at 1300 Hz and the compression ratio was programmed at 1:1 in the low band and 2:1 in the high band.

Figure 4 illustrates such a fitting. In this case, the Cf was programmed at 1300 Hz and the compression ratio was programmed to provide linear amplification in the low band (1:1) and nonlinear amplification in the high band (2:1). Figure 4 illustrates that for the low band, gain does not change as the input signal varies from 50-80 dB in 10 dB steps. However, in the high band, as the input intensity increases, the gain systematically decreases, showing greater gain for the softer input signal (50 dB) and progressively less gain as the input was increased in 10 dB steps from 60-80 dB.

The P^3 programmer allows the dispenser to program the Cf at 400, 600, 1300, 2000, 2800, 3700 or 4700 Hz. As the Cf is programmed higher, there is a widening of the low frequency band and a narrowing of the high frequency band. Also, as the difference between the gain requirements for soft sound (50 dB) and loud sounds (80 dB) becomes greater (up to 20 dB), the compression ratio becomes greater or more aggressive. With the P^3, the dispenser can program compression ratios between 1:1 (i.e., the gain for input levels of 50 and 80 dB is equivalent) to 3:1 (i.e., the gain for an 80 dB input level is 20 dB less than the gain requirements for a 50 dB input level) in the low and high band separated by the programmable Cf.

Other programmable hearing aids which allow the dispenser to program the Cf, dividing the frequency response of the hearing aids into two bands are the 3M MemoryMate and 3M SinglePro hearing aids and the Siemens 2004. On the other hand, the Siemens 3004 allows the dispenser to program two Cfs (***Cf1 and Cf2***) and divide the hearing aid into a ***low band*** (frequency region below Cf1), ***mid band*** (frequency region between Cf1 and Cf2) and ***high band*** (frequency region above Cf2). A recent report by Dirks, Ahlstrom and Noffsinger (1993) could not demonstrate any differences in preferred frequency response in nine subjects, utilizing two versus three frequency bands. That is, the authors could not demonstrate the advantage of programming two crossover frequencies to divide the bandwidth into three bands, in comparison to having one crossover frequency to divide the bandwidth into two bands.

3. Compression kneepoint

The intensity level at which a compression circuit is activated to reduce the gain is called the ***compression kneepoint or compression threshold.*** In a more technical sense, the threshold kneepoint is the point in the ***input/output curve (I/O curve)*** at which the slope digresses from ***unity gain (1:1),*** indicating the signal level at which nonlinear processing begins to take effect. For example, in hearing aids with linear amplification, for every 1.0 dB increase in input at the microphone there is a corresponding 1.0 dB increase in the gain and output at the receiver until the characteristics of the amplifier and receiver have reached their limits and the output is reduced via ***peak clipping.*** With hearing aids incorporating nonlinear amplification, there is a point at which the input level to the microphone (***input compression or AGC-I***) or output level from the amplifier (***output compression or AGC-O***) will activate the compressor to reduce the gain and output at the receiver. The major difference between AGC-I and AGC-O is that the compressor action is either before (AGC-I) or after (AGC-O) the volume control wheel. Therefore, for a hearing aid with AGC-I, the compression kneepoint will remain the same regardless of volume control setting, but the output will decrease when the volume control wheel is reduced and increase when the volume control setting is increased. On the other hand, for a hearing aid with AGC-O, the output will remain the same regardless of volume control rotation, but the compression kneepoint will increase when the volume control wheel is reduced and decrease when the volume control setting is increased.

For example, the upper I/O curve illustrated in Figure 5 for a composite signal reveals that amplification is linear between 50 dB to 75 dB (25 dB range of input) because there is a 26 dB

COMPOSITE I/O CURVE

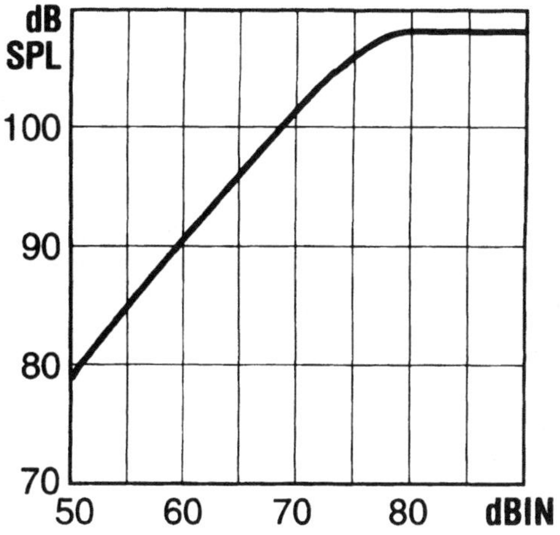

INPUT SPL	OUTPUT SPL
50 dB	79.7 dB
55 dB	85.1 dB
60 dB	90.6 dB
65 dB	96.1 dB
70 dB	101.5 dB
75 dB	105.8 dB
80 dB	107.9 dB
85 dB	108.0 dB
90 dB	108.0 dB

COMPOSITE I/O CURVE

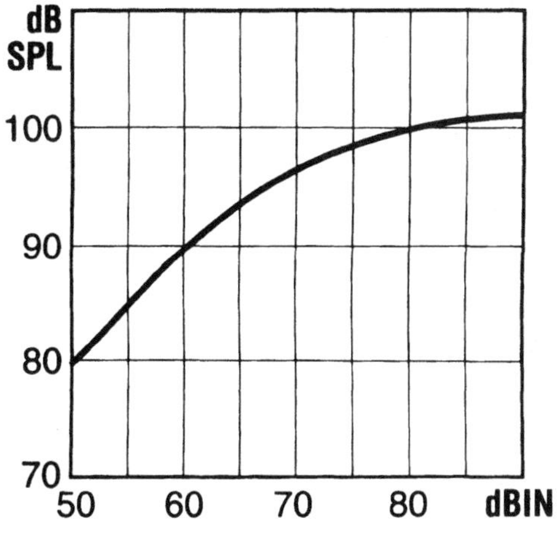

INPUT SPL	OUTPUT SPL
50 dB	79.9 dB
55 dB	84.9 dB
60 dB	89.4 dB
65 dB	93.4 dB
70 dB	96.4 dB
75 dB	98.1 dB
80 dB	99.4 dB
85 dB	100.4 dB
90 dB	101.3 dB

Fig. 5. Input/output (I/O) curves at input levels of 50–90 dB. The upper I/O curve is representative of a more linear response, while the lower I/O curve is representative of a more non-linear response.

(105.8 dB - 79.7 dB) increase in output. However, between 75 dB to 90 dB (15 dB range of input) there is only a 2.2 dB (108.0 dB - 105.8 dB) increase in output. Thus, the amplifier of the hearing aid has a compression kneepoint of 75 dB because this is the input level at which the input/output curve digresses from unity gain. The lower input/output curve illustrated in Figure 5 reveals that the amplification is linear between 50 dB to 60 dB (10 dB range of input) because there is a 9.5 dB (89.4 dB - 79.9 dB) increase in output. However, between 65 dB to 90 dB (25 dB range of input) there is only a 7.9 dB (101.3 dB - 93.4 dB) increase in output. Thus, the hearing aid has a compression kneepoint of 65 dB because this is the input level at which the input/output curve digresses from unity gain.

As can be seen in Table 1, several programmable hearing aids (Maico PHOX and Gamma, Starkey Star42, Starkey Eurostar, Starkey Resolution I and II and Unitron Sigma) allow for programming threshold kneepoint in a ***single-band.*** For example, the Unitron Sigma allows programming the compression kneepoint for the US-80s BTE (55-85 dB), Vista 4000 ITE (40-65 dB), IKON-S BTE (50-70 dB) and IKON-SD (52-72 dB). A compression kneepoint of 55-90 dB may be programmed in 2.7 dB steps for the Siemens Infiniti ITE, while a kneepoint of 60-90 dB can be programmed for the Infiniti BTE. Compression kneepoints of 55-70 dB may be programmed for the Starkey Resolution I and II ITEs and Resolution BTE in 5 dB steps, while a kneepoint of 53-81 dB may be programmed for the Starkey Eurostar and Star42 in 7 dB steps. The kneepoint for the Maico Gamma can be programmed between 30-78 dB and the kneepoint for the Maico PHOX can be programmed between 56-77 dB for the BTE series (P1 and P4) and between 56-70 dB for the ITE series (P20 and P30) in 7 dB steps.

Programmable hearing aids which allow the dispenser to program the Cf, dividing the hearing aid into two bands to program the compression kneepoint in two bands are the 3M MemoryMate and SinglePro hearing aids (50-92 dB) and the Siemens 2004 (55-90 dB in 5 dB steps). On the other hand, the Siemens 3004 allows the dispenser to program compression kneepoints in the ***low, mid and high bands*** between 55-90 dB in 5 dB steps. The new Siemens software for the PMC provides guidelines for the dispenser to select an appropriate" compression kneepoint in each of the three bands depending upon the listening environment for which the memory was intended to be used ("quiet", "party", "office"). However, as will be discussed later, the recommendations provided by the software is based theoretical data and has not been validated by well controlled research performed in the laboratory or field.

4. Compression ratio (CR)

Most programmable hearing aids provide automatic adjustment of the CR (1:1 to 10:1) as the input signal becomes higher (Mueller, 1994). Only ReSound allows programming the ***compression ratio (CR)*** (i.e., the ratio of the increment in input SPL to the increment in output SPL). When fitting the ReSound hearing aids, the dispenser can ***indirectly*** program the CR in eleven discrete steps from 1:1 to 3:1 in both the low ***and*** high bands by how the gain for the input levels of 50 dB and 80 dB are programmed. For example, if the gain for the input levels of 50 dB and 80 dB are programmed to provide equal gain, then the CR is 1:1. However, if the gain for the input level of 80 dB was programmed to provide 2 dB less gain than the gain for the input level of 50 dB, then the CR would be 1.2:1. Further, if the gain for the input level of 80 dB was programmed to provide 10 dB less gain than the gain for the input level of 50 dB, then the CR would be 1.5:1. Finally, if the gain for the input level of 80 dB was programmed to provide 20 dB less gain than the gain for the input level of 50 dB, then the CR would be 3:1.

Figure 5 will serve as an example for how the dispenser can calculate the compression ratio from the results of an ***input/output (I/O) test*** using a hearing aid analyzer. The upper I/O curve in Figure 5 reveals a CR of 1:1 from 50 dB to 75 dB, because the 25 dB increase in input results in a 26 dB increase in output. However, from 75 dB to 90 dB (15 dB range of input) there is only a 2.2 dB increase in output (108.0 dB - 105.8 dB). This would calculate into a CR of 6.8:1 (*CR = the range of the input divided by the range of the output;* or 15/2.2 = 6.8:1). This means that every 6.8 dB increase in input to the microphone will result in only a 1.0 dB increase in output. The lower input/output curve illustrated in Figure 5 reveals a CR of 1:1 from 50 dB to 60 dB because the 10 dB increase of input results in a 9.9 dB increase in output. However, between 65 dB to 90 dB (25 dB range of input) there is only a 7.9 dB increase in output. This calculates into a CR of 3.165:1 (25/7.9 = 3.165). This means that for every 3.2 dB increase to the microphone, only a 1.0 dB increase in output occurs.

5. Release time (RT)

Release time (RT) is the time (in milliseconds or msec.) it takes for the compressor to return to its original state of providing amplification. As one may see in Table 1, the Starkey Resolution I and II ITEs and the Resolution BTE (three choices between 9-330 msec depending upon the programmed kneepoint), Unitron Sigma (25-500 msec depending upon model) and 3M MemoryMate and

SinglePro (0, 20, 100 or 500 msec in the low band; 0, 7, 35 or 150 msec in the high band) allow for programming either the overall release time or the release time for the low and high band. The rationale for longer release times in the low band for 3M hearing aids is that vowels and low frequency noise tend to have longer durations, while the rationale for shorter release times in the high band for 3M hearing aids is that consonants and high frequency noise tend to have shorter durations. If the release time in the high band were longer, many of the weaker consonant sounds will not be amplified and speech intelligibility would be sacrificed (Stypulkowski, 1993; 1994; Stypulkowski, Raskind and Hodgson, 1992).

Several programmable hearing aids have, as a selection, ***adaptive release time*** where release time varies automatically. For example, the Widex Logo series has one choice of compression where the release time is fixed at 150 msec (***"AGC1"***). The dispenser can also choose "***AGC2"*** where the release time varies automatically from 150 msec to 2.0 seconds depending upon the duration of the input signal. For the Phonak PiCS, the dispenser has four output limiting options (called ***multi-mode limiting***). One of the options is ***SC+art (Super compression plus adaptive recovery time***) in which the release time varies up to one second depending upon the environmental situation (Bachler and Buerkli-Halevy, 1994).

6. Feedback notch filter

The presence of feedback is always detrimental to successful hearing aid fittings. There are numerous methods to reduce or eliminate feedback, but one of the most common is for the user to reduce the volume controls of the hearing aids. This will effectively eliminate the offensive "squeal", but may lead to insufficient amplification, particularly in the high frequency region. The Starkey Trilogy II allows the dispenser to electronically eliminate feedback by programming the hearing aids to reduce amplification at a "center frequency" within the frequency region (between 2500-5000 Hz in 500 Hz steps) causing the feedback. In addition, the dispenser can program the width of the frequency region (***narrow, medium and wide***) around the programmed center frequency. In the example shown in Figure 6 it was determined via real ear measures that feedback was a result of a sharp peak due to excessive gain at 2500 Hz. The dispenser programmed "2500 Hz" and "narrow width" in the feedback notch" menu and programmed the change to the hearing aid. After reprogramming, audible feedback immediately ceased and the REAR on the real ear monitor (Figure 6) revealed elimination of a small section of the frequency re-

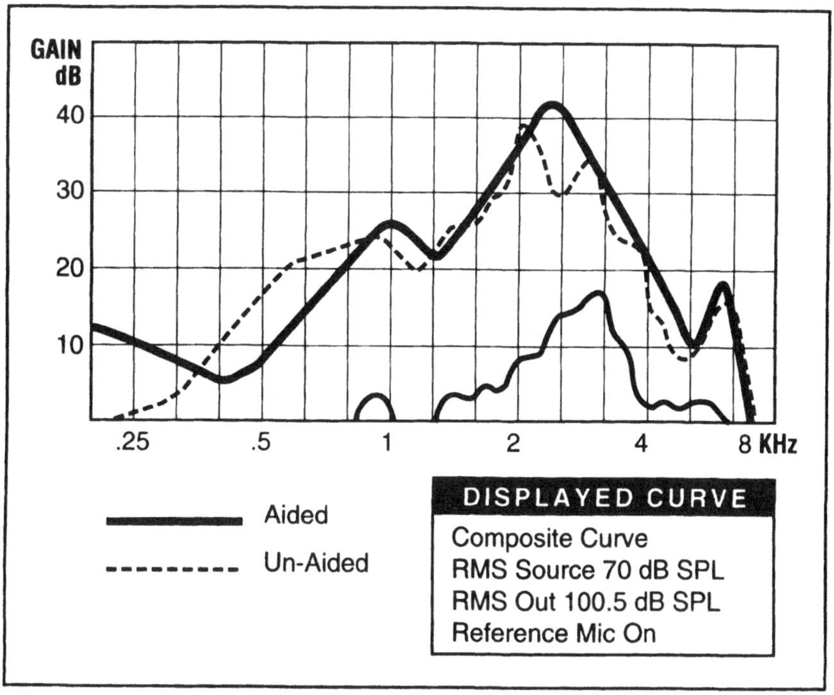

Fig. 6. Example of programming the feedback notch filter at 2500 Hz (narrow width) for a Starkey Trilogy II hearing aid.

sponse centered at 2500 Hz. However, the frequency response above and below 2500 Hz remained virtually unchanged. With this technology, the patient no longer has to reduce the volume control to eliminate the feedback and he can still maintain the required gain in the high frequency region.

7. Compensation at 3000 Hz

The Maico PHOX and Starkey Eurostar and Star42 can be programmed to add 6 dB at 3000 Hz and reduce the gain by 6 dB at 1500 Hz when the dispenser presses a button on the PX8 programmer (Figure 1) or interfaces with the Starkey ProConnect software. The purpose of this parameter is to compensate for the loss of the natural real ear gain which occurs when an earmold or hearing aid shell is inserted into the ear canal.

8. Resonant Peak Control (RPC)

The Starkey Trilogy I and the Siemens Infiniti allow the dispenser to change the high frequency response of the hearing aids. For the Siemens Infiniti, the rationale for the resonant peak control is to reduce high frequency gain to a) have better control over feedback; b) address subjective reports of intolerance to loud sounds (usually in the high frequency region where the dynamic range is typically narrower) or c) reduce the gain because the patient may have a rising configuration. The rationale behind the resonant peak control for Trilogy I is for the dispenser to have the ability to shift the peak gain of the frequency response to match the peak of the individual's ***real ear unaided response (REUR).*** This in turn would achieve a "***transparent amplifier***" which will reportedly improve sound quality (Libby, 1982). According to Libby (1982), achieving a "transparent amplifier" (i.e., the shape of the real ear aided response (REAR) "matches" the shape of the (REUR) will result in a smoother ***real ear insertion response (REIR)*** and "more natural" sound quality. The utility of this concept has never been substantiated and a small unpublished study at our clinic did not reveal improved user satisfaction when the resonant peak parameter was programmed to "match" the individual REUR, as opposed to when the peak was placed at the default setting of 2800 Hz.

9. *Balance between 500 and 2000 Hz*

The Maico PHOX and Starkey Eurostar and Star42 hearing aids have an ***high frequency emphasis (HFE)*** parameter which when programmed by the PX8 programmer or Starkey Pro-Connect software will reduce the gain at 200-500 Hz by approximately 6 dB relative to the gain at 2000 Hz. This parameter was developed based upon the reports by Skinner (1988) that the gain in the high frequency segment of the frequency response should not be greater than 35 dB of the gain in the low frequency segment of the frequency response. Skinner (1988) reported that if the appropriate balance between the gain in the low and high frequency segments were not achieved then the patient will complain that the amplification was "tinny" and sound quality will be reduced.

C. NUMBER OF ADJUSTABLE PARAMETERS

Potts and Valente (1995) surveyed eight manufacturers and found that the typical number of potentiometers on a BTE was two with a maximum of four. For an ITE hearing aid, the typical number of potentiometers was two and for an ITC the typical number of potentiometers was one, with a maximum of two. There are a few ITEs, such as the Argosy Three-Channel Clock which has as many as four potentiometers.

In contrast, the least sophisticated programmable hearing aid (see Table 1) has ***four*** adjustable parameters (overall gain, overall output, low frequency cut and high frequency cut) which is available for BTE, ITE ***and*** ITC hearing aids. Some programmable hearing aids have ten programmable parameters available for BTE, ITE, ITC and mini-ITC designs. Thus, all programmable hearing aids (BTE, ITE, ITC and mini-ITC) have at least four programmable parameters and some can have as many as ten to fifteen. This degree of flexibility is significantly greater than most nonprogrammable hearing aids.

D. RANGE OF ADJUSTMENT

Potts and Valente (1995) reported on the range of adjustments for overall gain, low frequency gain, mid frequency gain, high frequency gain, low frequency slope, high frequency slope and overall output for forty six programmable hearing aids from nine manufacturers. Across the forty six hearing aids, the range of adjustment for overall gain was from 15 dB for the Widex LOGO to 54 dB for the Phonak Sono Forte 331X. The range for adjusting low frequency gain was from 22 dB for the Oticon Multifocus to 51 dB for the Phonak Sono Forte 331X. When the mid frequency response was programmed, the range of adjustment was from 21 dB for the Oticon Multifocus to 53 dB for the Phonak Sono Forte 331X. High frequency gain could be adjusted from 14 dB for the Oticon Multifocus to 57 dB for the 3M BTE MemoryMate. The high frequency slope could be adjusted from 11 dB to 35 dB or from 12 dB/octave to 24 dB/octave. Overall output could be adjusted from 5 dB for the Oticon Multifocus to 42 dB for the Maico PHOX. Typically, overall output could be adjusted by approximately 25 dB.

All nine manufacturers involved in the Potts and Valente (1995) study reported that the range of adjustment typically provided by their programmable hearing aids were significantly greater than the range of adjustment available in their nonprogrammable hearing aids.

E. PRECISION OF ADJUSTMENTS

Usually, when rotating potentiometers on nonprogrammable hearing aids, the change is along a continuum from the minimum adjustment to the maximum adjustment. Oftentimes, the dispenser has little knowledge concerning the magnitude of the change in the response as the potentiometer is rotated in one direction or the other. With programmable hearing aids, the dispenser knows precisely if the change is 2 dB or 3 dB or 4 dB or 5 dB. In addition, each time the dispenser presses the keypad or clicks the mouse, he knows precisely the ***direction*** and ***magnitude*** of the change. The authors of this chapter have made endless real-ear and coupler measures and have been very pleased with the accuracy of the magnitude and direction of the measured changes in relation to the anticipated change expected from programming.

F. EASE OF FINE-TUNING

With nonprogrammable hearing aids, the dispenser will typically ask the manufacturer to select a matrix for an ITE, ITC or completely-in-the-canal (CIC) whose electroacoustic characteristics, measured in a 2cc coupler, match the requirements based upon the hearing loss and prescriptive target. When the hearing aids arrive, the dispenser will typically measure the ***real ear insertion response (REIR)*** to determine if the measured REIR closely matches the prescribed REIR. The dispenser may order a few potentiometers on the ITE or ITC (typically overall gain, low frequency cut or high frequency cut) to adjust the response so that the measured REIR arrives as close as possible to the prescribed REIR. At this point, the dispenser hopes that the delivered signal is perceived as comfortable (not too loud or too soft) and that the sound quality is "natural." If not, the dispenser has no choice but to send the hearing aids back to the manufacturer to redesign the circuit.

With programmable hearing aids, the dispenser can couple the hearing aids to the dedicated programmer, PC or remote control to program the hearing aids. Figure 1 shows the PX8 programmer which is used to program the Maico PHOX and Gamma hearing aids. Figure 2 illustrates the P^3 programmer which is used to program the ReSound hearing aids. Figure 7 illustrates the programmer which is used to program the Unitron US-80S, Vista 4000 and IKON hearing aids. Figure 8 illustrates the programmer which is used to program the Widex LOGO BTE, ITE and ITC hearing aids. Figure 9 depicts the PMC programmer which, among other hearing aids, is used to program the Siemens Triton and Infiniti hearing aids.

The trend of the future is using the PC to program hearing aids. Figures 10 and 11 illustrate PC programming of the Unitron and 3M hearing aids, respectively. Other manufacturers currently using the PC to program their hearing aids include the ReSound PC

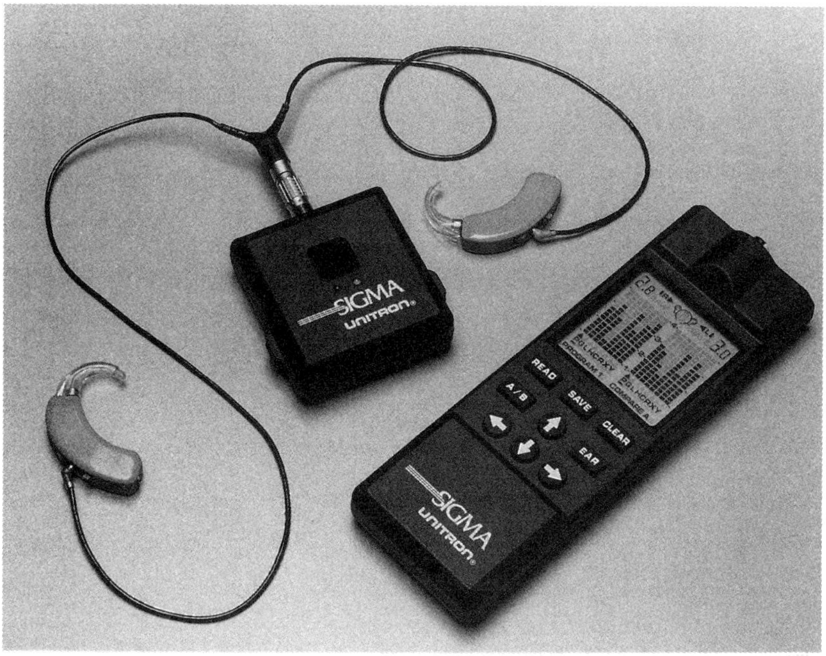

Fig. 7. Hand-held programmer to program Unitron programmable hearing aids (Reproduced with permission from Unitron Industries, Inc).

Expert, Phonak PiCS, Widex, and the Starkey Pro-Connect software to program Trilogy, Resolution, Star42 and Eurostar. Finally, Figure 12 illustrates the Widex Quattro remote which is used to program Quattro hearing aids. Widex also has a two-memory remote control, used to program their Duo hearing aids.

Once the hearing aids have been connected to the programmer, PC or remote control they can be reprogrammed using a greater number of adjustable parameters and with greater precision than is possible with nonprogrammable hearing aids. For example, one programmable hearing aid has as many as ten adjustable parameters. In addition, for some programmable hearing aids, each parameter can be adjusted in as small as 2 dB steps. With this degree of flexibility and precision, there is a greater possibility that the dispenser will achieve a final fitting which the user perceives as providing the greatest intelligibility and sound quality. A later section will discuss some methods which can be used to help the user determine which combination of parameters came closest to achieving the greatest speech intelligibility and sound quality.

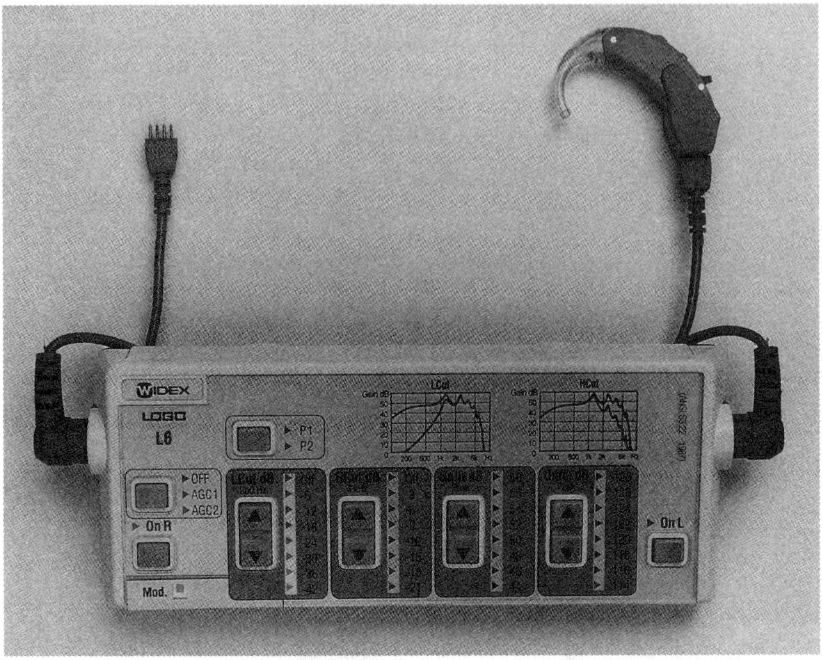

Fig. 8. Widex LOGO programmer with a L6 hearing aid attached for the left ear (Reproduced with permission from Widex Hearing Aid Co, Inc).

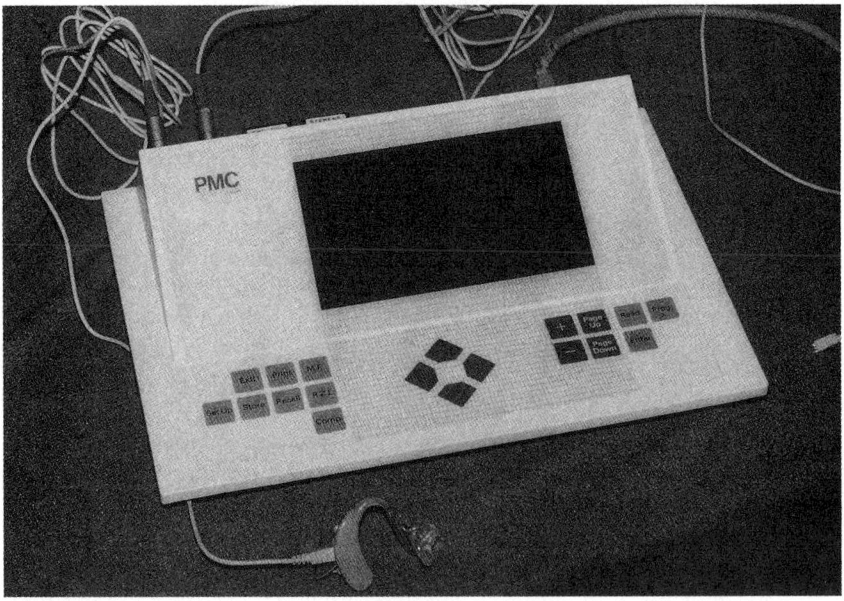

Fig. 9. The Programmable Multichannel (PMC) programmer.

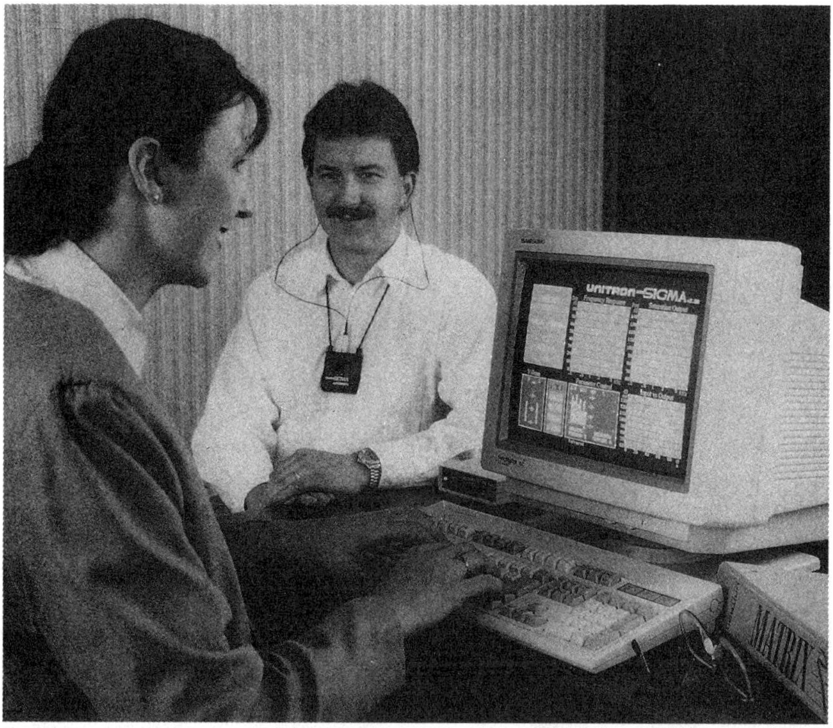

Fig. 10. Use of a personal computer to program Unitron programmable hearing aids (Reproduced with permission from Unitron Industries, Inc).

G. EASE OF PROGRAMMING

Another advantage of programmable hearing aids is the ability to efficiently and ***instantaneously*** forward changes in the adjustable parameters to the hearing aids and use real ear measures or other means of verification to determine if the change had the desired effect (i.e., the measured REIR is closer to the prescribed REIR). These changes occur simply by the dispenser pressing the "enter" key on the computer keyboard, clicking a mouse on the desired parameter within the software or pressing a button on the remote control or dedicated programmer.

This is in contrast to the requirement of rotating a potentiometer on the BTE case or the ITE/ITC faceplate. For those dispensers accustomed to changing the electroacoustic characteristics of non-programmable hearing aids by rotating potentiometers, the authors are sure the reader can remember observing the four or so unidentified potentiometers on the hearing aid and wonder which potentiometer controlled overall gain, overall output, low frequency or

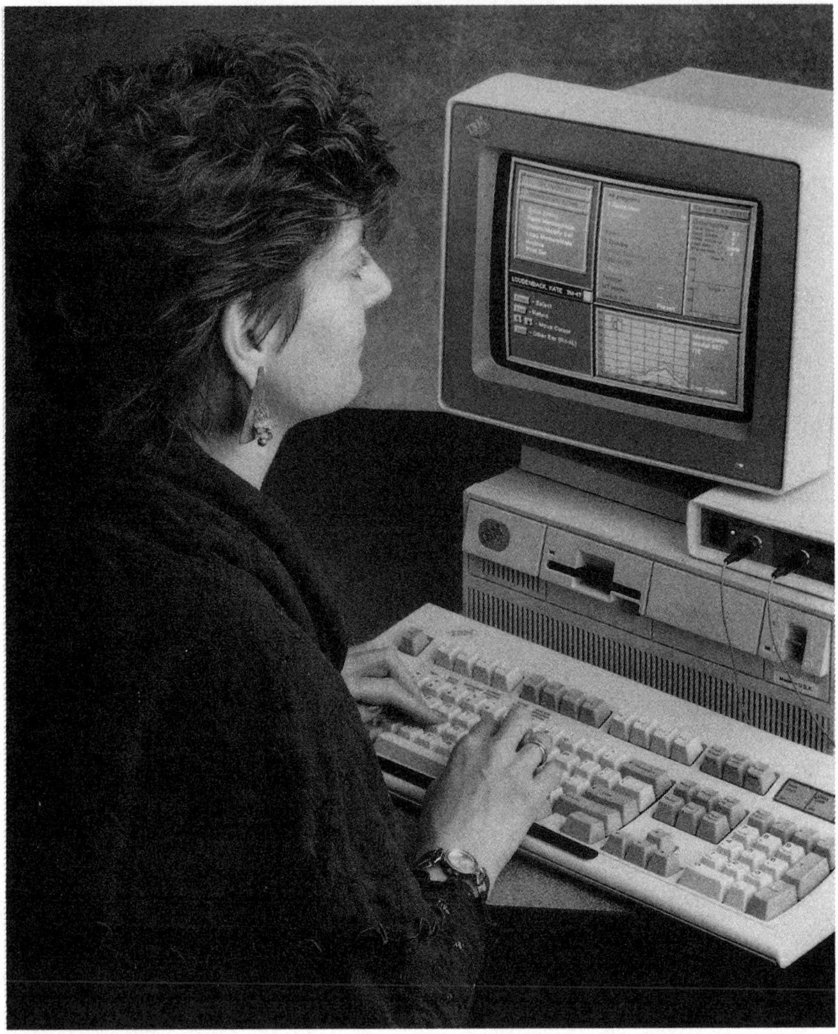

Fig. 11. Use of a personal computer to program 3M programmable hearing aids (Reproduced with permission from 3M).

high frequency response? The reader may have wondered if the desired change would occur if he rotated the potentiometer clockwise or counterclockwise? Occasionally, the reader would have liked to rotate the potentiometer, but the potentiometer was stripped! Or perhaps the reader may have rotated the potentiometer and the screwdriver slipped into a section of the ear or the side of the neck! The fact of the matter is that rotating potentiometers to achieve a desired response is inefficient and inaccurate relative to the technology which is currently available.

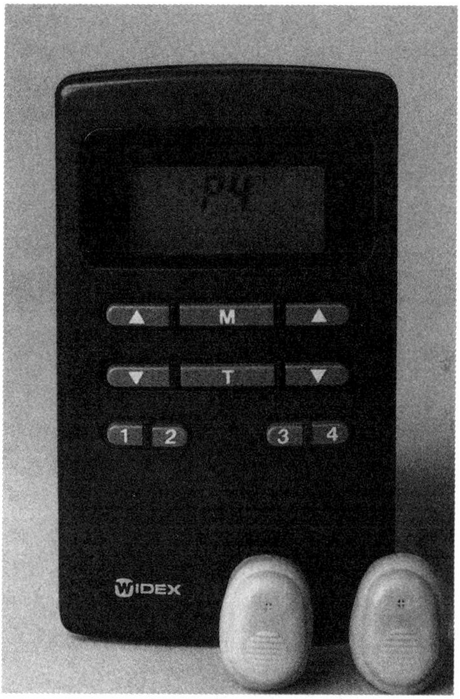

Fig. 12. Widex Quattro remote control and QX hearing aids (Reproduced with permission from Widex Hearing Aid Co, Inc).

H. TARGET SELECT

Several programmable hearing aids (i.e., Maico PHOX and Gamma via the PX8, 3M MemoryMate and SinglePro, PC version of the Unitron Sigma, PC version of Widex Quattro, Siemens PMC, Starkey Pro-Connect system and Phonak PiCS) allow the dispenser to enter the audiometric data and then select a prescriptive target. Then the dispenser presses the appropriate key on the programmer or PC and the software selects how the hearing aids should be programmed so that the measured REIR will "match" the prescribed REIR. Offering even slightly greater accuracy, the PiCS software allows the dispenser to also enter the individual ***real ear unaided response (REUR)*** as well as the characteristics of the ***earhook*** (damped or undamped), ***tubing*** (diameter) and ***earmold*** (3 or 4mm horn and the diameter of the vent) so that these effects can be corrected by the software to allow the measured REIR to arrive even closer to the prescribed REIR.

Using a different method, the ReSound P^3 requires the dispenser to enter the audiogram and then have the patient complete the LGOB. At this point, the dispenser can have the software of the P^3 select the programmable parameters based upon either a) the audiogram alone (***"audio plus"***); b) the LGOB alone (***"LGOB only"***) or c) the interaction of the audiogram and the LGOB (***"audio 1 LGOB"***). The experience of the authors finds that the ***"audio 1 LGOB"*** algorithm usually arrives very close to the response which the patient will ultimately select to be the most satisfying. Therefore, in our clinic, all patients undergo the LGOB prior to dispensing ReSound hearing aids and the "audio + LGOB" algorithm is initially placed into the hearing aids to begin the process of fine-tuning to arrive at the electroacoustic characteristics which the patient finds most satisfying.

As reported by Valente, Skinner, Valente, Potts, Jenison and Coticchia (1994) none of the "target select" programs for any of the programmable hearing aids yielded measured REIR which initially matched the prescribed REIR. However, if these programs are viewed as a good ***starting point*** from where to begin programming, then "target select" programs can be useful. If dispensers simply place their faith in the programmable parameters selected by the software, without external verification, then the success of the fitting is severely questioned.

I. SET-UP PROGRAMS

In the past, it was common for dispensers to have a wide selection of manufacturer "consignment" hearing aids to evaluate the benefits of amplification within the clinic. The need to maintain ***"consignment"*** hearing aids has been eliminated with several programmable hearing aids. For example, the Maico PX8 and Starkey Pro-Connect systems have eight manufacturer-selected hearing aid designs stored within the software. In addition, the dispenser can create four additional generic hearing aid designs. The PMC programmer has nine manufacturer selected hearing aid designs in one memory and the dispenser can create six additional hearing aid designs in another memory. The dispenser can retrieve any of these pre-set" hearing aid designs, in order to "fine-tune" and program the hearing aids to obtain the greatest user satisfaction.

J. MULTIPLE MEMORIES

Quite often patients will arrive at the dispenser's office with complaints that they have difficulty hearing in a background of noise. With nonprogrammable hearing aids, the dispenser attempts to select the electroacoustic response which will allow average conversational speech to be comfortable and audible. When the dispenser matches the measured REIR to a prescribed REIR, this is exactly what the linear hearing aid is designed to accomplish. If the input signal is softer or louder than average, the hearing aids will, for those moments, underamplify or overamplify, respectively. If the signal should be mixed with noise, then user performance will not be as satisfactory as it was when the signal was in quiet or at a level considerably higher than the noise level.

Some programmable hearing aids have several memories which the user may retrieve by the touch of a button on a remote control. For example, Figure 12 illustrates the Widex Quattro remote control which allows for storing and retrieving four memories. Figures 13 to 15 illustrate the remote controls for the Maico Gamma (two memories), ReSound (two memories) and Phonak PiCS (three memories). Other remote controls on the market are those for the Starkey Trilogy (three memories) and the Widex Duo (two memories).

For some patients, carrying a remote control to retrieve multiple memories can be both an inconvenience and an additional expense. For this reason, several manufacturers have multiple

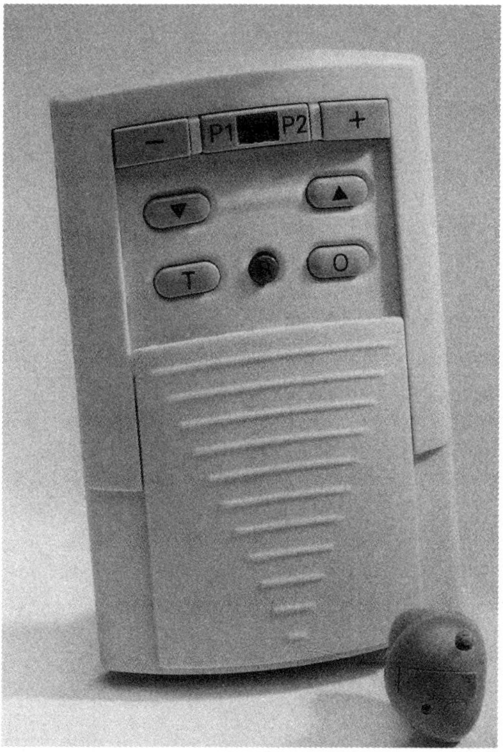

Fig. 13. Maico Gamma remote control and RD311 hearing aid (Reproduced with permission from Maico Hearing Instruments Inc).

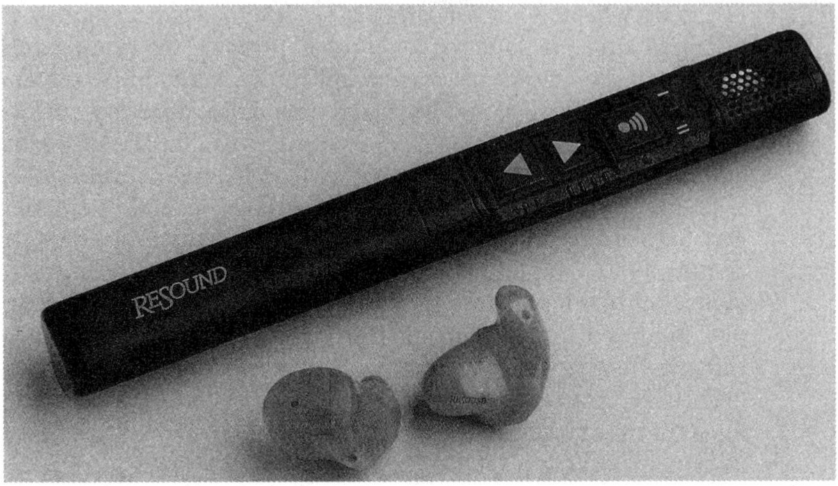

Fig. 14. ReSound remote control and ED3-HS hearing aids (Reproduced with permission from ReSound Corporation).

memory hearing aids where the individual memories may be retrieved by ***pressing a button*** on the case or faceplate. Figures 16 and 17 illustrate the presence of buttons on the 3M MemoryMate ITE (Figure 16) or BTE (Figure 17) to access each of the eight available memories. Siemens also uses a button on their 3004 and 2004 hearing aids to allow the user to retrieve four memories. Widex recently introduced their LOGO ITC series which requires

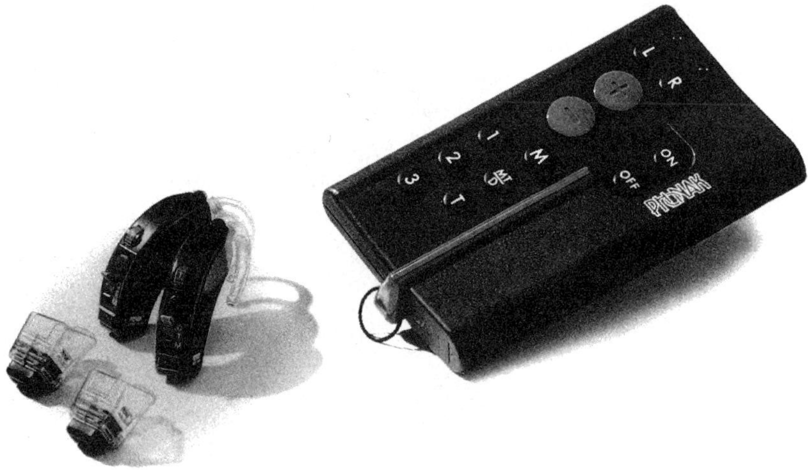

Fig. 15. Phonak PiCS remote control and Sono Forte 331X hearing aids and direct auditory input (DAI) boots (Reproduced with permission from Phonak, Inc).

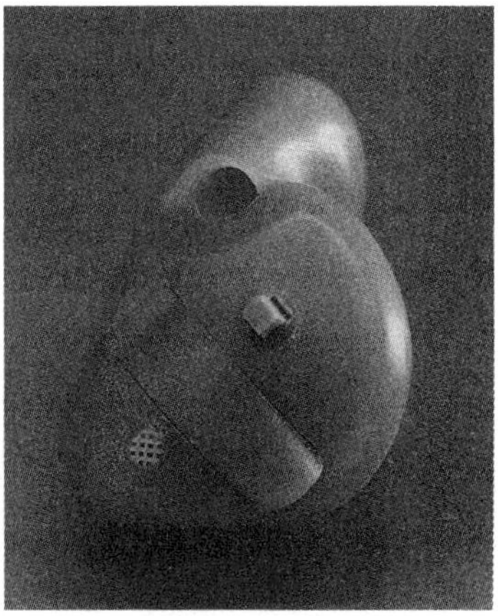

Fig. 16. 3M MultiPro ITE (Reproduced with permission from 3M).

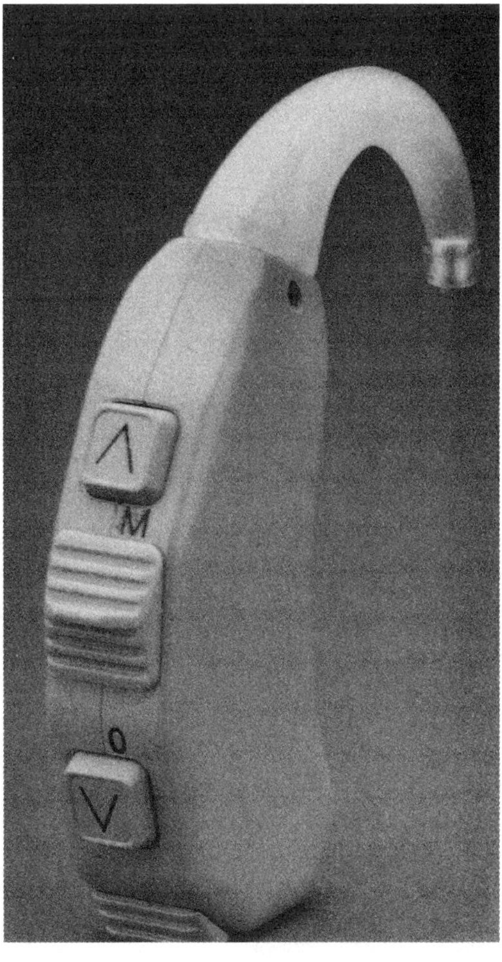

Fig. 17. 3M MultiPro BTE (Reproduced with permission from 3M).

the user to ***press the battery drawer*** to access the two memories. Finally, Figure 18 illustrates the Unitron US-80S where ***sliding a switch*** will allow the user to access one of two memories. Other hearing aids which use a switch to access memories include the Widex LOGO and Starkey Resolution II ITE and BTE.

In addition, with multiple memory hearing aids, the electroacoustic characteristics of each memory can be independently adjusted from the way in which they were adjusted in the other memories. Exceptions to this are the Unitron Sigma and Starkey Resolution II where only overall gain and low frequency cut can be programmed into the second memory relative to the adjustments which were programmed into the first memory. With programming limited to two parameters in the second memory, the authors question the decision by Unitron and Starkey to include overall gain as one of the programmable parameters in the view of the fact that both hearing aids have volume control wheels which allows the user to already control overall gain. It seems that a better choice would have been to allow the dispenser to program a

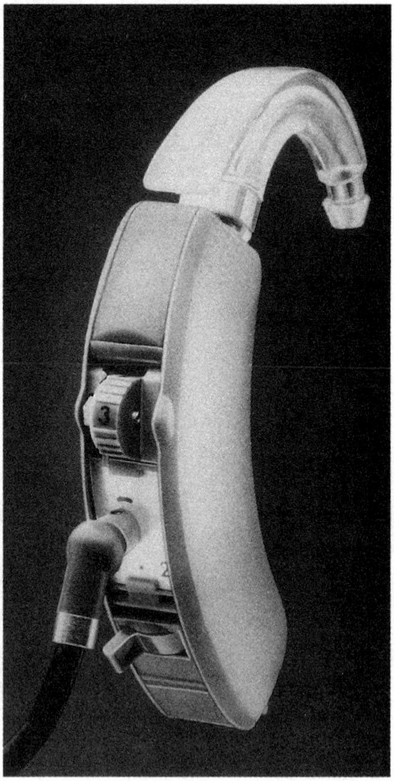

Fig. 18. Unitron Sigma US80-S hearing aid (Reproduced with permission from Unitron Industries, Inc).

lower compression kneepoint in the second memory which is usually programmed for easier communication in noisy environments. Our experience has shown that users with reduced dynamic range tend to prefer a lower kneepoint when listening in noisy environments" and a higher kneepoint when listening in quiet environments." Therefore, if the intent of the second memory is to provide greater user satisfaction in noisy environments, and we can only program two parameters into the second memory, then we would prefer to have the ability to program a lower compression kneepoint along with greater low frequency reduction relative to these same parameters programmed in the first memory. This, to the authors, makes greater sense than the current situation where only overall gain and low frequency cut are available to the dispenser for programming the second memory.

Figure 19 illustrates the measured REIR for two of the three memories of a Starkey Trilogy fitting. The upper REIR (light solid line) was programmed to match a prescriptive target (dark solid line), while the second memory (lower light solid line) was adjusted to provide less low frequency gain and slightly greater high frequency gain to theoretically enhance speech intelligibility in noisy environments. As will be explained later, a fitting strategy of providing reduced low frequency gain and increased high frequency gain in one memory, relative to a broader frequency response in another memory, to improve user satisfaction in noisy environments, may not be achieving the desired effect.

Usually the first memory is programmed for maximum benefit in "quiet" environments, while the other memories are programmed for improved understanding of speech in a variety of background noises (low frequency, high frequency, party). The other memories can also be programmed for greater user satisfaction when listening to music or using the hearing aid in the microphone position to more effectively communicate on the telephone (Figure 20).

Also available with some programmable systems having multiple memories is the option of having the software select parameter adjustments for the various memories. In these cases, the dispenser merely must communicate with the software how that particular memory is to be used by the patient. For example, Figure 21 illustrates the Phonak PiCS "***comfort programs***" screen for "***comfort program 2***" and "***comfort program 3.***" In this screen, the dispenser places the cursor over the proposed listening environments intended to be placed in *memory #2* (i.e., comfort program 2) and *memory #3* (comfort program #3). He can select a listening environment which is dominated by either low or high frequency

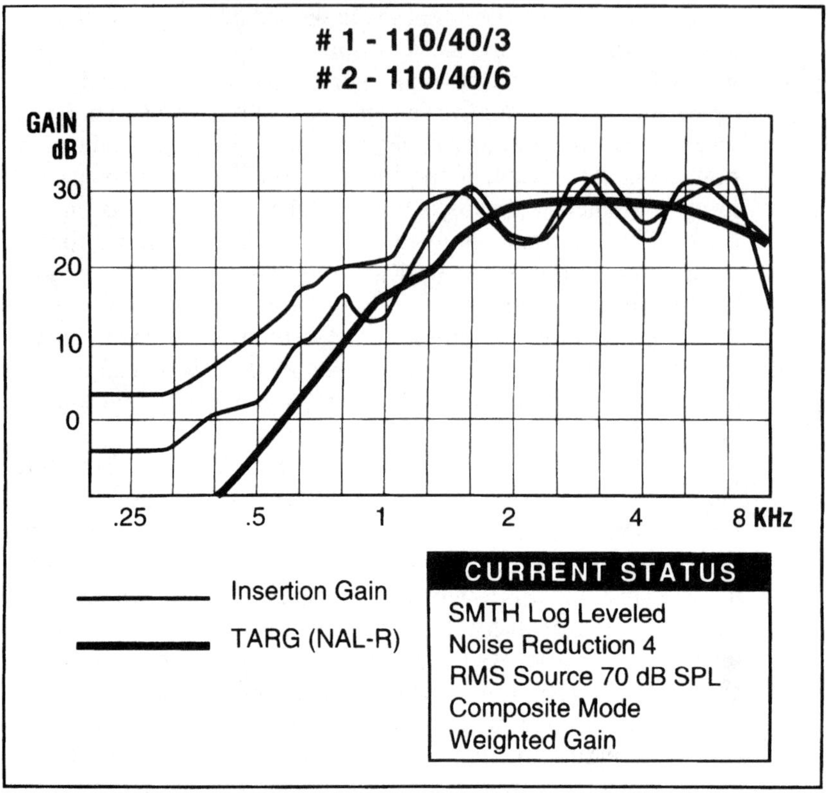

Fig. 19. Measured REIRs for a Starkey Trilogy I hearing aid. The solid dark line is the prescribed REIR using the NAL-R prescriptive target. The upper measured REIR is the response placed in memory #1 and the lower measured REIR is the response placed in memory #2.

noise. He can also select "party," "group conversation," music or an acoustic telephone response. Typically in this situation, the electroacoustic characteristics necessary to match a prescriptive target for "quiet listening" is placed in ***Program 1 (i.e, the "basic" or "comfort 1" program),*** while one "comfort program" is placed into the second memory and a different "comfort program" is placed into the third memory. For example, in Figure 21 party noise with activation of the dual microphones of the Audio Zoom was placed in program 2 (***party noise 1 zoom***) and comfort in noise with activation of the dual microphones was placed in program 3 (***comfort in noise 1 zoom***). Similar types of programming options for multiple memory hearing aids are available for the four memories of the Siemens 3004 or 2004, the four memories of the Widex Quattro and the eight memories of the 3M MemoryMate.

Unfortunately, none of the hearing aid responses programmed by the software for listening environments other than "quiet" has

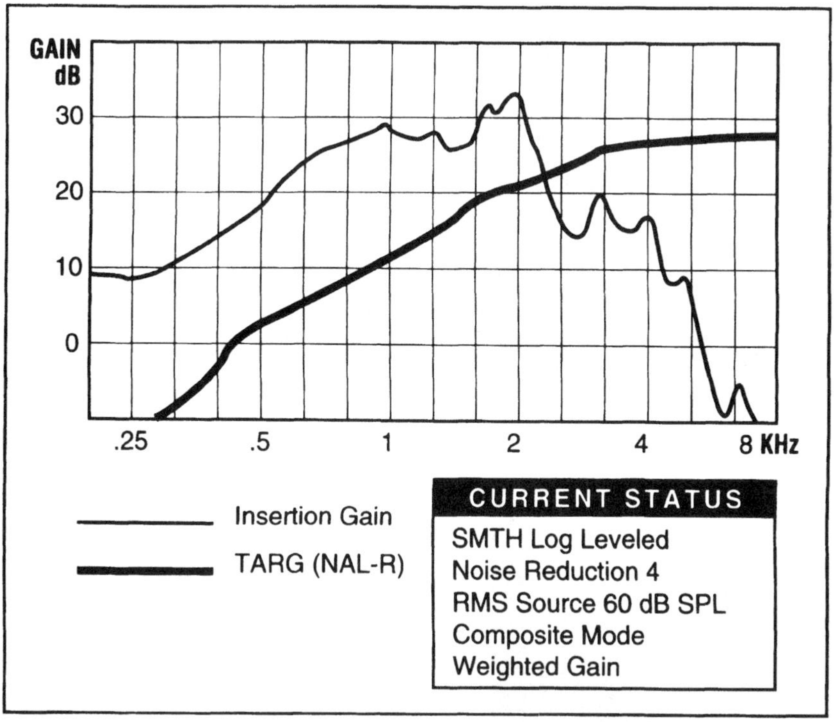

Fig. 20. Example of an acoustical telephone response programmed with the Starkey Trilogy I and placed in memory #3.

been validated. In addition, manufacturers have appeared very secretive in how decisions were made for selecting the suggested parameters to be placed in the various memories. It is the feeling of the authors that considerable research must be forthcoming before dispensers can accept these adjustments on blind faith. For example, in a recent study by Valente, Fabry and Potts (1995) there were no significant difference in signal to noise ratio when the program was switched between the "basic" and "party" programs. That is, reduction of low frequency gain in the "party" program did not provide significant improvements in background noise, in comparison to providing a broader frequency response to the subjects.

It is the experience of the authors that for the vast majority of users two memories have proven to be sufficient. In addition, it has been the experience of the authors that for the second memory to be useful, it must be programmed so that the amplified signal of one memory is significantly different than that of the other memory. Finally, it is the experience of the authors that a common strategy of reducing the low frequency gain in the second memory (re: the first memory) to enhance speech intelligibility in noise

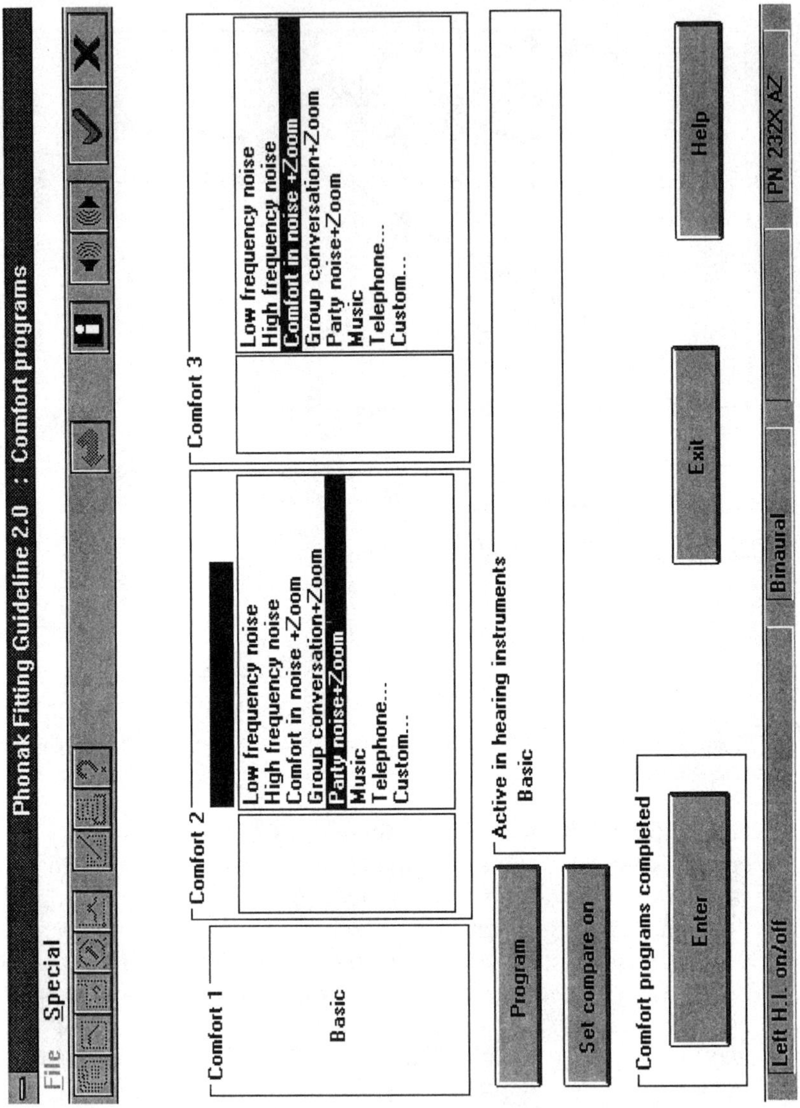

Fig. 21. "Comfort" programs screen for Phonak PiCS (Reproduced with permission from Phonak, Inc).

will prove ineffective in improving performance in noise (Fabry, 1991; Fabry, Leek, Walden and Cord, 1993; Valente, Fabry and Potts, 1995;).

K. PAIRED COMPARISONS

With many programmable hearing aids it is possible for the dispenser to place many variations of electroacoustic characteristics into memories within the programmer or PC for the user to determine which provides the greater satisfaction. For instance, the 3M, Phonak PiCS, Siemens Infiniti and Unitron Sigma will allow the dispenser to place a different hearing aid response into ***two memories*** to allow the user to toggle back and forth between the two memories to select the most acceptable response. The Starkey Trilogy I and II have the capacity to store and retrieve three responses in ***three memories,*** while the Maico PHOX and Gamma systems can store and retrieve six responses in ***six memories*** and the Siemens Triton can store and retrieve ***fifteen memories.***

To accomplish paired comparisons in our clinic, the patient is placed facing a loudspeaker at one meter's distance. For programs designed for listening in "quiet", we present female connected discourse at 58 dB(A) and multi-talker babble at 51 dB(A) resulting in a +7 dB signal-to-noise ratio. For programs designed for listening in "noise", the female connected discourse is presented at 68 dB(A) and the multi-talker babble is presented at 67 dB(A), for a +1 dB signal-to-ratio (Valente, Skinner, Valente, Potts, Jenison and Coticchia, 1994). While the patient is listening to either of the above stimuli, we program the hearing aids until the patient informs us that we have presented a combination of programmable parameters which results in the best sound quality (Gabrielsson, Schenkman and Hagerman, 1988) and speech intelligibility rating (Cox and McDaniel). These settings are then stored into the memories of the hearing aids or remote control. If we need to program a memory which is more appropriate for listening to music, we have at our disposal a number of compact disc (CD) recordings of classical, jazz and rock music. We also have at our disposal a number of excellent CDs from Widex (music, party, traffic, industry, office and high frequency noise), Oticon (office, home, beach, train, gas station, traffic, mall, birds, rain/thunder, football game, jazz, pop and classical), ReSound, Phonak (cafeteria noise, speech babble, high and low frequency noise plus dialogue at various signal-to-noise ratios, classical and pop music) and a four volume set of sound effect CDs from MicroSound Products. All of these CDs have been used at one time or another to help our patients decide which combination of adjustable parameters provides the greatest satisfaction.

The reader should refer to the excellent works of Kuk (1992; 1993; 1994) and Fabry and Schum (1994) for details in using paired comparison and subjective preference scales to evaluate the appropriateness of adjusting the various parameters of programmable hearing aids.

L. SUPERIOR SIGNAL PROCESSING

Although more research is needed to assess candidacy, benefits and fitting strategies for programmable hearing aids (Cox, 1993; Kuk, 1993; 1992; Stypulkowski, 1993; Preves and Sammeth, 1994) several recent studies have reported superior performance with several programmable hearing aids.

Benson, Clark and Johnson (1992) reported superior performance (functional gain at 500 Hz, 2000 Hz and for connected discourse, speech recognition for sentences at 50 and 65 dB SPL and a subjective questionnaire) for 18 experienced users fitted with hearing aids incorporating multiband compression (ReSound) in comparison to their linear hearing aids.

Moore, Johnson, Clark and Pluvinage (1992) programmed the two memory ReSound ED2 so that one memory was linear while the second memory was programmed for two band compression. They reported that two-band compression nonlinear listening resulted in better listener performance in improved signal-to-noise ratio than their performance with linear amplification. The listeners also reported subjective preferences for the two-band compression in comparison to the linear setting and to their own traditional hearing aids in everyday listening.

Johnson, Kirby, Hodgson and Johnson (1988) reported significant improvements in speech recognition (NU-6) in noise (multitalker babble at a signal-to-noise ratio which provided 50% intelligibility) for 27 experienced and satisfied users of linear amplification when fitted with a 3M MemoryMate hearing aid. Eighty five percent of the subjects revealed improved word recognition with the 3M hearing aid in comparison to their own hearing aid. The range of improvement was 3%-105% with a group average of 29%. Subjects also rated the quality of sound superior for the 3M when listening in quiet, noise and to music.

A recent study by Valente, Fabry and Potts (1995) reported that the dual microphones of the Phonak Audio-Zoom (Figure 22) re-

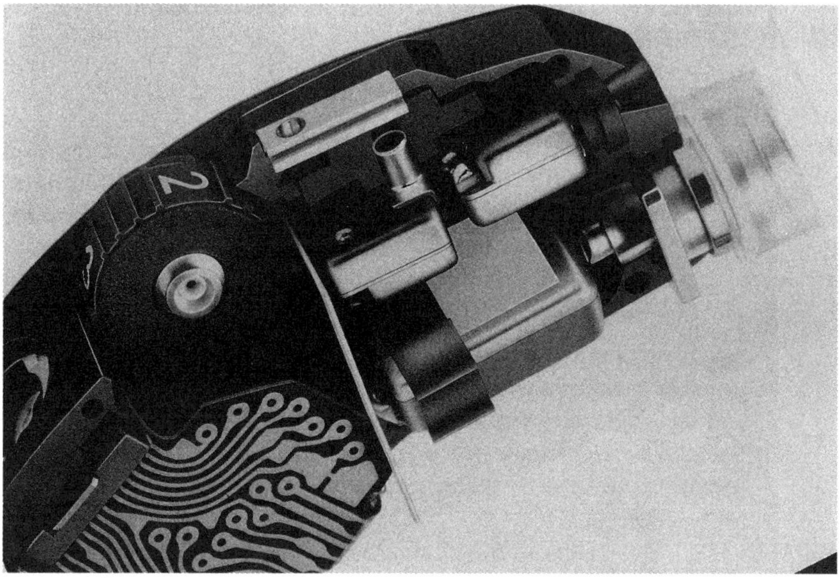

Fig. 22. Dual microphones of the Phonak PiCS Audio-Zoom (Reproduced with permission from Phonak, Inc).

sulted in an improved signal-to-noise ratio (SNR) of nearly 8 dB in comparison to omnidirectional performance using the same hearing aid. These results were nearly double the 3-4 dB improvement in SNR reported by Madison and Hawkins (1983) and Beck (1983). In addition, the benefit scores of the ***Profile of Hearing Aid Benefit (PHAB)*** (Cox and Gilmore, 1990) and ***Abbreviated Profile of Hearing Aid Benefit (APHAB)*** (Cox and Alexander, 1994) for the Audio-Zoom were significantly better than those reported by successful users of linear amplification.

M. INCREASED INTEREST BY CONSUMERS

The inescapable fact is that society is becoming more technologically oriented and there will be increased consumer interest in the more technologically advanced programmable hearing aids. Like any other healthcare field, it is probable that consumers will gravitate to dispensers providing programmable hearing aids because they will be viewed as having access to "cutting edge technology" and, therefore, as more qualified to provide hearing healthcare services.

ADDITIONAL FEATURES AVAILABLE IN PROGRAMMABLE HEARING AIDS

A. DUAL MICROPHONES

As mentioned earlier, the Phonak PiCS Audio-Zoom is the first hearing aid to offer dual microphones for improved listening in background noise. It is expected that this technology will be made available in the near future by other hearing aid manufacturers.

B. DATABASE MANAGEMENT

Aside from the ability to program hearing aids, the PC software programs accompanying the Unitron, Phonak, Starkey, Widex, 3M and ReSound hearing aids allow the dispenser considerable opportunities in database management. This includes storing and retrieving audiograms, fitting parameters, patient file management and marketing.

C. BINAURAL BALANCE

The Phonak PiCS allows the dispenser to program the hearing aids so that once turned on, the hearing aids automatically adjust to provide a sense of binaural balance and a comfortable loudness level.

D. REAL TIME LOW FREQUENCY ADJUSTMENT

The remote control of the Maico Gamma (Figure 13) has "an arrow up" and "arrow down" button. When pressing these buttons, the user is actively increasing or decreasing the low frequency gain in "real time" to find the setting which provides the greatest understanding of speech in the environment in which he is communicating.

E. REDUCE ACOUSTIC SIDE WHEN TELECOIL IS ACTIVE

The Phonak PiCS allows the dispenser to program the hearing aids so that upon activation of the telecoil, the gain of the hearing aid on the opposite "acoustic" side is automatically reduced by 6 dB to reduce the interference of ambient noise with the conversation on the telephone.

F. DATALOGGING

The 3M MemoryMate hearing aids (BTE and ITE) allow the dispenser to examine the use pattern of the hearing aids. This function is called ***Datalogging*** and allows the dispenser to know the percentage of time each program was used and the percent of switching between programs. Datalogging also allows the dispenser to know how many hours the hearing aids were used, the total number of switches between programs, when the programs were loaded and the number of days since the programs were loaded (Stypulkowski, Raskind and Hodgson, 1992; Stypulkowski, 1994).

G. STYLE OF HEARING AIDS

Initially, most programmable hearing aids were available only as a BTE and were most appropriate for patients with moderate to moderate severe hearing loss. Little attention was paid to the availability of this technology for patients with milder or greater hearing loss. This limitation has changed dramatically over the past two years. Recently several manufacturers have introduced products appropriate for patients with moderately severe to severe hearing loss. These include the ReSound BT2 and BTP power BTEs. Recently, ReSound introduced the BTP-A which has the capacity for direct audio input (DAI) and two telecoils. One telecoil is in a ***horizontal position*** for more effective use on the telephone and the second telecoil is in a ***vertical position*** for more effective use with loop systems. Each of the telecoils can be independently accessed via a switch on the case. Phonak recently introduced the Sono Forte power BTE and will shortly introduce the Sono Forte with Audio-Zoom (dual-microphone technology). Unitron has made available the US-80S, IKON-S and IKON SD with a directional microphone. Widex has had the Quattro 32 and Duo 32 available for a number of years and very recently introduced the LOGO L12 BTE. Starkey has had the Eurostar and Star42 available and recently introduced the two-memory Resolution power BTE. Finally, Siemens has the Triton 3004b and 2004b available for patients with more severe hearing loss. All of these BTE hearing aids have been used effectively, at one time or another, in our clinic with patients who have moderately severe to severe hearing loss and who are seeking the benefits provided by programmable technology. Finally, it must be mentioned that patients with moderately severe to severe hearing loss typically do not benefit from the advantages provided by multiple memory hearing aids. That is, the severity of the hearing loss limits the manner in which the dispenser can program the other memories in order for these patients to derive benefit.

Recently, the in-the-canal (ITC) programmable hearing aid has been widely introduced to accommodate patients with milder hearing loss and who prefer a smaller hearing aid's cosmetic appeal. ITC hearing aids are currently available from Siemens (Infiniti), Widex (LOGO LX series), Starkey (Trilogy I), 3M (SinglePro and Memorymate), and the Maico Gamma (RD311).

Siemens recently introduced another version of the Infiniti as the first programmable completely-in-the-canal (CIC) hearing aid, although the authors have no experience with this hearing aid.

H. READ STORED RESPONSE

How many times has a dispenser had to look at a specification sheet, if available, to determine the meaning of one potentiometer with the arrow at, for example, a 12:00 position and the other potentiometer at a 3:00 position? With every programmable hearing aid, the dispenser simply needs to connect the hearing aids to the programmer, remote or PC and ***to read*** how the hearing aids were programmed on the chips of the hearing aids. In addition, most programmable hearing aids have a ***print*** function which provides a hardcopy of what is stored on the hearing aid chips.

FUTURE DIRECTIONS IN PROGRAMMABLE HEARING AIDS

At this point, the authors will look into their "crystal ball" and predict what lies ahead for programmable hearing aids in the next five years. Due to rapid changes in hearing aid technology over the past year, the author would not be surprised if several of the following predictions may have been realized by the time this chapter appears in print.

A. PROGRAMMABLE COMPLETELY-IN-THE-CANAL (CIC)

One of the most exciting additions for the dispenser has been the recent introduction of the completely-in-the canal (CIC) hearing aid. At the time of writing this chapter, Siemens has introduced the first CIC and Maico has introduced a mini-canal (RD311) very close in size to a CIC. Several companies are currently working on introducing programmable CICs with the ability to be programmed in the same manner as their current BTE, ITE and ITC product lines.

B. DIGITAL HEARING AIDS

It is predicted that within five years, programmable digital hearing aids will be introduced. The authors are aware of several manufacturers who have been working on this technology for quite some time and field trials have already begun.

C. DUAL MICROPHONES

It is anticipated that manufacturers other than Phonak will introduce hearing aids with dual microphones or a single directional microphone with improved directionality. In addition, a better directional microphone will be introduced for ITEs and possibly ITCs.

D. NOAH SOFTWARE AND HI-PRO INTERFACE

Until recently, if a dispenser wished to be involved with programmable hearing aids, it required the purchase of a dedicated programmer from the manufacturer (cost of between $395 for an Infiniti programmer to $5500 for a PMC) or the purchase of a software package (cost of between $355 for the Phonak PiCS to $2995 for the 3M MD80) to run on a PC using a manufacturer interface box, software and cables. This has proven to be expensive, inefficient and a major stumbling block for many dispensers to enter into the programmable arena. For example, in our clinic we have interface boxes to communicate with a PC for ReSound (P^3), 3M, Unitron, Phonak, Starkey and Widex. In addition, we have dedicated programmers from Maico, Audiotone, Siemens (PMC and Infiniti), ReSound (P^3), Starkey and Unitron. Thus, when we need to program Phonak hearing aids, we must connect the Phonak interface box to the serial port of the PC. When we need to program 3M hearing aids, we must connect the 3M interface box to the serial port. In an effort to make this process less complex, we purchased and installed an A-B switch box to connect both the 3M and Phonak interface boxes to the same serial port. However, this method still requires numerous interface boxes to be placed near the computer. This method of programming has proven to be expensive and highly inefficient.

In the early 1990s, representatives from several major international hearing aid manufacturers (Danavox, Oticon, Phonak, Siemens and Widex) met to develop an industry-wide software standard to fit both programmable and nonprogrammable hearing aids. From those deliberations came the development of NOAH software through the ***Hearing Industries Manufacturer Software Association (HIMSA I/S) in Europe and (HIMSA/America) in the United States).*** Currently, ***GN Danavox, Oticon, Phonak, ReSound Europe, Starkey Europe, Unitron, Widex, Maico, Siemens, 3M Europe and Viennatone*** have agreed to develop

NOAH software modules for their dispensers (Grey, Rosner and Donnay, 1994; Jelonek, 1994).

NOAH is a comprehensive software package which will work most efficiently with a 486 IBM compatible computer having at least 8 megabytes (MB) of random access memory (RAM), Windows 3.1 or higher, DOS 5.0 or higher, at least a 120 MB hard drive and a VGA color monitor. It also requires the use of a single universal interface box (***HI-PRO)*** which is manufactured by Madsen and made available to dispensers from the participating hearing aid manufacturers (Figure 23). The HI-Pro is a plastic interface box

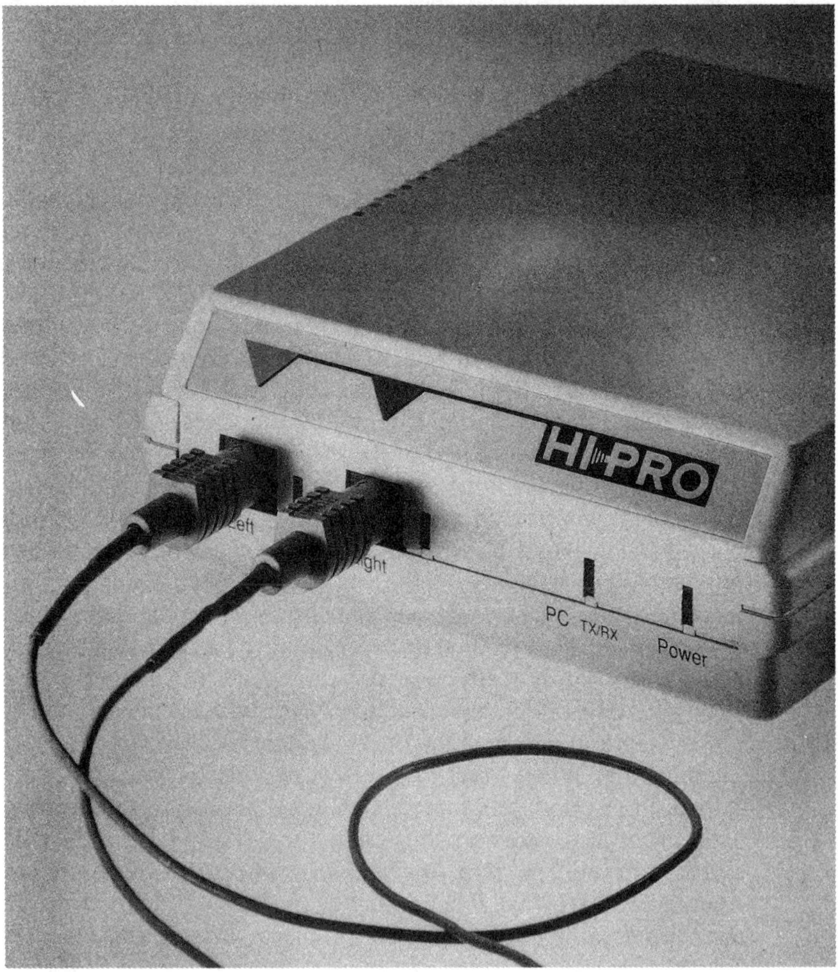

Fig. 23. Hi-Pro interface box (Reproduced with permission from Phonak, Inc).

which connects to the serial port of the PC. It has two slots in the front where cables from the participating manufacturer are connected for the right and left hearing aids. Thus, the NOAH software purchased from HIMSA and the individual software modules purchased from participating manufacturers are loaded onto the hard drive of the PC and the dispenser loads the software for the individual manufacturers from Windows (Figure 24) to begin the process of programming the hearing aids. With the NOAH system, the dispenser would require one PC, one interface box and the cables and software for the hearing aids he wishes to program. This would eliminate the need for multiple dedicated programmers.

NOAH will be available in two formats. One format is a ***stand-alone version*** which includes a basic client management module and the fitting modules from participating manufacturers. In this case, NOAH manages the storage, retrieval and transfer of data from NOAH to the fitting module for a manufacturer. Thus, the dispenser has to enter this data only once and the numerous manufacturer fitting modules will interface with NOAH to transfer the necessary file to the manufacturer fitting module. This will allow

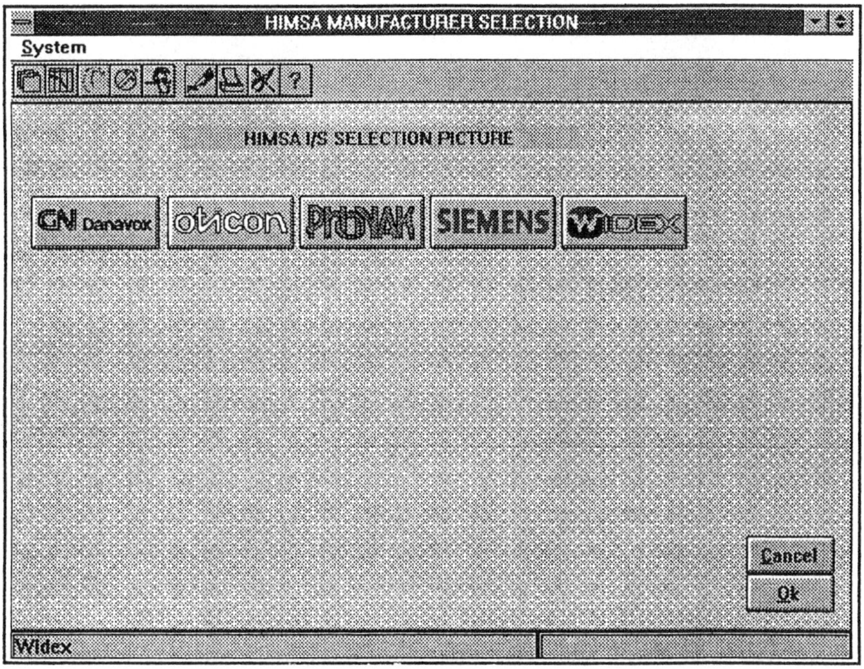

Fig. 24. Opening screen of NOAH.

the dispenser to access the client and audiometric data from NOAH and integrate that information with the numerous hearing aids available from the software modules provided from each manufacturer. The dispenser will have immediate access to the product information and fitting assistance for all the hearing aids (programmable and non-programmable). If it is a programmable hearing aid, the dispenser can use the software and HI-PRO to program and fit the hearing aids.

There will be also be a ***comprehensive version*** which includes the modules for the stand-alone version as well as a comprehensive ***Office Automated System*** which will include client management, database management, bookkeeping, accounting, inventory, marketing, scheduling, graphic interface and the ability to integrate audiometers, real ear systems and other audiologic equipment into one integrated system.

E. FITTING STRATEGIES FOR NONLINEAR AIDS

Another stumbling block for dispensers entering the programmable market may be their lack of comfort in making the necessary decisions on how to adjust the various programmable parameters to best suit the needs of their patients. While the efforts to find better ways to fit nonlinear hearing aids will continue, one major advancement has been the introduction, in 1994, of the ***Independent Hearing Aid Fitting Forum (IHAFF)*** comprehensive fitting protocol and software.

The IHAFF protocol includes both objective and subjective measures to assure that soft input levels are soft yet audible, loud input levels are loud, but not uncomfortable and average input levels are comfortable. In addition, the protocol specifies both coupler and real ear measures to assure the dispenser that the hearing aid is free of distortion and provides a smooth REAR.

One of the major components of the IHAFF protocol is a ***CONTOUR*** program which allows a computer to interface with an audiometer to automatically measure loudness judgments for pure tones of ***at least*** 500 and 3000 Hz. The dispenser can measure loudness judgments at 250, 500, 1000, 2000, 3000 and 4000 Hz, but he must measure loudness judgments for at least two frequencies. The use of 500 and 3000 Hz is the default settings with the CONTOUR software because, amongst other reasons, it allows for loudness judgments in both a low and high band to appropriately fit hearing aids containing two bands. If the dispenser does not have an audiometer with a RS232 port, then the CONTOUR test can be performed manually.

From these loudness measures, the ***VIOLA (Visual Input/Output Locator Algorithm)*** module of the IHAFF software calculates and creates three dots (Figure 25). These dots correspond to the loudness judgment for ***soft, average and loud speech*** as measured in a HA-1 2cc coupler corrected for the difference in loudness summation between pure-tones and a broad-band signal such as speech. At this point, the dispenser enters into the VIOLA program, the initial settings (see the upper boxes in Figure 25) for ***gain at 40 dB, first compression kneepoint, compression ratio from the first kneepoint and the second kneepoint, the threshold for second kneepoint, second compression ratio and maximum output.*** Once these settings are entered into VIOLA, the software immediately illustrates how close the 2cc coupler measures would be to the target of the three dots (solid line). As can be seen from Figure 25 the hearing aid would need to programmed in low band (centered at 500 Hz) with 25 dB of gain for a 40 dB input. In addition the output would be programmed to 125 dB SPL and the kneepoints would be set high at 80 dB and the compression ratio would be 1:0:1. The high band (centered at 3000 Hz) would need to be programmed with 45 dB of gain for a 40 dB input because of the greater hearing loss in the higher frequencies for this patient. In addition, the output would be reduced to 105 dB SPL and the kneepoints would be set lower at 40 dB and the compression ratio would be more aggressive at 3.2:1. It can also be seen by looking at the VIOLA graph that the dynamic range is much wider for the low band (nearly 55 dB) than the high band (nearly 25 dB). It is the narrower high frequency band which requires the lower kneepoint and more aggressive compression ratio.

In preparation for a presentation at the 1994 Jackson Hole Rendezvous, Valente and Potts (1994) rigorously followed the IHAFF guidelines and binaurally fit four patients using the CONTOUR and VIOLA modules of the IHAFF program. Interestingly, all four patients found the amplified signal produced by following this protocol to be very acceptable, although somewhat loud. The issue of loudness was attributed by Valente and Potts (1994) to be related to binaural summation. Unfortunately the IHAFF program was based upon monaural fittings and this will be corrected in future software updates.

Another fitting strategy which may be available in the near future is ***"real ear loudness mapping" (RELM)*** which combines loudness judgments using sound-field presentation and real ear measures to "map" the unaided loudness judgments (in dB SPL) near the eardrum (Pluvinage, Pavlovic and Humes, 1995). That is, the eardrum, instead of a 2cc coupler (i.e., IHAFF) is the reference

	500 Hz	3000 Hz
Gain at 40 dB	25	45
Comp. Threshold 1	80	40
Comp. Ratio 1	1	3.2
Comp. Threshold 2	80	40
Comp. Ratio 2	1	3.2
Max. Output	125	105
Gain at 60 dB	25.0	45.0
Slope (dB/oct)	7.74	

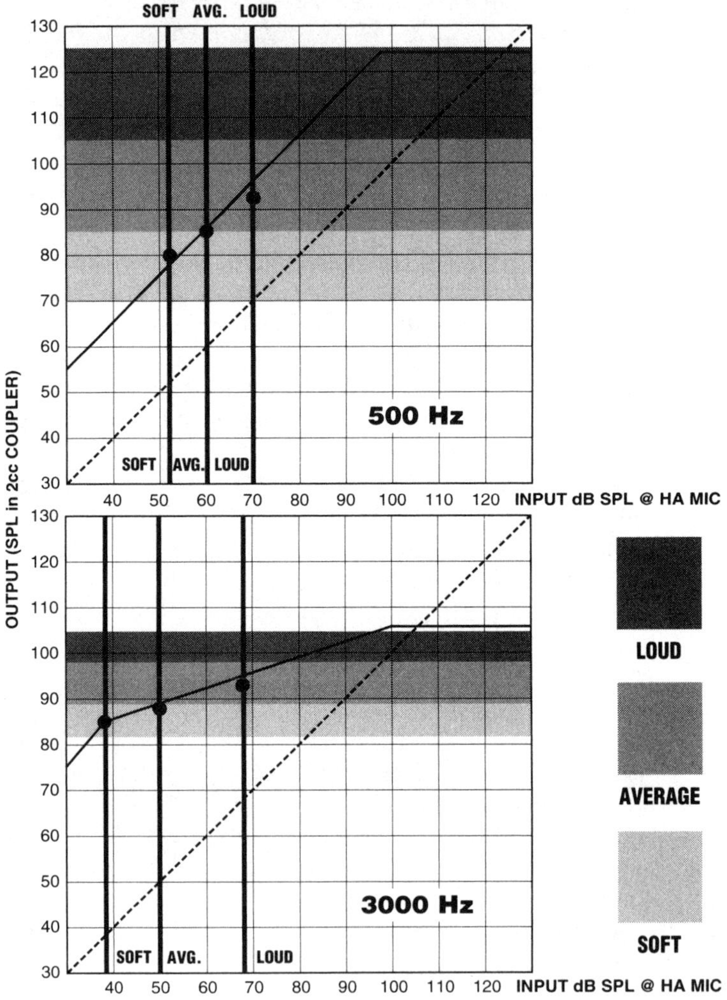

Fig. 25. Fitting screen of VIOLA at 500 and 3000 Hz. VIOLA is one software module of the IHAFF software package.

point for adjusting the parameters of the hearing aid. The goal of the RELM procedure is for the aided measure (i.e., REAR) corresponding to an input level for "soft speech" to be placed above the loudness judgment level for "soft"; the REAR for an input level corresponding to "average speech" to be placed near the loudness judgment for comfortable" and for the REAR for an input level corresponding to "loud speech" to be placed below the loudness judgment for "loud, but not uncomfortable." The first two authors of this chapter are currently collaborating with Pluvinage, Pavlovic and Humes to determine the effectiveness and efficiency of this fitting procedure.

SUMMARY

As mentioned in the introduction, the authors hope that the information within this chapter will be a catalyst for dispensers to recognize and utilize the significant advantages offered by programmable hearing aids. The authors have used programmable hearing aids in their daily practice for over five years and believe that when recommended and fitted appropriately, programmable hearing aids can offer significant advantages over nonprogrammable linear and nonlinear hearing aids.

GLOSSARY

APHAB (Abbreviated Profile of Hearing Aid Benefit) a twenty-four item subjective assessment scale of benefit from amplification developed at the University of Memphis. There are four subscales which include 1) ease of communication (EC); 2) reverberation (RV); 3) background noise (BN); 4) aversiveness of sounds (AV).

Adaptive Release Time automatic variation of release time (in milliseconds) dependent upon the duration of the signal.

Band division of the frequency response of a hearing aid into two or three frequency regions by one or two crossover frequencies.

Compression Kneepoint the point on an input/output curve at which the slope digresses from unity, indicating the signal level at which a nonlinear process begins to take effect.

Compression Ratio ratio of the change in output level resulting from a given change in input level in a compression amplifier.

Crossover Frequency the frequency or frequencies which present the cut-off frequencies of the filters used to separate the frequency range into separate bands. Analog signal manipulation of this type is limited by the steepness of the filter skirts. Consequently, there is some overlap of the bands on either side of the crossover frequency.

Dynamic Range residual hearing between hearing threshold and threshold of uncomfortable loudness.

Feedback Notch Filter programmable parameter which allows electronic elimination of a small section of the frequency response. This feature allows elimination of feedback without a dramatic reduction in high frequency amplification.

Input Compression compression amplification whose degree of gain reduction depends on the input level and the kneepoint. The volume control is positioned after the feedback loop so that an adjustment in volume creates a change in output but no change in kneepoint. A form of AGC-I.

LGOB (Loudness Growth of Octave Bands) a computerized loudness growth test developed by ReSound Corporation and integrated into their programmable fitting system.

Linear Amplification no change in gain for all input levels until the maximum output is reached.

Nonlinear Amplification a change in the overall gain and/or frequency response as a function of changing input signals.

Output Compression compression amplification whose degree of gain reduction depends on the output level and the kneepoint. The volume control is positioned before the feedback loop so that an adjustment in volume creates a change in kneepoint but no change in output. A form of AGC-O.

Paired Comparison a data collection technique whereby a listener compares two hearing aids (or settings) to decide on the one that meets the criteria set by the clinician and/or listener.

PHAB (Profile of Hearing Aid Benefit) a sixty-six item subjective assessment scale of benefit from amplification developed at the University of Memphis. There are seven subscales which include (1) familiar talkers (FT); 2) ease of communication (EC); 3) reverberation (RV); 4) reduced cues (RC); 5) background noise (BN); 6) aversiveness of sounds (AV); 7) distortion of sounds (DS).

Release Time the time required for a dynamic nonlinear process to reach its steady-state value once compression has been de-activated.

Resonant Peak Control a programmable parameter which allows the peak of the high frequency response to be adjusted.

REFERENCES

ALLEN JB, HALL JL, JENG PS. (1990). Loudness growth in ½ octave bands (LGOB)- a procedure for assessment of loudness. *J. Acoust Soc Amer* 88:745–753.

BACHLER F, BUERKLI-HALEVY O. (1994). Multi mode limiting: exploring the endless possibilities. *Hear Instrum* 45(3): 26,28–30.

Beck LB. (1983). Assessment of directional hearing aid characteristics. *Audiol Acoust* 22:178–191.

Benson D, Clark TM, Johnson JS. (1992). Patient experiences with multiband full dynamic range compression. *Ear Hear* 13:320–330.

Burton PL. (1992). Siemens Hearing Instrments, Inc.: Triton-Infiniti™. *Sem Hear* 13(2):161–169.

Burton PL. (1994). PMC and Triton: an expanding, comprehensive programmable product line. In: Sandlin RE, ed. *Understanding Digitally Programmable Hearing Aids.* Needham Heights: Allyn and Bacon, 67–86.

Cox RM. (1993). On The Evaluation of A New Generation of Hearing Aids. *J Rehab Res Devel* 30(3):297–304.

Cox RM, Alexander GC (1994). The abbreviated profile of hearing aid benefit (APHAB). *Ear Hear* (in press).

Cox RM, Gilmore C. (1990). Development of the profile of hearing aid benefit (PHAB). *J Speech Hear Res* 33:343–357.

Cox RM, McDaniel D. (1989). Development of the speech intelligibility rating (SIR) test for hearing aid gain prescriptions. *J Speech Hear Res* 32:347–352.

Curran JR. (1992). Trilogy system. *Sem Hear* 13(2):170–182.

Dirks DD, Ahlstrom J, Noffsinger D. (1993). Preferred frequency response for two-and three channel amplification systems. *J Rehab Res Devel* 30(3):305–317.

Fabry DA. (1991). Programmable and automatic noise reduction in existing hearing aids. In: Studebaker GA, Bess F H, Beck LB, eds. *The Vanderbilt Hearing Aid Report II.* Parkton: York Press, 65–78.

Fabry DA, Leek MR, Walden BE, Cord M. (1993). Do adaptive frequency response (AFR) hearing aids reduce "upward spread" of masking? *J Rehab Res Devel* 30(3):318–325.

Fabry D A, Schum D J. (1994). The role of subjective measurement techniques in hearing aid fittings. In: Valente M, ed. *Strategies for Selecting and Verifying Hearing Aid Fittings.* New York: Thieme Medical Publishers, 136–155.

Gabrielsson A, Schenkman B, Hagerman B. (1988). The effects of different frequency responses on sound quality judgments and speech intelligibility. *J Speech Hear Res* 31:166–177.

Grey H, Rosner M, Donnay L. (1994). Hi-Pro's mission: to help unlock the potential of programmables. *Hear J* 47(10):51–52.

Hall CM, Roth L. (1994). Dispenser programmable aids: is skepticism holding us back? *Hear Instrum* 45(5):16,18.

Jelonek S. (1994). Noah/Hi-Pro system offers industrywide standard for fitting programmables. *Hear J* 47(5):21–22.

Johnson JS, Kirby VM, Hodgson WA, Johnson LJ. (1988). Clinical study of a programmable, multiple memory hearing instrument. *Hear Instrum* 39(11):44–47.

KUK FK. (1992). Evaluation of the efficacy of a multimemory hearing aid. *J Amer Acad Audiol* 3:338–348.

KUK FK (1993). Clinical considerations in fitting a multimemory hearing aid. *Amer J Audiol* 2(3):23–27.

KUK FK. (1994). Use of paired comparisons in hearing aid fittings. In: VALENTE M, ed. *Strategies for Selecting and Verifying Hearing Aid Fittings.* New York: Thieme Medical Publishers, 108–135.

LIBBY ER. (1982). In search of transparent insertion gain hearing aid responses. In: STUDEBAKER GA, BESS FH, eds. *The Vanderbilt Hearing Aid Report.* Upper Darby: Monographs in Contemporary Audiology, 112–123.

MADISON TK, HAWKINS DB. (1983). The signal-to-noise ratio advantage of directional microphones. *Hear Instrum* 34(2):18,49.

Manual of the Independent Hearing Aid Fitting Forum (IHAFF). (1994).

MOORE BCJ, JOHNSON JS, CLARK TM, PLUVINAGE V. (1992). Evaluation of a dual-channel full dynamic range compression system for people with sensorineural hearing loss. *Ear Hear* 13:349–370.

MUELLER HG. (1994). Update on programmable hearing aids (with an assist from Yogi Berra). *Hear J* 47(5)13–20.

PLUVINAGE V. (1994). Rationale and development of the ReSound system. In: SANDLIN RE, ed. *Understanding Digitally Programmable Hearing Aids.* Needham Heights: Allyn and Bacon, 15–39.

PLUVINAGE V, BENSON D. (1988). New dimensions in diagnosis and fitting. *Hear Instrum* 39(8):28,30,39.

PLUVINAGE V, PAVLOVIC C, HUMES L. (1995). Real ear loudness mapping (RELM). Instructional course presented at the *Annual Meeting of the American Academy of Audiology,* Dallas: April, 1995.

POTTS LG, VALENTE M. (1995). Programmable hearing aids: applications for progressive and fluctuating hearing loss. *Semi Hear* (in press).

PREVES DA, SAMMETH CA. (1994). Some outstanding issues in hearing aid technology, fitting and research. *Hear Rev* 1(1):30,32–34, 37–38.

RUTLEDGE LF. (1992). Audiotone, Inc.: system 2000. *Sem Hear* 13(2):110–114.

SANDLIN RE. (1992). Widex Hearing Aid Co.: Quattro. *Sem Hear* 13(2):183–189.

SKINNER MW. (1988). *Hearing Aid Evaluation.* Englewood Cliffs: Prentice-Hall.

STYPULKOWSKI PH. (1993). Fitting strategies for multiple-memory programmable hearing instruments. *Amer J Audiol* 2(2):19–28.

STYPULKOWSKI PH. (1994). 3M programmable hearing instruments. In: SANDLIN R E, ed. *Understanding Digitally Programmable Hearing Aids.* Needham Heights: Allyn and Bacon, 97–121.

STYPULKOWSKI PH, RASKIND LA, HODGSON WA. (1992). 3M programmable hearing instruments and fitting systems. *Sem Hear* 13(2):135–142.

TREDE K. (1992). ReSound personal hearing systems. *Sem Hear* 13(2):153–160.

VALENTE M, FABRY DA, POTTS LG. (1994). Recognition of speech in noise using a new directional microphone. Submitted to the *J Amer Acad Audiol.*

VALENTE M, POTTS LG. (1994). Implementing the IHAFF protocol on four subjects. Presented at the *Jackson Hole Rendezvous,* Jackson Hole, WY (Aug, 1994).

VALENTE M, SKINNER MW, VALENTE LM, POTTS LG, JENISON GL, COTICCHIA J. (1994). Clinical comparison of digitally programmable hearing aids. In: SANDLIN RE, ed. *Understanding Digitally Programmable Hearing Aids.* Needham Heights: Allyn and Bacon, 203–255.

WALLACE BD. (1992). Maico Hearing Instruments, Inc.: PHOX. *Sem Hear* 13(2):127–134.

WESTERMANN S. (1994). Principles and applications of the Widex multiprogrammable hearing aid system. In: SANDLIN RE, ed. *Understanding Digitally Programmable Hearing Aids.* Needham Heights: Allyn and Bacon, 41–66.

X

POST-FITTING CARE AND PROCESSES

RAYMOND Z. RICH, BC-HIS
AND JAY B. MCSPADEN, Ph.D., BC-HIS

INTRODUCTION

Anyone can buy a high performance racing car. The act of buying such a vehicle does not make the person a driver. In the same way anyone can buy a Stradivarius or a Guaneri. The act of buying such a violin does not make the person a violin virtuoso. In some ways, getting hearing instruments is a similar activity. The modern hearing aid is the most advanced instrument ever developed for it's purpose. But, the act of buying them does not make an adept user. Nor does simply acquiring these instruments insure satisfaction or efficiency in their use.

The process of aural habilitation/rehabilitation requires cooperative effort, shared commitment, and an understanding that it is practice that makes perfect, it is perfect practice that makes perfect. Post fitting care and processes describe the activities of the professional in facilitating the adaptation of the patient/client to achieve the maximum benefit with the instruments. It is a long term commitment to ride the learning curve together to achieve positive, reasonable and realistic goals. The decisions to be tested, to consider the results of those tests and their impact, the choice to obtain the appropriate instruments, and the commitment to become efficient with them have all been completed. The impressions have been taken, the devices ordered and they have arrived and been fitted. Now, what processes are involved?

CHAPTER OBJECTIVES

This chapter asserts that successful post-fitting care is often the single most significant factor in hearing instrument acceptance and use. It encourages better understanding of those necessary processes in effective post-fitting care, such as assessing client response, counseling approaches and rehabilitation concepts, family member interaction and client instruction.

DEFINITION

It is critical for the student and/or professional to understand the integrated and integral nature of this work. We present this material in (hopefully) clear separate chapters as if the activities themselves were both differentiable and sequential. While this may make for coherent book chapters it does not represent the actual activity. In any effective habilitation/rehabilitation process there is an overlap of activities. At every step questions are asked and answered and instruction and counseling occurs.

It is important, in the pre-fitting part of patient/client education, the prospective user be made a part of the instrument selection process. Wearing hearing instruments is fundamentally an experiential activity and as such it cannot be completely understood intellectually. Therefore, acceptance of the idea of wearing hearing instruments is different than accepting the wearing of those same devices. A positive attitude is crucial not only about the instruments themselves, but, about the prospects for improved communicative efficiency based upon better understanding. When this kind of attitude can be generated or discovered, acceptance of the device and the benefits it can produce is vastly improved.

In simple terms, post-fitting care is the variety of procedures which make up the long term management of the client's need for amplification. In its most effective form, it is a process which never ends. The emphasis may shift over time as the patient/client uses his/her hearing aids. It is in this relationship that the professional will be a counselor, instructor, technician and evaluator. In a unique way the professional brings out the best aspects of the instrument and combines them with the "best effort" of the user in a synergistic relationship. When that combination is realized everyone wins!

We have described post-fitting care as a sequence of procedures whose success depends upon interactions between patient/client and professional as well as upon the success of the other steps in the process. The professional should exercise caution to insure that the post-fitting care does not conflict with pre-fitting activities. It is desirable to achieve a smooth transition from one phase of the fitting process to the next. Steps in the sequence do overlap and, as some elements of the fitting process fade out, other steps of the post-fitting care fade in. Timing is everything, as the saying goes and, in the case of the fitting of hearing instruments, it is critical here. All of the steps involved in the process are interactive, dependant, and synergistic. Together they enable the patient/client to obtain optimum benefit from the instruments and the process.

To the members of the Hearing Health Care profession, the term hearing aid fitting carries an connotation about which there is not always agreement. Fitting does, however, have a formal/legal definition which includes audiometry, earmold impression taking, sale, selection and adaptation. The five activities which make up this formal definition of "fitting" rarely take place at the same time. In the typical sequence of events, testing, instruments selection and impression taking occur early in the process. This is separated from the delivery and placement of the instrument by days and often weeks. Adaptation that is full and efficient can take some months. The reasons for this sequencing are easy to understand. Earmolds, ITE, ITC, or CIC aids have to be ordered and the instruments fabricated.

In practice, for many hearing instrument professionals, "fitting" is synonymous with the procedure defined as adaptation. It is the adaptation to hearing instruments that represents the next phase in the process of making amplification useful and worth while. While no one wants to need any prosthetic device, the critical aspects of patient/client behavior in response to the placement of the instrument are "driven" by the concept of received value. If the instruments do what you want them to do: Let you hear more; understand what you hear significantly better; and, reduce the strain and tension of communication for both the speaker and the listener, they are worth it no matter what they cost. If the instruments do not do those things they are not worth it no matter what they cost.

ASSESSING CLIENT RESPONSE

Often there are immediate and spontaneous expressions of response to amplified sound. Primarily, these are the patient/client's reaction to sudden auditory change. For new users of amplification, this is based upon the contrast to their unaided auditory memory or imagery. For the previous user of hearing aids, it is the difference between the perceived quality of the sound of the old instrument compared to that of the new. The process includes points that are multi-faceted. On the one hand, the hearing aid specialist correlates the subjective reaction of the patient/client with the test data which may include aided responses. Assessment must be made as to how the patient/client is affected by adjustments and modifications. At the same time the professional must keep in mind the envisioned goals and that a change in the quality of the amplified sound may be one part of that "learning curve". It is important that satisfaction be obtained. However, if satisfaction is based upon the precise reproduction of an older and less effective hearing aid device, the beneficial effects of the learning curve and of the new technology are lost.

The dialogue between the patient/client and hearing instrument professional includes instruction and counseling. The emphasis must now shift from the techniques of adaptation to these methods. Verification tests may be performed to be sure of the appropriateness of the elicited response. Further adjustments may have to be made. While these were features of the pre-fitting process (before), they will now also be part of the post-fitting process. As the focus of attention shifts to the answering of questions in great depth, there needs to be an agenda of specific points to be covered before the session is concluded.

There is little disagreement about the importance of answering the patient/client's questions when they occur. Throughout the rehabilitation process, it is counterproductive to postpone answering them. Often such dialogue may take the professional on what appears to be a tangential course. However, these questions are reflective of the thought processes of the patient/client and, as such, are organized in the way in which the patient/client understands them. Therefore, it may be of great benefit later as reinforcement of a particular point which needs repeated discussion. Moreover, it affords the hearing aid specialist useful clues and additional insight into the patient/client's attitude. Kodman (1973) stated that "The client who doesn't get the opportunity to talk about his problems is not likely to pursue counseling as an avenue of help."

COUNSELING AND REHABILITATION CONCEPTS

We repeatedly read or hear that the patient/client should be advised, or the patient/client should be counseled, or should receive instruction. What is the difference? Mindful of the risks of oversimplification, it may be helpful for our purpose to say that in instructing, the flow of information is predominantly one-way in nature. The communication of knowledge, facts and directions emanates from the person giving the instruction to the person to whom it is given. Counseling, in contrast, has a two-way orientation. Its definition refers to a mutual interchange of opinions, ideas and discussion. It is not enough for the individual seeking consultation to hear only the advice and opinions of the counselor. He/she must be a participant drawn into a mutual interchange of thought.

In advising, the patient/client is told what they should do based upon the experience of the professional. The only responsibility of the patient/client is to agree and follow the advise given to them. They do not, however, have a "vested interest" in the outcome, and, therefore, the responsibility is on the professional.

Counseling, on the other hand is the presentation of alternatives complete with a description of the consequences of each alternative from which the patient/client makes an informed choice. In this two-way interchange, the patient/client has a stake in the outcome, the consequences of the informed choice rest squarely where they belong, and the responsibility for a successful outcome is vested in the patient/client.

Repetition, inevitably, is part of the learning process and should not be avoided. We are taught that the most effective method for teaching is based upon the principle of fill, drain, and refill. The professional must not lose track of the agenda of items to be covered at any of the counseling sessions. Further, sharing the learning experience with a partner, caregiver, or relative is very important. When the patient/client leaves with the instrument there should be a reasonable understanding of their hearing and hearing loss, the hearing instrument(s), their operation and care, and reasonable expectations for the first few days of instrument use.

Before talking about specific applications of counseling techniques to the fitting of, and adaptation to, hearing instruments, it may be useful to say something about counseling itself. Kodman (1973) describes counseling relationships as an interaction between two persons, one desiring help and the other offering that help. He also points out that the counselor's success with a prospective hearing instrument user is greatly enhanced by the presence of three conditions: 1) accurate empathy, 2) unconditional positive regard and, 3) genuineness. The higher the degree to which the hearing instrument professional can integrate these requisites into counseling concepts and approach, the greater the effectiveness of these efforts.

Accurate empathy in Kodman's definition "is the degree to which the counselor understands the client's feelings." It requires readiness to listen even to the client's most innocuous feelings about the hearing problem and to respond to them fully. By so doing, the professional shows an understanding of the patient/client's point of view.

Unconditional positive regard means the acceptance of the patient/client as a person without restrictions or disapproval of behavior, and the extension of the best possible guidance the professional can render.

Genuineness relates to the personality of the hearing instrument professional. The capacity to be "real", not to be ill at ease, nor defensive, is critical. This genuineness is easily detected by the patient/client and establishes the basis for their working relationship. It requires the putting aside of facade and addressing the needs of the individual directly.

In agreement with Kodman's advising the counselor to avoid telling the client what to do in an autocratic manner, Sanders (1975) envisions the counselor's role as one which is aimed at helping the patient/client to find solutions to his/her problem. He advises the nondirective approach to counseling by, "assisting the client to make decisions rather than imposing them upon him."

In the summary of his report, Brooks (1979) states: ". . . . hearing aid users who receive counseling make better and more effective use of their hearing aids then those who are merely supplied with a hearing aid with basic operating instructions."

Counseling is the dominant factor in Zelski's (1979) seven point approach to guiding the hearing instrument wearer to the successful use of amplification. He believes that if patients/clients: "feel that the person fitting them with an aid cares about them and knows what is wrong with them, then that hearing impaired person begins to feel safe communicating with a fitter." It is crucial for the hearing instrument professional to "recognize the reaching out by the client, as opposed to just talking, and guide the client properly."

Sanders (1975) states that " . . . orientation and counseling of the potential hearing aid user should constitute the hub of the program to insure effective use of amplification."and that: "Support during the period of adjustment to the acceptance of the aid will be, in many cases, the factor that insures success."

A similar philosophy of combining amplification and counseling towards achieving maximum benefit from the hearing instrument was expressed years earlier in a different milieu by Reeve (1954). He found that there are those who adapt to amplification rapidly and succeed with relatively little guidance. However, for those whose auditory images had deteriorated by having adjusted to years of partial hearing, he strongly advocated aural rehabilitation. To counsel the first time hearing instrument user in the auditory re-education process, Reeve devised a manual in the form of a series of pre- and post-fitting letters of instruction for the patient/client and for a friend (or family member) acting as coach.

It is evident that the emphasis on counseling to maximize amplification benefits is not a new idea nor current trend. Depending on the person expressing the view, counseling ranges from unrelenting advocacy of an extensive and formal protocol of auditory rehabilitation to a minimum of written instruction. Gough (1976), believes that the basic difficulty with adult rehabilitation programs is due to the interpretation of the word rehabilitation by various professionals. He contrasts those hearing instrument professionals, who offer no counseling with those who recommend a formal and comprehensive program which begins with a hearing aid fitting.

Views vary considerably as to the true starting point of auditory rehabilitation. Perhaps it does begin, as Gough (1976) maintains, with the hearing aid fitting. Perhaps it actually begins when the individual makes the first inquiry into some form of hearing help. The information with the first elements of history taking and the counseling that follows the evaluation may be the modest beginning.

From time to time, an informed member of the hearing health care delivery team speaks of an idealized approach to aural rehabilitation. Such an approach would include all possible professional disciplines. Not just those with medical, diagnostic and instrumental skills, but psychologists, social workers, vocational counselors and others. Such programs are the exception rather than the rule and are available for only a very few.

Many hearing impaired persons, as viewed by hearing instrument professionals may not need a formal rehabilitation process. They clearly need to have individual needs identified and addressed. The emphasis is placed on the importance of providing the guidance and counseling the patient/client is willing to pursue. It is limited only by the level and complexity of material that the hearing instrument professional is willing, or able, to provide.

While this chapter is adult oriented, we recognize the differing needs and considerations that are age specific when it comes to counseling. The focus of this chapter is on the many facets of counseling which are common to all categories.

Rehabilitation of the hearing impaired child follows an observed professional protocol. The interaction of multiple disciplines from the moment of identification on the habilitative/rehabilitative process is the necessary ingredient. Exceptions, of course, do exist. In the unfortunate instances when they do occur they are often for geographic, social, economic or other reasons. Should the hearing instrument professional encounter a case in which a child's medical or educational needs have not been met, he/she should concentrate on providing informed guidance and referral to the appropriate professional team member.

The adult population, even in countries where hearing instruments and services are provided by the government, seldom avails itself of the counseling services that may enhance the amplification benefits. In the United States, private practitioners provide most forms of aural rehabilitation. It is the hearing instrument professional who provides most of the counseling that takes place, as well as the other post-fitting care.

It is essential that the hearing instrument professional recognize situations in which the help of other professional disciplines can be beneficial, and/or know where appropriate services are available. A current list of community resources is an important tool. While the patient/client may not be willing to pursue the recommended course, it remains the hearing instrument professional's task to make the best possible effort on their behalf.

FAMILY MEMBER INTERACTION

In the post-fitting process, a number of items need to be covered by counseling. The first to be discussed with a new hearing aid user, is the nature and severity of the hearing loss. While the patient/client is the principal participant, the role played by family and significant others, often has a direct bearing on the success of the aural rehabilitation. Much can be gained, if most of what is imparted to the patient/client is learned by the family. This is particularly true in regard to reasonable expectations. It is frustrating for the hearing instrument professional to have the rehabilitation progress negated by patient/client and family pulling in opposite directions. Therefore, let's review the role, participation and counseling of the family members and interested others.

Beginning with pre-fitting counseling and through the instrument selection process, including orientation, instruction, and follow-up sessions, it is advantageous to have a family member or caregiver present and involved. Often, it is the spouse or other family member who urges the hearing-impaired individual to do something about the problem. Frequently, though well intended, family members may be inconsiderate and create discord because they lack understanding of the problem. They can be a source of a great encouragement if they can learn about the hearing loss and understand its consequences. Only in this way can they adjust their expectations to reasonable goals and achievable results.

The negative attitudes of family members need urgent change if the patient/client is to make a successful adjustment to hearing instrument use. The family must learn that what they describe as "he hears when he wants to", is not capricious behavior but, rather, a consequence of the loss. They should understand the relationship between the degree and slope of the client's loss to his ability to hear at various distances. They should know how his speech discrimination skills influence his ability to understand in changing conversational environments. Above all, they must be counseled regarding those unrealistic expectations from hearing instruments so that they do not hinder the progress of the first-time user of hearing instruments.

Attitudes of family members regarding the hearing impairment of relatives include a variety of personal and subjective aspects. It often parallels the known biases and attitudes of society in general. How family members react to the one with hearing loss is influenced by other aspects of their relationship with that person. The difficulties hearing loss imposes on the patient/client and family have both general and specific effects on behavior. For the patient/client, the effects are often disproportionately magnified. Effects for family members may also be extensive. It would be folly to disregard the complex psychological makeup of patient/client and family interactions.

When the hearing instrument professional is aware of these human dynamics, it can be a significant help. It can enhance the effectiveness of the counseling efforts. In some cases, the emotional problems are beyond the professional's capabilities or scope of practice and the patient/client requires psychological referral. Being able to guide the patient/client and family in seeking additional professional help demonstrates both competence and a mastery of one's craft. In addition, to both the patient/client and family members gaining an understanding of hearing loss, it is useful if they learn about the operation (and care) of the instrument. They must also learn the specific "do's" and "don'ts" in communicating with a first time hearing instrument user.

By the time the point of post-fitting care is reached, both patient/client and family members should have learned something about hearing loss. As the patient/client begins to adapt to hearing instrument amplification, it is useful to make sure he/she has the facts straight. It helps the client and the professional, from the beginning, if the client knows how the ear works, how sound transmission and sensory components function and what parts of the auditory system are involved. This information will have been presented in a simple, straightforward manner in the discussion following the hearing evaluation.

Some individuals show considerable interest. Most do not. As a result, discussion of the subject has to be concise. The hearing instrument professional's answers to the most frequently asked questions can be made more satisfactory with such background information. The question, "What caused my hearing loss?" may have already been answered medically, but may come up repeatedly. Often the professional has to answer the question: "What percentage of my hearing have I lost?" Even though the question is simple, the answer is not. The difficulty arises from the lack of good information about what constitutes 0% hearing loss and what is 100%. In most cases, the question is based upon the relative idea: "Compared to what my hearing used to be, how much in percentages have I lost?". It is almost impossible to answer accurately, but, if you try to explain that difficulty, you sound like you are quibbling. The fact that hearing can be measured and expressed in numbers is both the source of the clarity - and the confusion.

PSYCHOLOGICAL CONSIDERATIONS

As important as it is for the hearing instrument professional to be able to deal with the measurable aspects of hearing loss, it is imperative to be aware of the psychological effects arising from that problem. These effects may not be measurable and may elude objectification (Nelson, 1969). To accurately identify the psychological aspects of hearing loss demands considerable time and effort. The hearing instrument professional and the patient/client should do their utmost to understand "the emotional and behavioral consequences of hearing loss" as suggested by Joensen and Saunders (1984).

In the initial stages of post-fitting care, the hearing instrument professional no longer views the patient/client as a stranger. From the history and other information obtained in previous encounters, the professional has a (general) picture of the patient/client's health and potential infirmities, as well as some observations of the individual's attitude regarding hearing loss. As these post-fitting sessions proceed, more of the emotional aspects may be revealed.

Joensen and Saunders (1984) describe them as "a range of difficult emotions that include fear, depression, frustration, insecurity and a sense of isolation." Misconceptions about hearing impairment nurtured through centuries have much to do with evoking these negative attitudes towards hearing loss. The word "absurd" means without hearing in Arabic. "Understanding them" concludes Joensen and Saunders, "can help the hearing handicapped person as he learns to live with his impairment."

The hearing instrument professional can contribute significantly to the outcome of these post-fitting sessions, if he/she can successfully modify the patient/client's ability to be constructive in dealing with their emotions. The professional must encourage dialogue in which the negative aspects of the patient/client's behavior can be revealed and related to their relationship with the hearing impairment. Assisting the patient/client to become aware of the relationship of his/her psychological and social response to the hearing loss is a significant step in helping them to accept methods of coping with the problem. "Will my hearing get worse?" is a question the hearing impaired ask those whose counsel they seek. Regardless of answers received from other professionals, this question will be asked repeatedly during post-fitting care.

The relationship of gain and output requirements of the hearing aid to the degree of hearing loss must be discussed. In addition, the question of progressivity and dealing with the needed amplification should be discussed. The hearing instrument professional must be prepared to explain the cause/effect relationship between an increase of needed acoustic power and the subsequent rise in sound awareness. The patient/client's understanding of this process will be helpful in later sessions as well as aiding in the psychological acceptance of the instrument.

In our experience, the expressed purpose of those who decide to pursue help through amplification is to "get the words"; to "understand speech", without appreciable interference of other sounds. The major problem with their hearing impairment that troubles them the most relates to communication: understanding what others are saying.

Ramsdell (1970) described three psychological levels of auditory function:(1) the symbolic level, which refers to sound used in the process of communication, (2) the warning level, which refers to hearing permitting one to respond to signals for action or danger;

and (3) and primitive level, which refers to the auditory background of all daily living at which we perceive the constantly changing incidental noises around us that connect us to the world.

Loss of any one level of these auditory functions has its psychological consequences. Ramsdell (1970), assigned the most pronounced emotional effects to the loss of background sounds he called the primitive level of hearing. Although the hearing impaired person may not be consciously aware of not hearing these sounds, the absence of this primitive level of hearing may, in part, constitute the reason for the depression which often accompanies certain types of hearing impairment.

In her book, *A Natural History of the Senses,* Diane Ackerman (1990) makes the statement: "Hearing loss disconnects one from life's logic". Having the client realize his emotional response to the loss of these auditory functions may facilitate adjustment to the abrupt change in these three hearing levels when so many sounds are "reinstated" through amplification.

Another item with major psychological implications is the onset of hearing loss. Questions about when the patient/client was first aware of hearing loss, and when did manifestations of its presence occur are important in getting to understand both the nature and impact of the problem. People who suffer from sudden loss of hearing are the exception in an hearing instrument practice. The majority of patient/clients come with a history of gradual decline in hearing acuity, often going back ten to fifteen years or more.

Many of these individuals insist that they have heard well until just about six months to a year ago. This self-assessment, inaccurate as it may be, frequently relates to the effect of the last decline which is remembered. The patient/client's belief regarding the onset of the loss cannot be ignored, because it may be one of the obstacles to be overcome. Minimizing both the extent and duration of hearing loss is common among the hearing impaired. It can become an obstruction to effective rehabilitation. The professional should be alert to this expression of client attitudes and bring it into the discussion. Another important part of the post-fitting counseling is that of discussing those elements of the hearing impairment which could impose valid limitations on benefits of amplification.

CLIENT INSTRUCTION AND POST-FITTING CARE

Counseling the patient/client regarding various aspects of hearing loss requires that certain points must be discussed in depth.

Consider, for example, the geriatric patient with mild-to-moderate hearing loss whose speech discrimination is extremely poor. These patients/clients may derive greater benefit from the use of hearing aids if they understand the relationship of aging and speech comprehension. The hearing instrument professional must make clear what hearing instruments can and cannot do. The professional should explain to the patient/client that lipreading (speechreading) is not limited to the deaf, and that a combination of training to improve visual skills coupled with amplification may produce greater benefits than either one of these alone.

Hearing loss and hearing instrument use, as they relate to the patient/client's occupation, warrant careful attention and should be thoroughly discussed. Effective on-the-job communication and occupational safety is a particularly important consideration. For example, the ability to tell where the sound comes from (localization), which is often impaired when hearing loss is present, has special significance in certain work situations. Pointing out an ordinary event that may turn into a matter of life and death may serve as a dramatic illustration of one's need to locate the source of sound. With careful attention to directional balance at the time of hearing instrument selection and fitting, significant improvement may be achieved in this binaural function.

In a few instances directional balance cannot be attained because of underlying central problems beneath the configuration of the hearing loss, or as a result of significant unilateral impairment. Much more commonly, however, insistence on monaural amplification, when bilateral loss is present, is the culprit. In either case, the more the patient/client can learn about the limitations of monaural hearing and the benefits of binaurality, the more realistic the expectations. Patient/clients will benefit from knowing why they may or may not achieve localization. They will appreciate the hearing instrument professional's explanation of some of the interaural relationships, such as the concept of "dichotic time difference as prime determinant of auditory localization" (Libby, 1980).

The immediate objective in post-fitting care is to prepare and guide the patient/client in the use of hearing aids in the work environment. It may be beneficial, therefore, to talk about the nature and level of noise at the work site. On one level, it may alert the patient/client to the possible need for some form of noise control. On another level, it may acquaint him/her with the existence of state and federal laws/regulations regarding environmental noise protection. He/she may also learn that there is a field of expertise which is available regarding these matters. It is possible that noise at the patient/client's work-place was a contributing factor to the advance of the hearing loss or, perhaps, even its cause.

In any event, the concern about the noise level at the work site is legitimate, since continued exposure to noise without adequate protection is detrimental to everyone. These concerns may increase when the individual's hearing is impaired and he/she is to use amplification for the first time.

Obviously, some instruction has already occurred. Once the initial adjustments and modifications of the instrument are complete, the focus of discussion should be on instruction of the patient/client in the operation of the instrument. This should be followed by instructions on how to use the hearing aid in various listening situations. The next step is the care of the instrument; and, the "do's" and "don'ts", which must be discussed thoroughly. The approach professionals follow in instructing the patient/client varies considerably. Some may follow a checklist of their own. Others may use the manufacturer's instruction booklet as a guide to cover essential points. There are those who prepare a list of their own instructions to augment those provided by instrument manufacturers.

If the professional provides written instruction material of his own, the manufacturer provided materials should be given to the patient/client as well. This suggestion has merit from practical as well as legal points of view. The material from the manufacturer generally contains the F.D.A. required statements. It also has diagrams and pictures, which provide the user with a quick reference to refresh his/her memory. Professionals should not forget about the legal requirements for appropriate referencing in the F.D.A. regulations, (801.420(c)), (801.421(b)).

If there is conflicting information contained in the two sets of instruction material, it should be pointed out and explained. In any event, it is important that the patient/client has instruction about the operation and care of the aid to which he/she can refer when the need arises.

One consideration, before proceeding with detailed instruction of instrument operation, is the language level of the patient/client. The hearing instrument professional and the patient/client will be helped by knowing that they have a common understanding when mentioning terms denoting parts of the instrument. (e.g., ear hook, switch, volume control, battery compartment, etc.,) One should use terminology that is common in the instruction booklet provided with the hearing instrument.

We have emphasized the importance of family members being present at these post-fitting sessions. It is helpful if those who live with, or are in frequent contact with the patient/client know something about the operation and care of the instrument. Family members may be called upon to step in and lend a hand to the very young and/or the elderly whose dexterity is limited. If the hearing instrument user becomes ill or needs to be hospitalized, aggravation and frustration may be avoided by a family member who knows enough to assist with effective hearing instrument care.

Counseling the patient/client in effective hearing instrument use should begin with instructions relating to the operation of the device. Start with the location and shape of the controls. Show the controls on the instrument, as well as where they are illustrated in the instruction booklet.

Having identified the location, position and shape of the controls (volume or gain control, on-off switch, telephone switch, battery compartment, etc.), explain what their functions are - and how to manipulate them. Go through several trials until the individual acquires some feel for using the controls. The hearing instruments are set commonly to a comfortable loudness prior to instruction on instrument operation. It is not unusual for the patient/client, in response to the professional's repeated questions about perceived loudness, to have asked "How do I make it lower?" It may be practical to repeat instructions relating to the volume control and to finding the position providing the point of comfortable loudness.

One of the most important areas to cover in this instruction is how the instrument is switched on and off. In some instrument designs the battery must be completely removed. For others, a partial or full opening of the battery compartment is required. There are models in which the volume control serves as the on-off switch. Many models use an O-T-M switch in which the O represents the off position. Switched to M, the aid is on and sound is picked up by the microphone. In the T position, the microphone is disconnected and the instrument is in the inductive telecoil, telephone pickup, mode.

Once the subject of telephone use is introduced, it is necessary to explain which telephones are and are not compatible with the hearing instruments telephone coil. In discussing telephone use, considerations should be given as well to hearing instruments which do not have telephone coils. The new hearing instrument user should be coached in the use of the telephone with such instruments. Some hearing aid users switch to the "T" position to "shut off" their hearing aids and often assume that it is thus turned off. The professional should explain the difference between not hearing environmental sounds on the "T" position and the actual "off" position.

There are other configurations in switch design. Some hearing instruments have a separate telephone switch. Others have a H-N tone switch. The "H" position reduces low-frequency amplification to a specific value. Sometimes, the "H" position is referred to as a noise suppressor switch. On some hearing instruments, it is actually a separate switch requiring practice to locate and use appropriately.

The location of the battery compartment should be discussed. This discussion should center on how it is opened and closed. The user needs to know what kind of battery is used and how it may be inserted and removed. Repeated practice is required if the battery compartment serves also as an on-off switch. Instruct the patient/client to inspect battery surfaces before insertion in the instrument's compartment, and demonstrate how these should be cleaned.

After the client is familiar with the position and handling of the controls, it is time to demonstrate and practice the insertion and removal of the aid or earmold, depending on the type of hearing instrument.

There are significant differences with insertion and removal methods for in-the-ear (ITE), in-the-canal- (ITC) and completely-in-the-canal (CIC) instruments compared to methods with devices using earmolds, i.e., behind the ear (BTE), and eyeglass or body worn instruments. There are marked differences, too, in several aspects of instruction about the role, handling and care of these instruments.

At this stage of instruction, the hearing instrument professional is concerned with instrument insertion and removal and assisting the new user of the instrument in doing both correctly. Written instruction may be of little help when ears, instruments and/ or molds are of such variety of shapes. This is especially critical when the patient/client's manual dexterity or spatial orientation may vary widely. Thus, the main thrust of instruction is experiential and practical: How to grasp and hold the mold (or instrument). What part of it is directed toward the canal? What should be the position of the hand holding the mold relative to the ear? What is the role of the other hand in assisting the process?

Another matter the hearing instrument professional should address is acoustic feedback. It is likely that acoustic feedback will occur during instruction of the patient/client about insertion and removal of the instrument or mold. The individual must be counseled about the cause of this whistling sound and recognize that it is not a sign of instrument malfunction. It is essential that the patient/client understand this aspect of acoustic feedback and be instructed in its avoidance.

One less frequent item of instruction is about "plugging in" and "unplugging" hearing aid receiver cords. This concerns only users of body type and some CROS and BICROS aids. In some instances, there may be different connector plugs on the ends of a cord and the polarity has to be observed, if they are to function properly.

Once initial instruction and practice in instrument operation is complete, a new set of instructions should follow: This set should deal with the effective use of the instrument. It should provide the client with guidance in how to get accustomed to amplification. It should describe how to handle various listening situations. The user must learn how to listen again with the hearing instrument.

Most instruction manuals advise beginning hearing instrument users to start their hearing instrument experience in quiet surroundings, preferably at home. Listening to one person only, with the volume set to a comfortably loud level, may be the initial step. Invariably, hearing instrument professionals advise that for the first few days the instrument should be worn for an hour or two, followed by a rest period. It is recommended that wearing time be increased and rest periods become fewer and shorter. The user should listen to background sounds and practice identifying them. This advice is practical and the caution is all to the good. Only a few years ago, a large percentage of professionals did not permit the patient/client to leave the office wearing their new instruments. Rather, they were put in the box following instruction and suggested that the use of the instruments begin at home.

When teaching the patient/client to use the instruments, one point requires considerable counseling skill and repeated effort from the professional. Namely, it is to impress upon the individual that learning gradual use of the hearing aid is VERY different from the concept of partial use of the instrument. That is, too many hearing instrument users find it emotionally comforting to rationalize their hearing deficiency by clinging to the reading glasses parallel for their use of hearing instruments. They feel a need to minimize their hearing loss by insisting on using amplification with moderation. Some hearing instrument patient/clients hold to this concept so strongly that they extend the advice intended for the first days of use to months or years. They insist that they are following the hearing instrument professional or physician's instructions. They declare themselves "slow learners" when in reality they become part-time wearers of the instruments and most likely no learners at all. If the person wears the instrument to church every week for a year they HAVE NOT worn hearing aids for a year. They have worn the hearing aids for one day, 52 times, with a weeks pause in between. No one learns how to live with amplification that way!

The literature suggests that most adult beginners wear their instruments for extended periods from the beginning. Most leave the professional's office wearing the device. With exceptions, this practice evidently works, but the professional should be alert to those cases where extended use is inadvisable. The professional should recognize those clients who require a gradual adjustment period. All new users of hearing instruments should be counseled about the world of sound they will encounter, i.e., street noise, wind noise, traffic noise, and other sounds of the environment. Properly forewarned, the majority will cope without difficulty. Preparing the hearing instrument user to cope with the distractions of new sounds in a positive manner is just as essential for those who adapt readily as for those who proceed in a gradual step-wise manner.

In keeping with our discussion of the psychological correlates of hearing loss, Goldberg (1977) offers an explanation. He describes the task of adapting to sounds which have not been heard for a long time by directing attention to the "auditory confusion" faced, regardless of whether one's hearing has been corrected medically or by means of amplification. He states that: "persons with hearing defects, unable to hear certain sounds, will develop an impaired auditory memory due to a lack of acoustical information." When these sounds suddenly become audible, a challenge to this impaired auditory image occurs. The abrupt confrontation with the heretofore unheard sounds - results in an auditory confusion. To many, this experience is difficult at first. Some become so frustrated they may refuse further experimentation with amplification. Yet, the secret of succeeding is just the opposite; to persevere and to keep using the hearing instruments tenaciously.

To reinforce the concept of adaptation, it is necessary to make every effort to keep the patient/client's expectations within realistic bounds. Frequently remind the hearing instrument user not to expect instant success - regardless of initial benefits. The patient/client should not assume that the hearing instrument will do the job by itself. Barnett (1974) suggested an appropriate bit of advice to give to the new hearing instrument wearer: "Just as he learned to ignore the insignificant sounds soon after birth, the wearer of a hearing aid must learn the same process over again. Admittedly it is harder to do this as an adult, but it can be done, and only by this process of re-education can one learn to be satisfied with a hearing aid, and to get all the pleasure and benefit possible from it."

It is reasonable to instruct the individual to concentrate first upon conversation with one person and gradually expand it to include more individuals. Nearly every instruction booklet has some directive on how to practice hearing instrument use in groups, at church, in theaters, and while listening to television and/or radio. There are basic rules common to developing listening skills in each of these situations. The ability to concentrate on the speaker against a background of noise can be acquired gradually and with consistent practice. Even then, there are limitations imposed on the hearing instrument wearer's ability to distinguish between similar, but not identical, speech sounds. In spite of missing some words, one should learn to follow the pace of the conversation, play or sermon. Much depends, too, on the range of the hearing function, such as loudness discomfort thresholds and the difference in threshold sensitivity between the two ears.

The subject of monaural versus binaural hearing is certain to come up in post-fitting counseling. Regardless of how thoroughly this issue has been discussed at the time of testing, hearing instrument selection and fitting, the professional will find it necessary and useful to explain, repeatedly, both the consequences and limitations of monaural hearing.

The main reason this subject surfaces frequently is based upon the difficulty beginning hearing instrument users encounter due to an absence of localization abilities (or a sense of directional balance). This is unavoidable when the new hearing instrument user is limited to monaural input (amplified or unamplified).

Some people have no choice but to learn to live with monaural hearing—CROS and BICROS notwithstanding—because one of their ears cannot be helped by amplification. However, since these (CROS and BICROS) are routing devices, there is the ability to capture all of the acoustic elements in 360 degrees of the auditory field. Hearing instrument users, with bilateral hearing impairment, who are wearing a single instrument by choice, need to understand the incontrovertible evidence of the past ten years. Studies on auditory deprivation (Silverman, 1993) have demonstrated that the ability of the unaided ear to retain it's capacity to discriminate speech deteriorates over a period of years. This is in contrast to the aided ear - in which there is almost no deterioration in discrimination skills. Further, after approximately 18 months, the difference in these discrimination scores remains, EVEN if the other ear is fitted with an instrument. In the auditory system it appears that if you do not use it, you will loss it.

This well documented effect is markedly accelerated in the elderly. Jerger (1993), suggests that the absence of hearing instrument fitting in some older hearing impaired citizens may be involved in the development of phonemic regression. There is clear evidence of the need for early identification of sensitivity shift (hearing loss) and prompt hearing instrument fitting to forestall permanent and irreversible effects.

An important aspect of instruction is that of counseling the hearing impaired individual in maintaining visual contact during conversation. "The eye is a natural ally to the ear. Spoken sounds which can be confusing to the ear may be distinguished by the eye." (Sonotone). In augmenting amplification with visual clues, one needs to observe not only the speaker's face and lips, but facial expressions and gestures as well. While the severely hearing handicapped may need formal training in lipreading, all hearing aid users benefit from combining hearing and vision into a more effective "listening attitude." Hearing instrument professionals need to know if the patient/client has visual problems which would limit or reduce their ability to use sight.

For many individuals, as it became more difficult to understand, and the effort of trying to understand words became more frustrating, the individual gradually stopped paying attention. Eventually, inattention may have become a habit. It requires considerable effort to train oneself to concentrate and to become a better listener.

The importance of having a member of the family present to learn the instructions given is stressed. The hearing instrument professional should try to convey through the person accompanying the patient/client, the key points of instruction to the rest of the family. This may be achieved by having printed instruction material available for that purpose. Urging the family to be understanding, encouraging and supportive are key points in family counseling. Another important point of instruction is to caution family members not to start talking to the new hearing instrument user, abruptly. Instruct them to start with a one-word "attention getter". Facing the person and speaking neither too loud nor too soft from a reasonable distance and without exaggeration are useful reminders.

An experiment that any one can perform consists of standing in front of a mirror and trying as hard as you can to shout and smile at the same time. It cannot be done. Therefore, EVERY TIME you raise your voice to someone—you ALWAYS convey—ANGER—whether you are angry or not. Sooner or later, the target of that anger will respond to perceived anger with real anger.

HEARING AID MAINTENANCE

Instructing the patient/client in the care of hearing instrument(s) is often done with a list of "do's" and "don't's." Instruction books include a variety of such directives which may be useful to the new hearing instrument wearer. If the professional finds it necessary to add to the instructions given, a list of the most frequently stated don'ts follows:

Do not drop, or throw a hearing aid.

Do not leave the instrument in a car parked in the sun, on a window sill, or near any heat source.

Do not allow the hearing instrument to be soaked by moisture.

Do not immerse it in water, swim or shower with it on. Do not expose it to steam bath, sauna or direct rain.

Do not apply hair spray, cold cream or similar items of beauty care while wearing the hearing aid. (They may either harm the plastic or clog the microphone opening.)

Do not leave spent batteries in the hearing instrument.

Do not dispose of spent batteries in an open fire, furnace or fireplace.

Do not carry batteries loose in pockets, purse or handbag as contact with keys, coins or metal objects will discharge them.

Do not refrigerate batteries. Keep them in a dry place at room temperature.

Do not use alcohol or cleaning fluid to clean the earmold or hearing instrument.

Do not lubricate the instrument or any of its controls.

Do not clean the hearing instrument with pins or other such objects.

Do not adjust or change settings of tone and output trimmers unless instructed to do so by the hearing instrument professional.

Do not take the hearing instrument apart or attempt to repair it.

Do not place the hearing aid within reach of pets or youngsters.

Do not keep a battery in the hearing aid if it is not to be worn for extended periods.

EARMOLD AND SOUND CHANNEL CARE

Keep the sound channel of the earmold free of wax and other debris. Demonstrate how the user is to do this and with what tools. In that a large percentage of instruments are ITE or ITC, it is important that the client be aware of the difference in handling the task of wax removal. While some instruction booklets have a separate section about ITE and other types of instruments, it is useful to point out differences in handling the earmold of a BTE instrument as opposed to the sound channel of an ITC.

There is considerable uniformity in the instructions provided by most manufacturers relative to how the sound channels of ITE and ITC aids can be kept free of wax. In almost every case, a small wax removal loop is provided for that purpose. It is relatively simple to instruct the user about cleaning the canal tip using the loop. The user should not clean the aid with any liquid and should be so instructed. Wiping the aid with a soft tissue or towel is the usual advice given to keep the earmold surface clean.

With respect to earmolds, there are instruction brochures which suggest cleaning the earmold with soap and water after it has been separated from the earhook of the instrument. The patient/client has to be sure that all moisture is removed from the tubing and sound bore before the mold is reconnected to the earhook. While there are many hearing instrument users who follow this procedure without difficulty, there are far more who do not. There are several risks in the frequent removal of the mold from the earhook. These are:

1) an accelerated reduction of the elasticity of the tubing.
2) a "loose" fit.
3) increasingly easy separation of the tubing from the earhook.

These, added to the probability of incomplete removal of moisture, make another less drastic method desirable. Providing the user with a wax loop to keep the tip of the sound channel of the earmold free of obstruction, and suggesting he/she clean the exterior, may be a wiser approach. Supplying the user with one of the disinfectant sprays which may be applied to a tissue or cloth to wipe the earmold is a practical addition to effective care. A more thorough cleaning of the mold can be done by the hearing instrument professional at the time of tubing change.

Clinical experience suggests that repeated instruction about the need for periodic change of the earmold tubing are often ignored by the patient/client. The "safest" and most effective practice is to have the hearing aid specialist replace the earmold tubing and earhook at regular intervals. This practice insures the best fit and coupling. If it is desirable for the user to be able to change the tubing, the earmold can have a variety of available connector elbows. It can make the task of tube change simpler and error free. Earmolds used with body aids can be separated from the receiver for cleaning, washing and drying. This is the safest and more practical method for the user to learn.

OTHER CONSIDERATIONS

Should the new hearing instrument user develop a skin irritation, rash or swelling where the plastics of the instrument come in contact with the skin, he/she should contact their hearing instrument professional or see their physician, immediately.

For most people, earwax (cerumen) is a normal occurrence. However, the wearing of any type of earmold, as well as an ITE, ITC or CIC instrument may accelerate the accumulation of that cerumen. It can be removed easily by a physician and one should be consulted, if the accumulation interferes with hearing.

There are still a number of older hearing impaired individuals wearing body instruments. Others wear a variety of instruments - such as CROS and BICROS configurations. A number of these instruments have receivers or connecting cords which can become intermittent or dead through wear and tear. Users of such devices should be reminded to keep a spare cord and taught how to plug and unplug it properly.

Hearing instrument users have been instructed not to expose their aids to moisture. Those who perspire frequently or profusely should be aware of the availability of dehumidifier kits and how these are used to remove potentially damaging moisture from the instruments.

Virtually every manufacturer's instruction brochure has a section devoted to trouble shooting for those instances when the instrument does not function properly. The patient/client should become familiar with these recommended procedures.

Ultimately, it is helpful to talk to patient/clients about the fact that hearing instruments can malfunction. An instrument of the highest quality can fail anytime and may need occasional service. How this situation is treated by the hearing instrument professional must be included in the discussion of care and maintenance of hearing instruments.

One of the most important items of concern, as the instruction session nears its conclusion, is that of arranging post-fitting visits. The professional should explain that he/she wants a report of the user's experiences, observations and questions. Inform the patient/client that this report is needed to determine what additional tests may be required to verify his/her performance with the instrument. Patient/clients will often want to know how many times they may have to come to the office. While there is no answer to how many times a certain person will need to be seen, there is no question about the "first" recheck and about projecting additional sessions as the situation may require. Stress, too, the importance of periodic visits. This gives one the opportunity to impress upon patient/clients the importance of post-fitting care and indicates the hearing instrument professional's interest in guiding and assisting them to achieve maximum benefit from their hearing instruments.

RECHECK SESSIONS

Through several preceding pages, we identified a list of situations and techniques about which to counsel and instruct the hearing instrument user and his/her family. Some of them were emphasized as musts for all cases. One of the most critical exercises that assists in the adaptation process involves reading. Insist that patients read ALOUD for 20 minutes per day during the first thirty days. The individual practices listening to the sounds of different phonemes in the language THROUGH the instrument. After one month, there is a major increase in discrimination ability and the effect is often marked improvement in both ability and confidence with the instruments.

The scenario was the fitting session - that major event is the aural rehabilitation sequence - at which the hearing instruments were fit and, if necessary, modified to meet the patient/client's acoustic requirements. It was the point at which the patient/client was about to leave the hearing instrument professional's office with the hearing aids in place and begin to experience a new sound environment.

The adaptation process, depending on the particular method used by the professional, may have included tests to ascertain if the aided response was near to the envisioned target goal. In many instances such verification measurements are done after the person has used the instrument for a few days or weeks.

In regard to instruction, there will be areas not yet touched upon because the client has not gained enough hearing instrument experience to benefit from some aspects of the counseling process. Consequently, points of emphasis and the depth to which some of these areas have been dealt with vary significantly from one case to another. There is merit in the hearing instrument professional reminding himself of this fact now that the fitting session is completed. The next event in the post-fitting care is of significance in guiding the patient/client in becoming a successful hearing instrument user.

One of the first things one should note is whether the patient/client arrives for the recheck session wearing the instruments. Though it could be expected that the client who comes without devices may be signalling rejection of their use, such is not always the case. It may be due to difficulty with inserting the instruments or earmolds. Possibly, it could be due to decreased manual dexterity. If the patient/client arrives wearing his/her instruments, the hearing instrument professional should note whether they are inserted properly, whether they are turned on and/or set to a certain gain position. Although these observations may tell one a great deal, they do not reveal how long, how frequently, or how regularly the instruments were worn prior to the post-fitting visit. Were the instruments worn full - time-from the outset - or was wearing time increased gradually?

While available statistics indicate that a large percentage of hearing instrument users wear their devices all or most of the time (Surr, et al, 1979) (Oja and Schow, 1984) (Broenen, 1983), there are those who use their devices only occasionally. Much can be done at this early stage to help channel the first time user in the right direction. If instrument use was sporadic, were the underlying causes predominantly auditory or attitudinal? Was instrument use limited to only desirable listening situations, avoiding their use in more distracting environments? Such a first time user may report fairly positive experience with his aids, but may become only a part time user. The patient/client is hardly in a position to present a true picture of his/her progress with amplification, if such is the case.

If the instruments were used mainly in acoustically difficult listening conditions such as restaurants, meeting rooms, church, etc., the reported experience would be most likely unpleasant and predominately negative. An individual having such experiences would be apt to conclude that all hearing experiences will be bad and that hearing aids make a lot of noise and have limited value. If that person continues hearing instrument use at all, he/she will probably be only a part time user.

The professional can learn much from listening to the patient/client's account of experiences with amplification, including early and developing habits in instrument use. At this point in the adaptation process, management of the new hearing instrument user truly becomes a practical science with a prime objective: doing! "Practical sciences," Griffing (1978) suggests, "are concerned with relationships between means and ends." The hearing instrument professional "is guided by results and adjusts the means to accomplish desired ends." The fundamental point is to achieve positive outcome.

Many useful clues are derived from analyzing the user's reported experiences and verbal comments. Some of these reveal "attitude" and may establish the direction in which the counseling should be heading. Other clues, coupled with data gained from verification tests, often result in modifications of the hearing aid and coupler (earmold) acoustic performance. These modifications can yield significant benefit and improve acceptance of the instruments. In many instances the patient/client's decision to keep the hearing aids is dependent on these acoustic modifications. Early post-fitting care presupposes the hearing instrument professional can identify and "sift out" those users showing evidence of making progress on schedule from those requiring more personal attention, counseling and instrument adjustments. In daily practice, hearing instrument professionals find ample evidence to support Kapteyn's (1977) findings which show that: the longer the process of an individual's adjustment to hearing aid use, the more his/her use of amplification decreases. Conversely, those whose progress is faster in adapting to hearing instrument use wear them more consistently.

It is in this first post-fitting session that information gathered by the professional establishes whether the user has made progress in the first weeks of hearing aid use. One must decide in what procedural order modifications, adjustments and reinforcement counseling are needed to achieve maximum benefit. The data needed to make these decisions may be derived from a review of how the user is doing with the instruments. Such a review may include:

1. Verification of performance;
2. Assessment of satisfaction;
3. Probing of client attitude.

MEASUREMENT CONSIDERATIONS

Determining the extent of hearing enhancement may include how the selected instruments improve hearing thresholds, aided discrimination and aided threshold of discomfort at target frequencies. These measures form some of the substance of the verification process. If the protocol included some form of these tests at the time of initial fitting, one may refer to the recheck session as re-verification. It provides data which show whether the desired aided thresholds were actually attained or approximated with the selected hearing aids.

Verification measurements will generally include sound field assessments for determining the difference between unaided and aided thresholds. That is, the "functional gain." The sound field procedure may be part of the particular fitting method the hearing instrument professional uses to select and fit the instruments. The concept upon which many of the fitting methods are based has been dealt with in other chapters. As such, the concept itself is not new and the variety of methods devised have a long history.

One could make a long list of the names of the methods their developers formulated. And, it is not our purpose to delve into a comparison of their merits. It is useful, nevertheless, to say that the effort(s) of these investigators had a number of objectives in common:

1) To establish a reliable and repeatable test to measure hearing levels by using or modifying existing equipment and procedures, or developing new ones;
2) To relate to these data a defensible formula to establish a goal to be reached by amplification; and
3) To verify how closely that goal was attained.

Lybarger (1978), in reviewing the history of selective amplification, describes eight fitting methods going back to Hutchinson in 1905. Keith and Sinninger (1978) review twelve different methods. Among those, Lybarger's method is considered to be the best. It bases its formulae on hearing threshold data.

Influenced by Lybarger's formulae, Berger's (1976) method is an example of calculating the desired goals of amplification based on the speech spectrum. Victoreen, (1973), and Pascoe, (1978), are noteworthy examples of relating a fitting concept to most comfortable listening levels. Both use test signals other than pure tones. Victoreen's damped wave train is the better known among these, particularly because he devised and marketed test equipment producing such a signal. Significantly, his method does not include speech audiometry, as he did not find it relevant to hearing aid selection or performance verification. The Carhart (1946) method is in a category of its own when evaluation concepts are discussed.

Test signals are of a variety, as are the equipment required and test environment. Pure tone and warble tone are the test signals employed in most instances. Readily accessible, well suited for office environment and/or field use, and with fewer measurement problems, are devices using narrow band noise, amplitude modulated pure tones, and damped wave train. With increased availability of computers equipment for office use, probe microphone measurements of insertion gain, a difference between unaided and aided sound pressures in the ear canal offer another means of effective assessment.

Before the hearing instrument fitting there is increasing utilization of this methodology in order to determine target gain information, measured canal resonance, and data about vent placement. After the instruments have been fitted, this method becomes even more important in the verification of the delivered sound pressure near the tympanic membrane.

It is important to provide information and materials to assist the new instrument user in familiarization with the device. In their post-fitting protocol, McSpaden-Hickok and Hickok (1994) describe the procedure. The use of lists of minimal contrasting pairs of words sharpens speech discrimination skills. Speech In Noise (S.P.I.N) testing under four conditions make a contribution to our understanding of performance. Those conditions are:

1. Low level presentations with continuous noise
2. Low level presentations with sudden onset impact noise
3. Presentations with moderate levels of noise
4. Presentations with high levels of noise

From these data, even before important subjective aspects are considered in the evaluation system, it may become evident that a particular feature of an instrument's response accounts for some of the irritation the new user encounters. Correlating this information with the client's reported experiences yields even more relevant clues suggesting need of instrument or coupler modification. It is an excellent method for cross checking the predicted benefits of a particular choice with perceived benefits.

INSTRUMENT MODIFICATION

Something should be said about what the "modifications" are to which these repeated references are made. The specifics of response modification have been discussed in other chapters of this book, particularly those dealing with fitting, earmold and shell management. Here, it may be sufficient to mention that changes which modify the instrument's response can be divided into two categories: Electronic and Acoustic.

Among the variety of hearing instruments, one can find models without trim-pots which markedly alter electronic response. Most models are available with two or more trimmer potentiometers, offering many possible combinations for electronic modification.

An instrument may have adjustments for gain, output, frequency, compression knee points and compression ceilings. The variety of acoustic modifications is quite large and includes several choices of dampers/filters of known acoustic properties, in addition to the shape, length, bore, tube diameter and other properties of the earmolds. Each of these electronic or acoustic adjustments can be used in combination with one or more of the others. Furthermore, virtually all of these modifications can be quantified by measurement. With this impressive number of available response alternatives, the hearing instrument professional has the means to accomplish change and refinements that can enhance the user's aided performance and improve satisfaction.

Correlating aided measurements with the user's reported experiences is not just a perfunctory process. Considering the functional or insertion gain of the instrument and modifying the response to conform with calculated or predicted aided thresholds, will not necessarily produce a "successful" fitting. The fitting philosophy of the professional will greatly influence the direction instrument modification and adjustment takes. To weigh the alternatives, the hearing instrument professional needs to assess the level of user satisfaction with the hearing instruments fitted.

The user's objections may be related to particular acoustic properties of the device and need to be considered, even if such instrument alteration may deviate from best aided performance. In a study of preference versus performance, Cafarelli (1981), has shown that less than half of the subjects chose the hearing aid providing the best aided response. Even fewer chose the best performing instrument when assessed in noisy environments. Little correlation was found between audiometric test results and user preference for any given instrument. In concluding, the author wisely indicates the need for careful consideration of the user's amplification preference. The successful hearing instrument is the one the patient/client will wear!

CLIENT EXPECTATIONS AND ACCEPTANCE

As the dialogue between patient/client and the professional progresses in the post-fitting session, more of the patient/client's attitudes about hearing instrument use will be revealed. The hearing instrument professional should probe any clues relating to social or emotional concerns that may influence attitude. Is the patient/client making progress in this area of adaptation to amplification? Is the professional making progress in modifying user attitude? If not, the reasons should be explored. Some client behavior may be difficult to understand.

Few hearing impaired persons accept hearing aid use with intelligent and prescient determination. Many yield, reluctantly, to the recommendation of their physician or the urging of family or friends. The lack of instant success, the early perplexing experiences of auditory confusion may be used to reinforce his/her negative attitude. Clients may have resisted or postponed the idea of hearing aid use for so long that they rationalize their resistance to amplification.

To minimize such a negative turn of events, the well motivated beginners need to receive, as a part of post-fitting care, reinforcement counseling. By discussing those difficulties experienced by the user, a positive atmosphere can be generated. The professional and the patient/client need to take an inventory of the positive benefits already achieved. The patient/client's efforts to use amplification must be supported by emphasizing advantages and stressing positive aspects associated with the continued use of his/her hearing instrument(s).

More difficult to assess is the attitude of immediate family or friends. Yet, their attitude influences the patient/client's acceptance of the hearing aid. Often their expressions of disappointment about a lack of normal hearing may have discouragingly negative consequences. Unreasonable expectations on the part of well-meaning family members or friends frequently retard progress toward achievable goals with amplification.

An example of failure due to family members' exaggerated expectations is described by Mynders (1982). He tells of a client who in her own judgement did hear better. Measured improvement was adequate for that hearing loss. However, those around her judged the results by how successfully each carried on a conversation with her. The results, falling short of their expectations, made the family members take the position that the aid offered no benefit. To avoid conflicts within the family, the client returned the aid to the professional. The hearing instrument professional must take every opportunity to contact and provide counsel to those close to the patient/client. The professional should emphasize to them the do's and don'ts in encouraging the beginning hearing instrument user. They have the ability to facilitate great acceptance and progress, but, they also have the ability to retard it.

The first post-fitting session presents an important opportunity for both the user and professional to agree to a method for obtaining successful use of amplification. Therefore, discussion of post-fitting care can be centered around that session. Reasonable expectations are a two-way street. Seldom is everything accomplished in one visit, nor is that even desirable. More sessions are usually required to resolve problems.

These sessions provide an opportunity to give more effective guidance to the user and increase the likelihood of developing rapport. After progress seems assured, it is necessary to continue with regular post-fitting sessions. With efficient management, a high percentage of persons are capable of adjusting to amplified sound and derive much benefit from it.

The professional must recognize that there will be instances in which efforts fail to bring together those factors which insure progress in the use of amplification. In such an event, the specialist should consider the possible contributions of some of the following:

1) A procedural flaw in the assessment of the hearing loss;
2) An error of judgment in the selection of the aid;
3) Misinterpretation of some aspect of the hearing problem. If such a possibility exists; retest, re-evaluate, rethink, readjust or refit.

In many instances, certain aspects of follow-up care, particularly performance verification, may be shared by the person who first evaluated the patient/client and the person who fitted the hearing instrument(s). Measured differences in the expected results and in the interpretation of derived benefits need to be constructively reconciled. The danger may be that conflicting opinion or advice given to the patient/client can damage a potentially successful fitting.

The best advice for those serving the hearing impaired is to maintain effective communication; a genial, intelligent and constructive two-way communication. It is not an option. It is a professional obligation.

SUPPLEMENTAL DISCUSSION

Emphasis throughout this chapter has been focused on the discussion of activities which help the new hearing instrument user to overcome obstacles encountered in learning to use, accept, and benefit from amplification. The importance of succeeding in that effort overshadows all other aspects of post-fitting care. Once the client becomes a successful hearing instrument user, other aspects of care become the subject of considerable consequence.

There are a variety of self-assessment questionaires and check-lists that are available. Our preference is for a hybrid "check-list" (see Appendices A and B). It was developed in Oklahoma by Hickok and McSpaden-Hickok using many different source materials. It addresses the proper questions without being an exhaustive listing of them. It reinforces the responsibility of the patient/client in the generation of answers.

Maintenance attains an importance the beginning instrument user could not appreciate. It should, therefore, become part of the instruction in post-fitting sessions.

The new instrument user should be made aware of routine points of maintenance such as periodic cleaning of the instrument or replacing discolored or hardened earmold tubing. The user should know that his/her hearing and the hearing instrument may go through gradual change. The user may adapt to negative changes without knowing it and regress to a far less effective level of instrument use. For that reason alone, periodic checks of the hearing instrument's performance and the user's hearing levels are advisable. The obvious value of such rechecks is that it alerts both the professional and the user to the need for adjustment, repair or medical attention.

The fit of the hearing instrument and/or the earmold needs to be carefully monitored. Excessive feedback may occur due to stretch or change of the ear canal tissue as well as aging or shrinkage of the plastics. New earmolds or hearing instrument shells may be needed to rectify the situation.

It is beneficial to include in post-fitting care periodic inspection of the physical condition of the aided ear. Among other things, inspection permits one to determine the presence of cerumen sufficient to interfere with sound conduction, visible irritation of the concha and ear canal that may indicate problems in maintaining normal hearing instrument use.

If a sudden change occurs in an instrument's acoustic per-ormance caused by malfunction of some component, the results are immediate and usually dramatic. The user is the first to know. The device may need to be sent to the factory for repair. The user should learn how the professional manages such a situation and what his/her policy is in regard to providing loaner instruments.

SUMMARY

Science and art converge from time to time aiding us in the advancement of our skills to provide an increasingly effective service to the hearing impaired and to achieve successful use of hearing instruments. In discussing post-fitting care through these preceding pages, we have intentionally emphasized concepts that shape thinking or influence our attitudes and actions. The critical one of these is that each of these aspects are integral parts of the concept of aural habilitation/rehabilitation.

We have tried NOT to produce a "cookbook" or give point by point instruction of what steps to take. Without being oblivious to the medical or organic difficulties inherent in various hearing losses, we have referred more to the behavioral and emotional correlates of hearing loss as they are understood today. Success, in these days of rapid change, is dependent upon the willingness to get aboard the learning curve and - to ride it - FOREVER!

GLOSSARY

Amplitude Modulated Pure Tone A coherent sound source with controlled variation in the amplitude of a carrier signal of a given frequency.

Counseling Guidance provided and obtained through discussion and mutual exchange of opinions and ideas.

Damped Wave Train A signal with a sequence of cycles of sound pressure in which the amplitude of the successive cycles is diminished progressively.

Dichotic Both of one's ears stimulated separately by the same signal at the same time.

Directional Balance A reciprocally equal ability of each ear to determine the position of the source of a sound.

Directional Hearing (Localization) The ability to determine the position of the source of a sound.

Functional Gain The difference between aided and unaided thresholds determined by sound field assessment.

Insertion Gain The difference between unaided and aided sound pressure in the ear canal determined by probe-microphone measurements.

Interaural Denoting the interaction of one's ears.

Listening Attitude The extent of a person's efforts to be attentive to what is being said; positioning oneself to best advantage to concentrate and training one's mind to listen carefully.

Narrow Band Noise A non-coherent signal with a critical band width of about 50 Hz centered around a test frequency generally with rolloff characteristics of 32 dB per octave.

Response (h.aid) The relative gain of a hearing aid through a range of frequencies when the input signal has been raised by any particular setting of the volume control.

Selective Amplification A hearing enhancement concept in which the response of a hearing instrument is adjusted to amplify certain frequencies more than others.

Sound Channel the pathway through which the sound passes from the receiver of the hearing instrument into the ear canal. It may be a combination of earhook, tubing, and sound bore of the earmold—as on behind-the-ear aids; of the mere sound bore of the earmold of a body aid, ITE or ITC aids.

REFERENCES

ACKERMAN, D. Chapter on "Hearing", in *Natural History of the Senses,* Random House Publishers, N.Y., N.Y., 1990.

AURAL REHABILITATION REVIEW FOR HEARING AID USERS, Starkey Laboratories, Inc., 1976.

BARNETT, G. A., "How to use a Hearing Aid," Sonotone Corporation, SA154, Reprint from *Journal of Lifetime Living,* N.C. (1974).

BERGER, K. W., HAGBERG, E. N. and RANE, R. L., *Prescription of Hearing Aids: Rationale, Procedure and Results,* Herald Publishing House, Kent, 1977. 5, 30–36.

BLACKSTONE, S., "Learning to Hear Again," Reprint No. 565. *The Volta Bureau,* Washington.

BROENEN, J. A., "A Hearing Aid Population Profile," *Hearing Instruments,* 34:10, 1983, 14, 16.

BROOKS, D. N., "Counseling and Its Effect on Hearing Aid Use," *Audecibel,* 28–4, 1979, 194–196, 198–204, 206.

CAFARELLI, D. L., "Hearing Aid Preference Versus Performance," *Hearing Instruments,* 32:4, 1981, 20–22.

CARHART, R., "Tests for Selection of Hearing Aids," *Laryngoscope,* 56, 1946, 780–794.

CURRAN, J. R., "Delivery of the Hearing Aid," *Hearing Aid Journal,* 29:12, 1976, 7, 30–31.

DODDS, E. and HARFORD, E., *"Helpful Hearing Aid Hints,"* A. G. Bell Assoc., Washington, 1970.

GOLBBERG, H., *"Psychological Adaptation to Hearing Enhancement,"* Dyn-Aura Engineering Laboratories.

GOUGH, K. H., "Rehabilitation of the Hearing-Impaired Adult," *Hearing Aid Journal,* 29:12, 1976, 9, 28–29.

GRIFFING, T. S., "Hearing Correction Is More Than a Hearing Aid, *Hearing Aid Journal,* 31:11, 1978, 6, 62–65.

HEARING AID CARE, Starkey Laboratories, Inc., Edina, 1981.

HEARING AID USER GUIDE AND INSTRUCTION BROCHURE, Marcon Hearing Instruments, Inc., Minneapolis, Revised, 1984.

HOW TO HEAR BETTER, Widex G-136-51, Denmark, N.D.

INSTRUCTION FOR YOUR RADIOEAR MODEL RE HP SERIES, Radioear Corporation, McMurray, PA, N.

JERGER, J., "Special Issue on Auditory Deprivation (Editorial), *Journal of American Academy Audiology,* vol. 4, no. 5, September 1993

JOENSEN, J. P. and SAUNDERS, D. J., "Psychological Correlates of Geriatric Hearing Loss," *The Hearing Journal,* 37:3, 1984, 39–41.

KAPTEYN, T. S., "Satisfaction with Fitted Hearing Aids, I. An Analysis of Technical Information." *Scandinavian Audiology,* 6, 1977, 147–156. II. "An Investigation into Influence of Psycho-Social Factors," 6, 1977, 171–177.

KEITH, R. W. and SININGER, L., "'New Ideas?' In Hearing Aid Selection," *Hearing Instruments,* 29:6, 1978, 6–8, 34.

KODMAN, F. JR., "Techniques for Counseling the Hearing Aid Client," *Audecibel,* 22, 1973.

LEARNING TO HEAR AGAIN, Audiotone, A Division of Lear Siegler, Inc. (Revised 1972).

LIBBY, E. R., "In Search of the Two Eared Man," in Libby, E. R. (Ed.): *Binaural Hearing and Amplification,* Chicago, Zenetron, Inc., 1980.

LYBARGER, S. F., "Selective Amplification—A Review and Evaluation," *Journal of the American Audiology Society,* 3:6, 1978, 358–266.

MCSPADEN-HICKOK, D. K., and HICKOK, R. L.: Personal Communication 1994.

MYNDERS, J. M., "Fact Versus Feelings: An Unsuccessful Fitting," *Hearing Aid Journal,* 35:6, 1982, 20–22.

NELSON, M., "The Psychological Aspects of Hearing Impairment," *Audecibel,* 12, 1963, 18–19, 41–42. Reprint from the Eye, Ear, Nose and Throat Monthly.

NEWBY, H. A., *Audiology,* (Third Edition), Prentice-Hall, Inc., Englewood Cliffs, 1972.

OJA, G. L. and SCHOW, R. L., "Hearing Aid Evaluation Based on Measures of Benefit, Use, and Satisfaction," *Ear and Hearing,* 5:2, 1984, 77–85.

PASCOE, P. P., "An Approach to Hearing Aid Selection," *Hearing Instruments,* 29:6, 1978, 12–16, 35.

RAMSDELL, D. A., "The Psychology of the Hard-of-Hearing and Deafened Adult," in Davis, G. and Silverman, S. R. (Ed.): *Hearing and Deafness (Ed. 3)* Holt, Rinehart and Winston, New York, 1970.

REEVE, J. W., "Letters to a New Hearing Aid User from the Old Hearing Aid Counselor," Knoxville, Author, 1954.

SANDERS, D. A., "Hearing Aid Orientation and Counseling," in Pollack, M. C. (Ed.), *Amplification For The Hearing Impaired,* Grune & Stratton, New York, 1975.

SILVERMAN, C., "Auditory Deprivation," *Journal American Academy of Audiology,* Vol. 4, No. 5, September 1993.

SIMPLE COURTESY AND THE HARD-OF-HEARING, St. Louis Hearing & Speech Center, F421-P, St. Louis.

SURR, R. K., ET AL., "Factors Influencing Use of Hearing Aids," *Hearing Instruments,* 30:1, 1979. Reprint from Archives of Otolaryngology, Dec., 1978, Vol. 104, p. 732–736.

10 KEYS TO BETTER LISTENING, Sonotone Corporation, SA-222, Elmsford, N.D.

TIPS FOR BETTER HEARING, Omni Hearing Systems, Dallas, N.D.

USER INSTRUCTIONS, Phonic Ear, Inc., 821-2755-1-10, 1980.

USER'S INSTRUCTION BROCHURE, Oticon Corporation, Somerset, 1980.

USER'S INSTRUCTION BROCHURE, Telex Communications, Inc., Minneapolis, 1982.

USER'S INSTRUCTION MANUAL AND GUARANTEE, Computer Hearing Aid Corporation, N.D.

VICTOREEN, J. A., "The Science of Hearing Prosthetics," Copyright J.A.V., 1978, 5–8.

ZELSKI, R. F., "Practical Approaches to Fitting and Counseling," *Hearing Instruments,* 30:11, 1979, 10–12.

APPENDIX A

CHECKLIST

____ Hearing Aid(s) received ______
____ Hearing Aid(s) tested.
____ Hearing Aid(s) passed electro-acoustic evaluation Y__ N__
____ Client notified within 24 hours of successful electro-acoustic evaluation of instruments.
____ Delivery scheduled for __/__/____.
____ Otoscopy done Y__ N__

Comments ____
____ Instruments fit—note any problems and/or changes needed:
____
____
____ Client can _______________________________________

Notes on adjustments made with tone controls, etc.: ______________
____

Notes on changes in venting: ______________________________
____
____

Notes on re-check of fit: _________________________________
____
____

Any other comments: _____________________________________
____
____

Client's signature: ______________________________________
Dispenser's signature: ___________________________________
License number: ____________________________ Date: __/__/__

APPENDIX B

DELIVERY CHECKLIST

____ Hearing Aid(s) received ______

____ Hearing Aid(s) tested.

____ Hearing Aid(s) passed electro-acoustic valuation Y__ N__

____ Client notified within 24 hours of successful electro-acoustic evaluation of instruments.

____ Delivery scheduled for __/__/____.

____ Otoscopy done Y__ N__ Comments: ________________

____ Instrument(s) fit-note any problems and/or changes needed:

____

____

____

____ Client can insert instrument(s): Y__ N__

____ Comments: ________________________________

____ Client can remove instrument(s): Y__ N__

____ Comments: ________________________________

____ Client can change batteries: Y__ N__

____ Comments: ________________________________

____ Client can adjust volume: Y__ N__

____ Comments: ________________________________

____ S/O Can insert and remove instruments Y__ N__; Can insert and remove batteries Y__ N__; Can adjust volume control Y__ N__

____ Comments: ________________________________

____ Hearing aids balanced.

____ Volume settings marked.

____ Questions/concerns with any of the following:

- ____ Feedback
- ____ Sound quality
- ____ Instrument noise
- ____ Volume level
- ____ Sound of client's own voice
- ____ Options (T-coil, switches, etc.)

Comments: ____

____

____

Notes on adjustments made with tone controls, etc.: ________________

____

____

____

Notes on changes in venting: ______________________________

____

____

____

Notes on re-check of fit: ________________________________

____

____

____

Any other comments: _____________________________________

____

____

____

Client's signature: ______________________________________

Dispenser's signature:____________________________________

License number: ___________________________ Date:__/__/____

APPENDIX C

CHECKLIST

I am hearing better with my new hearing aid(s). Y__ N__
If no, please explain:

____

____

____

____ I understand that wearing hearing aids will not restore my hearing to normal levels, but will help me to hear better.

____ I know that wearing hearing aids will not prevent further changes in my hearing, but may help me to retain my ability to understand speech.

____ I agree that the less time I wear my hearing aids, the less benefit I will receive from them.

____ I understand that I have a hearing loss in both ears, and that wearing one aid will not provide the best benefit for me.

____ I understand that the normal life of a hearing aid that is worn all day, every day, is 3–4 years.

____ I know that it is my responsibility to buy batteries for my hearing aids.

____ I know that eating batteries is hazardous to good health.

____ I know that hearing aids are mechanical devices and may break down.

____ I know that I will be hearing sounds that I have not heard for some time, and that I will need to adjust to that.

____ I understand that there may be changes in the sound of my own voice when I wear my hearing aids.

____ I understand that my ears may be tender for the first few days of wearing my hearing aids, and that I need to get this checked if it continues longer than that, or becomes sore.

____ I understand that I should try not to get my hearing aids wet; that I should keep them away from my pets; that I should avoid exposing them to excess heat, dust, hairspray, etc.

____ I know that I should find one place to routinely store my hearing aids at night.

____ I understand that it is best to not wear my hearing aids while asleep.

____ I know that if I cover my ears while wearing my hearing aids, they may whistle.

____ I understand that I should clean my hearing aids daily, and that I should not use alcohol, water, soap, or any other liquid to clean them with. I also understand that I should have my hearing aid cleaned by my dispenser every three (3) months.

____ I agree that hearing aids should not be used as earplugs in high noise situations.

____ I know that it is my responsibility to notify my dispenser of problems with my hearing aids.

____ I understand that these hearing aids were custom built for me and for my loss, and that they should not be used by other people.

____ I agree that the following are NOT good reasons for not wearing my hearing aids:

1. Hearing background noise.
2. Hearing loud sounds.
3. Cosmetic concerns.
4. Battery life (unless less than factory spec.).

I agree with the preceding statements.

______________________________ Date:__/__/____

(Client signature)

______________________________ Lic. # _________

(Dispenser signature)

XI

PSYCHO-SOCIAL PRINCIPLES OF HEARING IMPAIRMENT

MAX STANLEY CHARTRAND, Ph.D.

INTRODUCTION

Hearing instrument dispensing demands a thorough understanding of basic psychological behavior relative to human hearing. Indeed, as we learn more about how one interacts with the environs and copes with communicative challenges, the hearing instrument specialist begins to appreciate that the human sense of hearing—more than any other sensory input—provides a profound influence. It shapes one's personal sense of security, self-image, social relationships, and emotional responses to the external world. Albeit, specialists discover that while there are many serious maladies and deficiencies afflicting man, none is as insidious, transparent, and pervasive as progressive hearing impairment. In this vein, it is the ***insidiousness*** and ***transparency*** of unrecognized and uncorrected hearing impairment that is of particular interest here.

Otherwise, with all the hearing health empowerment so available for today's prospective hearing instrument user, why aren't more sufferers raising their hands in self-identification? Why is sales performance still mired in the statistical swamp of a rapidly growing market, which appears increasingly hesitant to seek out help? In this enlightened age in human history, why are consumers (and some professionals and government regulators) still grappling with so many misconceptions about hearing loss and its timely resolution?

Let's survey a large audience of older adults, and ask them to raise their hands in response to the following questions:

- ***How many of you hear, but have difficulty understanding some words?*** (A good many hands would go up).
- ***How many have difficulty understanding speech in the presence of background noise?*** (More hands would go up).
- ***How many have noises or ringing in their ears?*** (More hands yet).
- ***How many suffer from hearing loss?*** (No hands).

All the major symptoms of sensorineural hearing loss readily admitted, and *still* no hands raised when asked for self-assessment of the underlying *cause* of these symptoms! No hands. The skeptical statistician might point out that perhaps they were responding to the word "*suffering*", instead of the words "*hearing loss*", to which I rebut that in no matter which case, there is still an aversion in human nature toward first recognizing ***hearing loss*** as the sum of its symptoms, and secondly, recognizing that to experience hearing loss is to ***suffer its effects!***

On the threshold of the twenty-first century, why do so many suffer the symptoms of serious hearing impairment yet so few readily recognize or admit it for what it is? Are we only a little further in public education on hearing health than we were a hundred years ago, when hearing loss equated with mental infirmity or dementia in the public mind? Worse yet, why do so many, when informed of their malady and its logical resolution through prescriptive amplification, choose instead to:

- Turn radios and televisions louder?
- Struggle in poor noise competition environments?
- Struggle with strained family and marriage relationships?
- Be stifled in social, vocational, and education opportunities?
- Accept a diminishing lifestyle?
- Expect loved ones to change their world to accommodate an otherwise resolvable hearing problem?

"Oh, I don't have a hearing problem," say they. ***"I just miss some words."***

And about the time we think we've elicited a breakthrough admission, ***"If only people would speak a little plainer, and the***

noise in the background wasn't so loud, the preacher wouldn't mumble, the boss would speak a little slower. . . . "

If only.

CHAPTER OBJECTIVES

In this chapter we attempt to unlock some of the mysteries, challenge psycho-social barriers, and find ways to empower prospective hearing instrument patients to move forward to a timely resolution of their hearing impairment through the services and products of hearing instrument specialists. To do so, we must cover three major areas of exploration.

The first is ***a review of human auditory developmental principles*** and theories. To understand the *dysfunctional* system we must first have a foundational understanding of the psychoacoustic and neurophysiologic principles which inherently shape *normal* human auditory function.

Second, we will examine ***the fundamental psycho-social effects of hearing impairment on the prospective hearing instrument user.*** Looking at hearing loss through better defined prisms—type, degree, age of onset, and gender—we can then develop increasingly accurate paradigms of the *complexity* and *predictability* of hearing loss effects upon the lives of its sufferers and on those whose lives have been rearranged to accommodate its (mostly) avoidable aberrations.

Third, ***effective principles and concepts for professional intervention*** will be explored, including gearing our dispensing and counseling programs to the ***four stages of mourning*** to better assist hearing impaired patients in their timely acceptance of our professional guidance, products, and services. For it goes without saying that all the technological and rehabilitative wonders in the world will not be of one iota of help to one who does not take advantage of them. Hence, to do less than motivate the hearing impaired to partake of today's cornucopia of aural rehabilitation is akin to leading the hypothetical horse to water. . . . but being unable to persuade him to drink. His debilitation will be as sure as if the water had never been available in the first place. And, in the case of the unswayed hearing instrument prospect, another life stifled in opportunity, happiness, and good health.

INTRODUCTION TO HUMAN AUDITORY DEVELOPMENT

This section introduces fundamental principles in basic human auditory development. In addition, there will be a review of neurophysiological mechanisms wherein various auditory skills are developed, and some of the many psycho-social influences which shape human response to life through the sense of hearing. For the hearing instrument specialist to understand where he or she is taking their hearing impaired patients during the rehabilitative process they first must understand from whence they came.

EARLY AUDITORY DEVELOPMENT

Even before birth, the sense of hearing has a profound effect upon proper development of a personal sense of security, interpersonal bonding, cognitive and spatial development, goal-orientation, and language perception ability. The unborn infant is already familiarized with such things as mother's voice, musical patterns and background sounds, and things which both frighten and soothe. Invariably, by the end of this early period the stage is set for acquiring the needed skills for emotionally and cognitively adapting and dealing with life for years to come.

From a physiological standpoint, development of the hearing system during fetal gestation parallels many other structural and neurological developments. Parallels have been recently documented in the literature between *oto-osteo development* and *denticulation* (Johnsen, 1991); hence, a direct interrelationship exists between the development of baby's teeth and the bony structure of the middle ear. **Treacher-Collins-Franscetti Syndrome** (microsia, atresia, under-developed ossicular chain), for example, reflects closely the congenital underdevelopment of an infant's mandibulofacial features (Glanze, 1987) (Becker et al, 1989). To a lesser-documented degree come parallels in neurological development and the human hearing system, particularly those involving cortical language processing (Wills, 1993) and predisposition toward learning-disabilities (Vandenberg, 1967). Hence, many predictive patterns are set in the early developmental stages, including aberrations resulting from deprivation, trauma, and incomplete auditory development (Irwin and Marge, 1972) (Snyder, 1980).

At birth the baby is greeted with a harshness previously not experienced within the mother's protective womb, almost like reaching out on a limb in total faith, based upon past auditory and emotional memory, to the next stage of life's journey. The familiar sound of the mother's voice calms the agitated or startled newborn, assuring comfort, safety, and a sense of belonging (Horton, 1986). With the pattern having been set during the previous nine months of gestation, the baby is now equipped to adjust to the outside world environment and the challenges it brings.

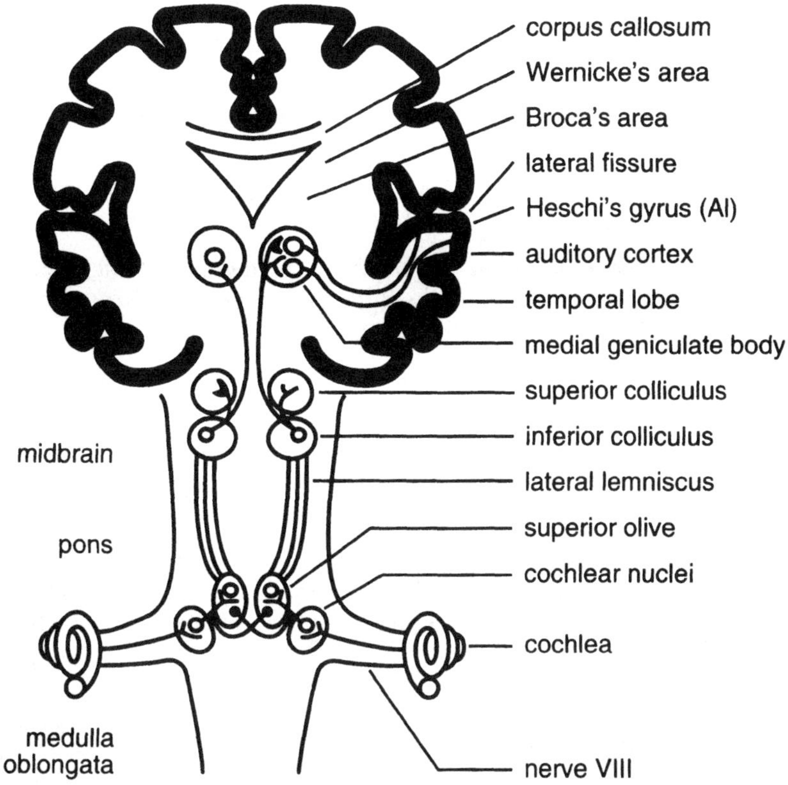

Fig. 1. Schematic of the human auditory projection system.

Fig. 1.

As the auditory projection system (see Figure 1) of the young child develops, the finer points of audition become "learned" or "acquired" (Hellige, 1993) (Ross, Brackett, and Maxon, 1991) (Briskey, 1980) (Harris, 1980). Below is listed just a small sampling of the developmental fine-tuning that occurs within the human auditory/language processing system (Pickles, 1992) (Graham, 1990) (Ross, Brackett, and Maxon, 1991) (Hellige, 1993) (Rose, 1992):

- ***Binaural squelch ability*** or the ability to binaurally suppress pervasive background noise in competition with discreet signals develops primarily from the thalamus of the auditory cortex to the efferent branch of the auditory nerve at the **cortical, central, and cochlear functional levels.**

- ***Sense of directionality and signal selectivity*** at the **Superior Olivary Complex.**
- ***Spatial mapping*** at the **inferior colliculus** of the central auditory process.
- ***Spatial/startle response*** via the **superior colliculus** and **limbic system.**
- ***Auditory attention*** or the ability to mentally focus listening skills develops primarily at the **thalamus** (the traffic controller of the auditory cortex or A1).
- ***Cortical tonatopical recognition*** develops at the **Heschl's Gyrus** of the A1.
- ***Short-term sequential memory*** (for sequences, patterns, and symbols) develops in the **A1 of auditory cortex** adjacent **Heschl's Gyrus.**
- ***Long-term memory, goal orientation, and cognition*** or stored auditory memory as well as goal-orientation develop in the **A2 of the auditory cortex,** and in the **M2 of the motor cortex.**
- ***Language comprehension*** develops in the left temporal lobe at **Wernicke's area.**
- ***Language expression*** forms in the left temporal lobe at **Broca's area.**
- ***Binaural summation*** or bi-hemispheric enhancement of signal develops via the **corpus callosum** which interconnects **right and left hemisphere** functions.
- ***Binaural fusion*** or the putting together of two auditory images into a whole develops via the **corpus callosum.**
- ***Development of the 3 perceptual levels of hearing*** (Primitive, signal, symbolic) which are described more fully later in this section.

The reader should keep in mind that just as the above-listed auditory/cognitive/language abilities are acquired during the prelingual and linguistic stages of a child's development, the adult who later experiences progressive hearing loss will, to varying degrees, experience a lessening of these acquired abilities. Hence, contrary to common understanding, to regain all that is possible during the rehabilitative process will take much more than the application of amplification. Instead, a carefully guided program for relearning and re-acquiring *lost auditory skills* will be necessary to truly return to a rehabilitated state. Albeit, in severe cases, additional compensating approaches—speechreading, assistive devices, and extensive aural rehabilitative counseling—will also be needed, **plus** a healthy dose of patient ***acceptance*** of unresolvable auditory limitations.

SEX DIFFERENCES IN AUDITORY DEVELOPMENT

Development of human hearing also indicates measurable patterns and differences in terms of sex of the child, some of which are transitory and others that become quite established (see figure 2). The ***female auditory system,*** as a rule, develops earlier (Waber, 1976) and tends to fall off much later in life than does the male auditory system (Davis and Silverman, 1970). Likewise, in the early development stage of human audition, females are more sensitive to loud sounds and have a more developed ***startle reflex***, which is closely tied to development of the interneural pathways between the ***limbic system*** (emotions) and the ***superior colliculus*** of the central auditory system (Pool, 1994). ***Males,*** on the other hand, exhibit greater interconnectedness at the more primitive (fight or-flight) ***amygdala*** portion of the brain and intuitive response to aurally-perceived danger signals (Naylor, 1994).

Female infants orient more readily to tones and subtleties of expression in voices (Hines, 1990). With increased ***skin sensitivity*** they are more proficient at early ***fine motor performance*** and, as a rule, are better than males at ***rapid sequential movements*** (Weinstein, 1968). Recent research points to the greater interconnectedness between the ***right and left brain hemispheres*** in females because of the greater dendritic mass at the ***corpus callosum,*** which connects both sides of the brain for greater simultaneous utilization (Pool, 1994). Males tend to use their left hemisphere exclusively for language processing and abstract thinking, often missing more aesthetic and holistic indicators in human communication. Thus, ***mimic of speech sounds*** (right brain/holistic ability) comes more readily in the early language development of females.

As children develop, females are more attracted to and attentive to ***social contexts*** such as facial expressions, speech patterns, and tones of voice which require near equal and simultaneous abilities from both the right and left hemispheres of the brain during human communication (Ley and Bryden, 1979). Females speak sooner, possess larger vocabularies, and rarely demonstrate ***speech defects.*** Stuttering and many other speech and learning-developmental

Auditory Development in Males / Females

FEMALES

- Early auditory/ language acquisition
- Utilize social contexts, nuances of speech
- Lowered spatial ability, re: right / left hemisphere
- Superior fine motor skills
- Earlier "ear-training" re: vocal music
- Use both hemispheres in communication
- Hearing declines later in life

MALES

- Late auditory development / early loss
- Early, lasting visual acuity bias
- Tend to be inquisitive, individual discovery
- Superior spatial ability re: right hemisphere
- Fast reaction, gross total body movements
- Listen primarily via left hemisphere

Fig. 2.

problems, on the other hand, occur predominantly among boys (Halpern, 1992) (Bloodstein, 1987). Because of earlier development at the tonatopical arrangement of ***Heschl's Gyrus*** in the auditory cortex portion of the brain (McGlone, 1980), females can sing in tune at an earlier age, and usually maintain superior ***linguistic bias*** throughout life. They also read sooner, learn foreign language easier, and often enter occupations involving superior ***language mastery.***

Males show early superiority in ***visual acuity*** and tend to compensate through vision for their initially lower auditory capacity (McGuinness, 1976). While more clumsy in situations involving fine motor performance, they generally excel in gross total body movements and skills especially those requiring fast reaction time (Burg, 1976). They are particularly superior in ***manipulating three-dimensional space,*** using their ***right hemisphere*** almost exclusively for spatial tasks.

Females, on the other hand, generally attempt to solve spatial problems with their left (abstract/logic/verbal) hemisphere of the brain, sometimes causing an ***interference phenomenon,*** a kind of log-jamming in which the use of words to solve a spatial problem results in slowed, incorrect, or absent responses.

Males tend to explore their environment and life experiences firsthand. Females, however, typically tend to gain such knowledge in a more ***communicative mode,*** asking others, taking advantage of others' experiences, sparing themselves the need to personally encounter all the objects in their environment.

The male's ability to focus on abstract language in the left hemisphere and to solve spatial problems in the right hemisphere—***hemispheric specialization***—allows them to more readily excel in abstract and spatial-manipulation occupations such as advanced mathematics, engineering, economics, medicine, athletics and computer programming. On the other hand, females naturally excel in subjects requiring use of both hemispheres: language, family counseling, the arts, and caregiving (Kimura, 1992).

In making these observations, however, it needs to be emphasized that there are myriad exceptions to the rule as today more and more women pursue academic studies and occupations requiring advanced logic and abstract thinking skills (Kimura, 1993) (U.S. Department of Education, 1992). In the other direction, one finds a great proportion of males that are leading musicians, artists, caregivers, and family counselors. The pattern of natural development, however, often proceeds along the lines suggested above (Springer et al, 1991).

Without a full discussion of what this author calls the ***"male psyche",*** it will have to suffice here to mention that because of long-established tendencies of males to deny frailties, physical weakness, or sensory shortcomings that, as a rule, such tendencies do not mix well with the types of hearing loss males typically develop over time, i.e. normal hearing in the lows accompanied with progressive and insidious high-frequency sensorineural loss. This admixture, therefore, presents significant challenges to the hearing care field in helping male patients as will be explained more fully in the next two sections.

THREE PERCEPTUAL LEVELS OF HUMAN HEARING

There are several ways we can look at human hearing and its uses in everyday life. Probably the best model was devised and expounded upon many years ago by Ramsdell (1970). His model, which I call *"the three perceptual levels of human hearing"*, has withstood the empirical test of time. The author, then, will base the following observations partially upon Ramsdell's model, from others' research, and from first-hand experience with patients. While the concept may be considered partially conjecture, it still provides an orderly and logical explanation of human auditory processing of sound from a psychological processing viewpoint. The order of the levels will be reversed from Ransdell's original model to better illustrate the developmental process (see figure 3).

The first (and most important) level of human hearing is called the **PRIMITIVE LEVEL**. Theoretically, we assume this to be the first level at which human perception is developed, for the ambient background represents the backdrop against which we interpret all other experiences around us. Our personal sense of security and environmental interconnectedness both result from the ability to hear and subconsciously distinguish background sounds. As mentioned earlier, it is this level at which an infant first connects with life and is able to define its interconnectedness therefrom.

The Three Perceptual Levels of Human Hearing

1. **Primitive Level: Background sounds**
   Origin of one's sense of security, interconnectedness with life around them, and general environmental awareness.
2. **Signal Level: Danger/attention sounds**
   Serves as 24-hour auditory "radar" system, involuntarily alerting to danger and other signals.
3. **Symbolic Level: Communication sounds**
   Language (verbal) and aesthetic (non-verbal) communication in which sounds become definitive symbols.

Fig. 3.

The next developmental level of hearing is tied closely to evolutionary human responses and reflexes at the autonomic nervous system level, and is called the **SIGNAL OR ALERTING LEVEL.** The author often refers to the signal level as an "auditory radar system" alerting to dangers and considerations demanding undivided attention, whether one is awake or not. Human response to most signals is learned over time, such as the telephone ring, alarm clock signal, fire alarm, or an approaching automobile as we proceed to cross the street. So broad are the range of these signals that it is nearly impossible to categorize them into a single specific frequency band, intensity level, or set of idiosyncratic characteristics.

Therefore, alerting or danger signals can exist at any frequency and at any audible intensity as they are monitored by one's subconscious. From the loudest siren at mid-day to the softest snap of a twig outside the bedroom window after midnight, the sounds that can be interpreted at this level are almost endless. Figuring heavily into the equation are situational and contextual determinants: location, time of day, customary routines, etc. Essentially, whatever gains our involuntary attention constitutes the very sounds that comprise this level of hearing.

It is interesting to note that when background sounds—due to hearing impairment—are no longer easily *distinguishable* by the listener, such sounds become perceived as *danger or alerting* signals, instead of routine background noise. Therefore, when one loses the ability to subconsciously discern background sounds from other sounds, what *is* heard demands attention, even to the point of affecting the autonomic nervous system. The ***hypothalamus*** at the mid-brain level provides the neural link between thoughts (cerebral cortex) and feelings (limbic system) to keep balance and perspective in response to environmental stimuli (Siegel and Pott, 1988) (Smith and DeVito, 1984). In the abnormal hearing system, this balance mechanism often goes awry (Chartrand, 1989), causing confusion and disorientation for the impaired individual.

The level of hearing of which people are most aware is the **SYMBOLIC OR COMMUNICATION LEVEL,** which comprises the conscious act of communicating and interacting with others. In addition, the communicative level is that which can best be objectively measured and evaluated in terms of auditory function. Therefore, we will focus on the basic principles underlying this level moreso than the previously-described levels of perception. This does not, however, diminish the importance of the previous two levels. Proper human auditory function requires that *all* *three levels* of perception be considered within the larger rehabilitative picture.

The symbolic or communication level represents the conscience use of ***language communication,*** both receptive and expressive. Language development is primarily characterized by sounds—or parts of speech—as ***language symbols*** which may comprise recognizable and similar meaning to both the speaker and the listener (Yule, 1985). In fact, the arbitrariness of language—or its lack of "natural" or literal symbolism but rather "contrived" symbolism—requires that the acquisition of language be arbitrarily "learned" over a great deal of time and practice. The learning process itself begins at the earliest attempts of the infant to orally express discomfort, hunger, or fright. Later, the preschooler learns by ***mimicking*** speech sounds—without actual phonetic symbolism. Then, the gradual life-long process continues building a growing vocabulary and verbal arsenal for effective interaction and manipulation in human communication, depending upon needs and aspirations. The process of acquiring language, therefore, requires years of vested time and effort, much of it taken in stride during the natural course of living and socializing.

In speech, the vowel sounds (ex.: a, e, i, o, u) often contain information exhibiting ***emotion, inflection, and intensity of expression,*** while consonant sounds (ex.: s, sh, st, k, t, th, d, m, n, l, etc.) provide the ***defining*** elements of language. Aleo (1995) likens this association to driving an automobile when explaining speech to prospective hearing instrument patients. In anecdotal form, he relates the vowel sounds of speech as the "engine" of a car, providing power, and the consonant sounds as the "steering wheel" which guides its course and gives it clarity. In this manner he is able to help patients understand that while they may still have the *power* (hearing acuity in the vowel region of speech) that they lack the *direction and clarity* that is most necessary for driving the vehicle because of their high frequency hearing loss. Understanding this basic principle is necessary to both motivate the prospective patient to action and to assist in their ultimate rehabilitation.

A related principle espoused by this author is:

> *The more advanced or scientific language becomes, the more reliant upon the more complex combinations of consonant sounds of speech it is, while emotional and less technical messages rely more upon the simpler vowels and diphthongs.*

Hence, the English language comprises almost endless volumes of words and terms in its behemoth dictionaries. The simpler, more primitive languages of the South Pacific and elsewhere, on the other hand, hardly fill a pamphlet-size dictionary. The point here is that the typical American adult vocabulary and, hence, their personal and professional ability to communicate, is heavily reliant upon the acquisition of consonant-laden vocabulary. The caveat, however, is that to acquire and utilize the English language through audition requires normal or near-normal hearing thresholds in the high frequencies . . . or at the very least, amplified correction of the impaired system accompanied by assistive devices and coping mechanisms as needed.

Likewise, the more scientific or technical one's field of endeavor, the more important becomes normal or near-normal hearing acuity in the high frequency region. Since most adult hearing loss is high frequency in nature, this poses a challenge especially for those involved with professions or fields which require language mastery or verbal technical communication. However, because the vowel sounds (under 500Hz) often remain near-normal long after the mid and high frequencies have degenerated, many of these cases are unaware that they suffer from hearing loss per se. Hence, a common complaint at even relatively advanced levels of high-frequency loss is, ***"I hear fine. . . . I just have trouble understand some of the words!"***

HEARING WITH BOTH HEMISPHERES OF THE BRAIN

From an interpretive standpoint, the "learning process" of language (or the symbols we come to know as language) becomes quite ***lateralized*** (specialized) to various and specific parts of the brain where the information is processed and responded to. In other words, language comprehension is actually composed of essentially two different "mental viewpoints", verbal and non-verbal. The *verbal viewpoint* is primarily processed in the **LEFT HEMISPHERE** of the temporal lobe in humans, as evidenced by the physical location of ***Wernicke's area*** (where language communication is received) and ***Broca's area*** (where language communication is expressed). Both of these vital language processing areas reside in the left hemisphere. Hence, the left hemisphere involves mainly ***abstract, logical, and technical interpretation*** of language, the "what and whereof". Since the right ear primarily lateralizes to the left hemisphere, we often refer to the phenomena of better speech utilization and retention in the right ear as ***the right ear advantage*** (Hellige, 1993). The right ear advantage aspect is particularly important in the rehabilitative process, in terms of fitting parameters and other considerations such as monaural vs binaural applications.

The **RIGHT HEMISPHERE**—via the left ear primarily—performs a different yet vitally important function in speech communication, albeit more subtly. From the right hemisphere, humans obtain ***spatial, holistic, contextual, and aesthetic interpretation of speech,*** the "non-verbal" meaning of communication. The right hemisphere is then more attuned to the emotions, and is able to "read into" language communication *how* a message was meant to be received, not getting lost in the logic (or lack of it) of it all. This ability, being the strong suit of the female of our species, is often referred to as "intuition" (Johnson, 1986). In actuality, though, it appears to be their more innate ability to listen with both sides of the brain. (Remember the larger ***corpus callosum*** in females?).

Another way to look at the interrelationship of the two hemispheres is this: To be verbally debating Einstein's Theory of Relativity vs Newtonian Physical Laws in one's left hemisphere while hanging, by fingertips, onto the edge of a sheer cliff, would come across as rather odd to the right side of the brain, which keeps an eye out for the "big picture" of events around us. Taking into consideration the "context" of the situation, the right (holistic) side of the brain then forces the left (abstract) side to take a momentary backseat while it sizes up the situation. Then, the right hemisphere—once its wits are collected—may "dole out" portions of the problem to be solved by the left hemisphere. But as adrenaline and other powerful "fight or flight" reactions come rushing to the rescue, the right brain will—in most cases—be fully in charge during the crisis! Once safely back upon solid terra firma, however, the left side of the brain tends to take charge in taking remedial action to the (now past) crisis.

A more anecdotal illustration of the right/left brain relationship was humorously put forth by Williams (1993):

> *. . . The hemispheres do not ignore each other or act independently, like the fictional Dr. Jekyll and Mr. Hyde. Our strong left brain doesn't drag our weaker right brain around by his gray matter—it wouldn't dare—the right brain would kick the heck out of him while he's sleeping.*
>
> *No, our hemispheres, although they are functionally biased, work together through many inner cerebral roads and connections. Each plays a special part in the reception, selection and perception of the uncountable stimuli that bombard us each millisecond of our lives. Life without one hemisphere or without full function of the other would be hazardous and dull indeed, and we would miss a lot of incoming stimuli.*
>
> *Now, can you think of a better argument for wearing hearing aids on both ears?*

IMPORTANCE OF BINAURAL RECEPTION

Since much of the acoustic information to the right hemisphere of the human brain is encoded and supplied from the left (contralateral) ear, we certainly cannot discount the importance of information from that ear. Together, the normal function of the right and left ears, primarily lateralized as they are contralaterally to opposing brain hemispheres, are needed for normal development of verbal and non-verbal language communication. The most successful rehabilitation program in bilateral hearing loss, at the symbolic level of hearing, would depend significantly upon ***binaural correction*** of the defective system.

Other binaural auditory functions, such as ***binaural summation, binaural squelch, binaural integration, spatial mapping,*** and ***localization*** are also vital bi-hemispheric functions. However, these do not come genetically, but are developed through time, exposure, and maturation in the ongoing process of hearing, listening, and communicating. In short, these are *learned skills.* For instance, as an adjunct skill to developing language communication ability, it is often not until the age of six or seven years that most normally developing children acquire sufficient ***attention and auditory focusing*** skills to function well in challenging listening situations such as in the classroom setting (Phillips, 1976). The ability to direct attention and to screen-out unrelated or unneeded sounds (or ***speech-in-noise ability***) is developed as a result of continuous ***bilateral exposure*** to the aural environment. Likewise, *deprivation of hearing acuity* (after language is attained) may cause a temporary central auditory processing condition called ***phonemic regression*** (Delk, 1991). This is a speech understanding problem that is either out of proportion to the degree of hearing loss, or which persists for a period of time after amplification is first applied. This is thought to be a most pervasive condition afflicting many long-standing and uncorrected sensorineural loss cases (Palmer, 1995).

OTHER END OF LIFE'S SPECTRUM

Recent research breakthroughs show the human brain has an amazing capacity to maintain function, even in the face of advancing age. In an unprecedented study currently underway by the University of Kentucky and the National Institute of Aging, on the effects of health habits and the aging process, 678 elderly nuns from the School Sisters of Notre Dame, a Roman Catholic order, opened their health records and gave permission for post-mortem examination of their brains (Chase, 1995). Thus far, evidence shows that the most intellectually active sisters suffer the *least* deterioration in brain function, even in minimizing symptoms of naturally occurring mental degeneration.

In the case of Sister Regin Mergens, a 102-year-old nun who recently passed away, researchers upon a post-mortem examination found her brain riddled with the expected protein plaque indicative of Alzheimer's. Yet all during her life—clear to the end—she had not shown any outward symptoms of the disease! Said researcher Dr. David Snowdon, "***She had one of the highest mental functions in the order. She was the gold standard.***" In fact, of the 678 nuns in this order—with an average age of 85—150 of them are retired. Moreover, researchers found that these sisters do not, as a rule, show signs of dementia or Alzheimer's Disease. ***Their secret?*** They watch carefully what they eat and drink, don't smoke, and stay ***exceptionally intellectually and culturally active.*** A daily routine for the retired nuns of the order consists of vocabulary quizzes, crossword puzzles, music lessons, reading and studying, card games, and volunteer work service. *But there was something else . . .*

At a lecture assignment in Minneapolis during the winter of 1994, this author met two of the sisters of the School Sisters of Notre Dame at a conference on hearing impairment. While their presence first led me to believe that they were attending solely out of interest in their own hearing impairment (both were hearing aid users), it turned out that they were there primarily to learn how to assist *other hearing impaired persons* in their more isolated community (further north in the state). Both credited their hearing aids, assistive devices, and myriad coping strategies with allowing them to maintain very active and productive schedules while helping others. Several letters and requests for hearing health reprint articles later, they are still going strong. In fact, just a few months after having met these outstanding ladies, I noticed that they were featured in the main story of July, 1994 issue of *Life* magazine. Below their photograph in the article ran the caption, "***The Nuns Who Wouldn't Sit Still.***" It turns out that the bold experiment for which their order has signed has been hailed by researchers the world over as the most revolutionary research in history on the human brain. And, with the healthy understanding these sisters exhibit toward the connection of mental health and good hearing, it is easy to see why!

Harvard's Dr. David Hubel, a Nobel prize winner, stated, "***The brain is much more modifiable than we ever suspected.***" He and many other researchers on the aging process have found that while every brain may be limited by ***genetic factors,*** that most ***contributing factors,*** which often determine the *rate* of degeneration and decrease of flexibility, are predominantly within the control of the individual. As we shall show near the end of this chapter, new evidence now points conclusively to a direct correlation between hearing health and mental health, long suspected by hearing health practitioners in the field, but only recently confirmed by scientific studies.

PSYCHOLOGY OF THE PERSPECTIVE PATIENT

One of the greatest pitfalls for researchers on the subject of psychology of hearing impairment has been the tendency to overgeneralize the hearing loss state, or to omit differentiation between types and degrees of hearing loss. Just as no two fingerprints are alike, so are no two hearing impairments. Add to the mix numerous differences extant in personality, skills, and experience. Because there are so many variables, hearing impairment as a single entity does not lend itself well to inferential statistical studies, but rather to *anecdotal* case studies. So, when a well-meaning university experiment (and they are legion!) attempts to record and analyze experiences of normal-hearing subjects who were merely mimicking hearing loss with ear-plugs, at best the data results constitute conjecture.

True, some repeatable patterns *do* surface. Cases of sudden hearing loss exhibit the most observable and dramatic effects (Menzel, Lovely, and Kisch, 1995). Subsequently, recognition of these effects, though more difficult, are especially more important when analyzing real-life situations with patients who have real-life hearing loss that developed over 10, 20, or even 30 years periods. In these less apparent cases, reports from the field by hearing instrument specialists often provide more reliable analyses of affected psycho-social behavior than do many formal studies. Moreover, individual social support systems, external stress factors, and occupations enter into the equation almost as much as the much-dissected hearing loss effects themselves. However, for rehabilitative reasons, we must explore the commonly accepted effects or rather ***tendencies***—in tandem with myriad other influences on one's life—caused by the impaired hearing system.

So while our discussion in the differences in effects of the various kinds of hearing loss must be somewhat definitive, it is most relevant to repeat a caution by Sandlin (Reiter, 1990):

> *". . . that by accepting a single definition of psychology of hearing impairment professionals run the risk of fitting the hearing impaired person into a particular personality subgroup and reacting accordingly to that individual . . . Each hearing aid candidate needs to be seen as a mini-study regarding the effects of hearing loss on his or her personality and psychological adjustment to hearing loss."* (pg. 5)

EFFECTS BY DEGREE OF IMPAIRMENT

Discussion here will center upon the psycho-social aspects typically incurred as a hearing impairment progresses over the passage of time. Also discussed will be the progressive stages of sensorineural hearing impairment (mild, moderate, severe, and profound). (see figure 4) Further noted will be perceptual changes that often occur at each stage between the prospective (uncorrected) patient and their significant others:

At the **MILD LOSS STAGE,** where pure-tone average (PTA) thresholds fall between 20 dB HL at best and 45dB HL at worst, there exists an almost unwinnable "great debate" about whether the person even has a hearing loss. Even among some professionals there seems to be misunderstanding about the importance of correcting mild hearing impairment, often arriving at a decision through dubious ***"candidacy criteria"*** which considers speech understanding under ideal conditions as the primary indicator of need. However, this author has always held to the belief that mild hearing loss:

1) Reduces auditory ability (especially in noise and at distances) significantly more than patients and family members can readily assess,
2) Results in many non-acoustic (and therefore unmeasurable) degradation effects such as stress levels, social dysfunction, and over-all well-being, and
3) Minimizes recognition of critical effects upon occupational, educational, and lifestyle demands.

Certainly, most mild loss sufferers are not ***conscious*** that their hearing is affecting their ability to function at optimum levels. However, the importance of having good hearing becomes crucial if one is a banker sitting in board meetings where "**m**illions" or "**b**illions" are being discussed, or a teacher, counselor, or sales person where the softer nuances of speech render important make or break clues, or retired individuals who wish to spend their golden years living a fuller and more socially active life, now that they have the time and means of doing so. In every case, lessened hearing diminishes function and well-being, though vaguely so.

Family members may notice that the impaired person is missing some of the conversation, but it is common to attribute the problem to mental or personality factors (***"John just doesn't pay attention", "Her mind is off somewhere else", "He isn't interested in me anymore",*** or "***He hears when he wants to"***). These accusations are so common that the experienced hearing health professional can almost lip-sync them with third parties who accompany the prospective patient to their offices. And, the trip-switch for the timely close of a hearing instrument fitting is so often the third party who still does not empathize with the person's hearing loss. But, there's more than just mildly affected speech discrimination scores in these cases . . .

When related to the three levels of hearing discussed earlier mild hearing loss is usually ***most*** affected at the ***primitive or background level,*** where common ambient noises are less discernible. The discernment of background is closely tied to one's sense of security and connection with life itself. When these sounds cannot be easily recognized at the subconscious level they instead tear away at one's sense of security and become annoying and distracting. This, in turn, subconsciously adds to one's stress level in a somewhat vague and unexplainable way. Rather than being able to sit and relax while sitting in public gatherings or events, the sufferer of mild loss must "***sit up and pay closer attention***" to receive the same amount of auditoy informaton as the normal hearing person relaxing beside them. This adds to stress levels, and makes the typical day seem longer and longer as the loss progresses. As an illustrative way of explaining this concept to patients and third parties, the author often describes the phenomena in this way:

> *"We tend to think of a 24-hour day as being the same for everyone, but in some cases that is not necessarily true. For those with hearing loss, the stress experienced over a given 24-hour period is much greater than for those with normal hearing. Mild loss, then, brings a mildly longer day; moderate hearing loss, a moderately longer day; and severe loss, a much longer day. Most disease is caused or exacerbated by higher levels of stress.*
>
> *One of the non-acoustic benefits of proper hearing correction is that stress levels can be lowered significantly. Then, the greatest*

benefits realized from proper hearing correction could be less stress, more relaxation, and better health."

One of the best paradigms for correcting hearing loss in its earliest stages lies in the ***auditory deprivation*** factor. That is, as hearing impairment continues to progress from mild to moderate, and from moderate to severe, those who begin their rehabilitative program during the earliest stages are the least apt to be affected by their hearing loss as it continues its downward progression. They are better able to not only ***preserve speech understanding,*** but their own speech, as well. They are ***less bothered by the stress*** caused by hearing loss and enjoy life more, and ***relationships are less affected*** as hearing changes. This rather unscientific paradigm was one of the debates at the heart of the recent controversy over proposed FDA rule changes in hearing aid advertising (Kirkwood, 1995). Yet, this paradigm is real and unchallengeable when placed under the bright light of user reports and experiences. Hence, better hearing ***does*** bring better living. The real question then becomes, "***How much does one's quality of life need to diminish before it is considered worthwhile to correct a hearing loss?***"

Empirical evidence suggests, "***The sooner the better.***"

When uncorrected hearing impairment progresses to the **MODERATE LOSS STAGE**, comprising PTA thresholds between 45-65dB HL, the effects become more marked and more evident to observers. However, by this time, without correction, definite tendencies in behavior change become more deeply rooted. For instance, its' a hostile world out there to one who cannot hear well. Regular exposure to (perceived) hostility brings ***defensiveness*** and a tendency toward shifting blame in social misunderstandings. Detachment from bonded relationships brings ***feelings of isolation and rejection.*** Lessened auditory clues in the environment which are ordinarily used by hearing individuals to stimulate short- and long-term memory bring ***depression, frustration, and auditory memory loss.***

A strong propensity toward either ***withdrawing or dominating conversation*** is not uncommon for the moderate loss sufferer. Instinctively, there develops an ***avoidance of group situations,*** especially where background levels interfere with conversation. These tendencies cause one to ***turn inward, limit social contacts,*** and ***feel unappreciated*** or ***misunderstood***. The composite effect of these tendencies work to thwart the best efforts in getting this person to seek help. In other words, the psycho-social anomalies created by the hearing impairment tend to prevent the seeking of hearing help to be forthcoming.

Progressive Stages of Sensorineural Hearing Impairment
(in uncorrected state)

Mild Loss (20-45dB)

1. "Hears when wants to"
2. "Not paying attention"
3. Mild frustration in S/N situations
4. Denial of impairment/slight defensiveness
5. Little desire to seek help for loss

Moderate Loss (45-65dB)

1. Marked frustration in some social settings
2. Personality changes
3. Defensive, deep denial
4. Lessened creativity/intellectual stimulus
5. Tends to dominate conversation or withdraw
6. Lessened desire to seek help on own

Severe Loss (65-90dB)

1. Social isolation, anti-social behavior
2. Sense of loss/depression
3. Insecure/aggressive/socially withdrawn
4. Falling quality of life/doubted self-worth
5. Least of all motivated to seek help

Profound Loss (95dB+)

1. Fewer psycho-social dilemmas
2. Social separation and isolation
3. Difficult to bond in relationships
4. Severely lessened environmental awareness

Fig. 4

Therefore, it is important for loved ones to realize that a person with moderate or greater hearing loss needs their support and encouragement in arriving at a positive decision regarding hearing correction. For the third party to shrug their shoulders with "***It's up to them***" or "***I'm not going to make up their mind for them***" is akin to pushing a person who cannot swim out on a rubber raft into swirling rapids. In truth, if the moderately hearing impaired individual could have done something about their loss on their own, they would have done so long before now.

In cases of uncorrected impairment at the **SEVERE LOSS STAGE** (65dB HL to 90dB HL), usually a great deal of time has elapsed since the earliest signs of hearing loss and, therefore, effects upon one's life are quite established. Signs that were almost transparent at the mild stage have now become magnified larger than life. For example, attempts to mask the hearing loss in social situations has largely given way to ***avoiding*** those situations altogether. Feelings of distrust have often given way to ***social paranoia and isolation***. Frustration has often given way to ***anger and an ill-defined belligerence.*** The fear of being called upon in groups leads to ***avoidance of eye contact*** or feigned ***disinterest;*** stress to ***resignation and boredom.***

Probably the most tragic of all is the breaking of life-long bonds in human relationships. Those close to them have—except for a few unheralded saints—long given up rearranging their own world to accommodate the sufferer's severe hearing loss. Therefore, in this group we find increased incidence of ***divorce, alcoholism, drug abuse, and dependency.*** Of course, the age of the person—and their relative life experiences leading up to this point—play a significant role. In other words, an elderly person whose hearing acuity gradually deteriorated will likely not be subject to the forces of divorce, alcoholism, and drug abuse. But most certainly many in their number have been overdiagnosed for ***dementia*** and ***Alzheimer's***. Many of their number live largely isolated lives away from others, in nursing care facilities where social interaction and lifestyles are too often considered secondary to life itself.

The tragic truth is that, for nearly every one of these cases, their suffering is essentially avoidable if only interested third parties and caring professionals would take the time to see that they receive proper aural rehabilitation and correction. Hearing aids are a God-send to most of these people. And, under new FDA-approved guidelines, the more advanced cases could also benefit from cochlear implants. The life improvement qualities of either hearing instruments or cochlear implants in such cases is astounding, behooving any reasonable person to ask why modern society still has a good number of people suffering from unmitigated severe hearing loss.

PROFOUND HEARING LOSS, with pure-tone averages greater than 90dB HL, will only be commented upon here. Profound loss, while not anyone's choice of personal status, appears not to be as psycho-socially and emotionally debilitating as some of the stages leading up to it. The deaf community is comprised of many such persons who seem to lead relatively functional and fulfilling lives. Even in the best cases, limitations in functioning in the hearing world through the visual mode are still enormous challenges; hence, the strong propensity to separate out of society's mainstream.

Therefore, it is a virtual near-miracle that modern technology has brought unprecedented assistance to the profoundly deaf through cochlear implants, TDDs, TDD Relay Service, Closed Caption, vibrating and flashing alerting systems, and a host of other devices and methods for joining the hearing world. One concern of this author has long been that some in this group actively resist these technologies and empowering strategies and, worse, insist that ***other*** deaf persons should do likewise (Bonillas, 1995). It is hoped that such thinking will eventually be neutralized, as more and more deaf persons successfully join the hearing world to lead happier, more productive and successful lives. While many of these subjects suffer substantially from auditory sensory deprivation and exhibit physiologically underdeveloped central and higher brain function in the auditory format, recent studies show promise of successful later development of these systems for both children and adults even long after the ***critical development period*** has past (Ross, Brackett, Maxon, 1991).

Today, great debate swirls in professional circles over hearing vs deaf culture, as if the subjects are part of a protected minority or lifestyle choice. Somehow, in this line of thinking, if one chooses to join the hearing world by using hearing instruments, cochlear implants, speechreading, and assistive devices, they are considered a "traitor" to the "cause" of deafness . . . as if anyone would consciously choose to be deaf by their own volition. 1995 Miss America Heather Whitestone and others who've struggled and smashed through the wall of deafness could well lead the way for other deaf persons to finally take advantage of all the new technological and therapeutic treatments available today. Furthermore, as more and more hearing instrument specialists become involved in cochlear implants, tactile and frequency transposition devices, and associated deaf rehabilitation strategies, we will witness a dramatic reduction in the number of persons who voluntarily choose to remain in the "deaf" world.

PSYCHO-SOCIAL EFFECTS BY TYPE OF LOSS

It is widely accepted that, statistically, ***sensorineural impairments*** comprise between 90 to 95% of all adult hearing loss in the United States and Canada (IHS, 1993). Likewise, this figure is often reversed for children, indicating the widely-held belief that about 90% of hearing loss in children is ***conductive.***

The author's experience indicates that lost in this statistical over-simplification are the myriad exceptions which have elements of *both* conductive and sensorineural. For the older adult population, we must also add the prevalence of ***mild central auditory processing problems*** in the mix (Cooper and Gates, 1992) (Willott, 1991) (Stach, Loiselle, and Jerger, 1991). With these exceptions in mind, then, we will proceed to list the most identifiable psycho-social effects of hearing impairment by type and degree.

Conductive impairment is chiefly characterized by the physical blockage of sound in an otherwise normal hearing system. In this day and age of modern medicine and micro-surgical procedures it seems almost redundant and unnecessary that a text written near the start of the twenty-first century would include psycho-social effects of such a predominantly resolvable malady. But this misconception is where the distinctions for varying types of conductive loss become crucial to our discussion. Effects on human behavior are quite dependent upon site of lesion, the length of time since onset, and degree of severity, whether mild, moderate, severe, or (very rarely) profound (see figure 5).

To differentiate such effects, we must first categorize by ***duration and etiological aspects:***

Transient conductive impairment: Cerumen impaction, middle ear effusion, external otitis, acute mastoiditis, foreign object, membrane perforation, and/or air pressure equalization dysfunction. These conditions tend to produce the most traumatic short-term psycho-social and cognitive effects upon sufferers of conductive loss. Tendencies include: ***pronounced feelings of isolation and disorientation, marked loss of sense of security and depression, a state of dread or mourning, and a lessened feeling of self-confidence.*** Admittedly, a significant portion of these reported effects stem indirectly from fluid accumulation, occlusion, and interaural attenuation. Over time, however, many eventually subside or resolve—if the physical disease itself is not treated—to resemble more closely those of longer-term pathologies. Our primary concern, in this category of conductive impairment, rests mostly with the millions of school-age children who lag behind in school by a year or more because of widespread ***chronic otitis media.*** Evidently, most of these cases result from increasing trends in inhalant allergy and prevalent reliance upon immune-destroying antibiotics. More will be covered on this population further on.

Longer-term pathological disease: Adhesive otitis media, cholesteatoma, glomus tumor, chronic mastoiditis, and/or ossicular disarticulation. These conditions can last for many years without treatment giving the sufferer longer periods of time in which to accept and acclimate to the imperfect auditory state. Especially notable is the absence of pain in most cases; hence, these conditions—with the exception of ossicular disarticulation—tend to be life-threatening because of the lack of sense of urgency to seek medical intervention. ***Occlusion***—or rather, amplified conduction of one's own voice via interaural attenuation—added to unabated ***feelings of isolation*** mark this type of conductive impairment. ***Frustration and anxiety*** in verbal communication are commonplace. ***Tinnitus*** is most often characterized by "heart beat" or pulsation, which can induce varying degrees of ***psychosis and insomnia*** (McSpaden, 1993). It is imperative that observant dispensing professionals always be on the lookout for the tell-tale signs of serious ear disease in cases of conductive impairment: ***pulsating tinnitus, pressure or fullness, adhesive otitis media, "blue drum" or visible tympanic membrane abnormalities during otoscopy, and a history of ear disease.***

Degenerative conditions: otosclerosis, tympanosclerosis, epithelial atrophy, neuritis, and/or necrotizing vasculitis. Because of the progressive nature and long-term effects of these auditory conditions—added to the fact that prognosis is not always good after medical or surgical treatment—most of these cases become intermingled within the general condition we conveniently call ***presbycusis***. Therefore, in cases of older adults, few of these cases are purely conductive but have an integral sensorineural component. Therefore, the reported psychosocial effects derived from presbycusis are more closely identified with those of sensorineural loss.

Congenital malformations: microsia, atresia, and/or ossicular malformation. As a general rule, the greater the longevity of the lesion (congenital conditions representing the largest segment of conductive loss cases in the deaf community), the less effect upon cognition and emotion. This could explain why there is still a sizable portion of conductive cases within the deaf community who choose not to ameliorate their problem through medicine or surgery (or even amplification). From a medical standpoint, these losses are increasingly treatable with successful outcomes. From a psycho-social standpoint, long-standing congenital deafness is typified by ***social isolation, lessened environmental awareness,*** and ***development of alternative psychoneurological pathways for spatial and cognitive function.*** In such cases, the applicable designation is ***habilitation,*** as their auditory systems likely do not have enough auditory memory or established neurological auditory functions for ***rehabilitative*** treatment per se. In late-treated cases, the habilitative road could be long and difficult, requiring more specialized professional and clinical care.

In the ***intensity domain,*** conductive cases of all etiologies usually do not exhibit recruitment or other loudness-growth distortions, since the cochlea is intact and "protected" from overly loud sound. Elevated noise apparently does not adversely effect these patients until intensities are great enough to cause actual cellular or molecular damage (approximately 130dB SPL). In fact, if the conductive impairment is less than 65dB, these patients generally

Psycho-Social Aspects of Conductive Impairment
(in uncorrected state)

1. Sense of social isolation/lessened awareness
2. Depression/anxiety/social withdrawal
3. Ill effects of occlusion/interaural attenuation
4. Fair to good function in poor S/N situations
5. Relatively normal dynamic range/loudness growth
6. Usually open to medical/rehabilitative intervention

Fig. 5

do quite well in noisy circumstances where otherwise normal hearing individuals seem to have difficulty. This is because the person communicating to them must raise their voice over the general noise level of the environment, and since the hearing impaired person does not hear most of the background noise they are left with a less cluttered speech-in-noise (SiN) scenario. Therefore, the attendant Pavlovian-like social responses so often observable in sensorineural loss cases appear nearly absent in comparable levels of conductive impairment.

Sensorineural impairment presents the proverbial Pandora's box of psycho-social manifestations commonly referred to as ***the psychology of the hearing impaired*** (Chartrand, 1988). Of course, it should be noted that our primary discussion here centers upon the *uncorrected* and uncompensated state, not necessarily patients who have received corrective amplification and proper rehabilitation. However, for those patients who wear hearing instruments, but have not had the benefit of proper counseling and other rehabilitative strategies, a certain degree of application of these principles may still hold.

Perplexing elements in discerning sensorineural aspects of psycho-social problems stem from the ***transparency and insidiousness*** inherent in the vast majority of sensorineural cases. *Insidious* because of the extremely gradual decline in threshold sensitivity over time, and *transparent* because of spectral bias in retaining low frequencies while losing sensitivity in the highs. A good allegory of this phenomena is that of a person intently watching the minute hand of a clock move the span of seven minutes while not keeping track of the starting point. Detection of movement and its intervening distance without a starting reference are humanly impossible to determine, yet time continues to march on. ***Hence, by the time most sufferers are aware of the existence of hearing impairment via self-assessment, the loss of high frequency acuity has already often travelled to the severe state.*** Waiting until "*it gets bad enough*" represents a form of illusory self-delusion, at best. For when that self-assessed state is finally arrived at, ideal correction has already become impossible because of the resulting:

- Severe cochlear distortions at the hair cell level, especially in the highs.
- Significant loss of horizontal bandwidth sensitivity, making discrete frequency resolution difficult.
- Marked loudness growth abnormalities, both at suprathreshold and in upper limit discomfort levels.

Psycho-Social Aspects
Sensorineural Loss
(in uncorrected state)

1. Denial/Fear of "being found out"
2. Distrust/paranoia/anti-social
3. Pavlovian-like responses re: loudness growth
4. Depression/withdrawal/isolation
5. Defensiveness/frustration/anger
6. Phonemic regression/speech degradation
7. Speaks loudly in moderate noise environment

Fig. 6

Psycho-social effects (see fig. 6) of sensorineural impairment include ***denial*** of the hearing loss, ***defensiveness, paranoia,*** and the ***fear of being "found out."*** This last one might strike the reader as odd, for it implies that the sufferer has something to hide. For instance, untreated sensorineural sufferers may rarely understand the punch-line of a joke, but they certainly will give it the hardiest laugh. On this point, the author was once asked why I laughed so hard at a joke I didn't understand, to which I replied, "***Because it sounded so funny!***".

Other situations, such as receiving verbal directions, instructions, or technical information require a great deal of *guess-work* and *blank-filling,* skills for which many long-time sufferers of sensorineural impairment develop an uncanny ability. But, again, they are still afraid of "being found out" because they didn't receive their information the old fashioned way through clear, phonological communication. Overall, sufferers of sensorineural impairment *try to hide their malady* because of the *awkwardness* it presents for others around them (such as in knowing when to repeat, when to speak up, or if something is even worth repeating). So, often, a *po-*

lite smile, a nod of the head, and utterances of agreement ensue, even when the communication being spoken by the other party is incoherent, incorrect, or ill-considered. *Trial and error,* hit and miss, eventually teaches the sufferer to avoid such situations or risk "being found out"; hence, it is not uncommon to find a lessening in one's sense of humor, especially in group settings. Normal hearing people from foreign lands who are not fluent in the language of those around them, of course, have a similar challenge. If they are seeking employment or social acceptance, they too are in fear of "being found out". Once, when a foreigner was introducing himself and apologized that he did not understand English very well, I shot back, ***"That makes two of us! I don't either."***

Loudness growth abnormalities bring a host of dilemmas for those with sensorineural loss. Unlike their conductive loss counterparts, sensorineural cases do not have a built-in earplug, nor, in the more serious stages of loss, do they enjoy some of the neurophysiological loudness protective mechanisms enjoyed by normal hearing persons, such as ***stapedial reflex*** and ***tensor tympani contractions*** at the handle of malleus, both of which serve as the auditory system's shock absorbers. So, not only are loud sounds more uncomfortable (once they exceed UCL), but impact noise actually tends to cause even greater damage to the sensorineural-lesioned ear. These loudness growth distortions often render ***Pavlovian-like psychological responses*** which tend to develop for the sufferer in various acoustic settings, such as in crowds of people, at dances, and at large social gatherings where speech-in-noise skills (SiN) are a must for social survival. ***Avoidance of such situations*** becomes almost automatic when the sufferer is given a choice, and may cause them to appear ***anti-social*** or ***socially withdrawn.*** Add to this the tendency to deny or cover their hearing loss, and it is easy to see why they lack the motivation on their part to seek out hearing help. Note back in figure 4 how the desire to seek hearing help tends to diminish as the loss worsens over time. Without a "face-saving" way in which to attribute a long, steady history of unhappy social experiences, the desire to seek help tends to diminish proportionately.

Social Paranoia has long been recognized as an integral aspect of hearing loss, in general, and in moderate to severe sensorineural hearing impairment, in particular. This form of so-called "paranoia" actually stems from:

- ***Loss of spontaneity*** in verbal and non-verbal communication.
- ***Loss of "small talk"*** which is how humans bond with one another.

- ***Feelings that one is being "talked about".***
- ***Distorted perspectives*** re: difficult listening situations.
- ***Denial and the fear of being "found out".***

These and more all contribute to what appears to be *paranoia,* when in actuality what we are looking at is the result of societal breakdowns in verbal and non-verbal communication. The admixture of ***loudness growth distortions, paranoia,*** and the ***fear of being found out*** present a dilemma for normal hearing persons around those with uncorrected sensorineural impairment. *As an illustration:* The normal hearing person raises his voice to be understood, only to be told, "***You're hurting my ears. You don't have to shout!".*** In turn, the normal hearing person begins to form a conflicted assessment of the sufferer's true problem (i.e., not paying attention, not interested, distracted, slow-of-mind, etc.).

The unspoken analysis may be, "***If you really have a hearing problem, why can't you hear me better when I speak up?".*** Or, an even more jaundiced analysis—but one painfully aligned with logic—is, "***If you really have a hearing problem, why don't you wear a hearing aid?".***

"But," mentally replies the hearing impaired person, "***I don't have a hearing problem, I just miss some words. My problem is that people mumble, the background music is too loud, and, besides, I'm worried that people will notice I'm different."*** (Fear of being found out, anyone?).

What makes it difficult for the hearing impaired person to overcome these seemingly unfair assessments is the strong tendency to cover the hearing loss, making others think it is anything but a hearing problem. Add to that the tendency to strenuously avoid the one solution that is available: ***prescriptive amplification and aural rehabilitation.*** Such intrapersonal roadblocks make for a difficult rehabilitative road down which to travel. In the other words, by putting off seeking hearing help, the sufferer only reinforces the lack of empathy on the part of observers. On the other hand, if after the acquisition of hearing instruments, speech understanding difficulty is still experienced, the public's perception of the patient will often change from criticism and doubt to one of empathy and understanding.

This author, as both a hearing aid and cochlear implant user, can personally attest to receiving better treatment by the public in general when a hearing aid is visible even when speech discrimination problems still persist, than if no instruments were worn at all. To the public mind, obtaining hearing help is simply a demonstration of common courtesy.

SENSORY DEPRIVATION & IMPAIRMENT IN CHILDREN

While the subject of children with hearing loss may seem out of the domain of hearing instrument specialists, the reality is changing as more and more audiologists enter the dispensing field, and the two disciplines (dispensers and audiologists) work increasingly as a team. As the population of hearing impaired children continues to grow, the need for more dispensing and rehabilitative professionals is also increasing, evidenced most by the fact that most public school programs are currently overwhelmed in screening for and ameliorating increasing numbers of hearing impaired children, both transient and permanent. Therefore, a developing trend presents a unique opportunity for traditional dispensing professionals to become better grounded and skilled in assisting parents, teachers, and other professionals in meeting the needs of hearing impaired children.

When reviewing hearing loss among children it is important to point out that, unlike adults who lost hearing ***post-lingually,*** children most often are ***pre-lingual.*** This means the professional's effort is not so much to restore a function or ability that has already been established as it is in assisting the development itself of the missing, yet to be realized, auditory function. We call this process ***aural habilitation.*** Therefore, a deprivation and developmental view is in order for our discussion here. For literally millions of pre-school and school-age children who suffer from ***mild and intermittent hearing loss*** occurring from chronic otitis media (approximately 10 million cases per year in the U.S.), recent research has shed light on the debilitative effects of ***sensory deprivation*** (Ruben and Rapin, 1980). Of particular interest are the myriad data from animal sensory deprivation research pointing toward a correlation to human auditory function. From these data come the proposition that **binaural** auditory deprivation causes serious developmental problems during a child's first few years of life, particularly in the speech, language, academic, and psycho-social disturbances domains.

For example, when newborn rats were temporarily deprived of sound, they were later unable to differentiate complex sound patterns or time differences. ***These are the two most important components needed for development of speech understanding.*** Other studies show decreased auditory sensitivity twice to three times the norm in early audition-deprived rats (Clopton and Winfield, 1976). Still other studies show ***structural changes in the brainstem auditory nuclei*** when subjects were deprived sound stimulation over a significant time period (Webster, 1983). **Monaural deprivation** also presents difficulties in the auditory brainstem, such as ***localization of sound sources, selectivity of signals in competing background noise, and suppression of unwanted sounds*** (Kirkwood and Kirkwood, 1983). Moreover, it should also be noted that these are the very problems repeatedly reported by adults who either have uncorrected hearing loss in one ear, or, if they have bilateral hearing loss, were fitted only in one ear!

Data from studies on children with hearing impairment confirm the above observations, so much so that Ross et al (1991) have observed:

> *"These results have been interpreted to suggest that there is a critical period for the acquisition of auditory learning skills, and that the hearing loss secondary to otitis media could cause irreversible damage to the ability to process auditory input."* (Pg. 8)

The above conclusion was drawn relative to children with mild and intermittent hearing loss resulting from chronic middle ear effusion. Further on, however, they offer this revealing comment about children who are without meaningful or useful hearing in the early years of life:

> *". . . that if the auditory system is not stimulated with some critical quantity of meaningful sound at an early period after birth, then that system may display structural and physiological abnormalities that can forever limit its capacities below its original potential . All we can state with any sense of assurance is that the earlier we begin* (with treatment or amplification), *the more likely it is that we can reduce or eliminate the occurrence of auditory sensory deprivation."* (Ibid. above)

Children with hearing impairment exhibit several psycho-social tendencies, depending upon the degree of their loss and the adequacy of correction and habilitative treatment. As a general rule, however, children tend to exhibit:

- Fear of non-conformity (i.e. resistance to hearing aid use)
- Poor human relationship bonding and socialization skills
- Reduced intellectual creativity
- Lagging academic performance
- Passive/aggressive personality traits

The sad fact is that misdiagnosis of hearing impairment in children can lead to false assumptions suggesting ***mental retardation, partial or mild autism, general learning disability, and attention deficit disorder (ADD).*** Significant effort is currently underway to improve both the frequency and quality of screening for hearing loss in children. But, as mentioned earlier, most public school systems are overwhelmed and woefully insufficient in seeking out and addressing hearing loss. This could explain the huge variations in studies about the actual number of children with hearing impairment (from 16 to 30 per 1,000)! One of the truths of many children's audiology programs is the obvious lag in up-to-date technological and habilitative application. For instance, most programs still perpetuate the myth of monaural amplification; hence, few children enjoy binaural amplification. Plus, many children are fitted according to an outmoded ***"candidacy criteria"*** that is almost wholly dependent upon arbitrary thresholds and speech data (ex. 35dB HL, >50% aided discrim, etc.). However, mountains of evidence show that losses as little as 16dB PTA can deter speech and psycho-social development, and the probability of falling behind one or more years in school increases several-fold over children who hear normally (Quigley, 1978) (Oyler et al., 1988).

Children today still are rarely fitted with smaller, less physically limiting (and imposing) instrumentation, though the cost of shell remakes of custom instrumentation barely exceeds the cost of earmold updating. Advanced evaluative applications such as real ear, video otoscopy, electroacoustical analysis, and programmability (used regularly in private practice) are rarely available in children's public programs. And if the child is profoundly deaf, there are a legion of advocates against the child using amplification (oral/aural habilitation) or receiving a cochlear implant for fear of depriving them of the "choice" to be deaf.

The above is certainly not meant to denigrate the many fine children's programs, but as one who has come up through the system, here I am several decades later, noting as an educator in the profession the distance we still must travel to provide our children with at least the same level of hearing health care routinely offered the private adult population! A growing chorus of educators, professionals, and parents are saying,

> *"The time* is now *to change this tragic oversight by the hearing health profession!"*

PRINCIPLES AND CONCEPTS FOR PROFESSIONAL INTERVENTION

The purpose of this section is to introduce hearing instrument specialists to practical applications and strategies for removing psycho-social barriers to hearing health care. In this way, more hearing impaired persons can step forward and take advantage of the technological and rehabilitative near-miracles available to them. Most of the recommendations could be classified as "tried and true" but certainly do not, in and of themselves, claim scientific proof of their effectiveness. Oftentimes, the best laboratory is the "laboratory of real life", and that is the laboratory from which this section of the chapter will most heavily draw.

OVERCOMING MISCONCEPTIONS THROUGH PRE-COUNSELING

It is imperative that hearing instrument specialists recognize the significant impact of their advertising on their market. In this profession, advertising is actually public education which forms and shapes public opinions about hearing impairment and professional intervention approaches. Public education, in turn, becomes pre-counseling to the prospective hearing instrument patient, motivating or deterring them toward positive decision to seek resolution of their problem.

For example, over the past decade and a half, the industry has been in a virtual crash program to resolve the loudness growth/signal-to-noise dilemmas which plague so many adult hearing impairments. Huge sums of research and development dollars and a foray of technological breakthroughs have produced breathtaking accomplishments in taming this problematic challenge. In attempting to trumpet these accomplishments to the hearing impaired market, however, industry advertising has inadvertently painted ***background noise as public enemy #1.*** The difficulty with this is that the real culprit of most impairments is ***poor signal-to-noise or speech-in-noise ability,*** not nefarious ambient background. So that, when hearing instruments fail to eliminate or substantially reduce background noise (whatever that is to the listener), credit returns pile up at the factory and public regulators launch another assault against the industry.

When patients ask about the elimination of background noise, it is important that the specialist explain the importance of background sounds as a requisite for one's sense of security and interaction with the world around them. For what might be considered background one minute can be lifesaving or invaluable information the next. The *real* goal is ***improved speech-in-noise ability,*** or the proper spectral balance between frequencies. As the patient enjoys restored focusing and squelching abilities, they will find that their hearing instruments perform well in complementing their residual hearing. The key is to focus on the positive benefits of signal-to-noise capabilities instead of the unwieldy nature of a noisy world over which no one can exert control.

Another misdirected focus is the implicit and sometimes explicit assurance of "**clear hearing**", a tenuous goal at best for the hearing impaired market at-large. Rather, ***improvement*** or ***best use of residual hearing*** is the desired and attainable goal. By implicitly or otherwise promising "clear hearing" the specialist is setting the stage for disillusionment and failure. A standard phrase that the author has used successfully in counseling hearing instrument patients at the time of evaluation goes something like this:

> *"After we have done all we can do to correct your hearing, you will still have some hearing loss, albeit considerably less than you would have without correction. For that reason it is important for you to learn to make the most of the new sounds and to use every available coping strategy and device needed to achieve complete rehabilitation."*

The patient who accepts the fact that hearing instruments are merely the "foundation" to their aural rehabilitation program and that other help is available will be more likely to keep better perspective during the acclimation and adaptation process. Specialists can further assist the patient significantly by providing a clear, methodical ***wearing schedule.*** In this way, new hearing instrument patients can be taught to at first focus upon things near and easily discerned. Then, as their ability to recognize sound improves they may extend their listening range and focus to more challenging sound sources.

Third parties can make or break a hearing instrument fitting by not being aware of the above counsel. Their over-expectations can frustrate even the most determined patient. Likewise, third parties must be counseled:

> *"Just because they now have hearing aids does not mean they will be able to hear perfectly. In fact, at first they will be overwhelmed by all the forgotten or unfamiliar sounds. Please, be understanding and patient and help them limit their initial listening environments until they are more familiar with the new sounds. Usually, it takes up to 12 weeks to fully acclimate, and even after that, there may be steady improvements in their hearing and understanding ability."*

Where many hearing instrument specialists seem to short-change themselves and their patients is in the failure to point out the many ***value-added services*** they offer. It is important that patients know, up front, that in the price of a hearing instrument fitting there are many important and necessary services. For instance, if evaluative and post-fitting services are included in the price of the fitting, a listing of each specific test and/or the equipment used may be advisable. The same goes for other services, such as:

Video otoscopy

Screening Tympanometry

Real ear probe-mic

Soundfield (discreet tone and speech)

Electroacoustic analysis

In-house repair and modification lab

Speech-language and speechreading services

Clinical audiological evaluations

Medical referrals

Battery programs

Maintenance schedules

Post-fitting programs

Assistive Devices

The challenge lies in the fact that the prospective patient has no basis of comparison as to the true value of your services and products. On a results-oriented basis, properly fitted hearing instruments and counseling provide the highest cost/benefit advantage of any healthcare service available today. Moreover, the many value-added features of today's dispensing services have been too long neglected in consumer advertising and public education, making it what this author calls ***"one of the best kept secrets in healthcare today."*** These value-added services need to be listed in advertising (where feasible), on retail or waiting room price lists, and disseminated in newsletters, etc. Then, when the patient is quoted a given price, there will be some realistic basis for judging attendant value.

Another area that will go far in dispelling consumer misconceptions about specialists is in displaying, where possible, ***the level of training and education of the specialist.*** During the Senate Subcommittee on Aging Hearings held during 1993, panelists were surprised to find the high level of formal and professional education achieved by the average hearing instrument specialist (Cohen, 1993). Relative uniformity among state licensure examinations was only the tip of the iceberg. National Board for Certification (NBC-HIS) represented another dimension in competency assurance, as well as the fact that over three-quarters of practicing dispensers today have college degrees, most at the post-graduate level (Skafte, 1995). As a professional body, no healthcare group currently matches the level of ongoing continuing education as hearing instrument specialists. Many specialists attend 30 or more hours each year, though state licensure and certification requirements demand far less.

Thc relevancy of the above information is that it is not being made known to a skeptical market that increasingly wants to know. Dissemination requires more than just hanging framed diplomas and certificates on office walls. It involves news releases, with photo, about recent attendance at major training courses, seminars or trade shows, published works, and achievement awards. Using the NBC-HIS and/or IHS symbols (where appropriate) on business cards and in advertising are other ways to get this information out, as well as personnel profiles in patient newsletters. As pre-counseling tools such information is invaluable in assuring the patient that they can trust the abilities and skill of their caregiver.

Other pre-counseling tools and dispellers of misconception are:

- Focus advertising messages toward the debilitating effects of hearing impairment and the enhancement of quality of life and health through better hearing. Use testimonials by patients and celebrities.
- Advertise value-added services and capabilities, professional qualifications, and other information that will let the market know of your trustworthiness, value orientation, and competency.
- Invest in time and materials to train receptionists and others who will be handling prospective patients on the telephone. Teach them how to get callers to "open up" about the life effects of their hearing loss. Build trust in that crucial initial contact. In many cases, it is difficult to tactfully yet convincingly convey the importance of the spouse being present at the evaluation. As will be discussed further in this section, many men insist on not bringing their spouses with them. The author has found that the conquering of this persistent difficulty can literally double sales of hearing instruments!
- Clear out all reading material in the waiting room that is unrelated to hearing health and keep an ample supply of informative, motivating material out for patients and others to read while sitting in the waiting room. In fact, it is advisable to build

about 10-15 minutes into each appointment so that valuable time can be spent reading such material before going in for an evaluation. Request your receptionist to point out or hand material to those waiting.

- Don't despair if the patient is not ready to be fitted at the initial evaluation. Remember the "four stages of mourning" (see the Rich/McSpaden chapter in this text) and gear your program to assist the patient through each stage. Make sure, however, that they continue to make forward movement by reading material that is relevant to their case. Reprint articles from consumer and professional journals, sections of this textbook, and other materials have been found effective in getting patients to the next stage of readiness.
- After first contact (whether by telephone or in person) continue to develop a growing relationship with the prospective patient through an effective patient management and marketing program. Their hearing loss is not going to go away and the effects upon their lives will continue to plague them without correction. As they step into that last stage of motivation, they should know who to see.

MEN & WOMEN: FITTING PATTERNS

At risk of being "politically incorrect", the author makes some observations, based upon professional experience, which have too long remained unspoken about the hearing instrument market and the growing gap between those who need help versus those who actively seek it out. To unlock the secret of this roadblock in reaching a growing market of hearing impaired persons, the professional must first address and ameliorate obvious yet often unspoken societal factors in market response to the availability of hearing help.

For instance, high frequency sensorineural loss with normal and near-normal hearing in the low region tends to be the ***classical male pattern of loss,*** albeit a most transparent state (Moscicki et al, 1985). Flatter or more gradual audiometric patterns are more common among females, often maintaining relatively near-normal mid-to-high frequencies until much later life when high frequencies begin the precipitious fall similar to, but later than men, in general (Staab, 1990). Traditionally, it has been assumed that this age-lag difference was solely the result of occupational and recreational noise exposure differences. While much of that assumption certainly holds, there is an interesting study that sheds more light on sex differences in hearing loss and reinforces the hypothesis that actual physiological differences do exist between the sexes. This particular study (JASA, 1995) screened out external exposure differences so that both groups had experienced relatively similar exposure levels. Their conclusion was that men as a statistical group still lose their hearing acuity at a rate earlier than women, and especially in the high frequencies.

More important than audiometric pattern differences, though, are the way men and women tend to approach hearing impairment. As mentioned earlier, men tend to put off hearing correction longer than women with similar thresholds. This would explain why, though there are many more males with hearing impairment than females, the proportionate number of male and female hearing instrument users is roughly equal. In addition, upon first time hearing examinations, the severity of the loss tended to be significantly greater among male patients than females (Chartrand, 1989). But since females are more attuned to the auditory and communicative mode they tend to voluntarily seek out help for their hearing problems at an earlier stage of loss.

In addition, based upon years of experience working with hearing impaired adults, the author found that males, in the role of third party, tend not to be as empathetic with their spouse's hearing loss and the need to invest in correction. Females, on the other hand, generally made more empathetic and supportive third parties for their spouses. So there appears to be a dual psycho-social deterrent pattern in that men, as a rule, are most resistant to seeking and accepting help with their hearing, while they also tend to be less empathetic with their own spouse's hearing loss when it comes time to make a decision of forward movement.

To alleviate these challenges, it is suggested:

- Require, where possible, for spouses of married persons to be present at the initial evaluation and at delivery, especially when the husband is the patient.
- Work toward developing empathy in third parties by making them active participants in evaluation and delivery sessions. Get them *emotionally* involved and work with them as a team in resolving the patient's problem.
- Help patients and third parties prioritize the importance of better hearing when compared to other material possessions. Stress non-acoustic and "quality of life" benefits of amplification.

COUNSELING FOR OVER-EXPECTATION

When the sufferer of serious sensorineural loss finally seeks out corrective amplification as a solution to his malady, the dispensing practitioner is many times held (often unfairly) to a level of corrective expectation that may be physically impossible to meet. As it appears that ski-slope and severe high frequency cases are statistically on the upswing (as recreational noise exposure and proliferating ototoxicity cases accelerate unabated), these misperceptions are expected to continue to increase in the future. So, in the more and more commonplace severe-to-profound high frequency configurations—ongoing technological breakthroughs in loudness growth capability notwithstanding—the challenges to the profession are to:

1) Improve counseling methodology to better assist the patient in the acceptance of limitations, which are beyond everyone's control, and better recognition of the resulting incremental benefits of amplification. This includes counseling in regard to the diminishing returns trade-off between meeting best target use-gain level while accommodating loudness tolerance limits. Or, in the more aberrant split-band losses, the occasional difficulty in suppressing gain in the near-normal midband, without destroying gain levels at either side of the audiometric peak. While multi-band programmables show promise in accommodating many of these cases, there still exists today a significant challenge in the trade-off between tolerance and gain/output parameters.

2) Take the pressure of unrealistic expectations off hearing instrument amplification by effectively motivating patients to obtain and use appropriate assistive devices, and to accept aggressive rehabilitative strategies such as speechreading and other visual compensatory skills.

3) During the initial 60-90 day post-fitting period, assist the patient in taking the proper amount of time in developing better listening skills with the new instruments by expanding their "circles of hearing" gradually over an extended period of time while avoiding listening experiences in which they are not yet ready to handle (Aleo, 1994). Anyone familiar with the aggressive and lengthy rehabilitative strategy used for cochlear implant patients will understand the crucial importance of this concept.

A unique concept explored by Gatehouse and Killion (1993) can be effectively utilized in educating patients as to realistic expectations. Their assertion is that "***there is a fundamental perceptual process whereby a hearing aid listener, when presented with a range of speech information which had been previously unavailable, can take considerable time to make optimum use of the new set of speech clues and thereby derive optimal benefit from the amplification.***" (p. 30). Their contention is that it takes an average of 4-6 weeks after the initial fitting ***before*** measurable improvement actually begins!

Supporting this concept, and making it visually relevant to patients, is a graph by Gatehouse (1992) represented in Figure 7. The reader will note that the graph's primary purpose was to show timed speech-in-noise (SiN) comparisons between amplification with flat response and with shaped (prescriptive) response. But the

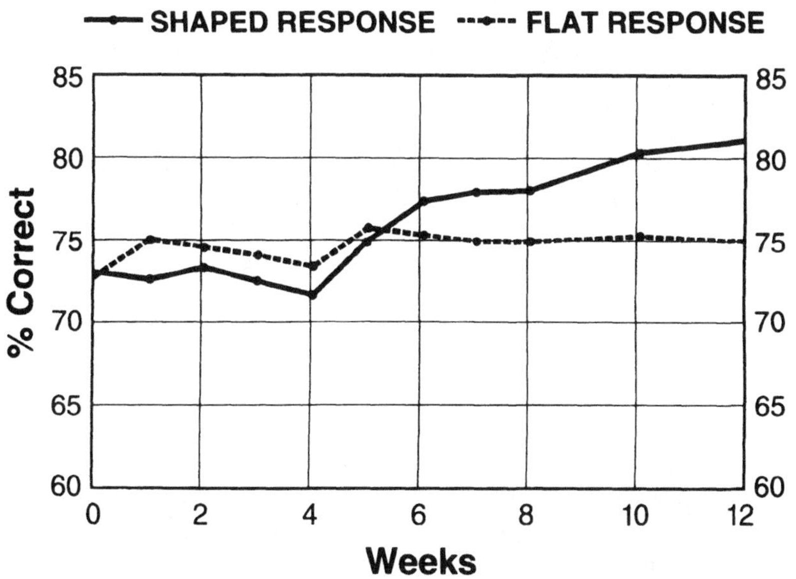

Fig. 7. Time-based speech-in-noise (SiN) score comparisons from Gatehouse (1992) in fitted patients with flat and shaped responses in amplification. Used by permission of Gatehouse & Killion, from an article on HABRAT.

real story behind the story is that although the SiN-scores of patients with shaped response instruments actually ***declined*** during the first four weeks, later weeks showed a dramatic ***increase of SiN ability*** through the 12-week period of acclimation! (So much for the efficiency of 30-day trials!).

Their theory, supported by plentiful empirical and anecdotal evidence, is that during the acclimatization period the brain of the new user is "rewiring" itself to recognize and better utilize new acoustic information. A side-note to this is that while many users erroneously preferred the flat response over the more advantageous shaped response, lack of speech understanding scores failed to show substantive improvement over the same 12-week period. This concept can be a powerful counseling tool in assisting patients to have realistic expectations relative to new amplification equipment. Expressing this concept to patients and third parties can be thus:

> *"At first, when you wear your new hearing instruments, you may actually experience a slight decrease in speech understanding while in difficult listening situations. Don't be alarmed if that happens. This is a normal response.*
>
> *"After a few weeks, however, your brain will have had time to accommodate the many new and forgotten sounds. Then, you will begin understanding better, while the most dramatic improvements will eventually be in less-than-ideal listening situations. The process for reprogramming your brain may take up to 12 weeks before you enjoy optimum benefit of your new instruments.*
>
> *"In the meantime, take it a day at a time, try not to get into difficult listening situations, and most of all, religiously follow the wearing schedule I am giving you. Over time, you will do much better."*

PATIENTS' ATTITUDES MIRROR PROFESSIONAL RESPONSES

Professional influence over attitudinal factors in evaluative and rehabilitative settings can be easily underestimated. The most important use of information relative to psycho-social factors in hearing impairment is for the professional dispenser to help "lift" the patient and accompanying third parties from out of the quagmire in which they find themselves. This requires some independence and candor on the part of the dispenser. It also requires that they not reinforce the patient's negative psycho-social behavior by reflecting that behavior themselves. Instead, the patient needs to feel that the dispenser is the one person they can trust in opening up about their impairment and its effects upon their life.

Try these exercises:

If the patient arrives . . .	***You respond by being . . .***
Angry, distrustful	Warm, trusting
Stand-offish, uncomfortable	Friendly, old-hat
Nervous, impatient	Relaxed, patient
Insecure, bashful	Confident, approachable
Will not listen	Listen, listen, listen
Insincere, skeptical	Sincere, forthright

A similar exercise might be used with third parties, as well. Keep in mind that the third party who is not empathetic with the one suffering from the hearing loss may feel internally that they have good reason for feeling that way. Perhaps they are resentful about having had to change their own life around to be the patient's "hearing aid". Or perhaps they have interpreted the patient's psycho-social responses to hearing loss in a personal way. Indeed, the wife who has been encouraging her hearing impaired husband for the past fifteen years to "do something" will have some strong emotional responses to let go of once he finally takes that step. To assist third parties in the release of their own negative psycho-social emotional attachment to the spouse's hearing loss state, the dispenser may do several things:

- As the pure-tone evaluation proceeds, have the third party sit close by you so they can be apprised of the findings as they unfold. Make soft verbal comments and observations, such as:

  "Look at this. No wonder he feels he doesn't have a hearing loss. He hears the lows almost normal, but look at these high frequencies . . . they're practically off the chart!"

  "How long has he been suffering with this hearing loss?"

  "Can you hear that? That's almost as loud as my audiometer will go, yet he can barely hear it!"

- Involve the third-party during the demonstration portion of the evaluation by having them read sentences, ask questions, and be part of the decision.

  "Mrs. Brown, would you please read your husband the following questions and let's see if he understands you better?"

  "Now, we would like to try different frequency responses on your husband. Would you please read these sentences,

> *repeating them twice, while he listens to various hearing aid responses?"*
>
> *"It's time to make a decision on the style and model of instrument he will need. We need your help in arriving at the best decision."*

At this point, some third parties tend to "jump ship", leaving the patient "stranded" to make the decision alone. This, of course, unloads a bigger burden than most hearing impaired persons can carry. In fact, it is at this point that the third party who has been waiting years for this moment will need most to drive their effort to finality. ***Now*** is the time for them to encourage the hearing impaired person to make a positive decision. In such cases, the dispenser may have to reinforce the third party's involvement in the decision process. This has been done a number of ways. With so much now written on this subject, this author often gives the doubting or reading third party something to read (briefly) on the importance of helping the patient with the decision. Some highlighted passages from this chapter would be appropriate for that purpose.

On the other hand, the dispenser will want to refrain from making the choice of "closing options" too difficult for the patient. In other words, choices of recommended models and circuits should be clear enough to be distinguishable by the untrained person. The author has long subscribed to the "either/or" close approach, raising not the question of "if" but of "which" style or model they would prefer. The decision of whether or not to accept hearing correction should have been decided long before this point. Now, should be the "easy part".

MENTAL HEALTH AND HEARING LOSS

No up-to-date text on psychological behavior of hearing impairment would be complete without reporting some unfolding research findings re: ***the close correlation between hearing impairment and cognitive dysfunction*** (HJ, 1995).

Cognitive development is defined as the "***process of acquiring skills in perception, imagination, conception, memory, judgment, and reason, which are the foundation for cognition.***" (Delk, 1991, pg. 29). Note that a wide array of mental functions, from attitude to memory, are included in this rather broad definition. In essence, cognition represents one's relationship with life and humanity. When we talk of depression and despair, we are referring to the most common form of cognitive dysfunction. When we are talking of a memory loss, short or long term, we are again referring to cognitive dysfunction. Cognitive dysfunction has long been associated with hearing loss, albeit secondarily. Because hearing loss is so prevalent among older adults, however, its effects can exacerbate and over-promote the diagnosis of any existing organic forms of cognitive dysfunction—such as Alzheimer's disease, senile dementia, senile psychosis, and Pick's disease. Uncorrected hearing loss, then, cause outward symptoms to be more pronounced and render the patient less respondent to medical treatment.

One such study was performed by researchers at the University of Washington and Harborview Medical Center in Seattle (Uhlmann et al, 1989). There they found that hearing impairment was twice as prevalent among older adults with diagnosed Alzheimer's disease than with non-demented individuals. Furthermore, the greater the hearing loss, the greater the symptoms of dementia. Their findings were that while hearing loss may not be a causal factor in dementia that it most certainly exposed and exacerbated its symptoms. Thus, as patients were aurally cut-off from communication and their environment they suffered "increased disorientation". Making them more susceptible to depression and cognitive dysfunction, severe loss cases appeared to suffer the most. The researchers concluded that

> *". . . correction of hearing impairment would not prevent the pathophysiological progression of dementia, but it could potentially ameliorate the symptoms of dementia. This would make the correction of hearing impairment a promising opportunity for the treatment of cognitive dysfunction in elderly persons, particularly since there are currently no means of altering the pathophysiological progression of common dementias such as Alzheimer's disease."*

In another study, it was found that hearing aid use can lead to such dramatic outcomes as reduced depression and improved mental function (Pickerill, 1991). Says Cynthia Mulrow, M.D. at the University of Texas Health Science Center in San Antonio:

> *"Many physicians don't routinely screen elderly people for hearing loss, and we thought they may not realize how much hearing aids help."*

They studied 188 patients over 64 years of age who had varying levels of hearing loss. From that group, half were given hearing aids. At the end of a four-month period, the hearing aid group exhibited marked improvements in social, emotional and communication functioning. Some even improved in measured mental score testing. Mulrow concluded:

"Many of the people with new hearing aids reported that they started going to the movies or that they spent more time with families and friends than when they could not hear as well. In general, more of the people with new hearing aids were happy, and fewer were depressed."

CONCLUSION

In our practices, we have assessment tools to observe the individual human hearing system from myriad vantage points. Causal factors, site(s) of lesion, and courses of intervention—both medial and rehabilitative—are no longer the mystery they once were. The average hearing instrument specialist today can perform a plethora of sophisticated assessments that were merely wistful thinking only a short decade ago. In addition, hearing instrument technology has escalated in capability far in excess of our ability to adequately convey breakthrough advantages to the market. Likewise, the ability of the specialist to assess and make timely medical and clinical referrals based on pre-medical screening skills re: FDA regulation has been empirically demonstrated in competency examinations and in actual practice.

Without a skillful grasp of the underlying psycho-social fundamentals which accompany decreased hearing acuity, all of these achievements will provide little benefit to the larger market. The key to unlocking access to that ever-growing market is in the touching of hearts, minds, and emotions, not in hardware, software, and flow-charts. It is now time to awaken those who've not noticed their world fading away to the fact that dedicated men and women have toiled non-stop to make hearing impairment one of the least excusable maladies in modern times.

GLOSSARY

Alzheimer's disease Most common form of *senile dementia,* characterized primarily by memory loss, disorientation, and personality change. Alzheimer's has been shown to be exacerbated or over-diagnosed when accompanied by unresolved hearing impairment.

Amygdala Part of the *diencephelon* (mid-brain) that stores information (genetic and learned) for involuntary emotional responses to external stimuli, particularly things to approach or avoid.

Auditory sensory deprivation Referring to functional and/or organic changes or underdeveloped as a result of one being deprived of auditory stimulus or adequate hearing acuity.

Binaural fusion Binaural psychological perception that dichotic signals are one. Necessary ability for balanced auditory perception, localization, and spatial mapping ability.

Binaural summation Interhemispheric auditory sensation created when the psychologically-perceived sum of two monaural signals is greater by 3-6 dB than either monaural signal alone.

Binaural squelch Learned ability to neurologically squelch or suppress unwanted ambient noise while focusing on a specific sound source. Functional only in dichotic hearing state.

Broca's area Portion of the *left cerebral cortex* where speech is formulated for language communication expression.

Candidacy criteria Set of arbitrary parameters (pure-tone, speech discrim, etc.) applied to human hearing loss to determine if one is a candidate for hearing instrument correction.

Cognitive dysfunction Breakdown in mental functions which affect attitude, social interaction, and mental organization. Most common symptoms are depression and memory loss.

Corpus Callosum Intermedial dendritic mass that connects the right and left hemispheres of the human brain.

Dementia Disorders of organic breakdown in mental function. Most often revealed in depression, loss of memory, and personality changes which grows worse over time.

Hechl's gyrus Auditory reception center of the *auditory cortex* comprised of lines of cells organized tonatopically to decode neural responses from the periphery mechanism for higher brain interpretation.

Hemispheric specialization Innate or learned ability to focus various psychological functions—spatial, verbal and non-verbal communication, etc.—primarily in one hemisphere.

Hypothalamus Part of the *diencephelon* (mid-brain) which acts as mediator between thoughts (*cerebral cortex*) and feelings (*limbic system*).

Insidiousness Refers to the gradual progression of sensorineural hearing impairment without the sufferers' awareness.

Interference phenomenon Mental log-jamming when one has difficulty giving verbal response to a spatial or emotional problem.

Left hemisphere Portion of the human brain which focuses primarily upon verbal communication, logic, and abstract thinking.

Long-term memory Ability to maintain goal orientation, memory of the past, procedures, semantics, and stored logic and emotional response. Primarily seated in the A2 of the *auditory cortex.*

Mimicking Method of acquiring language by the involuntary repetition of words or phrases heard from others.

Paranoia Delusions of persecution, social rejection, and distrust.

Pavlovian-like Refers to conditioned mental or emotional responses to environmental, in this case auditory, stimuli associated with experiments on dogs by Russian physiologist Ivan Pavlov.

Phonemic regression Speech discrimination ability out of proportion to the degree of pure-tone auditory loss of acuity. Temporary central auditory condition in most long-standing, unresolved sensorineural losses that is usually corrected during the adaptation to amplification.

Primitive level First developmental level of hearing perception which assists humans in establishing sense of connectedness and security to background and ambient noise around them.

Right hemisphere Portion of the human brain which focuses primarily upon non-verbal communication, spatial orientation, wholistic perspective, and aesthetic interpretation.

Short-term memory Ability to recognize sequences, patterns, and symbols in hearing. Seated in the auditory cortex adjacent to Heschl's gyrus.

Signal level Level of auditory mental perception associated with alerting involuntarily to signals, danger and otherwise.

Spatial mapping Innate or learned ability to assess physical movement and location of objects in the environment, especially in relation to one's position.

Speech-in-Noise (SiN) Similar to signal-to-noise except denotes ability to understand speech in noise.

Stages of mourning Rehabilitative stages (i.e., *numbness, denial, despair, and acceptance*) through which many hearing impaired persons travel before hearing help is accepted.

Startle reflex Involuntary psychoneurological response at signal level of hearing. Controlled at the *amygdala* in the mid-brain via the *superior colliculus* from the *central auditory projection system.* The defective hearing system diminishes control of this reflex.

Superior Olivary Complex Early analytical junction within the *central auditory projection system.* Comprised of two analytical sectors: The *lateral superior olive* (interaural intensity differences) and the *medial superior olive* (interaural time differences).

Symbolic level Level of auditory mental perception associated with speech and language, primarily in the parts of the left temporal lobe known as *Wernicke's and Broca's areas.*

Thalamus Comprises the floor of the A1 of the *auditory cortex.* Acts as traffic controller and assists in the focusing voluntary *auditory attention.*

Tonatopical recognition The ability to perceive discrete pitch at *Heschl's gyrus* in the *auditory cortex.* Most often associated with short-term memory and sequential functions.

Transparency Refers to the patient's lack of self-assessment as to severity of their high frequency loss, because of normal or near-normal acuity in low frequency thresholds.

Wearing Schedule Refers to a specially-designed schedule of daily wear of hearing instruments assigned by the specialist to assist the user in the adaptation and rehabilitation.

Wernicke's area Portion of the *left temporal cortex* responsible for speech reception and understanding.

REFERENCES

ALEO, E., *The Aquinas Method: The Four-Gear Sales Presentation,* Aquinas Rehabilitative Services, Inc.: Kingston, NY, 1994.

ALEO, E., *The Aquinas Method: Treat With Care,* Aquinas Rehabilitative Services, Inc.: Kingston, NY, 1994.

BECKER, W., NAUMANN, H. and PFALTZ, C., *Ear, Nose and Throat Diseases,* Buckingham, R., ed., Thieme Medical Publishers: New York, 1989.

BLOODSTEIN, O., *A Handbook on Stuttering,* National Easter Seal: Chicago, 1987.

BONILLAS, P., "On the Other Hand", *Hearing Health,* 11:4, 1995, Pg. 50.

BRISKEY, R., "Selecting and Fitting a Hearing Aid: Binaurally", in *Binaural Hearing and Amplification,* Vol. II, ed., E. Robert Libby, Zenetron, Inc.: Chicago, 1980, pp. 187-204.

BURG, A., "Visual Acuity as Measured by Dynamic and Spatial Tests: A Comparative Evaluation", *Journal of Applied Psychology,* No. 50, 1966, pp. 460–466.

CHARTRAND, M., *Human Signal Processing,* CE Course for National Institute for Hearing Instruments Studies, 1989.

CHARTRAND, M., *Psychology of the Hearing Impaired,* Unimax Professional Education Series: Gainesville, TX, 1988.

CHARTRAND, M., *Hearing Instrument Counseling: Practical Applications for Counseling the Hearing Impaired,* National Institute for Instruments Studies: Livonia, MI, 1990.

CHASE, M., "Feed Your Brain, And It May Thrive in Old Age", in "Health Journal", *Wall Street Journal,* October 12, 1994.

CLOPTON, B., and WINFIELD, J., "Effect of early exposure to patterned sound on unit activity in rat inferior colliculus", *Journal of Neurophysiology,* No. 39, 1976, pp. 1081–1089.

COHEN, SENATOR WILLIAM, in telecommunications with the author re: the Senate Subcommittee on Aging Hearings, 1993.

COOPER, J., and GATES, G., "Central Auditory Processing Disorders in the Elderly: The Effects of Pure Tone Average and Maximum Word Recognition", *Ear and Hearing,* 13:4, 1992.

DAVIS, H., and SILVERMAN, R., *Hearing and Deafness,* Holt, Rinehart and Winston, Inc.: New York, 1970.

DELK, J., *Comprehensive Dictionary of Audiology,* Laux Co.: Maynard, MA, 1991.

GATEHOUSE, S., "The time course and magnitude of peripheral acclimatization to frequency responses: Evidence from monaural fittings of hearing aids", *American Journal of Acoustical Science,* No. 92, 1992, pp. 1256–1268.

GATEHOUSE, S., and KILLION, M., "HABRAT: Hearing Aid Brain Rewiring Accommodation Time", *Hearing Instruments,* 44:10, 1993, pp. 29-32.

GLANZE, W. D., ed., *The Signet/Mosby Medical Encyclopedia,* Penguin Books USA: New York, 1987.

GRAHAM, R., *Physiological Psychology,* Wadsworth Publishing Co.: Belmont, CA, 1990.

HALPERN, D., *Sex Differences in Cognitive Abilities,* Lawrence Erlbaum Associates, Publishers: Hillsdale, NJ, 1992.

HARRIS, D., "My Love Affair with Ruth Bender: A History of Binaural Hearing Aids for Babies", in *Binaural Hearing and Amplification, Vol. II,* ed., E. Robert Libby, Zenetron, Inc.: Chicago, 1980, pp. 259–274.

HELLIGE, J., *Hemispheric Asymmetry: What's Right and What's Left,* Harvard University Press: Cambridge, MA, 1993, pp. 285–293.

HINES, M., "Gonadal Hormones and Human Cognitive Development", in *Hormones, Brain and Behaviour in Vertebrates,* ed., Jacques Balthazart, Karger: Basel, 1990, pp. 51–63.

HJ, "Hearing Loss and Mental Health", *Hearing Journal,* 48:6, 1995, pg. 8.

HORTON, P., *Solace: The Missing Dimension in Psychiatry,* University of Chicago Press: Chicago, 1986.

IHS, "Written testimony of the International Hearing Society before the Special Committee on Aging, United States Senate", September 15, 1993, pg. 4.

IRWIN, J. and MARGE, M., *Principles of Childhood Language Disabilities,* Meredith Corporation: NY, 1972.

JASA, *Baltimore Longitudinal Study of Aging,* Journal of the Acoustical Society of America, 1995.

JOHNSEN, DAVID, "Studies on primary tooth enamel defects and hearing loss", Case Western Reserve University, Department of Otolaryngology—Head & Neck Surgery, School of Medicine, 1991.

JOHNSON, G., *Machinery of the Mind,* Tempus Books: Redmon, WA, 1986, pp. 254–56.

KIMURA, D., "Sex Differences in the Brain", *Scientific American,* September, 1992, pp. 118–125.

KIMURA, D., Kimura's reply to Melissa Hines' "Sex Ratios at Work", *Scientific American,* February, 1993, p. 12.

KIRKWOOD, D., "We've Made Our Move", *Hearing Journal,* 48:6, 1995, pg. 4.

KIRKWOOD, C., and KIRKWOOD, M., "Otitis media and learning disabilities: The case for a causal relationship", *Journal of Family Practice,* No. 17, 1983, pp. 219–227.

LEY, R., and BRYDEN, M., "Hemispheric Differences in Recognizing Faces and Emotions", in *Brain and Language* No. 7, 1979, pp. 127–138.

MCGLONE, J., "Sex Differences in Human Brain Asymmetry: A Critical Survey", in *The Behavioral and Brain Sciences,* No. 3, 1980, pp. 215–263.

MCGUINNESS, D., "Away from a Unisex Psychology: Individual Differences in Visual Perception", *Perception,* No. 5, 1976, pp. 279–294.

McSpaden, J., *How Grows Loudness,* CE Course for National Institute for Hearing Instruments Studies, 1993.

Menzel, O., Lovely, S., and Kisch, B., "Sudden Deafness: After the Crash", *Hearing Health,* 11:4, 1995, pp. 25–28.

Moscicki, E., Elkins, E., Baum, H., and McNamara, P., "Hearing loss in the elderly: an epiodiologic study of the Framingham Heart Study Cohort", 1985:6:184–190.

Oyler, R., Oyler, A., and Matkin, N., "Unilateral hearing loss: Demographics and educational impact", *Language, Speech, and Hearing Services in the Schools,* No. 19, 1988, pp. 201–209.

Palmer, C., "Deprivation, Acclimatization, Adaptation: What Do They Mean For Your Hearing Aid Fittings?", *Hearing Journal,* 47:5, 1995, pp. 10, 41–45.

Phillips, P., *Speech and Hearing Problems in the Classroom*, Cliff Notes, Inc.: Lincoln, NE, 1975.

Pickerell, M., "Hearing Good News", *Health,* January, 1991, pg. 14.

Pickles, J., *An Introduction to the Physiology of Hearing,* Academic Press: London, 1992.

Pool, R., *Eve's Rib: Searching for the Biological Roots of Sex Differences,* Crown Publishers: New York, 1994.

Quigley, S., "Effects of hearing impairment on normal language development", in *Pediatric Audiology,* ed., Fred Martin, Prentice-Hall: Englewood Cliffs, NJ, 1978.

Ramsdell, D., "The Psychology of the Hard-of-Hearing and Deafened Adult", in *Hearing and Deafness,* ed., Davis, H., and Silverman S., Holt, Rinehart, and Winston: New York, 1970.

Reiter, R., "Psychology of the Hearing Impaired and Hearing Aid Use", in *Handbook of Hearing Aid Amplification, Vol. II,* ed., Robert E. Sandlin, College-Hill Press: Boston, 1990, pg. 5.

Rose, S., *The Making of Memory,* Bantam Doubleday Dell Publishing Group, Inc.: New York, 1992.

Ross, M., Brackett, D., and Maxon, A., *Assessment and Management of Mainstreamed Hearing-Impaired Children: Principles and Practices,* Pro-Ed: Austin, TX, 1991.

Ruben, R., and Rapin, I., "Plasticity of the developing auditory system", *Annals of Otology,* No. 89, 1980, pp. 303–311.

Siegel, A., and Pott, C., "Neural substrates of aggression and flight in the cat", *Progress in Neurobiology,* No. 31, 1988, pp. 261–283.

Skafte, M., "A Review of the 1994 Hearing Instrument Market", *Hearing Review,* March, 1995, pp. 16–40.

Smith, O., and DeVito, J., "Central neural integration for the control of autonomic responses associated with emotion", *Annual Review of Neuroscience,* No. 7, 1984, pp. 43–65.

SNYDER, L., "Have We Prepared the Language Disordered Child for School?", *Topics in Language Disorders,* 1:1, 1980.

SPRINGER, S., and DEUTSCH, G., *Left Brain, Right Brain,* W. H. Freeman and Company: New York, 1989.

STABB, W., "Hearing in the Elderly, Part II", *Audecibel,* Spring, 1990, pp. 16–22.

STACH, B., LOISELLE, L., and JERGER, J., "Special Hearing Aid Considerations in the Elderly Patients with Auditory Processing Disorders", *Ear and Hearing,* 12:6 Suppl., 1991.

UHLMANN, E., LARSON, T., REES, T., KOEPSELL, and DUCKERT, L., "Relationship of Hearing Impairment to Dementia and Cognitive Dysfunction in Older Adults", *JAMA,* Vol. 261, 1989.

U.S. DEPARTMENT OF EDUCATION, *Digest of Education Statistics 1992,* Office of Educational Research and Improvement.

VANDENBERG, S., *Louisville Twin Study,* Univ. of Louisville Medical School, Dept. of Pediatrics, 1967.

WABER, D. "Sex Differences in Cognition: A Function of Maturation Rate?", *Science,* No. 192, 1976, pp. 572–573.

WEBSTER, D., "Effects of peripheral hearing losses on the auditory brainstem", in *Central Processing Disorders: Problems of speech, language, and learning,* ed., E. Lasky and J. Katz, Pro-Ed: Austin, TX, 1983, pp. 185–202.

WEINSTEIN, S., "Intensive and Extensive Aspects of Tactile Sensitivity as a Function of Body Part, Sex, and Laterality" in *The Skin Senses,* ed., D. R. Kenshalo, Charles C. Thomas: Springfield, IL, 1968, pp. 195–222.

WILLIAMS, H., "Thinking about our 'thinkers'", *Hearing Instruments,* 44:4, 1993, pg. 50.

WILLOTT, J., *Aging and the Auditory System: Anatomy, Physiology, and Psychophysics,* Singular Publishing: San Diego, CA, 1991.

WILLS, C., *The Runaway Brain: The Evolution of Human Uniqueness,* BasicBooks, Div. Harper Collins Publishers: NY, 1993).

WOOD, F., FLOWERS, D., and NAYLOR, C., "Cerebral Laterality in Functional Neuroimaging", in *Cerebral Laterality: Theory and Research,* ed. Kitterle, Frederick L., Lawrence Erlbaum Associates: Hillsdale, NJ, 1991, pp. 103–115.

YULE, G., *The Study of Language,* Cambridge University Press: Cambridge, MA, 1985.

XII

GERIATRIC CONSIDERATIONS IN HEARING AID FITTING

ARAM GLORIG, M.D. AND ROBERT NOVAK, M.D.

INTRODUCTION

The fact that hearing is important to well-being cannot be disputed. The order of importance is a relative matter, however. For example, the loss of hearing in early childhood is infinitely worse in its effects on well-being than when this loss occurs late in life.

World history records, in one form or another, depict a lack of care for the senior citizen. In fact, some cultures put the elderly out to die when they had outlived their usefulness. I suppose in a society constrained by the lack of food, space, and health services, there was not much else to do. As society and cultures developed through the ages and the availability of food, space, and health services improved, the older citizen achieved a more secure position and with it more respect and responsibility. As more food, better management of space, and infinitely better health care became available, longevity increased in leaps and bounds and consequently, the relative proportions of old to young changed drastically. In the United States the percentage of people over 65 years of age has increased from 4.1%, in 1900, to 10.5%, in 1975. According to the Department of Health, Education and Welfare, this will change to 11.7% by the year 2000 (Cutler, 1975).

CHAPTER OBJECTIVES

In this chapter the reader will be aware of the need for extended use and adjustments over a period of time before a geriatric patient can adjust to hearing amplification. This must be accompanied by pretrial and post-trial counseling. Counseling of this sort for patient and close associates is imperative. It is essential for all hearing aid candidates, but is imperative for the senior candidate. The reader is reminded of the differences between geriatric clients and other, younger clients, who require hearing aid devices to carry out activities for more active daily living.

THE PROBLEM

It is well known that hearing disorders in the aged are a problem that is long overdue for attention. Numerous studies show that hearing loss increases with age to the extent that 30% of people over 65 years of age have enough loss to need assistance for everyday communication. In terms of the statistics quoted above, that is about one-third of the total number over 65, or approximately ten million people. It is further estimated that about 25 million people have enough hearing impairment to need amplification. About 40% of that group are over 65 years of age. Such statistics point out the enormity of the problem of hearing disorders in our aging population and illuminate the increasing burden to the aging citizen and society itself (Glorig, 1965).

Hearing loss tends to increase with age; 33% of persons between 65–74 years, 45% of those between 74–84 years and 62% of those over 85 years of age (NCHS 1987) have a communication problem related to decreased auditory acuity.

DISORDERS OF THE EAR IN THE AGED

A short discussion concerning these disorders is not out of place at this point. Perhaps the most important of these disorders is really not a disorder but a natural consequence of aging, i.e., presbyacusis. The definition of presbyacusis is somewhat ambiguous in the general literature and in the mind of the clinician at this point. Because of this ambiguity, it is frequently used as a "wastebasket diagnosis" for a hearing loss in someone over 60 or 65 that cannot be related to any specific disease or causative factor. It is commonly misspelled. I believe it should be spelled "presbyacusis" and not "presbycusis." The origin of the word is "presby," or age, and "acusis," or lack of hearing. I expect, however, I shall lose in favor of our American habit of promoting brevity. In my opinion, presbyacusis strictly defined should describe the effects of normal physiological aging on the auditory system from the external canal to the auditory cortex.

There are numerous studies of the effects of aging on the auditory threshold of pure tones, discrimination of speech, pitch perception, impedance changes in the middle ear, and auditory brainstem responses. When studying the auditory effects of aging, we are confronted with an insurmountable problem. That environmental effects are present is indisputable and any attempt to separate normal physiological changes from changes due to auditory environment is doomed to failure.

There is evidence that when environment is controlled the effects of physiological aging appear to be measurably less. When various population studies are done, differences in hearing are found as a function of the environment from which the group came (Glorig, 1962). Figure 1 shows a group of audiometric curves that can be used to estimate group median hearing losses as a function of age.

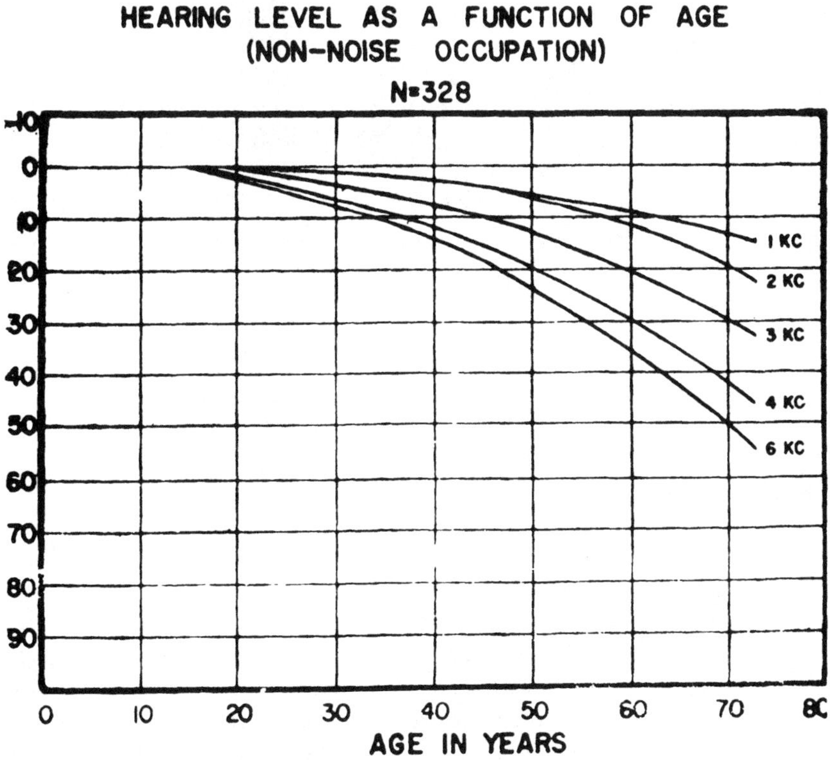

Fig. 1. Hearing loss as a function of age.

AUDITORY EFFECTS OF AGING

The auditory system sustains effects that follow the general changes of aging but are peculiar to the auditory system. This is not the place to discuss the basic pathophysiology of aging, however. We will confine our discussion to known effects on the performance of the auditory system and the coincident effects on the aged person.

In general, the auditory system can be compared to an electronic device whose purpose is to receive sound waves, transmit them efficiently to a transducer, analyze them and convert them into meaning. Anatomically, the ear and its neural connections can be divided as follows: external, middle and inner ear, eighth nerve, midbrain and auditory cortex.

The external and middle ear can be compared to a mechanical transformer whose purpose is to gather sound waves and present them to the inner ear or electrical transducer properly matched, i.e., with the least loss of energy when the inner ear fluids are inserted into the circuit. The external and middle ear functions are strictly mechanical: they act to prevent a mismatch at the point where sound has to be transduced from mechanical energy or vibration to electrical energy or current. An analogy would be an audio device using a low impedance microphone with a high impedance amplifier (Rubin, 1971). The device would need an impedance matching transformer for the efficient transformation of mechanical energy to electrical energy. As sound continues through the auditory systems, it is transduced in the cochlea or inner ear and carried via the eighth nerve to the brain where analysis takes place. Another way of saying it is the inner ear codes the sound into electrical pulses as a function of intensity, duration and time pattern and the brain decodes these pulses into meaningful messages.

The effects of aging occur over the entire auditory system. I will discuss the principal components separately (Glorig, 1961).

EXTERNAL EAR

There are many things that can happen to the external ear, but I will confine my discussion to those that effect hearing. Perhaps the most common of these is impacted cerumen. The amount of wax produced does not seem to change with age, but it appears to be more inspissated and consequently packs and becomes extremely dry and hard. It affects hearing only if the cerumen entirely blocks the canal and/or contacts the drumhead. The loss in hearing can be

Lesson 2
796, 797

considerable if the canal is completely blocked. When the loss that accompanies impacted cerumen is superimposed on the effects of presbyacusis, it is quite noticeable and, consequently, when the wax is removed the individual notices a distinct improvement. Removing the wax can be difficult, and, if not done expertly, it may damage the canal wall or even the drumhead itself. (Maurer 1979)

Another not uncommon problem is a collapsed canal. Frequently, as age increases, the cartilage of the pinna and outer third of the external auditory canal becomes soft and floppy and may partially close the external canal. This can produce a minor change in hearing, particularly when earphones are used for a hearing test. The pressure of the earphone collapses the canal and blocks the transmission of sound. Such cases need special care, especially when testing hearing. (Schow 1980)

Obviously, the external ear is subject to infection and tumors of the soft tissue and bone. Hearing loss is frequently the first symptom of a tumor of the ear and/or the upper nasopharynx. Anyone over 65 years of age with a unilateral hearing loss should be thoroughly studied before a final diagnosis is made. There are changes in the drumhead and middle ear related to aging. Frequently, the drumhead thickens and loses is normal luster and transparency. It also becomes stiffer and slightly less compliant. When the tissue of the middle ear is examined microscopically, the ossicular joints are somewhat arthritic and the ligaments show loss of elastic tissue. All these combine to make high frequency transmission less efficient and add to other changes to show the elevated high frequency thresholds in the older person.

MIDDLE EAR

Diseases of the middle ear in the aged are more or less the same as for middle age, i.e., infection, tumors, otosclerosis and trauma. Acute and chronic middle ear disease may result in acute or chronic mastoiditis which, if not treated properly, may result in brain abscesses which, by the way, is the most common cause of brain abscess in the aged. Otosclerosis is primarily a disease of the middle ear but not exclusive to the middle ear. Its clinical manifestations are evident in the third decade but become troublesome in the fourth decade and it is more common in women than men (Balle, 1984). It is a hereditary disease that promotes bony changes in the oval window area which ossify and freeze the footplate of the stapes. As the stiffening increases, the air conduction threshold is elevated but the bone conduction threshold remains unchanged until years later when it also begins to become elevated. The mechanism that causes the sensorineural hearing loss after a period of time is not understood. Hearing tests in patients with otosclerosis show what is called an air-bone gap. That is, the air conduction threshold is higher than the bone conduction threshold. Furthermore, the audiogram has a flat configuration showing nearly equal losses at all frequencies. People with otosclerosis usually have low, modulated voices and complain they cannot hear well when chewing celery or other noisy food. Until a few years ago, it was thought that otosclerosis did not affect the cochlea without first affecting the stapes. Recently, it has been shown that otosclerosis does affect the cochlea only and sometimes produces a severe sensorineural hearing loss (Balle, 1984). When the air-bone gap is found, surgery is the treatment of choice. On the other hand, when the loss is more severe than would be expected in uncomplicated presbyacusis, one should suspect cochlear otosclerosis. For some time now, sodium fluoride has been used to arrest cochlear otosclerosis. There is a real evidence to support this form of treatment. Temporal bone studies indicate that cochlear otosclerosis is not uncommon in the aged. Paget's disease and osteogenesis imperfecta may produce middle ear and cochlear changes. Unexplained progressive conductive hearing loss may indicate either of these diseases (Reuben, 1971). Paget's disease, also known as osteitis deformans, is a disease of the bones which may affect the temporal bone and the ossicles and produce a conductive hearing loss much the same as otosclerosis. The cause is unknown. It is usually found in adults over 40.

INNER EAR

The aged inner ear also is subject to the same problems of middle age. Noise is a very important factor. Noise, except for unusually loud noise, takes years to produce a significant effect on the ear. Anyone who is over 50 or 55 years of age may suffer the effects of noise. This effect is principally on the hair cell population and produces mainly a high frequency (above 1000 Hz) loss (Glorig, 1980).

Ototoxic drugs are a very important cause of sensorineural loss in the aged. Indiscriminate use of these drugs should be avoided. They can and do produce serious hearing losses. Acoustic neurinomas (eighth nerve tumors) are not uncommon in the aged. If hearing tests show one ear to be significantly worse than the other, the physician should suspect an eighth nerve tumor. Recourse to surgery in the aged tumor patient depends on the size of the tumor and the severity of symptoms, such as, hearing loss, tinnitus, and dizziness. These tumors are usually slow growing and surgery may not be indicated. Hearing loss, particularly unilateral loss in the aged patient, should alert the examiner to the possibility of a metastatic tumor as well (Brackmann, 1984).

CENTRAL NERVOUS SYSTEM

The central nervous system is the final component in the auditory system and it plays a very important role in the aged hearing impaired person. It appears that the central nervous system, or the decoder of the auditory input, in the aged is not able to handle the complex information contained in speech and language. We know that there is a reduction in brain cell population, which could certainly be one explanation of this inability (Birren, 1959). Even when the pure tone audiogram shows only minor changes, aged people have difficulty understanding speech. Discrimination of speech, particularly in the situations with competing signals, such as noise and group conversations, is very difficult for the older person (Jauhianen, 1983).

PATHOLOGY OF THE AGING EAR

Numerous studies of hearing in the general population have been reported. In general, they agree rather well in regard to threshold as a function of age. Figure 1 shows a set of curves taken from a study in the late 1950s.

One of the most insurmountable difficulties encountered in such studies is separating physiological aging from environmental aging. Most populations in today's culture sustain a certain amount of auditory wear and tear created by the environment. How can one be sure that aging thresholds are free of the effects of environment? The data in Figure 1 represents the results from a study designed to eliminate any obvious environmental influences. They are a reasonable representation of the median threshold changes due principally to physiological aging. The following figures are a diagrammatic representation of thepathology found in microscopic studies of the temporal bones in individuals over 65 years of age. Note that they are accompanied by pure-tone air conduction audiograms and discrimination scores as obtained by PB words.

Figure 2 shows the findings in a patient whose audiogram shows normal thresholds except for a slight change at 4 kHz. This particular patient had a 100% discrimination score. Each rectangle shows the relative amount of pathology in the organ of Corti (hair cells), the spiral ganglion (nerve fibers), and the stria vascularis (the source of the chemicals in the endolymph necessary for the hair cells to function). Note that the organ of Corti shows some pathology in the basal turn and a very small amount of pathology in the apical turn (dark areas).

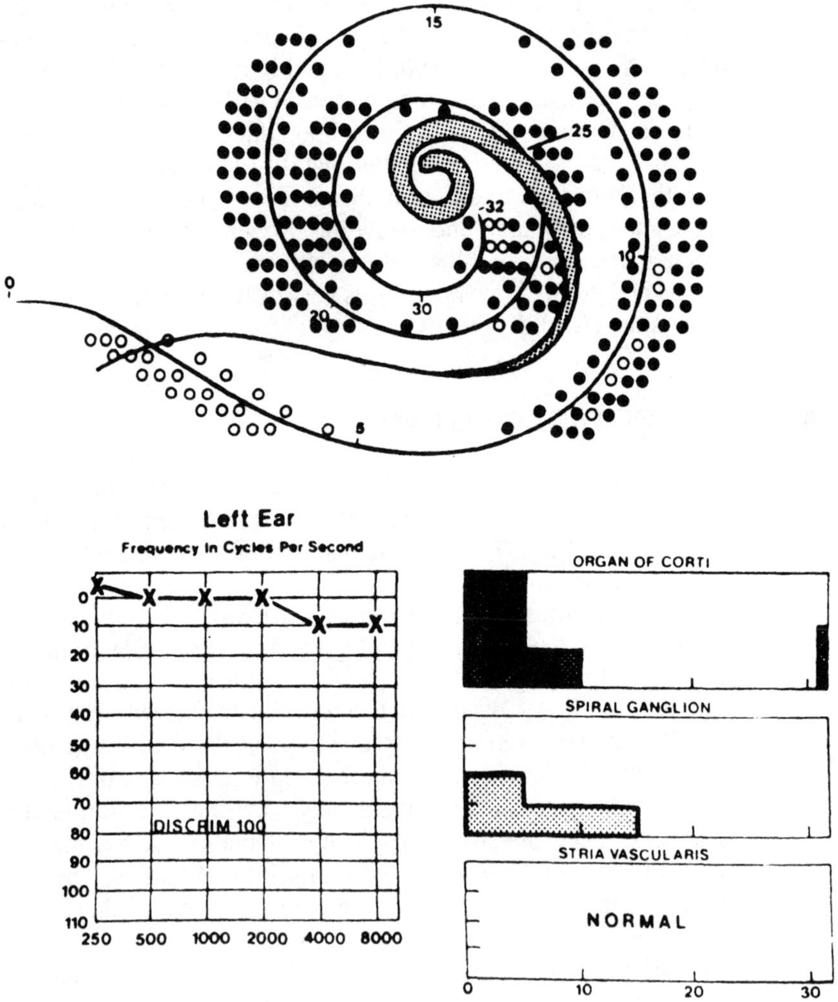

Fig. 2.

The diagrammatic cochlea shows the hair cell rows. The open circles indicate those cells that are pathological. Note the correlation with the dark areas in the organ of Corti as shown in the rectangles.

Figure 3 shows the findings in a patient with a flat loss of 50 dB and a 100% discrimination score. Note that the organ of corti and the spiral ganglion show only minimal pathology but the stria vascularis is severely damaged.

Figures 4–7 show cases with differences in threshold and discrimination scores. Note the pathology in each of these. It appears

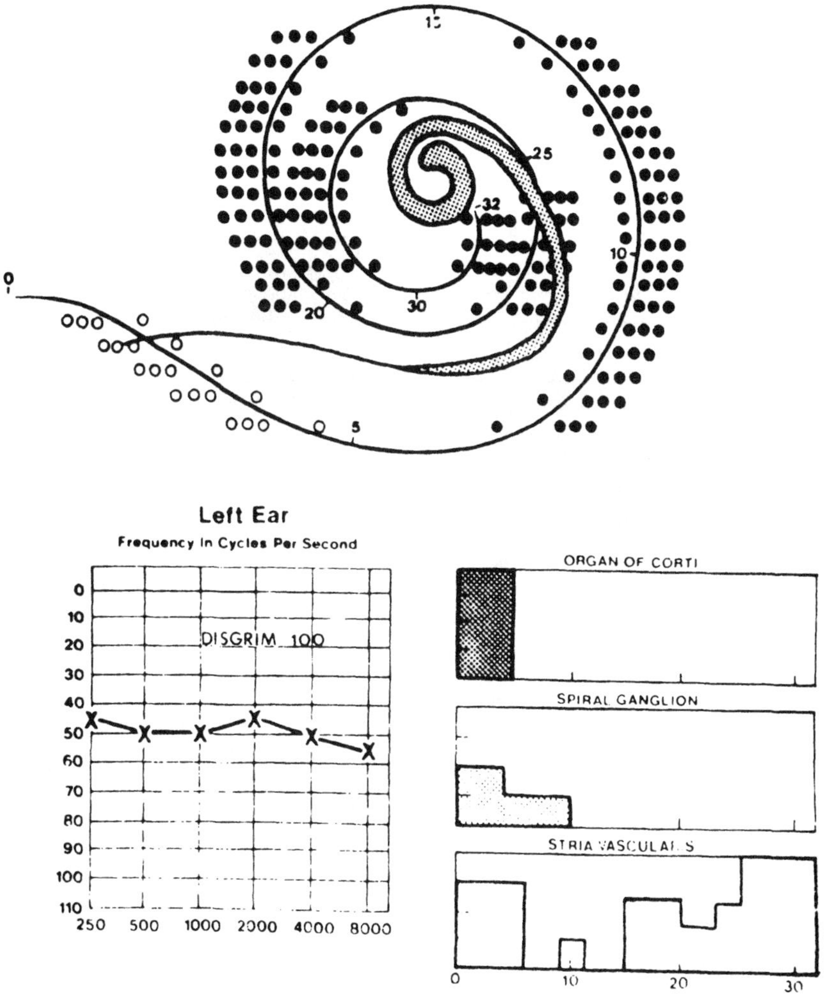

Fig. 3.

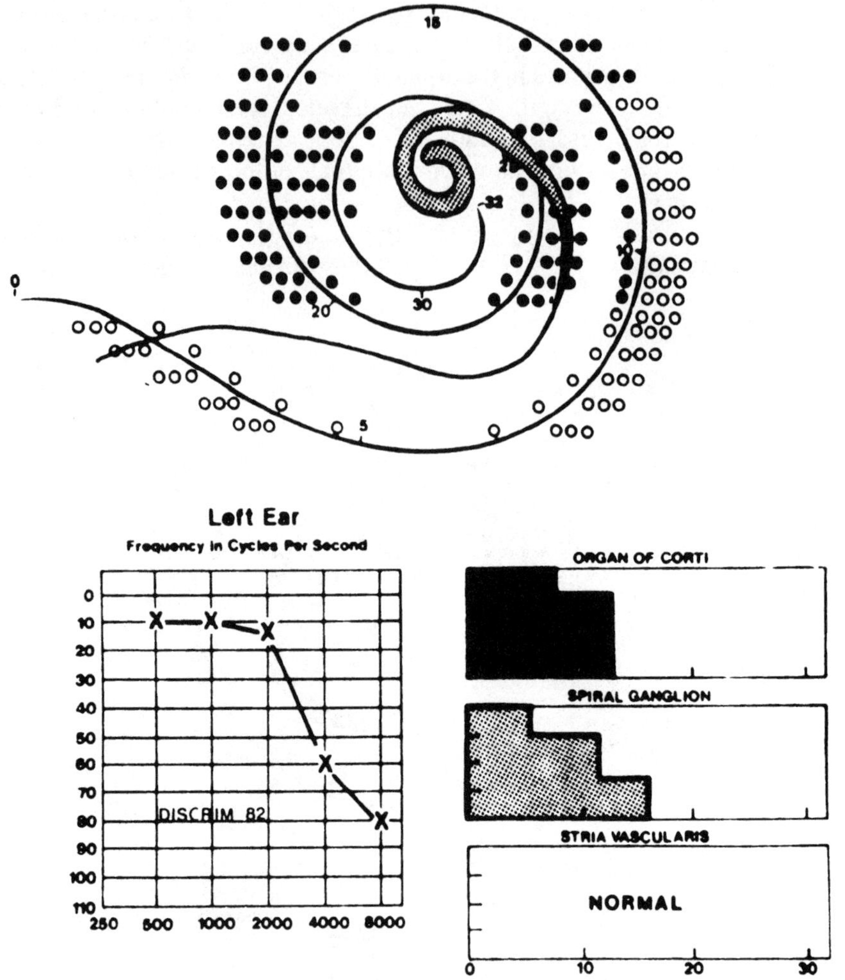

Fig. 4.

from studies of this kind that the success of fitting hearing aids in these cases would be correlated at least to some degree with the pathology, and until we devise tests of hearing which will indicate these differences in pathology, fitting hearing aids will be based on trial and error methods.

Such studies of pathology of the ear serve to point out that we need to know much more about these changes and their relation to performance before we can develop a signal processor that will adequately compensate for them. These studies are supportive of Schuknecht's Classification (1974) of types

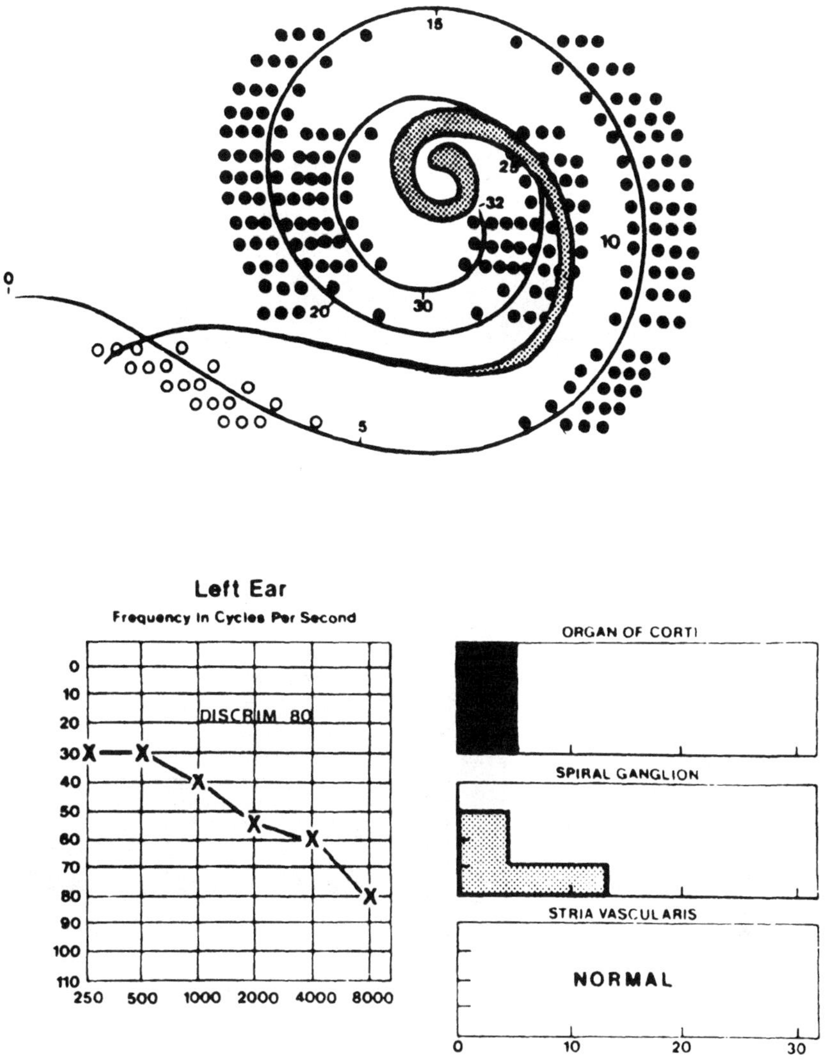

Fig. 5.

of pathology seen in presbyacusis. He has divided his classification into:

1. Sensory presbyacusis, due to changes in the hair cells.
2. Neural presbyacusis due to changes in the cochlear neurons.
3. Strial presbyacusis, due to changes in the stria vascularis.
4. Cochlear conductive presbyacusis, due to changes in cochlear mechanics.

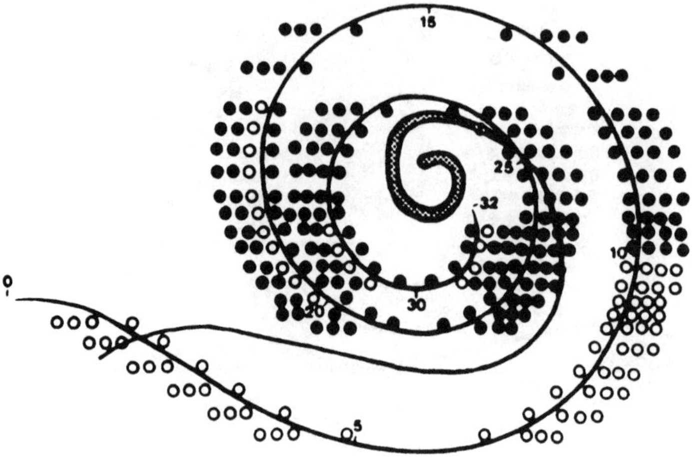

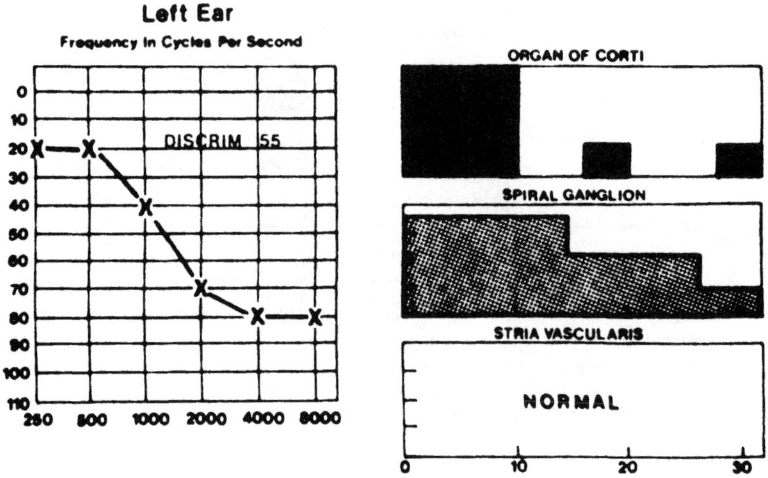

Fig. 6.

MEDICAL TREATMENT OF PRESBYACUSIS

When diseases of the aged ear exist, the medical and surgical treatment is no different than as in younger ears. Such a statement should be qualified somewhat depending on the real age of the person and the general physical condition. Any decision about the presence of pathology must be left to the physician to decide. This

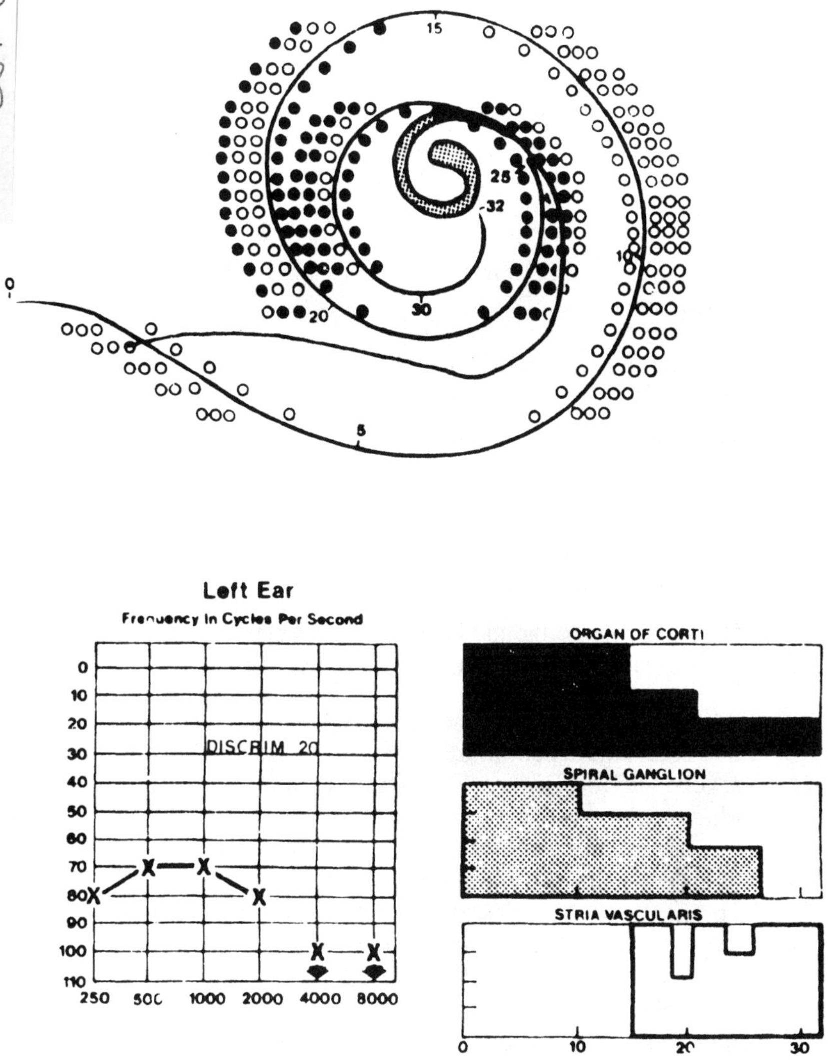

Fig. 7.

emphasizes the point that no rehabilitation procedures should be considered without a thorough medical workup. Older citizens are just as apt to have tumors, otosclerosis, general neuropathies and ear infections as middle age or younger individuals. Not infrequently, hearing loss, particularly a monaural loss, is the harbinger of some other pathology which may have serious consequences. It is important for the person dispensing the hearing aid to remember this.

PSYCHOLOGICAL PROBLEMS

Be aware of the fact that hearing loss in the older individual usually comes on gradually. Partial compensation for this has been taking place gradually. This combination of factors makes the presbyacusic person partially unaware that he is having a problem even if he is willing to admit it.

Remember that there is considerable redundancy in communication skills that come to his aid as his hearing loss progresses. For example:

1. The dynamic range of within-normal performance limits extends from zero to about 25 dB in the speech frequencies.
2. The individual does not notice real difficulties in communication until this level reaches 35–40 dB.
3. Conversational voice is about 60–65 dB.
4. Conversational speech has many redundancies in context and content.
5. Speech reading and body language (visual speech) add much valuable information.

All contribute to compensating for changes in auditory sensitivity and to a large extent to maintaining communication at acceptable levels. Obviously, there is a point in auditory sensitivity that precludes these benefits.

In the meantime, the older citizen may have experienced changes in life style which cause him to withdraw from active communication circles. Any attempts to bring his communication skills back to normal are resisted. How many of you have heard the older listener say, "Why should I worry about my hearing. I've heard everything that is worth listening to already?" Remember that the need for communication skills even though modified with age is still present, but the demand for these skills may be reduced or lacking. Before any attempts to improve communication skills in the aged are made the demand must be present and this demand is directly proportional to motivation. These factors are principally psychological.

What of the physiological factors? This process of withdrawal from auditory activities is very gradual. With the change in auditory sensitivity comes intolerance to sound both psychologically and physiologically. Psychologically because of the frustration and physiologically because of decreased dynamic range. Psychological intolerance must be counteracted by the professional in cooperation with the supporting persons whether they be family or friends. On the other hand, physiological intolerance must be compensated for by the professional, i.e., the dispenser of hearing aids. In many, especially the older person, the threshold of discomfort is such that he or she complains that the sounds are too loud when they are barely above threshold. This may or may not be due to recruitment. Recruitment is not necessarily present in presbyacusis.

In any case when there is a narrow dynamic range, it is difficult to prevent exceeding the physiological intolerance level. Speech itself has a dynamic range of about 12–14 dB. Add to this the variability of levels due to other reasons and it is easy to see why the person with a limited dynamic range has difficulty becoming accustomed to the severe changes in loudness. Consequently, physiological intolerance must be controlled by such circuits as peak clipping, automatic volume control, automatic gain control and compression.

The physiological threshold for discomfort does not change with the change in threshold; therefore, the frequency of intolerance may be more directly related to psychological intolerance. If this is the case, and I feel that it is, proper application of amplification can at least partially compensate for it in time. I believe time is the crux of the matter. If you expect to fit a hearing aid to such an individual without making allowances for accommodation you will be disappointed. I believe this is one of the most important causes of rejection of rehabilitation, especially the hearing aid component of the rehabilitation program.

SOCIOLOGICAL AND PSYCHOLOGICAL PERSPECTIVES

In addition to changes in sensory and neural processes, aging may be accompanied by modifications in adjustment strategies, problem solving capacities, emotional states, perception, and memory (Mauldin, 1976). These changes are not consistent across the elderly population and may also vary as a function of race and culture. The focus of this portion of the chapter is on the relationship these modifications have to the rehabilitation of hearing loss and specifically to the successful fitting of amplification devices in elderly populations.

Successful utilization of amplification by the geriatric population is dependent on a number of factors including the magnitude of loss in threshold sensitivity, reduced tolerance for loud sounds, and the subsequent reduction in work identification skills. Although a large percentage of hearing aid candidates have these problems, many hearing health professionals are not fully aware of other age-related factors that contribute to acceptance and use of amplification systems. Therefore, some of the behavior manifested by the elderly are reviewed here and their importance in the consideration of hearing aid use is assessed.

Cultural influences, coupled with the aging process and the changes that accompany it, are often major determinants of the elderly adult's behavior. Social, physical, and economic conditions also may affect attitudes, assessment of need, and ability to afford hearing aid use and care in the face of other, sometimes more pressing, economic realities. The need for hearing amplification is a physical reality. The use and acceptance of any amplification system, however, is tempered by a number of other concerns.

The stereotype of the elderly as physically feeble, severely hearing impaired, partially sighted, and demented fits less than three percent of the aged population. This stereotype would be true if survival to the maximum life span of 110 years was typical (Eisenberg, 1985). Aging can be viewed as both positive and negative, as growth and decline (Birren, Imus, & Windle, 1959; Gottlieb, 1983).

Higher neurologic functions are often largely preserved in normal aging (Posner, 1982). For example, self-esteem scores of older persons living independently in the community have been found to be nearly double those of high school students (Atchley, 1983). However, older individuals admitted to retirement homes have been found to have more latent pathology than elderly subjects who remain in the community (Busse, 1965).

Seeking help for hearing loss is influenced by economic constraints. The U.S. Department of Commerce (1975) reported that one in six persons over 65 years of age lives in poverty versus one in 10 under the age of 65 years. Maulding (1976) observed that certain consequences of aging present problems because they directly impact on the older person's consumer needs. Digestive metabolic changes may require changed diets. Changes in sensory processes, such as eyesight and hearing, may require eyeglasses and hearing aids; physical disabilities may require medical services, medical products, and institutionalization. The hearing health care professional must determine whether the hearing loss is considered a problem by the aged individual and, if it is a problem, where the remediation of hearing loss fits into the older person's priorities of consumer needs. Elderly hearing aid candidates may be ill, poor, without resources, and surrounded by people who avoid them. They are often described as rigid, conservative, cautions, and uncertain. However, as Gelfand (1982) has stated, these characteristics may be cohort effects related to how individuals were parented and their struggle to achieve security in first- or second-generation

Americans. Subsequent generations of elderly individuals may have improved quality of hearing care, better nutrition, higher long-term socioeconomic status, and better educational level thus influencing these characteristics.

CULTURAL CONSIDERATIONS

In American culture, if one can generalize, the aged often have not been given, or allowed to assume the esteemed role given to elders in some other societies (e.g., China). Rather, they are often treated with impatience and patronization. Approximately 6 percent reside in extended care facilities. For a significant subset of the older Americans, as their life expectancy increases, they are given less reason to live (Parenti, 1978). Chinese psychiatrist Wer Chen-I contended that depression in the elderly is found more often in western cultures because "the west extrudes older citizens, they lose place in the family, industry, community, their sphere of influence collapses as does their morale, leaving them vulnerable to disability and disease" (Greenblat & Chien, 1983). When hearing loss exists in the older American client, great potential for depression and low morale must be assessed as possible etiologies of lack of desire to communicate and to pursue use of amplification and aural rehabilitation.

It is very difficult to make generalizations about older Americans due to ethnic diversity of the population in the United States and the existence of relatively pure ethnic and cultural subgroups, such as Asians, native Americans, and "neighborhood" Hispanics and blacks. The sociological ramifications of group membership, sexual differences, and educational and economic levels in each of these subcultures relative to hearing help-seeking behaviors of their older members are complex and should be assessed. For example, Cheng (1988, interview) described three subgroups of Asians and America: new immigrants; refugees, including those from Indochina, Vietnam, Laos, and Cambodia; and second-generation Asian-Americans.

New immigrants are defined as people who came to the United States as young people after 1950. If they have hearing problems, they are the most likely to seek help. Refugees may rely on remedies from nontraditional health care providers for various ailments, including hearing loss. There are many sheltered, protected, and isolated older people in this subgroup who do not speak English and who live with their extended families. Barriers to the pursuit of hearing health care and hearing aid use in this group include:

- Fear of American culture
- Illiteracy in their own language and lack of knowledge of English
- Lack of knowledge of available help
- Psychological maladjustment to life in the United States

The third subgroup is American-born Asians. Cheng described two subgroups within this group. The "Chinatown ghetto" group whose members are born, raised, and never leave the Chinatown area is limited in its understanding of hearing problems and in access to audiological services. On the other hand, individuals who left Chinatown early and established their own life-styles typically have their own English-speaking physicians and may seek help if they have a hearing problem.

For all groups, Asian cultural themes affect behavior in response to significant hearing loss. A general Asian belief that aging is a natural process that does not require intervention is common. In Asian cultures, for example, the young show respect for hearing-impaired aged by either speaking loudly or nodding to the elder during conversation, even when they cannot hear or understand the speech. In this case the elders may not feel a need to improve communication because they are consistently acknowledged during family conversations. If they purchase a hearing aid and it does not work satisfactorily, they will simply not wear it rather than seek confrontation. When asked if a problem exists, they will deny it ("How can the audiologist or the dispenser be wrong? It must be me"). Cheng (1988) asserted that these problems will not subside through acculturation in the foreseeable future because increasing numbers of immigrants from Hong Kong and mainland China are expected in the coming decades. Culturally specific issues related to hearing help-seeking behaviors and application of amplification devices in all ethnic subgroups of the American population demand further investigation.

DEMOGRAPHICS

Hearing impairment ranks second only to arthritis (Maurer & Rupp, 1979) as a chronic disability affecting the aged. In 1971 the American Speech and Hearing Association reported that at least 2.5 million U.S. citizens over the age of 65 years had significant bilateral hearing loss (Alpiner, 1982). Of persons 65 years and over with bilateral hearing loss, 7.2 percent had onset of loss before 21 years of age. Of that 7.2 percent, 10.2 percent could at best hear shouted speech unaided, and 4.8 percent could hear normal conversational speech. The remainder had varying degrees of difficulty understanding speech (Gentile, 1971). Persons over 70 years of age represent only 5.2 percent of the hearing population, but 30.2 percent of the population with hearing loss. Forty-nine percent of the total population with serious hearing loss (able to hear only shouted speech unaided) are over 70 years of age (Feller, 1981). Ries (1982) examined the hearing ability of older persons as a function of the socio-demographic characteristics of sex, family income, and level of education. Table 1 summarizes his findings for persons over the age of 64 years. McCartney (1977) found that 84 percent of nursing home residents in a Sacramento study had significant bilateral hearing loss. In 126 older residents in nursing homes in San Diego, Novak (1980) found mean pure tone thresholds in the best ear were 47 dB HL (re: ANSI, 1969) at 500 Hz, 46 dB at 1000 Hz, 51 dB at 2000 Hz, 61 dB at 4000 Hz, and 69 DB at 8000 Hz. Ries (1982) found that of persons with serious hearing loss who lived independently, 49 percent of those 30 to 44 years old cited hearing loss as the main cause of limited activity, whereas only 6 percent of the same age group with normal hearing said they were limited in activity. In contrast, only 6 percent of those over 64 years old with severe hearing loss said that hearing loss was the main cause of limitation in activity. Ries concluded that younger, severely hearing-impaired people have few other limitations of activity and therefore view hearing loss, when it is serious, as a primary deficit.

Older people, however, have a greater array of causes of limited activity and view even severe hearing loss as minimally responsible

	Sex		Race		Family Income			Years of Education		
Hearing Ability	**M**	**F**	**White**	**Black**	**<7K**	**7K-14.9K**	**>15K**	**<12**	**12**	**>12**
No trouble hearing	38	62	90	10	53	30	17	60	22	18
All levels of loss	49	51	94	6	60	26	14	68	18	14
At best hears shouted speech (71-91 dB HL)	50	50	95	5	61	24	15	76	14	10

*All data in percent of total population over 64 years
Adapted from Ries (1982) with permission.

TABLE - 1 Hearing ability of persons over 64 years of age as a function of sex, race, family income and level of education.

for limitations of activity. Ries (1985) concluded that hearing impairment is generally overrepresented in the elderly population, with highest incidence occurring in individuals who are low income, poorly educated, and ill. These groups may view even a serious hearing loss as insignificant.

Novak and Ybarra (1988) found that perception of handicap can vary across ethnic subgroups. In correlating perceived hearing handicap with objective measures of hearing loss, they found that, although the relative prevalence of varying degrees of hearing loss was similar for their nonaudiology clinic samples of older urban black and native American subjects, the native Americans, regardless of degree of hearing loss, tended to perceive greater hearing handicap. In fact, several native Americans with clinically normal hearing (audiometric thresholds better than 25 dB HL for 500–3000 Hz) perceived significant hearing handicap. A possible explanation for this is that the older native Americans were hunters and gatherers and thus relied on a keen sense of hearing for their success and safety. In this study, the older blacks had less cultural emphasis on the importance of hearing as an isolated sense.

THE NURSING HOME POPULATION

Of elderly individuals living in the United States at any one time, only 5 to 6 percent live in extended care facilities. The nursing home subpopulation consists of four subgroups:

1. Residents who are in nursing homes for rehabilitation with the realistic expectation of again living independently in the community, depending to various degrees on community-based services and their own resources
2. Residents who have physical limitations that prevent them from living independently but otherwise are mentally intact
3. Residents who, like group 2, are limited physically and are also mentally impaired
4. Residents who are critically and terminally ill

Nursing home residents, like all older people, have an increased desired for privacy. The paradox, however, is that institutional living reduces the ability to maintain privacy. For a significant subset of hearing impaired, long-term nursing home residents, hearing loss may be their source of privacy, their insulation from the ever-present intrusions on their personal space. Ulatowska (1985) cited gestures, degree of eye contact, gaze, and orientation of body parts as methods used by nonambulatory nursing home residents to declare their territory and desire for solitude. Even a slight movement of the body or chair away from a fellow resident or staff member can indicate the termination of a conversation (Lipman, 1968). With this in mind, the hearing health care professional must ask what maintenance-of-privacy function the hearing loss serves for each of the subgroups of residents, and how truly motivated each group is to improve hearing for purposes of communication.

Specific hearing-air related services that the hearing health care professional might provide for each of these subgroups include the following:

GROUP 1. Maximization of electroacoustic function of existing hearing aids and assurance of proper use and application of the hearing aids by the patient and nursing home staff, respectively. Electroacoustically appropriate loaner hearing aids or new hearing aids should be provided in cases where patients need amplification and do not have their own hearing aids.

Maximum use of residual hearing by members of this group is of paramount importance if they are to have optimum receptive and expressive communication during the rehabilitation process.

GROUP 2. Maximization of long-term life quality in the nursing home by allowing the hearing-impaired resident the option of using appropriate amplification when they desire to communicate. The ability to succeed in communicating when they desire to and when others must "get through" is imperative to the quality of life for this population of nursing home residents. The hearing health care professional, therefore, must ensure that the residents have optimum access to and use of:

- Appropriate amplification
- Ongoing staff inservice instruction in the use of amplification systems including personal hearing aids and assistive listening devices
- Regular follow-up with residents using hearing aids on site
- Hearing aid assessment and fitting procedures that ensure valid application of amplification
- An in-house loaner hearing aid bank to ensure access to amplification for new and experienced hearing aid users

The hearing aids in the loaner bank can be donated by former residents, their families, and staff members, and electroacoustically analyzed and catalogued for appropriate use. Supportive aural rehabilitation programs and the availability of trained resident peer support and hearing-impaired patient advocate groups are also important for the optimum use of hearing aids by this subgroup.

GROUP 3. Maximization of functional mentation through the enhancement of meaningful sensory stimulation. The questions the hearing health care professional must answer for this group are: To what degree is inadequate and inconsistent sensory input responsible for the resident's impaired mental health? Are the symptoms displayed by this subgroup indicative of true chronic brain degeneration (dementia) or can the symptoms in part be described as signs of pseudodementia with the etiology of those symptoms being reduced meaning of sensory input (e.g., remediable auditory dysfunction)? To the extent that the latter is true, the hearing health professional is challenged to determine and fit appropriate amplification and optimize successful use through effective staff involvement and support. The availability of portable auditory brainstem evoked potential equipment for assessing hearing loss and probe tube microphone systems for assessing the insertion gain provided by hearing aids can be very helpful in working with this subgroup.

One in five persons over 65 years of age exhibits dementia at varying stages of severity; 25 percent are severely demented, and 75 percent have mild or moderate intellectual impairment (Mortimer, Schuman, & French, 1981). "Dementia must be greeted as a diagnostic challenge, not as an inevitable harbinger of death or a cause for nihilistic despair" Cummings, 1985, p. 55).

GROUP 4. Maximization of receptive and expressive communication through the final stages of the terminally ill resident's life. The hearing health care professional may be critical in facilitating meaningful communication of the terminally ill hearing-impaired resident with his of her family physician, clergy, nursing staff, and friends. If hearing-impaired members of this subgroup are not currently hearing aid users, they are logical candidates for use of hearing aids provided from the facility's loaner hearing aid bank or use of institutionally owned assistive listening devices.

The hearing health care professional often must act as a vocal advocate for access of this patient subgroup to hearing aids and associated improved receptive communication function. Access to the hearing-impaired nursing home resident, in most cases, is determined by requests for services by the patient, nursing home staff, patient's physician, or family. Extended care facilities should have nonexclusive contracts with appropriate health care professionals to whom referrals for medical and audiologic intervention can be made. In most states, however, it is only with the consent of the resident's physician that these referrals can be consummated. Therefore, it is imperative for the nursing staff and personal physicians of extended care facility residents to be educated as to the potential benefit of appropriate intervention (e.g., hearing aids, assistive listening devices, aural rehabilitation therapy, otologic medical and surgical treatment) by hearing health care professionals.

PHYSICALLY IMPAIRED ADULTS LIVING AT HOME

Ten percent of the elderly individuals who live at home are as functionally impaired as individuals who live in nursing homes. Mutual access of this subgroup of the aged population to the variety of hearing health care services is limited by the individual's motivation to seek help for hearing problems either because of low priority in the list of more fundamental human needs or because of minimal demands for communicative efficacy (i.e., few visitors, no television or radio, no telephone use, or use of communication devices at high volume to compensate for the individual's hearing loss). Access is also limited by the person's ability to get hearing health care services for initial and necessary follow-up appointments. The logistical problems of follow-up may be so overwhelming to the individual that it may seem impossible to overcome them; therefore, the person does not try. If services are to be provided to this group they must be more accessible to them than they typically are to the more flexible ambulatory hearing-impaired consumer.

INDEPENDENT AMBULATORY ADULTS

Eighty-five percent of the older population live independently in varying stages of wellness and well-being. This group by far contains the majority of aged hearing-impaired persons. The total population of aged hearing-impaired individuals constitutes 55 percent of adults with hearing losses severe enough to interfere with receptive communication (Berkowitz, 1975). Of this hearing-impaired population, Maurer and Rupp (1979) asserted that four out of five individuals are probably experiencing some communication problems in listening. Less than 25 percent of the hearing impaired persons over age 65 who need and could benefit from amplification have purchased hearing aids (Skafte, 1986). The reason for this, surmised from clinical experience, include:

- Lack of acknowledgment of hearing loss as a problem
- Lack of desire to rehabilitate acknowledged hearing loss

- Lack of knowledge of available services and technology
- Lack of appropriate support system and ability to manage use of hearing aids
- Financial inability to purchase hearing aids
- Erroneous understanding of what hearing aids can do and dissatisfied testimony from other hearing aid users or their own dissatisfaction with previous hearing aid use
- Inadequate audiometric and psychosocial assessment of the residual auditory function and communication needs of the hearing-impaired aged
- Amplification that was inappropriately applied because of electroacoustic and personal style preference inappropriateness
- Lack of or poor supportive aural rehabilitation services for the first-time hearing aid user

PSYCHOLOGY OF ADULT ONSET HEARING LOSS

The emphasis of this chapter is on the application of amplification systems to the post-lingually hearing-impaired older adult, particularly adults who experience progressive hearing loss through middle and into old age. For this population, psychological adjustment to hearing loss and the ability to accept responsibility in the rehabilitation process are of profound importance in attaining maximum aural rehabilitation.

Becker (1980) stated that prelingually deafened adults have created a society in which group membership allows them a nonstigmatized personal identity and normalized social relationships. "These factors stand them in good stead throughout the life cycle. It is when they become old however that these factors are especially useful in coping" (p. 98). For this population, hearing loss, which can be so catastrophic to the socialization of the aged post-lingually hearing impaired, is of no concern.

Glass (1985) suggested that there are two distinct older populations, the deaf who are growing old and the old who are growing deaf. She asserted that each group is affected similarly by the physical changes of aging but that the two populations undergo very different social, emotional, and behavioral effects related to hearing loss.

Factors important to the assessment of the effects of adventitious hearing loss include age at onset of loss, degree of impairment, rapidity of onset, and audiometric configuration. The earlier in adult life the loss is acquired, the more abnormal and catastrophic it is perceived as being. Hearing health professionals typically assess severity of loss through tests of pure tone sensitivity, word identification, and binaural auditory integration. Weinstein and Ventry (1983), however, concluded that hearing handicaps in the elderly are more appropriately measured by a self-report format than audiometric test data. This is discussed further in a later section of this chapter.

Sudden adult-onset hearing loss is most traumatic. Mulrooney (1973) described grief as an overwhelming response to sudden deafness. Ashley (1985) used adjectives such as "thunderbolt," "devastating," "shattering," "desolating sense of loss," and "lifelong burden" to describe his reaction to adventitious hearing loss.

Depression and withdrawal with resultant isolation are the most prevalent responses to significant hearing loss (Myklebust, 1964). Although Myklebust found this to be more true of "deafened" adults who are of employment age than older adults and equally true of the moderately and severely hearing impaired, it is a common clinical finding in the hearing-impaired elderly population. They assess themselves as withdrawing unwillingly from the mainstream of their social lives. Other symptoms found in adventitiously hearing impaired adults are nervousness, anxiety, heightened fearfulness, irritability, embarrassment, and fatigue from trying to communicate (Meadow-Orlans, 1985; Oyer & Oyer, 1979).

Myklebust (1964) reported that hearing-impaired men were less well adjusted than hearing-impaired women; however, this may be a cohort effect reflective of the work status of men versus women, relative demands on communication, and the concomitant effects of retirement and accompanying isolation. Although paranoia is frequently ascribed to the adventitiously hearing-impaired adult, this has not been empirically substantiated (Myklebust, 1964; Thomas & Gilhome-Herbst, 1980).

Severe social effects of adult onset hearing loss have also been reported. There may be loss of some old friends who will not struggle with labored communication or who are threatened by the intensity of the hearing-impaired person's feelings (Luey, 1980). In a group of newly severely hearing-impaired adults, Hunter (1978) found that 86 percent made new friends, 50 percent divorced, and 68 percent changed career objectives. In spite of the seeming advisability of socialization with people with similar problems, elderly hearing-impaired individuals are not likely to join organizations for the hearing impaired, especially if they lose their hearing late in life (Miller, 1975). As a result, hearing loss can render the elderly "prime candidates for needless senility" (Maurer & Rupp, 1979). Hearing loss accentuates social isolation, dependency, and loss of status (Beattie, 1981). Group aural rehabilitation sessions run by hearing health care professionals and Self-Help for the Hard of Hearing (SHHH) organizations, available in many cities nationally and internationally, can be critical factors in determining successful use of amplification systems and optimum aural rehabilitation of elderly individuals.

Although there is abundant evidence, particularly when hearing-impaired adults are asked to discuss the concept in aural rehabilitation settings, that older hearing-impaired adults believe that they are stigmatized by hearing persons, the nature and degree of the stigma is imprecise (Meadow & Orlans, 1985). It seems to be related to hearing-impaired persons' negative projections of what others think when they see a person wearing a hearing aid and normal hearing people's inability to understand the variability in the hearing ability of hearing-impaired persons in different listening situations.

Some adult clients believe that wearing a hearing aid elicits negative reactions in others, who consider a hearing aid a sign of old age and lack of intelligence. The negative stigma attached to hearing aid use, called the "hearing aid effect," has been demonstrated for normal hearing and speaking adolescent boys rated by college students (Blood, Blood, & Danhauer, 1978), geriatric patients rated by nursing home personnel (Knoll, 1979), and normal hearing and speaking preschool-age boys rated by audiologists, speech language pathologists, and college students (Danhauer, Blood, Blood, & Gomez, 1980). Iler, Danhauer, and Mulac (1982), however, found no differences in peer ratings of elders either wearing or not wearing hearing aids, using factors such as achievement, personality, or appearance. More recently, the wearing of hearing aids by the former president of the United States, Ronald Reagan, has served to reduce the self-perceived stigma of hearing aid use by the elderly.

ADJUSTMENT TO ADULT HEARING LOSS

Kyle, Jones, and Wood (1985) presented a model that described the phases of acquisition and adjustment to adventitious hearing loss in adults. It is important to assess which stage an individual is in when hearing aid assessment and fitting is being attempted. Phase 1, acquisition of hearing loss, is described as the period when the loss is not acknowledged. It may last less than a month or go on for 20 years or more. It is the time period between initial onset of loss and the first visit to a hearing health care provider. Up to 75 percent of the population with acquired hearing loss may be in this phase at any time (Medical Research Council, 1981). During this phase the unaided person receives feedback from the environment that he or she is talking too loud, the television or radio is too loud, he or she has misheard important information, and so on. During the initial stages of this phase, the hearing-impaired person ascribes the inability to hear to the faulty speech of others and other problems external to him- or herself. The initial visit to a hearing health care professional for evaluation may be made only in acquiescence to the demands of family members. Since realization of the existence of the loss is fundamental to initiation of help-seeking behavior. Kyle and colleagues suggested that when persons are forced to be in situations where they cannot control the volume of speech (e.g., lectures, church), they are apt to more quickly realize the extent of their impairment than if their time is spent in listening activities where they can control the volume of speech (e.g., watching television) or ascribe their inability to understand to faulty connections (e.g., using the telephone).

Phase 2 is described as the time between first contact with a professional and diagnosis of permanent hearing loss and the receipt of a hearing aid. Kyle and colleagues found that in England, where hearing aids are provided at no charge, this phase lasted a few months. In the United States, where the cost of hearing aids represents a significant financial investment, this phase may last a year or more. It is marked by uncertainty as to the ramifications of the newly identified hearing loss, and the resolution of this phase in large part is dependent on the accommodation and support of the person's family and friends. The resolution of this phase is also dependent on the person's willingness to accept responsibility for his or her own successful use of assertive communication techniques and speechreading skills taught in supportive aural rehabilitation sessions.

Phase 3 is the period of subsequent accommodation to the hearing loss. This phase is characterized by the individual's realization of the level of control he or she can expect to have in various communication settings. The ultimate goal of hearing aid fitting and supportive rehabilitation is to maximize the independence and control of the hearing-impaired individual in all desired communication environments. Kyle and colleagues cited maladaptive behaviors in this phase as behavioral changes resulting in (1) excessive introversion and control of conversations with minimal listening and (2) withdrawal from communication situations that threaten control and independence.

An acceptable resolution of Phase 3 is dependent on how the individual adjusts to the hearing aid, to personal and social situations, vocational and avocational demands, and the dynamics of family life. Fundamental to adjustment to the hearing aid is acceptance of its physical appearance, optimum electroacoustic compatibility with and compensation for the hearing loss, independence in the use of the amplification system, acknowledgment of the use of a less than perfect amplification system to others with whom communication is initiated, and realistic expectations of others regarding the aided benefit the new hearing aid user can derive in a variety of listening environments. Kyle and Wood (1983) found that, although 89 percent of their aided respondents had difficulty with street conversations, 79 percent would not tell people that they had a hearing problem. This is also typical of the reactions of new hearing aid users in the United States. If audiologists and dispensers were able to perfectly match the hearing aid configuration to the psychophysical needs of the client, there would be no need for public acknowledgment of the loss and the use of hearing aids.

However, given the as yet imperfect match of electroacoustic hearing aid parameters to clients' psychophysical needs and our incomplete understanding of the optimum psychophysical measures needed to adequately define the aidable parameters of the hearing loss, acknowledgment of the hearing loss and use of hearing aids remains critical to the successful resolution of the aural rehabilitation process.

The remainder of this chapter deals with assessment and intervention strategies.

AUDITORY ASSESSMENT FINDINGS IN THE AGED POPULATION

This section concentrates on threshold and suprathreshold auditory function in the aged listener. This information is, of course, most important when considering appropriate assessment and intervention strategies to amplify the older hearing-impaired client.

Marshall (1981) suggested the following hypotheses in the clinical evaluation of the older hearing-impaired listener: (1) Aging listeners are no different than young listeners with equal degrees of hearing loss and (2) Aging listeners will show auditory function problems in addition to those shown by younger listeners with similar hearing losses, possibly due to peripheral problems associated with presbycusis, which are not adequately assessed by the pure tone audiogram, central auditory nervous system degeneration, cognitive differences, or a combination of all of the above.

ASSESSMENT PROBLEMS RELATED TO AGE

The incidence of excessive impacted cerumen is higher in the older versus younger population (Fisch, 1978; Schow, Christensen, Hutchinson, & Nerbonne, 1978). Otoscopy must be performed prior to auditory and hearing aid evaluation.

Collapsing ear canals with the application of earphones has also been found to occur more frequently in older listeners (Zucker & Williams, 1977; Schow & Goldbaum, 1980) and may explain the high frequency conductive loss cited in several studies (Rosen, Plester, El Mofty, & Rosen, 1964). The implication is to assess the anterior posterior relationship of the tragus to the cavum of the concha and the relative collapsibility of the tragus and cartila genous portion of the external auditory meatus. If circumaural earphones or canal inserts are used to eliminate this problem, calibration of the audiometer must be completed with the modifications in place. As described earlier, collapsing ear canals also present a challenge for the fabrication of earmolds and ITE hearing aids.

It has been suggested that aged listeners are more conservative in their threshold criterion than younger listeners when they are asked to respond yes or no to the presence of an auditory signal (Rees & Botwinick, 1979; Potash & Jones, 1977). Clinical observations indicate that aged listeners may be less willing to guess in their discrimination of suprathreshold auditory signals if only a portion of the signal is heard (as with a suprathreshold single-word identification task). This symptom may be representative of older listeners or it may be endemic only to the current aged population as a consequence of low self-esteem and the low value generally placed on the aged by our society. In either case, the implication for the hearing health care professional is to reduce auditory test anxiety and reinstruct the older client regarding the clinician's expectation that errors in signal identification are expected, and in fact necessary, if an accurate evaluation is to be obtained. Implications for the test procedures include changing the threshold response to a two-interval forced choice task (eliminating the possibility of a nonresponse) and using closed-set, forced choice suprathreshold speech identification tests, such as a Modified Rhyme type test, the Synthetic Sentence Identification Index, or a comparison of closed set (high redundancy) to open set (low redundancy) word identification performance using a tool such as the Speech in Noise test (SPIN).

LOUDNESS AND ADAPTATION

Because of the bilateral symmetry of most hearing losses in the aged population and the difficulty of comparing loudness levels of very different frequencies in the same ear, it is not possible to use the alternate binaural loudness balance test (ABLB) or the monaural loudness balance (MLB) test to behaviorally assess loudness recruitment. Short Increment Sensitivity Index (SISI) results are equivocal (Jerger, Shedd, & Harford, 1959) or similar to those shown with cochlear hearing losses of non-age related etiologies. Since this test is typically done in a yes or no paradigm, given the potential for conservative response, it may also be inappropriate as a measure of recruitment in the older client. "Other than using uncomfortable loudness thresholds as a recruitment measure, there is currently no behavioral test of recruitment for elderly listeners" (Marshall, 1981). It has been suggested by clinical audiologists that uncomfortable loudness measures using speech and pure tones lack validity as representations of the levels of sound a person will truly accommodate when they are motivated to do so (i.e., in social or vocational situations).

In spite of this perception it is important to assess frequency specific tolerance limits, known by various names such as uncomfortable loudness levels (UCLs), upper limits of comfortable loudness (ULCL), loudness discomfort levels (LDLs), and most comfortable listening levels (MCLs), in each ear for each subject in order to make the most appropriate initial decisions regarding the appropriate frequency-specific gain and saturation sound pressure level (SSPL) characteristics of hearing aids.

Adaptation, or reduction in the loudness percept of suprathreshold continuous pure tones, has been assessed in older individuals using Bekesy and conventional tone decay tests. Bekesy tracings are usually consistent with normal hearing or a cochlear site of lesion (type I or II tracings, respectively) (Jerger, 1960; Harbert, Young, & Menduke, 1966), and tone decay is typically less than 30 dB, also consistent with cochlear site of lesion (Olsen & Noffsinger, 1974; Ganz, 1976).

Implications for Amplification

The primary behavioral assessment of recruitment for the aging listener is loudness tolerance for pure tones, warble tones, or speech. The dynamic range from threshold to these levels is reduced in all persons with sensorineural hearing loss. Although the usable auditory dynamic range is not inordinately reduced for aged hearing impaired listeners, they often have a decreased ability to ignore the presence of loud environmental noise, which interferes with their understanding of important auditory input.

The aided listener with sensorineural hearing loss requires a comparatively wide range of input signal intensities to be amplified to suprathreshold levels and maintained within the compressed suprathreshold dynamic range of the individual. These findings suggest that, if maximum hearing aid benefit is to be achieved for the elderly and all persons with sensorineural hearing loss, SSPL90 values that closely correspond to obtained frequency-specific UCLs must be utilized, while at the same time providing enough gain to boost important auditory stimuli to the person's MCLs. Depending on the separation in dB between the person's MCL and UCL at each frequency, these criteria may be met without the use of a compression circuit in the aid. However, as MCLs approach the levels of the UCLs, reducing the dynamic range, it may be possible only to provide adequate gain for lower level input signals in order to keep all amplified signals below the UCLs. This situation would necessitate the use of a compression circuit. If compression is utilized, it is therefore important to keep the "knee" or threshold of compression as high as possible in order to maximize gain for speech input (particularly for frequencies at and above 1000 Hz). The audiologist or the dispenser who uses frequency-specific stimuli to determine MCLs and UCLs should also evaluate whether MCLs and UCLs for more complex signals (e.g., speech and environmental noise) might be somewhat lower due to loudness summation resulting from the simultaneous presentation of the multiple frequency components contained in these stimuli.

FREQUENCY DISCRIMINATION

Reduced frequency selectivity in persons with sensorineural hearing loss has been shown using difference limens for frequency (DLF) (Zurek & Formby, 1979). DLFs have been shown to increase with increased magnitude of loss and for low frequencies as well as high frequencies in persons with only high frequency pure tone loss. It has not been established whether aged hearing-impaired listeners have inordinately greater DLFs than their younger counterparts when learning effects and potential age-related criterion effects are controlled (Marshall, 1981).

Psychophysical tuning curves for listeners with sensorineural hearing loss, obtained by fixing the level and frequency of a probe tone and measuring the level of a second tone at various frequencies required to mask the probe, have shown abnormal broadening, abnormal shape, and loss of the tip in regions of hearing loss (Zwicker & Shorn, 1978; Tyler, Fernandes, & Wood, 1984) and abnormality in regions of normal hearing sensitivity (Mills, Gilbert,

& Adkins, 1979), especially in the presence of significant high frequency loss (Nelson, 1979). It is not clear whether these results differ in older versus younger persons with similar audiograms (Marshall, 1981).

It has been suggested that each frequency is surrounded by its own critical bandwidth of frequencies and that all frequencies within the critical band of a probe frequency are processed equally. Thus, formants in the speech signal that are separated by a critical bandwidth are perceived as different frequencies; however, environmental noise located within the critical band of each formant frequency is processed along with the speech signal. A widening of critical bandwidths, or loss of frequency selectivity, has been found with the advent of sensorineural hearing loss (deBoer & Bowmeester, 1974, 1976). The widening of critical bands may be due to cochlear changes (efferent olivocochlear neuron degeneration) not related to afferent input, and frequency discrimination may be independent of loss of pure tone hearing threshold sensitivity (Bienvenue & Michael, 1979). It has not been definitively shown, however, that the widening of critical bandwidths in aged listeners with sensorineural loss is in excess of that for young hearing-impaired listeners. Bienvenue and Michael (1979) listed four functions of critical bands: (1) to band limit the effect of background noise on the target signal serving to enhance the signal-to-noise ratio; (2) to determine ability to perceive harmonic content and formant content (in the case of speech) of complex signals; (3) to determine ability to perceive phase relationships among tone complexes; and (4) to sharpen frequency discrimination beyond that which can be described by basilar membrane mechanics.

Critical ratios (signal-to-noise ratio at masked threshold) and upward spread of masking have been assessed in aged listeners and are a reflection of critical bandwidth. Critical ratios have been demonstrated to increase for higher frequencies in both normal hearing (Reed & Bilger, 1973) and high frequency noise-induced hearing impaired listeners (Tyler, Fernandes, & Wood, 1984). Margolis and Goldberg (1980) concluded that critical ratios are not a simple reflection of auditory filter bandwidth in aged listeners. Upward spread of masking in aged hearing-impaired listeners has not been shown to be any greater than for younger cochlear hearing-impaired counterparts. Although upward spread of masking has been found to be detrimental to speech discrimination of normal hearing listeners at high signal intensities (95–100 dB SPL) (Danaher, Osberger, & Pickett, 1973), it has not been shown to be abnormally broad in all listeners with sensorineural hearing loss (Jerger et al., 1960; Leshowitz & Lindstrom, 1979).

Implications for Amplification

It is quite possible that peripheral deterioration of the frequency selectivity of the cochlea accounts in large part for the reduced understanding of speech in noise in the aged hearing-impaired listener. It is also possible that aged persons with different audiometric configurations and etiologies of hearing loss have varying degrees of alteration in critical bandwidths and cochlear-based frequency specificity.

Once a reliable data base is established regarding the frequency discrimination of older versus younger hearing-impaired listeners with controls for loss configuration, etiology, and task response criterion effects, it seems imperative that tasks that assess frequency discrimination be included in the hearing aid assessment process. The information obtained would make it possible to severely band limit the amplified signal, based not only on the audiometric configuration of the pure tone loss, but also on the extent of abnormality of frequency selectivity across the frequency range, even in the presence of what appear to be normal pure tone thresholds. This would be quite possible with the use of digital filtering which, unfortunately, is not currently available in the majority of hearing aids.

SPEECH DISCRIMINATION

From the previous discussion of the importance of peripheral frequency selectivity to the discrimination of complex signals (speech) in noise, it can be argued that if population-specific information was available, much of the responsibility for reduction in speech discrimination in noise demonstrated by significant numbers of aged hearing-impaired listeners could be described on the basis of impaired frequency selectivity at the level of the cochlea. If this were true, particularly with the advent of digital processing technology, algorithms could be designed into the hearing aid to compensate specifically for abnormal cochlear function. An additional portion of the reduction in speech understanding in aged listeners can be explained on the basis of inadequate sensation levels, particularly of high frequency speech sounds and high formant frequencies within those speech sounds.

To determine age-only related changes in auditory temporal processing, Blackington, Novak, and Kramer (1988) examined NU-6 word identification in normal hearing young and elderly subjects with 0 and 60 percent temporal compression of the speech signals. The authors compared these data to forward masking threshold results using 500 and 2000 Hz as the target stimuli with wide band noise as the masker. The older subjects, ages 60 to 79 years, obtained 70 percent correct identification on the compressed speech presented at 40 dB H L compared to 82 percent correct identification for the young controls. There was no difference in word identification scores between the two groups for non-compressed speech stimuli (97–99% for all subjects). Blackington, Novak, and Kramer also found that, for separations between the masker and target stimuli of 0 to 250 ms, the older subjects required higher tone sensation levels in order to achieve the same 70 percent correct detection level as their younger counterparts. This was particularly true for the 2000 Hz stimuli.

A common clinical observation from aged hearing-impaired listeners is that their understanding of speech improves with a mildly reduced rate of speech. The results of many of the altered speech studies have showed excessively reduced performance in aged hearing-impaired listeners. The results of Blackington, Novak, and Kramer (1988), which showed the same reduction of performance in normal hearing aged listeners, suggest that the critical causal factors are age-related central factors that are not dependent on changes in pure tone sensitivity.

BINAURAL INTEGRATION

Binaural auditory fusion and release from masking tasks have been used to assess central auditory nervous system integrity. Binaural auditory fusion compares word identification when high and low frequency information is presented monaurally versus when high-pass filtered speech is presented to one ear and low-pass s filtered speech to the other. Breakdown in the former task can be attributed solely to abnormal cochlear filter effects, whereas breakdown in the dichotic high pass-low pass task can also be impaired by brainstem pathology and bilateral and diffuse cerebral pathology (Lynn & Gilroy, 1976). Investigators have found that the aged listener's binaural fusion ability is not significantly poorer than younger listeners with similar pure tone thresholds (Harbert et al., 1966; Palva & Jokenen, 1970). In fact older listeners often perform more poorly on the monaural task than on the dichotic speech fusion task, which is consistent with peripheral auditory system pathology. Franklin (1975) also found this to be true with young (13–23 years) listeners with sensorineural hearing loss.

The binaural masking level difference (MLD) is a psychophysical task which also relies on intact lower brainstem function for maximum MLD results. Many studies that have reported MLD results for presbycusic listeners have concluded that MLDs are generally smaller for the presbycusic 1 population (Olsen, Noffsinger, & Carhart, 1976; Warren, Wagener, & Herman, 1978), in spite of considerable overlap of MLD values between young normal hearing and older hearing-impaired groups. Novak and Anderson (1982) were the first to attempt to systematically control for age, degree of hearing loss, bilateral symmetry of loss, shape of loss, and central auditory integrity in the evaluation of the MLD in older hearing-impaired listeners. They found that, for older listeners, MLD magnitudes for 500 Hz were significantly reduced only for the neural presbycusic (Schuknecht, 1964, 1974) group. The authors concluded that central auditory system function as measured by the MLD task was significantly different only for the neural presbycusic group with high frequency sloping sensorineural hearing loss and single-word identification scores less than 70 percent. These binaural speech fusion and MLD studies support the contention that binaural integration is intact for many aged hearing-impaired listeners.

Implications for Amplification

From the results of the studies cited in the previous two sections, it must be concluded that, although problems of speech understanding in the aged hearing-impaired listener can be attributed in large part to cochlear filtering effects due to pathology at the level of the cochlea, even older normal hearing listeners show poorer performance than their younger counterparts on temporal masking tasks (compressed speech identification, forward masking signal detection). In this case, age appears to be a critical factor in determining the ability to understand rapid speech. On the basis of the recent forward masking data of Blackington, Novak, and Kramer (1988), even normal hearing older listeners may benefit from mild high frequency emphasis amplification in order to improve their detection and processing of rapidly presented auditory information.

In the case of bilaterally symmetrical hearing loss and PB word discrimination scores in excess of 80 percent, binaural fitting of aids must not be ruled out solely on the basis of concern for inability to binaurally integrate dichotically presented information (typical sound-field listening). Age, in and of itself, does not appear to be a significant factor in reduction of binaural auditory fusion or binaural release from masking abilities in older persons with cochlear-based hearing loss. The implications of all of the psychoacoustic findings with aged hearing-impaired listeners are that:

- The population is indeed composed of subgroups as defined by different peripheral and central auditory system function.
- The pure tone audiogram, in and of itself, is not an adequate descriptor of important auditory psychophysical abilities.
- The onus is on the audiologist to develop a valid, reliable, and efficient test battery that will delineate cochlear versus retrocochlear function as it relates specifically to the specification of hearing-aid parameters.

This test battery must differentiate between improved auditory function that can be expected based solely on differential hearing aid design and benefits from "appropriate" amplification predicted on the basis of psychosocial motivational parameters unique to each aged listener.

HEARING EVALUATION PROCEDURES SUGGESTED FOR USE WITH THE AGED LISTENER

The audiologist must apply hearing aids that (1) have the electroacoustic characteristics most appropriate for the client's residual auditory function and (2) are acceptable to the client. Satisfaction of the first requirement does not always ensure satisfaction of the second. Barford (1979) stated that user satisfaction across clients, as measured by speech perception ability, can be high or low with similar sudden significant changes in aided versus unaided auditory sensitivity. High satisfaction results if the additional frequency information provided to the "recognition device" is indeed meaningful and useful. Low satisfaction results when enhanced aided sensitivity for high frequencies relative to low frequencies causes a "mismatch of the recognition device and the input code." A degradation in speech perception ability at the time of initial hearing aid use "will result if the latter effect dominates." Barford suggested that, "this mismatch will gradually decrease as a result of adaptation, if adaptation is possible." However, the length of the adaptation is not easily predicted (re: age of client, type of loss, and a variety of psychosocial variables) for each individual client and may last from a few days to 6 months or longer. Because of the potential existence of this very real paradox between self-assessed user benefit and objectively measured improvement in aided versus unaided sensitivity, recent investigations indicate that it is important to include client self-assessment of aided versus unaided hearing handicap (Alpiner, 1982; Weinstein & Ventry, 1983; Demorest & Erdman, 1984a; Hawkins, 1985) as well as objective measures of auditory ability in order to maximize appropriate application of hearing aids to the hearing-impaired older adult population.

The steps in the geriatric hearing aid evaluation can be divided into measurements required for:

- Selection of client-specific optimum hearing system (hearing aid plus acoustic coupler) electroacoustic characteristics
- Assessment of client's perception of the communication handicap imposed by the hearing loss
- Assessment of the client's auditory, psychological, and physical ability to benefit from amplification
- Assessment of the reduction in handicap afforded by appropriate application of amplification as measured by objective and subjective procedures

SELECTION OF ELECTROACOUSTIC PARAMETERS OF HEARING AIDS

Many articles have been written on procedures for determining appropriate gain, frequency response, and SSPL90 characteristics of hearing aids, as well as the need for directional microphones, compression amplification, binaural fitting, and acoustically modified earmolds or ITEs. It is not at all obvious, however, that the typical auditory measures of thresholds, MCLs, and LDLs for pure tones and speech measured under earphones versus the same measures made in the sound field for aided versus unaided assessment are sufficient to model the auditory needs that must be accommodated by the hearing aid. For example, might it not also be beneficial to assess critical bandwidths? This could be done for high as well as low frequencies and differential discrimination of frequency across the critical auditory spectrum (500–6000 Hz) in order to better identify the signal processing parameters that would maximize use of these auditory abilities in the hearing-impaired client. This information would tell us if the older client can discriminate between target frequencies in the hearing aid response curve, thereby helping the hearing aid provider to determine which frequency response curve modifications are most meaningful. For example, attempting to increase gain for frequencies above 3000 Hz would be unnecessary if the client is unable to discriminate differences between frequencies in the 4000 to 6000 Hz target range. These considerations are crucial to optimum design of future "speech processor" type hearing aids but are beyond the scope of this chapter.

Efficiency, speed, validity, and reliability of test procedures are critical when assessing auditory function in aged clients in order to select appropriate electroacoustic characteristics available in current hearing aids.

AUDITORY EVALUATION

It is recommended that, at a minimum, the following parameters should be assessed:

1. Pure tone thresholds and MCLs under earphones in order to specify general frequency response characteristics and absolute gain requirements. Methods for calculation of desired frequency specific gain values on the basis of pure tone audiometric data (thresholds or MCLs relative to assumed frequency specific values for the long-term speech spectrum) have been described by Berger, Hagenberg, and Rane (1977); Pascoe (1978); Skinner, Pascoe, Miller, and Popelka (1982); McCandless and Lyregaard (1983); Cox (1985, 1987); Byrne and Dillon (1986); Libby (1986); Byrne (1987); and Skinner (1988). In applying audiometric data to determinations of frequency response requirements and preselection of specific hearing aids, it is important to realize that 2 cc coupler values indicated on manufacturers' specification sheets may under-represent desired functional gain (aided versus unaided thresholds for warble tones or narrow band noise) or insertion gain (aided versus unaided ear canal sound response level) (Hawkins & Schum, 1984). The difference will be greater for BTE than for ITE hearing aids, particularly for frequencies above 1000 Hz. Lower insertion and functional gain will also be seen in persons with large ear canal volumes medial to the tip of the hearing aid on the earmold and with very flaccid middle ear systems.
2. Immittance testing with special attention to the physical volume measure and the Peak Y amplitude value of the tympanogram.
3. Frequency specific LDLs for those frequencies for which amplification is desired in order to specify SSPL90 values to which the aid should first be adjusted. It is suggested that the client's own ear mold coupled to an external hearing aid receiver, which is coupled to the output of the audiometer (Hawkins, 1984), used in order to arrive at LDL values in dB SPL that correlate directly to hearing aid specification data. Etymotic insert earphones, available through the Etymotic Re-

search Lab, calibrated in the cc coupler are a less cumbersome alter native. LDLs should be obtained for both frequency specific and broad band stimuli (speech or speech noise) to determine the extent to which loudness summation may necessitate the lowering of the SSPL90 requirements.

4. Word identification scores using the receiver described by Hawkins (1984) on the etymotic earphones with speech presented at precalculated frequency specific gain levels (as afforded by a master hearing aid-type audiometer). This enables assessment of speech perception that is less contaminated by the upward spread of masking and distortion, which might be created by the overamplification of lower frequencies and underamplification of higher frequencies when using the typical flat spectrum speech audiometer set to the client's MCL.
5. DLFs for frequencies needing significant amplification in order to determine the individual's ability to discriminate between adjacent frequencies. This is particularly helpful in determining how important it really is to try to achieve significant target gain values for 3000, 4000, and 6000 Hz.

In a less than optimal testing environment, the effects of background noise are reduced for persons with thresholds > 40 dBL at or above 500 Hz. Methods utilized include assessment of pure tone thresholds, UCLs, and MCLs under earphones using a portable audiometer, and identification of recorded words under earphones using a tape recorder with dB HL settings marked on the dial, as determined by previous 6 or 2 cc (depending on the earphones used) coupler calibration of the speech levels. Probe microphone measures are invaluable in allowing a quick and reliable comparison of aided versus unaided ear canal sound pressure levels (insertion gain) to assess adequacy of hearing aid gain without requiring subjective judgments from the client. Aided versus unaided speech identification can be assessed in the sound field at a pragmatic distance of 3 feet with the clinician's speech being monitored at 55 to 60 dBA at the patient's location using a sound level meter. The speech stimuli used will vary with the abilities of the client (standard word lists for more intact clients or abbreviated word lists emphasizing high frequency words, the Ling 5 sounds test incorporated into real words [e.g., shaw, she, shoe, saw, see, sue], and more meaningful questions about the client and his or her environment for less intact clients). Speech testing, aided versus unaided, should also be done with and without the use of lip cues in order to show the older client the importance of enhancing hearing aid use by watching the speaker's face.

ASSESSMENT OF SELF-PERCEIVED HANDICAP IMPOSED BY THE HEARING LOSS

There are a variety of self-assessment inventories designed to allow clients to rate the psychological, social, vocational, and emotional handicaps imposed by their hearing losses. These include the Hearing Handicap Scale (High, Fairbanks, & Glorig, 1964), Hearing Measurement Scale (Noble & Atherley, 1970), Social Hearing Handicap Index (Ewertson & Birk-Nielsen, 1973), Denver Scale of Communication Function (Alpiner, Chevrette, Glascoe, Metz,. & Olsen, 1974), Hearing Performance Inventory (Giolas, Owens, Lamb, & Schubert, 1979), Revised Hearing Performance Inventory (Lamb, Owens, & Schubert, 1983), Hearing Problem Inventory (Hutton, 1980), Hearing Handicap Inventory for the Elderly (Ventry & Weinstein, 1982), McCarthy-Alpiner Scale of Hearing Handicap (McCarty & Alpiner, 1983), Communication Profile for the Hearing Impaired (Demorest & Erdman, 1984).

Use of the Hearing Handicap for the Elderly (Weinstein & Ventry, 1983) is recommended because it has been used and validated with hearing-impaired older persons typically seen in speech and hearing clinics. It is relatively short and assesses the critical concerns of the emotional and social and situational effects of the hearing loss. Weinstein and Ventry found that older clients with pure tone averages of 0 to 25 dB HL (500, 1000, 2000 Hz) almost never described their hearing losses as handicapping. Half of the clients with pure tone averages of 26 to 40 dB HL perceived the hearing loss as a handicap and half did not. Older clients with hearing losses greater than 41 dB HL very often (88–92%) perceived their hearing loss as handicapping. There was, however, considerable variability even for the greater-than-40-dB loss group in the degree (mild to significant) of perceived handicap. Results for older persons were very similar to the results for younger persons, and audiometric data (e.g., pure tone averages, speech reception thresholds, and speech discrimination scores) accounted for less than 50 percent of the variance in self-assessed hearing handicap. These results are consistent with the recommendation that, although pure tone thresholds are important for the description of the desired hearing aid electroacoustic parameters, they do not adequately describe the functional deficits imposed by a given hearing loss, particularly for losses less than 40 dB HL for the three-frequency pure tone average.

The Demorest and Erdman (1984) Communication Profile for the Hearing Impaired is also recommended for use in problematic cases that require very specific aural rehabilitation procedures. The test battery allows assessment of adequacy of communication in the individual's social environment. Problem awareness, communication need, physical environment, attitudes and behaviors of others, maladaptive behaviors, verbal and nonverbal communication strategies, self-acceptance, acceptance of loss, anger, defensiveness, guilt, discouragement, stress, withdrawal, and denial are also assessed. Some items from this tool are not appropriate for retired adults and would therefore have to be deleted. Most aged clients who admit that they are having communication difficulties secondary to hearing loss complain that with previous hearing aids sounds were often too loud, and speech was difficult to understand when background noise was present (e.g., informal group gatherings). If bilaterally impaired, sounds originating on the unaided ear were often difficult to initially detect and process if relocation was not easy (e.g., when seated in a car). Mueller, Hawkins, and Sedge (1984) suggest that, for the majority of the hearing-impaired population, who have potential for bilateral amplification, it is preferable to use compression, directional microphones, and binaural fitting. If the client is over 70 years of age and a first-time hearing aid user, the recommendation for binaural fitting might be qualified, based on the person's ability to physically and mentally cope with, at first, just one new hearing aid and then, at a later time, possibly a second hearing aid.

PREDICTION OF ABILITY TO SUCCESSFULLY USE AMPLIFICATION

The Rupp Feasibility Scale for Predicting Hearing Aid Use (Rupp, Higgins, & Maurer, 1977) differentially weighs factors of motivation, fault, initial impression, age, vision, significant others, self assessment, functional gain for speech, adaptability, manual dexterity, and financial resources and, accordingly, allows for scoring of each client from poor (0) to excellent (100) prognosis for successful use of hearing aids. Hosford-Dunn and Baxter (1985) found that in a group of 95 clients ranging in age from 20 to 89 years old (mean age, 65 years) with mild to severe hearing losses at 1000 to 4000 Hz, clinician-assessed "motivation" and "initial subjective impressions of amplification" to be the two best predictors of long-term (first 3 months of aid use) satisfaction. As Hosford-Dunn and Baxter suggested, for clients older than 70 years of age, other factors of this instrument may have predictive value as well and should not be eliminated for that population. Hosford,

Dunn and Baxter also examined the predictive value of standard audiometric measures relative to the successful use of amplification. Only aided versus unaided single syllable word identification scores in quiet were found to be of predictive value. Although predictive studies with aged hearing aid users have not been reported using data from the Communication Profile for the Hearing Impaired, the completeness of the range of parameters assessed by this test battery would make it very useful in identifying problems that could interfere with an otherwise seemingly good prognosis for successful hearing aid use. The length of the test battery and scoring time may preclude its use in some clinical settings.

ASSESSMENT OF REDUCTION OF HANDICAP AFFORDED BY AMPLIFICATION

Audiometric indications of a successful hearing aid fitting are aided versus unaided functional gain for warble tones and narrow band noises, allowing for aided thresholds from 1000 to 6000 Hz of 30 to 35 dB HL with aided speech in quiet for words presented at 50 dB HL in excess of 88 percent, and aided conversational to loud speech levels reported by the listener to be comfortable and within their tolerance limits, respectively. Coupled with discrimination scores greater than 88 percent for speech in environmental noise with +10 dB or poorer signal-to-noise ratios and tolerance of all ranges of aided environmental noise levels, these results should assure most hearing aid dispensers that their fitting of the aid was successful. However, it is rare for all of these conditions to be met in more typical cases of aged hearing aid users. As stated earlier, even with optimum electroacoustic matching of the hearing aid to the hearing loss with near normalization of aided auditory sensitivity for important speech frequencies, aged hearing aid users may reject hearing aids. Rejection may occur because the aided auditory signals are too different from the internal auditory code they have used to previously encode the auditory speech signal (Barford, 1979). With the aged client, therefore, it is advisable to include pre- and post-aided self-assessment inventories of handicap, as discussed earlier, to validate audiometric suggestions of a successful hearing aid fitting. This might be accomplished through pre- and post-administration of the Hearing Handicap Inventory for the Elderly (Weinstein & Ventry, 1982) or, as Hosford, Dunn and Baxter (1985) have done, pre- and post-fitting administration of the Hearing Performance Inventory (Lamb, Owens, & Shubert, 1983) using only the 38 items (HPI_{38}) related to speech understanding. Lamb and colleagues measured HPI_{38} scores of clients in their sixties and seventies with primarily moderate losses prior to hearing aid fitting and 3 months post-fitting. They concluded that if the difference score was in excess of 10 percent, there was "no chance of dissatisfaction" with the aid. It would be ideal if this type of assessment could be done within the currently mandated 30-day trial period. However, since adjustment to the hearing aid may take in excess of 6 months for an older first-time user, it might be argued that this type of pre-post assessment within the current 30-day trial period would not give a valid reflection of the client's ability to benefit from hearing aid use. This period may be dramatically affected by intensive aural rehabilitation counseling immediately post hearing aid fitting. The critical question, however is: How do age when first amplified, degree and slope of hearing loss, amount of change in unaided versus aided sensitivity, and nonauditory psychosocial and cultural factors interact with the amount and type of counseling necessary to optimize adjustment within the 30-day trial period? Even with daily rehabilitation sessions, 30 days may not be long enough for some aged hearing aid users to adapt to hearing aid use.

The aged hearing-impaired population presents infinitely complex diagnostic and rehabilitative challenges to hearing health care professionals. Older hearing aid candidates may have a variety of physical changes in addition to hearing loss, which provide a complicated backdrop to problems created by hearing loss, or hearing loss may be their only significant disorder. Aged clients may present themselves alone with no one to assist in the aural rehabilitation process, or they may be warmly supported by a child, a spouse, or a friend in their adaptation to the use of hearing aids and new assertive communication skills. They may have predominantly cochlear-based sensorineural hearing loss and seem no different than their younger counterparts, or they may have more difficulty understanding aided speech than would be predicted on the basis of their pure tone audiograms. They may present themselves at hearing aid clinics because they truly realize the extent of their disability and desire rehabilitation or may come only to appease a significant other with no acknowledgment of responsibility for the communication problems they are having.

Knowledge of appropriate psychophysical data necessary to discretely describe the auditory function of presbycusic subgroups is incomplete. Our ability to model "normal" auditory function is each aged hearing-impaired client with uniquely appropriate amplification is, therefore, also imperfect. The procedures that are used in the assessment of the aged client for use of amplification should specifically define unique cochlear versus retrocochlear function in presbycusic subgroups. The resultant data should be adaptable to a prescriptive approach for the recommendation of hearing aids to minimize the time spent in hearing aid evaluation and fitting.

In the final analysis, the clinician is best advised to listen to elderly clients and to understand, as much as possible, the orientation (cultural, social, psychological) of the client with respect to the hearing aid and aural rehabilitation process. Successful aural rehabilitation of the older client is possible only if there is mutual respect and honesty between the client and the hearing health care professional. The onus is on the individual professional to recommend the most appropriate hearing aid, or aids, to provide supportive aural rehabilitation counseling to the aged client, and to involve the client in a manner that will maximize independent use of all the equipment and communication strategies offered.

REHABILITATION PROGRAM

There is no doubt, if one believes the literature, that a rehabilitation program enhances communication skills in the hearing impaired when coupled with wearing a hearing aid. I believe the most important reason for failure in fitting hearing aids is the lack of understanding on the part of the wearer and the professional. Past experience has convinced me that some sort of structured informational training program must be part of the package. This is especially true for our senior wearers. Believe me, there is no substitute for this component of treatment for the older hearing impaired person. Any structured rehabilitation program should include at least the following: A frank discussion about hearing loss designed to give the individual a better understanding of the function of hearing and its dysfunction when impaired. This must include the disadvantages of hearing aids as well as the advantages. No one should be led to believe that a hearing aid will provide normal hearing. The goal of the rehabilitation program is to provide usable communication skills, not "normal hearing." During any discussions, the patient must be convinced that you are there to assist him to attain these goals. It must be evident to him that his efforts in this direction must be strong and sincere and that success is directly proportional to the strength of his efforts. You must make it clear that you cannot bring about success without his help. Teamwork including the patient, his family and friends, a professional rehabilitation counselor, and you is the keyword. I promise you that time spent in this sort of discussion is time well spent. The patient must be made to understand that the hearing aid is just the beginning.

He should learn that the hearing aid only provides louder sounds and that he must take advantage of his audiovisual system to partially makeup for the elements lacking in his auditory system.

It is becoming constantly more evident that hearing aid dispensing must include some form of instructional component if rehabilitation of the hearing impaired older population is to be successful. The forward-looking dispenser of hearing aids must prepare to make this available if he is to be competitive (Garstecki, 1981).

Such programs must include information designed to acquaint the patient with his problem; assist him to develop realistic expectations; inform him of the importance of amplification; convince him of the need for his serious participation coupled with the education of his immediate supporters such as family and friends; train him in communication skills including visual and auditory techniques and, equally as important, counsel him concerning the problems that will arise as a result of his impairment.

HEARING AIDS

Properly fitted modern hearing aids can enhance communication skills enough to be given serious consideration for use by the older hearing impaired individual. The modern hearing aid is an electronic marvel in terms of amplification, frequency response, gain control, and compression circuitry. It is, however, a limited signal processor when compared to the normal cochlea. Any attempts to build a signal processor for aiding impaired hearing are frustrated from the start, since at present we are unable to measure the various parameters of human signal processing properly. I have frequently been told by very competent engineers that if we (the biologists) will tell them what we need they have the technology to provide it.

Our shortcoming is a lack of measurement tools to determine just what the impaired cochlea needs to rectify the problems. Our present measurement techniques are far from satisfactory and until we develop better methods for quantifying normal and impaired performance, fitting any prosthetic device, hearing aids in particular, will remain a trial-and-error procedure.

"Hearing" is probably our most complex sensory process. Measuring sensitivity to pure tones and responses to speech gives us very little information. In fact, none at all about pitch discrimination, pattern recognition, and phase relationships. I mention this merely in passing. Recent information on the cochlea appears to show that the outer hair cells act as a fine tuning mechanism to integrate the incoming information, at least partially, prior to passing it on to the inner hair cells which seem then to pass it on to the eighth nerve and the cochlear nucleus which acts as a gate to the mid-brain and higher centers.

When an impaired cochlea is examined carefully it is obvious that many outer hair cells are missing which cause the fine tuning process to be distorted. Present clinical testing methods provide no information on what effect this has on the final signals as they reach the higher centers for processing. This could well be the explanation of the problems associated with hearing in noise or in the presence of competing signals. It is highly probable that fine discrimination tasks are related to this fine tuning function: until we are able to evaluate and assess the loss of this function, we will be unable to device a means of compensating for it. If our assumption is correct about the functions of the outer hair cells, it is easy to see why we encounter so many problems when fine auditory processing is needed. One of the most obvious findings in sensori neural hearing loss is the loss of outer hair cells. (Wallott 1991)

We must begin to examine and devise better methods of testing the effects of sensorineural hearing loss on the signals which finally reach the higher auditory centers for processing. It is especially important to examine and devise methods of testing aided hearing. Our present techniques of devising information on aided hearing provide us with only intensity changes. Further testing to include pitch discrimination and pattern recognition is imperative. (Berkowitz 1975)

This chapter is not a "how to" chapter but an attempt on my part to outline some general guidelines concerning the application of amplification to hearing-impaired people over 65.

When one of our older citizens decides to try a hearing aid, he has made a decision to do so after much mental agony. He has had to overcome his desire to hide his physical frailty which is another reminder that he is getting closer to the inevitable. He has had to suppress his vanity which has been no mean battle. His admission to himself means also that he must admit it to his friends and family. It means that he will no longer be able to comfortably resolve his communication problems by resorting to isolation. He must say to himself and others that he is no longer a top contender in life's competitive market, that he must step aside and allow his younger competitors to take over. Admission of hearing impairment and seeking assistance for it in the form of artificial correction of the defect does not necessarily correct many psychological personal problems that accompany it. It should be obvious that the solution of this person's problem cannot be handled like the proverbial "bull in a china shop."

Heretofore, I have mentioned "tolerance" problems. Any attempt to bring these individuals to close-to-normal threshold sensitivity should be approached with care. Trying to get the best "hearing threshold" at the first, or even the fifth, sitting will not result in success with most of them. Try and determine what they will accept and are willing to live with then give them just a slight push in the direction of your final goal. Bring them back in a month or six weeks. If they appear to be happy or at least not dissatisfied give them another slight push toward your eventual goal. I believe the secret is "underfitting" until their psychological tolerance threshold has been raised, then they will accept more gain. Remember they have had the loss for many years so don't try to correct it in a few hours or even weeks. Let them get "broken in" to wearing the aid gradually.

Another problem relates to self-consciousness concerning hearing loss. Wearing hearing aids, no matter how "invisible" they are or appear to be, lets everyone know the person has a hearing loss. I supposes "vainity" is the principle factor of resistance to wearing hearing aids. Many individuals, particularly the aged, are resistant because of the so-called "social stigma". Perhaps this is best summed up be the statement; "move slowly, cautiously and sympathetically" when recommending a hearing aid.

There is no doubt that binaural aids are better than monaural aids. Binaural fitting should be thoroughly discussed, but if the person is somewhat adamant about not wearing two hearing aids tell him or her you will grudgingly agree to wearing one if he or she will promise to try two. Remember the ultimate goal is two hearing aids, so don't give up too easily. Of course, some judgment should be used about how aggressive you are in this respect. Determine just how much this person will be using his/her hearing. If he or she is somewhat confined and will be listening to only one or two people in a quiet environment, the need for binaural hearing is small. Don't ever forget that you are not fitting ears, you are fitting an individual and responses to hearing aids are as individual as the person who wears them.

The most obvious factor one is confronted with where the senior citizen is concerned is related to hearing aid size and motor ability. In general, fine motor control is somewhat decreased in persons over 65. This varies with the individual but is generally the case. Consequently, in-the-ear and canal hearing aids may cause some problems, especially when controls are very small and in awkward, hard-to-reach positions. A good example of this is the replacement of a battery. This is sometimes difficult even for the younger person with normal dexterity. Some attempt should be made to determine whether a prospective wearer can successfully manipulate the hearing aid controls before advising its use.

The choice between an ear level aid and a body aid in older wearers is critical. Ear level aids should be used whenever possible. The ear level advantages are particularly important for older wearers since they need all the information they can get. Ear-level listening has the advantages afforded by head shadow and ear lobe configuration. Remember that unless ear level aids are used, true binaural hearing is impossible. I am firmly convinced that binaural hearing is of particular importance in the older person.

Changes in the cochlea and the eighth nerve system materially effect the information reaching the central nervous system. Couple this with the slowing down in central processing and sensorineural hearing loss and you produce a handicap of considerable proportions.

If one examines the binaural system carefully, it is evident that the nerve fibers which carry contralateral information are able to, and do, carry more information than the ipsilateral fibers. It seems, then, that the contralateral information must add a great deal to the final processing and organization of the incoming information before final output instructions are completed. Again I stress the importance of binaural hearing aids.

SUMMARY

In the United States the number of individuals 65 years of age and over is increasing and constitutes a sizeable citizen group which may require hearing aid devices.

There are hearing disorders peculiar to this age group and the specialist should be familiar with them. In addition he should be aware of neurologic, physiologic, pathologic and psychologic changes if he is to be successful in the fitting of hearing aid devices.

The hearing aid specialist is admonished to organize his procedures permitting the geriatric patient the time necessary to experiment with and adapt to hearing aid amplification. In most instances, binaural amplification is essential to achieve maximum performance with hearing aid amplification.

GLOSSARY

Air bone gap A difference between air conduction and bone conduction thresholds.

Central nervous system The part of the auditory system that begins where the eighth (acoustic) nerve enters the midbrain and extends to the cortex.

External ear The auricle or pinna and external auditory canal.

Inner ear The part of the ear housed in the temporal bone that contains the cochlear and semicircular canals.

Middle ear The cavity enclosed by the drumhead externally and bony medial wall internally.

Presbyacusis (Presbycusis) Changes in hearing related to physiological aging.

Spiral Ganglion Area in the cochlea where the hair cell nerve fibers are gathered before becoming the acoustic nerve.

Stria vascularis A sponge-like organ in the cochlea which acts as a filter to supply the cochlear fluids.

Transducer A device that transforms one form of energy to another.

Viz Microphone or earphone.

REFERENCES

ALPINER, J. G. (1982). *Handbook of rehabilitative audiology.* Baltimore: Williams & Wilkins.

ALPINER, J. G., CHEVRETTE, W., GLASCOE, G., METZ, M., & OLSEN, B. (1974). *The Denver Scale of Communication Function.* Denver, CO: University of Denver.

ASHLEY, J. (1985). A personal account. In H. ORLANS (Ed.), *Adjustment to adult hearing loss.* Boston: College-Hill Press.

ATCHLEY, R. C. (1983). *Continuity and change.* Belmont, CA: Wadsworth.

BALLE, V. LINTHICUM, F. H., JR., "Histologically Proven Cochlear Otosclerosis with Pure Sensorineural Hearing Loss," *Ann Otol Rhinol Laryngo, 1984 Mar-Apr, 92(2 PT 1), 105–111.*

BARFORD, J. (1979). Speech perception processes and fitting of hearing aids. *Audiology 18* 430–441.

BEATTIE, J. A. (1981). *Social aspects of acquired hearing loss in adults.* Report on research project, 1978–1981 (summary of contents and findings). Bradford, England: Post Graduate School of Applied Social Studies, University of Bradford.

BECKER, G. (1980). *Growing old in silence.* Berkeley: University of California Press.

BERGER, K., HAGENBERG, N., RANE, R. (1977). *Prescription of hearing aids.* Kent, OH: Herald Publishing.

BERKOWITZ, A. (1975). Audiological rehabilitation of the geriatric patient. *Hearing Aid Journal,* 8, 30–34.

BIENVENUE, G., & MICHAEL, P. (1979). Digital processing techniques in speech discrimination testing (critical bandwidth measurements for use in hearing aid testing). In P. YANECK (Ed.), *Rehabilitative strategies for sensorineural hearing loss.* New York: Grune & Stratton.

BIRREN, J. E., IMUS, H. A., & WINDLE, W. F. (1959). *The process of aging in the central nervous system.* Springfield, IL: Charles C. Thomas.

BIRREN, J. E., "Sensation, Perception and Modification of Behavior in Relation to the Process of Aging." In BIRREN, J. E., IMUS, H. A., WINDLE, W. F., *The process of aging in the Nervous system,* Springfield, Ill., Thomas, 1959, 143–165.

BLACKINGTON, B., NOVAK, R. E., & KRAMER, S. A. (1988). Temporal masking effects for speech and pure tone stimuli in normal hearing aged subjects. Unpublished masters thesis, San Diego State University, California.

BLOOD, G. W., BLOOD, I. M., & DANHAUER, J. L. (1978). Listeners' impressions of normal hearing and hearing impaired children. *Journal of Communicative Disorders, 11,* 573–578.

BRACKMANN, D. E., "Review of Acoustic Tumors" 1979–1982, *Am J. Otol,* 1984 Jan 5(3):233–244.

BUSSE, E. W. (1965). Research on aging: Some methods and findings. In M. A. BAREZIN & S. H. CATH (Eds.), *Geriatric psychiatry.* New York: International University Press.

BYRNE, D. (1987). Hearing aid selection formulae: Same or different. *Hearing Instruments, 38,* 5–13.

BYRNE, D., & DILLON, H. (1986). The National Acoustic Labs (NAL) new procedure for selecting gain and frequency response of a hearing aid. *Ear and Hearing, 7,* 257–265.

CHENG, L. R. (1988). *Personal interview with R. E. Novak.* San Diego, CA.

CORSO, J. F. (1963). Age and sex differences in pure tone thresholds. *Archives of Otolaryngology, 77,* 53–73.

COX, R. (1985). A structured approach to hearing aid selection. *Ear and Hearing, 6,* 226–239.

COX, R. (1987). The MSU hearing instrument prescription procedures. *Hearing Instruments, 39,* 6–10.

CROWE, S. J., & GUILD, S. R. (1934). Observation of the pathology of high tone deafness. *Johns Hopkins Hospital Bulletin,* 54, 315–380.

CUTER, N. E., HAROOTYAN, R. A., "Demography of the Aged," in WOODRUFF, D. S., BIRREN, J. E. (Eds.) Aging: Scientific Perspectives and social issues, Philadelphia. D. Van Nostrand, 1975, 31–69.

Danhauer, J. L., Blood, G. W., Blood, I. M., & Gomez, N. (1980). Professional and lay observations of preschoolers wearing hearing aids. *Journal of Speech and Hearing Disorders,* 45(3), 64–71.

Danaher, E. N., Osberger, M., & Picket, J. (1973). Discrimination of of formant frequency transitions in synthetic vowels. *Journal of Speech and Hearing Research, 16,* 439–451.

deBoer, E., & Bowmeester, J. (1974). Critical bands and sensorineural hearing loss. *Audiology, 13,* 236–259.

deBower, E., & Bowmeester, J. (1975). Clinical psychophysics. *Audiology,* 14, 274–299.

Demorest, M., & Erdman, S. (1984a). Applications of self assessment inventories. *Hearing Instruments, 35,* 32–40.

Demorest, M., & Erdman, S. (1985a). A database management system for the communication profile for the hearing impaired. *Journal of the Academy of Rehabilitative Audiology, 17,* 87–96.

Eisenberg, S. (1985). Communication with elderly patients: The effects of illness and medication on mentation, memory, and communication. In H. K. Ulatowska (Ed.), *The aging brain and communication in the elderly.* Boston: College-Hill Press.

Ewertson, H., & Birk-Nielsen, H. (1973). Social hearing handicap index: Social handicap in relation to hearing impairment. *Audiology, 12,* 180–187.

Fabini, G. (1931). Regarding morphological and functional changes in the internal ear arteriosclerosis. *Laryngoscope,* 4, 663–670.

Feller, B. (1981). Prevalence of selected impairments. *United States, 1977* (Series 10, No. 134) National Center for Health Statistics. Washington, DC: U.S. Government Printing Office.

Fisch, L. (1978). Special senses: The aging auditory system. In J. C. Brocklehurst (Ed.), *Textbook of geriatric medicine and gerontology.* New York: Churchill Livingstone.

Fisch, U. (1972). Degenerative changes of the arterial vessels of the internal auditory meatus during the process of aging. *Acta Otolaryngologica, 73,* 259–260.

Franklin, B. (1975). The effects of combining low- and high-frequency pass bands on consonant recognition in the hearing impaired. *Journal of Speech and Hearing Research, 18,* 719–727.

Ganz, R. P. (1976). The effects of aging on the diagnostic utility of the roll over phenomenon. *Journal of Speech and Hearing Disorders,* 41, 63–69.

Garstecke, D. C., "Aural Rehabilitation for the Aging Adult," in Beasley, D. S., Davis, G. A. (Eds.), *Aging: Communication Processes and Disorders,* Grune & Stratton, 1981, 267–280.

Gelfand, D. (1982). *Aging: The ethnic factor.* Boston: Little, Brown.

Gentile, A. (1971). Persons with impaired hearing. *United States, 1971* (Series 10, No. 134). Washington, DC: U.S. Government Printing Office.

GIOLAS, T. G., OWENS, E., LAMB, S., & SCHUBERT, E. (1979). Hearing Performance Inventory. *Journal of Speech and Hearing Research,* 44, 169–195.

GLASS, L. (1985). Psychosocial aspects of hearing loss in adulthood. In H. ORLANS (Ed.), *Adjustment to adult hearing loss.* Boston: College-Hill Press.

GLORIG, A. "Noise: Past, Present and future," *Ear Hear,* 1980 Jan-Feb 1(1) 4–18.

GLORIG A., & DAVIS, H. (1961). Age, noise and hearing loss. *Annals of Otology, 70,* 556–571.

GLORIG, A., & NIXON, H. L. (1962). Hearing loss as a function of age. *Laryngoscope, 27,* 1596–1610.

GLORIG, A., ROBERTS, J., *Hearing Levels of Adults by Age and Sex: United States 1960–1962,* (Vital and Health Statistics: Data from the National Survey. Ser. 11, No. 11) Washington, D.C., US Dept of HEW, PHS, 1965, 1–34.

GOLDMAN R. (1971). Decline in organ function with aging. In I. ROSSMAN (Ed.), *Clinical geriatrics,* Philadelphia: Lippencott.

GOTTLIEB, B. H. (1983). *Social support strategies.* Beverly Hills, CA: Sage.

GREENBLAT, N., & CHIEN, C. (1983). Depression in the elderly. In L. BRESLAU & M. HAUG (Eds.), *Depression and aging Causes, care and consequences.* New York: Springer-Verlag.

HARBERT, R., YOUNG, J., & MENDUKE, H. (1966). Audiological findings in presbycusis. *Journal of Auditory Research, 6,* 297–312.

HAWKINS, D. B. (1984). Selection of a critical electroacoustic characteristic: SSPL-90. *Hearing Instruments, 35,* 28–32.

HAWKINS, D. B. (1985). Reflections of amplification: Validation of performance. *Journal of the Academy of Rehabilitative Audiology, 17,* 87–96.

HAWKINS, D. B., & SCHUM, D. J. (1984). Relationship among various measures of hearing aid gain. *Journal of Speech and Hearing Disorders, 49,* 94–97.

HIGH, W. S., FAIRBANKS, G., & GLORIG, A. (1964). Scale for self assessment of hearing handicap. *Journal of Speech and Hearing Disorders, 29,* 215–230.

HOSFORD-DUNN, H., & BAXTER, J. H. (1985). Prediction and validation of hearing aid wearer benefit: Preliminary findings. *Hearing Instruments, 36,* 34–41.

HUNTER, C. C. (1978). *A pilot study of late deafened adults.* Unpublished master's thesis, California State University, Northridge.

HUTTON, C. (1980). Responses to a hearing problem inventory. *Journal of the Academy of Rehabilitative Audiology, 12,* 133–154.

ILER, K., DANHAUER, J. L., & MULAC, A. (1982). Peer perceptions of geriatrics wearing hearing aids. *Journal of Speech and Hearing Disorders, 47,* 433–438.

JAUHIANEN, T., "Investigations of Disorders of Hearing," in HINCHCLIFFE, R., (ed.) *Hearing and Balance in the Elderly,* Edinburgh, NY, Churchill Livingston, 1983, 74–96.

JERGER, J. (1960). Bekesy audiometry in analysis of auditory disorders. *Journal of Speech and Hearing Research, 3,* 275–287.

JERGER, J., SHEDD, J., & HARFORD, E. (1959). On the detection of extremely small changes in sound intensity. *Archives of Otolaryngology, 69,* 200–211.

KNOLL, C. (1979). *The influence of the hearing aid on the attitudes of nursing home personnel.* Master's thesis, Wichita State University, Kansas.

KRMPOTIC-NEMANIC, J. (1971). A new concept of the pathogenesis of presbycusis. *Archives of Otolaryngology, 93,* 161–166.

KYLE, J. G., JONES, L. G., & WOOD, P. L. (1985). Adjustment to acquired hearing loss: A working model. In H. ORLANS (Ed.), *Adjustment to adult hearing loss.* Boston: College Hill Press.

KYLE, J. G., & WOOD, P. L. (1983). Social and vocational aspects of acquired hearing loss. Final report to MSC School of Education, Bristol. (Reported in KYLE, J. G., JONES, L. G., & WOOD, P. L. [1985]. Adjustment to acquired hearing loss: A working model. In H. ORLANS [Ed.] *Adjustment to adult hearing loss.* Boston: College-Hill Press.)

LAMB, S. H., OWENS, E., & SCHUBERT, E. D. (1983). The revised form of the Hearing Handicap Inventory. *Ear and Hearing, 4,* 152–157.

LESHOWITZ, B., & LINDSTROM, R. (1979). Masking and speech-to-noise ratio. *Audiology and Deaf Education, 6,* 5–8.

LIBBY, E. R. (1986). The 1/3-2/3 insertion gain hearing aid selection guide. *Hearing Instruments, 3,* 27–28.

LIPMAN, A. (1968). A socio-architectural view of life in three homes for older people. *Gerontologica Clinica, 10,* 88–101.

LUEY, H. S. (1980). Between worlds: The problems of deafened adults. *Social Work in Health Care, 5,* 253–265.

LYNN, G. E., & GILROY, J. (1976). Central aspects of audition. In J. NORTHERN (Ed.), *Hearing disorders.* Boston: Little, Brown.

MARGOLIS, R., & GOLDBERG, S. (1980). Auditory frequency selectivity in normal and presbycusic subjects. *Journal of Speech and Hearing Research, 23,* 603–613.

MARSHALL, L. (1981). Auditory processing in aging listeners. *Journal of Speech and Hearing Disorders, 46,* 226–236.

MAULDIN, C. R. (1976). Communication and the aging consumer. In H. J. OYER & E. J. OYER (Eds.), *Aging and communication.* Baltimore: University Park Press.

MAURER, J. F., & RUPP, R. R. (1979). *Hearing and aging: Tactics for intervention.* New York: Grune & Stratton.

MAYER, O. (1970). Das Anatomische *Substrat der Altersschwerhovigkeit. Arch. Ohren-Nasenu-Kehlkopfh., 105, 1313.*

MCCANDLESS, G., & LYREGAARD, P. (1983). Prescription of gain/output (POGO) for hearing aids. *Hearing Instruments, 1,* 16–21.

MCCARTHY, P. A., & ALPINER, J. G. (1983). An assessment scale of hearing handicap for use in family counseling. *Journal of the Academy of Rehabilitative Audiology, 16,* 256–270.

McCartney, J. (1977, November/December). A look at hearing loss. *Perspectives on Aging,* 10–11.

Meadow-Orlans, K. P. (1985). Social and psychological effects of hearing loss in adulthood: A literature review. In H. Orlans (Ed.), *Adjustment to adult hearing loss.* Boston: College-Hill Press.

Medical Research Council Institute of Hearing Research. (1981). Population study of hearing disorders in adults. *Journal of the Royal Society of Medicine, 74,* 819–827.

Merluzzi, F., & Hinchcliffe, R. (1973). Threshold of subjective auditory handicap. *Audiology, 12,* 65–69.

Miller, L. V. (1975). The adult and the elderly: Health care and hearing loss. *Volta Review, 77,* 57–63.

Mills, J. H., Gilbert, R. M., & Adkins, W. V. (1979). *Some effects of noise on auditory sensitivity, temporal integration and psychophysical tuning curves.* Paper presented at Second Midwinter Research Meeting of the Association for Research in Otolaryngology, St. Petersburg, FL.

Mueller, H. G., Hawkins, D., & Sedge, R. K. (1984). pg. 651 onal Center for Health Statistics (NCHS) Current estimates from the National Health Interview Survey: United States 1987. Vital & Health Statistics. Series 10. Public Health Service, Washington. U.S. Government Printing Office 1987.

Nelson, D. A. (1979). *Frequency selectivity in listeners with sensori-neural hearing loss.* Paper presented at Second Midwinter Research Meeting of the Association for Research in Otolaryngology, St. Petersburg, FL.

Nixon, J. C., & Glorig, A. (1962). Changes in air and bone conduction thresholds as a function of age. *Journal of Laryngology, 76,* 288292.

Noble, W. G., & Atherley, G. R. (1970). The Hearing Measurement Scale: A questionnaire for the assessment of auditory disability. *Journal of Auditory Research, 10,* 229–250.

Novak, R. E. (1980). *Demographics of hearing loss and staff awareness of hearing loss in primary and secondary care nursing homes in San Diego.* Unpublished study.

Novak, R. E., & Anderson, C. V. (1982). The differentiation of types of presbycusis using the masking level difference. *Journal of Speech and Hearing Research, 25,* 504–508.

Novak, R. E., & Ybarra, S. (1988). Hearing loss. Hearing handicap and help seeking behaviors in American Indians and Black elders. Unpublished master's thesis, San Diego State University, California.

Olsen, W. O., & Noffsinger, D. (1974). Comparison of one new and three old tests of auditory adaptation. *Archives of Otolaryngology, 99,* 94.

Olsen, W., Noffsinger, D., & Carhart, R. (1976). Masking level difference encountered in clinical populations. *Audiology, 15,* 287–301.

OYER, H. J., & OYER, E. J. (1979). Social consequences of hearing loss for the elderly. *Allied Health and Behavioral Science., 2,* 123–137.

PALVA, A., & JOKENEN, H. (1970). Presbycusis V. Filtered speech test. *Acta Otolaryngologica, 70,* 232–241.

PARENTI, M. (1978). *Power and powerlessness.* New York: St. Martin's Press.

PASCOE, D. (1978). An approach to hearing aid selection. *Hearing Instruments, 6,* 12–16, 2627.

POSNER, J. D. (1982). Particular problems of antibiotic use in the elderly. *Geriatrics; 37,* 49–54.

POTASH, M., & JONES, B. (1977). Aging and decision criteria for the detection of tones in noise. *Journal of Gerontology, 32,* 436–440.

REED, C. M., & BILGER, R. C. (1973). A comparative study of S/NO and E/NO. *Journal of the Acoustical Society of America, 53,* 1039–1044.

REES, J. N., & BOTWINICK, J. (1971). Detection and decision factors in auditory behavior of the elderly. *Journal of Gerontology, 26,* 133–136.

RIES, P. W. (1982). Hearing ability of persons by sociodemographic and health characteristics. *United States* (Series No. 10, No. 140). National Center for Health Statistics. Washington, DC: U.S. Government Printing Office.

RIES, P. W., (1985). The demography of hearing loss. In H. ORLANS (Ed.), *Adjustment to adult hearing loss.* Boston: College-Hill Press.

ROSEN, S., BERGMAN, M., PLESTER, D., EL MOFTY, A., & SOTTI, M. (1962). Presbycuses study of a relatively noise free population in the Sudan. *Annals of Otolaryngology, 71,* 727–743.

ROSEN, S., PLESTER, D., EL MOFTY, A., & ROSEN, H. High frequency audiometry in presbycusis. *Annals of Otolaryngology, 79,* 18–32.

RUBEN, R., "Aging and Hearing," in ROSSMAN, I., (Ed) Clinical Geriatrics, Philadelphia, Lippincott, 1971, 247–252.

RUPP, R., HIGGINS, J., & MAURER, J. F. (1977). A feasibility scale for predicting hearing aid use (FSPHAU) with older individuals. *Journal of the Auditory Rehabilitation Association,* 10, 81–194.

SCHOW, R. L., CHRISTENSEN, J. M., HUTCHINSON, J. M., & NERBONNE, M. A. (1978). *Communicative disorders of the aged.* Baltimore: University Park Press.

SCHOW, R. L., & GOLDBAUM, D. E. (1980). Collapsed ear canals in the elderly nursing home population. *Journal of Speech and Hearing Disorders,* 45, 259–267.

SCHUKNECHT, H. F. (1951). Lesions of the organ Corti. *Transactions of the American Academy of Ophthalmology and Otolaryngology, 57,* 366.

SCHUKNECHT, H. F. (1955). Presbycusis. *Laryngoscope,* 65, 42.

SCHUKNECHT, H. F. (1964). Further observations on the pathology of presbycusis. *Archives of Otolaryngology,* 80, 369–382.

SCHUKNECHT, H. F. (1974). *Pathology of the ear.* Cambridge, MA: Harvard University Press.

SKAFTE, M. (1986). Communicate for a longer life. AMPLIFICIATION FOR GERIATRIC ADULTS 165. *Hearing Instruments,* 37, 4.

SKINNER, M. (1988). *Hearing aid evaluation.* Englewood Cliffs, NJ: Prentice-Hall.

SKINNER, M., PASCOE, D., MILLER, J., & POPELKA, G. (1982). Measurements to determine the optimal placement of speech energy within the listener's auditory area: A basis for selecting amplification characteristics. In G. STUDEBAKER & F. BESS, *The Vanderbilt hearing aid report: Monographs in contemporary audiology.* Upper Darby, PA.

THOMAS, A., & GILHOME-HERBST, K. (1980). al or psychological implications of acquired deafness for adults of employment age. *British Journal of Audiology,* 14, 76–85.

TYLER, R. S., FERNANDES, M., & WOOD, E. J. (1984). Masking temporal integration and speech intelligibility in individuals with noise induced hearing loss. In G. TAYLOR (Ed.), *Disorders of auditory function III.* New York: Academic Press.

ULATOWSKA, H. K. (1985). *The aging brain: Communication in the elderly.* Boston: College Hill Press.

U.S. DEPARTMENT OF COMMERCE. (1975, February (10). Reported in U.S. *News and World Report.*

VENTRY, I. M., & WEINSTEIN, B. E. (1982). The Hearing Handicap Inventory for the Elderly: A new tool. *Ear and Hearing,* 3, 128–134.

WARREN, L. R., WAGENER, J., & HERMAN, G. (1978). Binaural analysis in the aging auditory system. *Journal of Gerontology,* 33, 731–736.

WEINSTEIN, B. E., & VENTRY, I. M. (1983). Audiometric correlates of the Hearing Handicap Inventory for the Elderly. *Journal of Speech and Hearing Disorders,* 84, 379–383.

WALLOTT, JAMES F., Aging and the Auditory System: Anatomy, physiology and psychophysics, Singular Publishing Group Inc., 1991.

ZUCKER, K., & WILLIAMS, P. S. (1977). *Audiological services in extended care facilities.* Paper presented at the American Speech and Hearing Convention, Chicago, IL.

ZUREK, P., & FORMBY, C. (1977). *Frequency discriminability of sensorineural listeners.* Paper presented at the Second Midwinter Research Meeting of the American Speech and Hearing Association, Chicago, IL.

ZWAARDEMAKER, H. (1891). DerVerlust an Horen Tonen Mit Zunehemendum Alter: Ein Neues Gesetz. *Arch Ohr Nas.-Kehlk-Heilk,* 32, 53.

ZWICKER, E., & SHORN, K. (1978). Psychoacoustical tuning curves in audiology. *Audiology,* 17, 120–140.

XIII

MANAGEMENT CONSIDERATIONS IN HEARING INSTRUMENT DISPENSING

R. DAVID NELSON, M. A.

Contributors: Galen Berry, William Campbell, Kenneth Lowder, Greg Moore, Jerry Smith, Patricia Stark, Charlie Stone, and Paul Woodard

INTRODUCTION

The practice of dispensing hearing instruments varies throughout the United States, with respect to training and experience, testing equipment, and products and services offered to the public. The diversity of each dispensing office reflects the owners personality and the social, economic, and competitive nature of the community. The common thread among successful dispensers is that of good management.

Managing or owning your own hearing instrument dispensing business can be personally rewarding, stimulating, interesting, satisfying, and frustrating all at the same time. There is no question that the perspective manager or owner must have dedication and feel a real desire to help the hearing impaired.

There are thousands of hearing aid dispensers in the world and the successful ones benefit from good management skills. There may be differences in individual training, education, sales techniques, products and equipment but the successful dispenser receives referrals from doctors, nursing homes, and, most important, other patients. Good management results in satisfied customers, congenial employees and sales people who are willing to go the extra mile.

There is increasing evidence that successful hearing aid businesses of tomorrow will be those using management techniques today. Prior to 1980 only a few isolated articles on management existed. Since then, professional journals have devoted more attention to this dimension of the business. Certainly, without adequate planning or direction, a business will fall short of its true potential. Good management considers the methods necessary to properly implement plans for achieving success.

CHAPTER OBJECTIVES

The purpose of management discussion is to provide hearing dispensers and specialists with the necessary tools for a successful business. In discussing these broad aspects of management, we provide an overall view of the many necessary skills it takes to effectively run a hearing aid dispensing organization. Our intent is to focus on information for individuals who derive the major portion of their income from the dispensing of hearing aids. Regardless of title, those engaged in this activity are dispensers and as such, must be knowledgeable about effective management practices.

CHOOSING A NAME AND LOGO

The selection of a name for the business is a personal endeavor. Many select their own name as the business identity. Others will select the name of a state, town, manufacturer, or prominent geographical attraction. Some will select a more general service or product identity such as Better Hearing Aid Services, or Professional Hearing Aid Services. In selecting a name for the business, several general factors should be considered. Whatever you ultimately decide to call your business, keep in mind that is must be an overall, general description of the services you offer.

The name should be simple so that letterhead, advertisements, and other promotional items can be easily developed. The name should allow easy recognition and recall by the public. The name should identify the product or service. John Doe and Company does little to inform the public of either the product or service. Finally, consideration should be given to the future prospect of selling the business. Doe Hearing Aid Service will not be particularly attractive to Mr. Smith. Name identity with a manufacturer may be unwise in the event the owner wishes to select from multiple manufacturers, or if his manufacturer goes out of business.

A logo is used to create an association to a business. Usually, it is a graphic image designed to enhance the quality of the name. It is wise to choose a neutral logo (such as an ear) or a logo that promotes positive images. Choosing a negative logo (such as of hearing aids) can promote an image which is not pleasing to the potential client. Many businesses do not use a logo in their practices. A logo should be developed with the purpose of facilitating a quick one glance public recognition of your business.

Each business owner should carefully consider the benefits or necessity of a logo against the cost of development. The relative value of a logo in the overall success of a business may be important as a centralized theme which ties together your location, name tag, business card, letterhead, vehicles, forms, signs and envelops of future mailings. However, if time, energy, and cost must be rationed, as is normal in most businesses, other details of the marketing plan should take precedence.

LOCATION OF BUSINESS

The location of an office will have a direct effect on retail activity. Consequently, several factors should be considered in choosing the location for an office. What factors or conditions will favor the geriatric customer? Should the office be in a downtown area or in a residential setting? Should the office be on a side street, major highway, shopping center, or mall area? What competition exists in the immediate area? Are the surrounding stores prosperous? Is the neighborhood shabby or in good repair? Is the street traffic too busy for the customer to have easy access? Is the office convenient to pedestrian traffic? Is public transportation available? Is there sufficient parking near the office for the customer? Are sidewalk conditions favorable? Will handicapped individuals have easy access to your office? Is street lighting adequate? If the office is rented or leased, will the terms and lease duration be favorable? Last of all, will your customers feel comfortable in coming to this location? You are selecting the location for your customers and not for your own personal convenience or other personality factors. Remember that the success of your business depends upon what your customers think not what you think. This particular sentiment should prevail in all your decision making.

The answers to the previous questions require little time or research. Each question, however, should be carefully considered when choosing an office. Generally the office should not be moved to a new location more frequently then is absolutely necessary. Establishing another location involves a disruption in work activity and forces the dispenser to revise or change many office forms involving address and other location information. Relocating also forces the consumer to make a special effort to find your new location and to remember your address change. In this type of business it is important to choose a location that can be permanent. Relocation is not only confusing but may result in loss of business. If you rent a building, make sure you read the terms of the lease very carefully to avoid later "surprises".

OFFICE IMAGE AND DESIGN

Both the interior and the exterior design and physical condition of an office has an effect on business activity. Interesting, yet functional, design and decor can have a positive influence in creating a warm, friendly, and relaxed business climate for both office personnel and clients.The physical design or arrangement of each office should consider the availability of restrooms, door opening sizes, hallway traveling space, and accessibility of examination or fitting rooms for the geriatric or handicapped client. Office space should include a reception or waiting area, a private office or consultation area, fitting rooms, work room, testing rooms, and a space for the normal transactions of business. The size and physical location of each area should fit the overall design consideration of client flow and work utility. Careful design of work space and placement of equipment can reduce significantly needless work movements and duplication of effort.

Most people desire confidentiality in consulting with the hearing aid specialist. Consequently, the reception area should be physically separate from the fitting or consultation area. If this is not possible, music might be introduced into the reception area to provide sound isolation. The lighting, selection of furniture, and the physical travel in the office should accommodate the needs of the geriatric client. Geriatric customers require furniture of adequate height, which provides good support and adequate arm rests. Office design, furniture selection, and interior design should reflect client requirements and not the personal tastes of the owner. Magazines and other reading materials in the waiting area should also be selected with the client in mind.

Careful consideration should be given to the amount of initial space and the requirement for future growth. Individual circumstances will dictate the total number of square feet required for adequate space. Most offices can utilize about 1000 square feet for the total operation for a single dispenser. Additional space will be required if the services offered are in addition to the dispensing operation.

A dilemma exists for all businesses that are new or expanding. This dilemma is the anticipated need for additional space and cost of under-utilized space. Abundant space is always desirable, but high rent costs could cripple other areas of an expanding business if cash is not available to the owner.

POPULATION DENSITY AND COMPETITION

An office must be located in an area that has an adequate population of hearing impaired to support its retail activity. Offices will have a natural trade boundary. In rural areas, people have a town where they normally trade. Traveling to an unknown facility in an unfamiliar town may be difficult and create apprehension. Similarly, residents in a large metropolitan area may not travel easily to another section of the city. Many specialists increase their trade area by locating service centers away from the main office. Each owner should be aware of the trade boundaries and the population base for the area. Skafte (1984) computed the number of potential hearing aid users in the United States to be 11,205,000 or about 5% of the general population. Each owner could use these values in estimating market potential. Skafte also estimated the market penetration or sales in 1983 to be about 8%. The growth of population in the senior citizen category is likely to increase the market and sales in the future.

Offices located in large concentrations of geriatric persons may require a smaller population base. This type of population information is available from the Bureau of Census in the United States Department of Commerce or from local Chamber of Commerce offices. Determining the population necessary to support retail activity is complex. Starting a new business in an area with established successful businesses will result in a difficult business environment.

MANUFACTURER RELATIONSHIP

Selection of manufacturers is an important step in developing a business enterprise. Important considerations in selecting a manufacturer are: quality of the product, manufacturer reliability, credit arrangements, discount on volume purchases, repair services, brand recognition, and marketing assistance. Manufacturer support for an individual starting a new office was available in the past when franchise operations and single brand dispensing were common practice. Although the hearing aid specialist support system has diminished in some aspects, there is important ongoing information available from manufacturers. The relationship that hearing aid specialists have with their suppliers will influence the marketing assistance available to them. Remember that your continued success is important to the manufacturer.

Persons new to the hearing aid business may want to limit the number of suppliers to avoid the confusion arising from having to become familiar with different credit policies, volume discount schedules, repair policies, insurance forms, product familiarity, marketing support systems, and other related problems. Limiting the number of suppliers also simplifies the number of accessory items necessary, such as earhooks, battery compartments, filters, cords, and other repair or replacement parts.

How do you plan to take care of your customers? Will you have the correct repair part when they visit your office or will they have to wait while you order the needed item? Established offices that have well developed service programs for their customers, will have hundreds if not thousands of dollars invested in repair and accessory items. Basically, as you increase the number of manufacturers and models, the larger your repair and accessory inventory. Not only do these small value items involve an investment cost but they also require more inventory control.

CONSUMER BEHAVIOR

Knowing the purchasing behavior of the consumer is important. Advertising strategies can be planned to meet the needs of the buyer. Knowledge of consumer buying practices will increase the owner's ability to influence the consumer's decisions in the purchasing process. Consumers have several considerations in mind when purchasing hearing aids. Price, brand name, size, style, warranty, insurance, and reliability are factors for most individuals. Some will purchase because they like the specialist, or because a close friend or relative recommended a particular specialist, model or style. Some will purchase because of a professional recommendation. Most consumers follow a predictable buying pattern. The following steps have been identified by Fox (1983): First, there is a basic need; second, a recognition of that need; third, a decision to act; fourth, a search and evaluation of the product; fifth, choosing the particular product; and sixth, a post purchase evaluation period. These six steps are neither artificial nor abstract theoretical steps but are common steps in the purchase of nearly every commodity. A child buying a candy bar, for example, would follow these six steps as would a potential house buyer. Understanding each of these steps in creating a favorable climate for the customer is of great importance.

CONSUMER PROTECTION

Many regulations affecting the business person are located at federal and state levels, and in codes of ethics of professional associations. During the past decade or two, increased activity has been evident at both federal and state levels. At the federal level the Food and Drug Administration (FDA) completed and published in the Federal Register the Regulations of Hearing Aids (Amendment to Federal Food, Drug, and Cosmetic Act: Section 801.420 and 801.421). These regulations, effective August 15, 1977, require manufacturers of hearing aids to provide uniformity in manufacturing, labeling, and instructing the prospective hearing aid candidate. These regulations set forth medical contraindications for the use of amplification (the eight red flags) for all consumers; a medical evaluation within six months preceding the sale, and a mandatory medical clearance statement from a physician for all children under the age of 18 years. An optional waiver to the medical evaluation requirements was allowed for individuals 18 years or older. Currently the FDA is revising its Regulations of Hearing Aids. These new rules although not known at this time are thought to be more restrictive than the earlier version.

State laws for regulating hearing aid dispensers were nearly nonexistent twenty years ago. Now most states have some form of regulations. These laws have been designed to provide competency for those licensed. Regulations are similar in most states.

A recent development in verifying the credentials of the hearing instrument specialist is that of specialty level accreditation through a competency examination that is national in scope. As a member of the National Commission for Health Certifying Agencies (NCHCA), the National Board for Certification in Hearing Instrument Sciences (NBC-HIS) provides this independent credentialing.

Codes of ethics developed by the International Hearing Society and through state hearing aid specialist organizations should be honored as they are in the best interest of both the consumer and the hearing aid specialist.

Advice from legal counsel should be sought for the application of federal, state, and local requirements for business operation. Clear, concise, and accurate contracts are a necessity for both the owner and the buyer.

CONSUMER INFORMATION

Several types of information should be considered for the consumer. Pamphlets are effective methods for describing specific policies and procedures for a particular office. Zupko (1982) describes the areas of information to be included in an office brochure. They are specialty and type of service, appointment times, office hours, telephone numbers, fees, billing, collection, and insurance information. Other areas that should be considered are the normal business days, the location of the business (a map may be helpful if the business is difficult to find), a picture of the office building (if distinctive), a picture of the owner or manager, and a list of the other personnel in the office. Others could be added or deleted to meet specific demands of the consumer or business practice.

Product and service information can be presented through the advertising media. More detailed information can be given at the evaluation and at the time of fitting. Finally, additional post-fitting information can be given at office appointments, in newsletters, or similar informative literature.

CUSTOMER SERVICE

A satisfied customer is the by-product of good service. Customers are most likely to desert their dispenser if they perceive that there is a service problem. A satisfied customer will tell one other person and a dissatisfied customer tells an average of three other people about their negative experience. Employees who are skillful in resolving customer complaints can reduce the number of dissatisfied customers. As a hearing aid dispenser, your employees must have the ability to lend a sympathetic ear. Lack of attentiveness can reduce your business if your customer's needs are ignored. Encourage your employees to ask questions: Where do they work? Are they exposed to high levels of noise? Do they just see people on Sundays in church? Do they have a job? Does one person in particular give them difficulty? Questions like these show the customer that you generally care about their well being and that you are making a commitment to their better hearing, not a commitment to a thirty-day trial period.

CUSTOMER SERVICE CONTRACTS

Our journals have classified dispensers into three categories: 1) the physician-based office, or hospital dispensaries; 2) independent audiology dispensers; and 3) the traditional hearing instrument dispensers. Service is delivered in either a bundled or unbundled approach. Traditionally the first category utilizes an unbundled approach, while category 2 and 3 are more frequently bundled. The bundled approach does not differentiate between products and services and lumps the two together. The unbundled approach separates the pricing of products and services.

Service contracts make the assumption that there should be some separation of goods versus services. The professional's knowledge and wisdom in resolving problems and recommending solutions is a service that is separate and consequently should have an assessed value. To accomplish this separation of goods versus services some form of contractual arrangement must be made between the dispenser and individual being served. These controls are referred to as service contracts or extended service agreements.

These service contracts have the following goals:

1. Gradually convert your clients or patients from a service-for-free to a fee-for-service orientation.
2. Provide patient retention while increasing utilization of goods and services.
3. Add additional revenue to your business.
4. Add to enhance your professional image.

At the delivery you explain that the instrument is covered by XYZ manufacturer for one year for defects in workmanship and material. The warranty, however, does not cover office calls, new impressions if needed, office modifications, routine maintenance checks and annual checks of their hearing levels. These services are covered by a service contract which is included in their purchase price at no additional charge for this first year. These services and other benefits of this service contract can be renewed annually. By presenting the concept that the instrument and the professional services are separate, you can establish in the patient's mind that a charge is assessed for your professional services that can be waived or reduced if they are on your service contract. The objective of a service contract should be to retain patient loyalty and increase utilization of your goods and services, a long-term profit enhancer, not a short-term sales producer. The lower the renewal price the higher the percentage of renewals. It may be better to offer one or two different options for what is covered at different prices rather than to try to include too much at a higher price.

When patients renew their service contracts, this ensures payment in advance for those services. If a customer does not renew, a reason exists to contact them to see why they dropped your contract. This lets you know which patients feel you are doing a good job and which ones feel you are not. Some people may feel you are doing a good job but that the service contract is not that beneficial. They know, however, that when they come in to your office they will be charged if they do not renew the service contract. These service contracts may be implemented by outside professional services such as ESCO. These firms assist the dispenser in developing the service contract and in the routine paperwork necessary for renewal.

Service contracts also help with your marketing activities. The patients who renew have essentially committed themselves to your practice for another year. Most service contracts call for at least two office visits per year and because the individual has prepaid for this benefit, they almost always keep their appointments. This gives the practitioner face-to-face opportunities to present the newest procedures and latest technology. You do not need to direct mail or solicit loyal patients, you need to increase the number of loyal patients you have.

DATA AND INFORMATION MANAGEMENT

COMPUTER SYSTEMS

Naisbitt (1984) states that our society is currently involved in a new major revolution: a change from an industrial society to that of an information society. Information processing has been assisted by development of the computer. Recent advances in computer applicability to small business operations have induced many owners to consider the utilization of the computer in their hearing aid business practice. There is little doubt the computer is and will continue to be an important component in a business operation.

Existing hardware is already well established, operational, and available. Software for hearing aid businesses is developed and is emerging in a usable format. Standardization is not complete but the computer has application for many business functions such as accounting, general ledger, payroll, accounts receivable, and other management-related functions. Audiometric testing, hearing aid selection, and hearing aid fitting are now routinely augmented by computers. Many of the more advanced technological hearing instruments cannot be dispensed without the assistance of a personal computer.

For those individuals contemplating leasing or purchasing a computer, Axelson (1978) lists several considerations of importance. Although 1978 is "light years" in the past for the computer industry the following are still important considerations in computer selection.

1. Should the system be able to hook up to computers in other locations?
2. Should there be more than one input and output terminal?
3. Should the computer have potential for telephone transmission?
4. Does the manufacturer or representative furnish system and programming assistance?
5. Is backup equipment available in case of breakdown?
6. What is the cost of the instrument and is it economically feasible?
7. What is the speed of processing and printout and will they meet future demands?
8. What is the risk of obsolescence?
9. What physical size and storage capacity are needed?
10. What is the availability of maintenance service?
11. Is training available from the manufacturer?
12. Should the computer be leased or purchased?
13. Are the computer and associated software 'user friendly'?

Additional questions that concern each decision maker are:

1. Will the computer be in the fitting room or in the business office?
2. Should the system be designed for networking?
3. Can the system be used for digitally programmable products?

Those having practical experience with computers are aware that the computer, in and of itself, provides little benefit unless appropriate procedures are developed to utilize the information stored in the computer. Perhaps one of the most valuable benefits of computer use is that it forces the owner to organize and systematize existing information. Once these tasks are performed, the computer allows rapid recall, sorting, and analysis of data.

DATA PROCESSING PRINCIPLES AND PRACTICES

What types of information should be gathered and how should this information be stored? Duplication of effort is a continual battle in establishing effective office practices. Gathering, storing, and outputting information in a readily accessible form will save both time and effort. The design of audiometric data sheets, audiometer calibration records, and hearing aid registry sheets are examples of where time and effort should be spent in developing an economic and usable form. In the construction of each form or computer record, the following questions should be addressed:

1. Is the form really necessary?
2. Will duplicate copies be necessary?
3. Is all the information on the form necessary?
4. Can some forms be combined?
5. Have all manual operations been incorporated in the form, i.e. numbering, return address, etc.?
6. What is the most efficient design for the form?

Other forms that should receive equal scrutiny are shipping, inventory control, purchasing, receiving, market research, sales analysis, advertising, budgeting, payroll, accounts receivable, acounts payable, general ledger posting, and personnel records. Special attention should be given to the development of a case history form and client service records, primarily because these two forms are used extensively on a daily basis and, as such, offer an excellent opportunity to reduce redundancy and routine manual duplication.

FINANCIAL MANAGEMENT

When building a professional practice, there are so many details to be taken care of, it seems the list becomes endless. After getting the office located and furnished, employees hired and opening the door for business, you would think all had been accomplished.

There is, however, one very important aspect left, financial management.

For most small business, the initial area commanding the greatest importance will be the cash control or cash flow. As the practice grows, other areas such as general and tax accounting, credit management of receivables, budgets, capital expenditures and others will require attention as well. As the business expands, detailed information from each area will be required. Since each area may require periodic review, techniques to systematically bring these areas to review becomes valuable.

For small businesses, financial management considers areas of cash control, bank relations, financing, tax accounting, insurance, general accounting, credit management, budgetary control, capital expenditure control, real estate management, purchasing, and investments. The complexity of each of these areas can be elaborate or simple to meet the needs of the owner. As the size and complexity of the business operation grows, the requirement for more detailed information in each of these areas increases. The specific steps in financial management will vary from owner to owner. Each of the areas mentioned requires some degree of financial management and should be considered on a periodic basis. A file or other simple technique to systematically bring these areas to review is valuable.

Access to business financial matters must be in the hands of one responsible individual who has the ability to keep these matters confidential. You must decide if it is you or your bookkeeper that makes financial decisions. Work together to set up a satisfactory process in which money is to be distributed and how bills are to be paid.

Understanding your balance sheet and profit and loss report is essential to proper business analysis. A balance sheet tells how business stands at one given moment in the business year. A profit and loss statement sums up the results of operations over a given period of time.

In and of themselves, these two financial documents are a collection of mute figures. But when the assembled financial symbols are interpreted and evaluated, they begin to tell a story.

A single balance sheet is like the opening chapters of a book. It gives the initial setting. Thus, one balance sheet will show how the capital is distributed, how much is in the various accounts, and how much surplus of assets over liabilities exists. One lone profit and loss statement indicates the sole volume for a given period, the amount of costs incurred, and the net profit or loss after allowing for all expenses.

When a series of balance sheets for regularly related intervals, such as a fiscal or calendar year ends, is arranged in vertical columns so that the same items may be compared, the changes in these items begin to disclose trends. The comparative balance sheets are no longer snapshots, but become X-ray photos of the structure of all basic management actions and decisions.

With the information in the above documents much knowledge can be ascertained. These are referred to as "Financial Ratios", a proven way of keeping score. Comparatively, ratios tell where a firm has been, where it stands, and where it is going.

A company can get an indication of its strengths and weaknesses by using these measures. They are a way for management to track a company's performance, spot danger signals, and make financial decisions. Analyzing the financial ratios management can determine how outside lenders will evaluate business.

By analyzing profitability, turnover and various other financial ratios, managers can get a pretty good idea of a company's ability to meet short and long-term debt. It is important for a manager to remember that ratios can not stand by themselves because they are only meaningful when used comparatively. Ratios should be used in reference to past, present and future activity as compared to budget expectations, previous ratios, the ratios of competitors and published industry averages.

Ratios generally fall into six major categories: those of profitability, trading, turnover, liquidity, leverage, and solvency. Four of the most common ratios are listed in the glossary. Additional ratios as well as the four listed will be most meaningful to any manager when these are generated and explained by your CPA.

The properly managed business should crate an operating budget or projection sheet on an annual basis. These projections should be derived from past history with consideration of current trends. Your financial advisor can provide the necessary form and assist you in personalizing the information to your business.

Given the above information, you may manage the business, however, without this information, the business manages you. Proper preparation makes the difference.

ACCOUNTING, COST ANALYSIS AND CONTROL

The most common causes of failure of small businesses is poor or nonexistent accounting procedures. Any person preparing to own and/or manage a hearing aid dispensing practice should obtain a working knowledge of accounting procedures. If you do not already have this knowledge, excellent courses in business accounting are frequently offered by local colleges, adult education programs and business schools.

Often the person who is a successful hearing aid dispenser will not have a similar interest in business accounting. It is important to recognize this fact and make plans to obtain a person or firm who will provide you with record keeping and reports about how your business is progressing. Just like selecting any other professional, it is important to find a Certified Public Accountant (CPA) who is competent and who will earn your trust.

Utilizing the services of a CPA will help insure that financial records are available for purposes of analysis and tax reporting. These records can provide financial planning and analysis for the business. Financial planning generally is concerned with budgeting for the operation of the business. Most business owners find it difficult, if not impossible, to supply a detailed financial plan for their business. Some areas such as major equipment acquisitions can be anticipated and planned accordingly. However, financial plans for equipment repairs and other unexpected expenses can never be adequately anticipated. Most owners deal with business planning on an item by item basis as they occur. Prudent and common sense decisions are, for most, the key to success. Murphy's Law (if anything can go wrong, it will) is dealt with periodically in any business operation.

Financial analysis is concerned with reviewing sales, expenses, and profits. Most accountants recommend periodic financial statements. Whether this is done on a monthly, quarterly, or yearly basis will depend upon the amount of financial records needed for good control. Knowing what records you should maintain can assist in meeting tax obligations on time. A formal plan for setting aside money to meet various federal, state, and local tax obligations is an important function. It is important to understand that CPA's can detect if business expenses are excessive or profit margins inadequate. This analytical information, however, has little bearing on where potential future sources of revenue can be obtained. This is the sole responsibility of the owner and explains to some extent why the badges of maturity (ulcers, gray hair, and worry lines) are the province of the owner.

BUDGETS

The key word in financial planning and management is budgeting. Budgeting provides a plan of action and serves as a control device for expenditures. Budgeting involves the projected cash needs of the business. Business expenses to be considered include projected costs of personnel, advertising, auto expenses, dues and subscriptions to professional organizations and journals, insurance, interest payments to the bank, legal and accounting expenses, office supplies, postage, rent or office payment, equipment rent, repairs and maintenance, operating supplies, payroll taxes, telephone, entertainment and convention expenses, educational expenses, utilities, and miscellaneous expense. A reliable estimate of these expenses can be very difficult. Numerous factors can increase or decrease the magnitude of these expenditures. Individuals new to business will almost always underestimate expenses and overestimate sales. The most realistic estimate of expenses can best be derived from determining actual expenses from a business of approximate size operating in a similar geographical area.

Capital investment requirements are classified as those financial needs that extend beyond one year. These expenses may include building purchase, office furniture, business office equipment (typewriters, computers, postage machines, adding machines, duplicating equipment, paper folding machines, etc.), audiological testing equipment, hearing aid fitting equipment, automobile, work room repair equipment, and loaner stock. Budgeting for capital investment expenditures is more easily estimated because of the relatively fixed cost of each item

CONTROL SYSTEMS IN MANAGEMENT

A good way to manage your money is to compare projected cost with actual cost. A comparison of weekly, monthly and yearly costs can tell you which business decisions were financially sound and which ones were not.

Without being able to use the past as a reference point, it is extremely difficult to protect the future. To establish guidelines for activities and expenditures, it's suggested that you establish a projection sheet monthly and annually.

Financial managers should establish long term goals. To acquire prudent information for this task, you should anticipate trends, local population base, composition, change in services and future costs of financing your business.

For most small businesses, budgeting does not entail necessarily lengthy complication formulas, tables, or computations. A simple comparison of purchases is often sufficient for budgeting. A comparison of projected cost with actual cost provides valuable information for future projects.

CREDIT MANAGEMENT

Small businesses in the first years of development are usually underfinanced for capital expenditures. During this period, good credit management is necessary as cash flow will be restricted. Temporary credit or long term term payment reduces needed funds for payment of capital expenditures and general operating expenses. Credit requests result in subsequent borrowing from a lending institution. Unpaid accounts have a way of mushrooming if not controlled. A credit check may be desirable for some clients. Bank references and information from national and local retail credit bureaus are helpful and necessary. If the business person decides to provide credit themselves, they must decide whether or not to charge interest on the unpaid balance. If interest is charged, then legal counsel should be consulted to determine if the contract contains all of the pertinent information and disclosures as required by law.

The extension of credit to a consumer will increase the complexity of a business operation. Geographical and business environments will affect the requirement for credit management. Rural areas, where the customer's credit rating and past history are known, will require less formalized procedures as contrasted to a metropolitan area where customer identity and credit rating may be unknown. Many dispensing businesses require payment when the product or service is delivered unless the customer asks for special terms. This method of collection is common in both retail stores and professional offices.

Credit cards such as Master Charge, Visa, Discover or American Express are utilized in payment of products and services. This procedure places the burden of payment on the consumer and not the business. The payment process is quick and can be easily monitored.

Third party payments from federal, state, or private sources such as insurance, comprise another area for credit management. Unfortunately, the policies are established by the third party and, consequently, neither the conditions of the sale nor the method or schedule of reimbursement is controlled by the hearing aid specialist. Additional paperwork is frequently required, which places additional burdens on office staff.

Any business owner with a few year's experience can provide illustrations of customers who were slow in paying, who left the area, or who required legal action to collect their accounts. There is a danger in allowing isolated cases to unfavorably influence future credit policy. Each business owner must remember that credit policies too stringent or harsh may adversely affect all future customers and result in less favorable attitudes toward the business, or worse, a loss of sales.

BANK RELATIONSHIPS

The bank views each business account as a means of revenue from fees, interest on loans, and reinvestment of deposits. The irony of most bank relationships is that establishing credit is most difficult during the early period of business operation. This is a time when the business owner must depend most heavily on loans from the bank. It is necessary to provide the bank with well prepared financial statements, clearly defined capital needs, and cash flow or profit statements. This will promote a favorable relationship with the bank. Banks value their customers as the hearing aid specialist values hard of hearing persons. Consequently, owners should ask for their credit policies, interest rates, checking account charges, and other pertinent information. A comparison of several lending institutions in these areas will allow the owner to make a favorable choice for banking needs.

WORKING CAPITAL

Working capital is defined as the finances required in the normal daily operation of a business. The amount of working capital will vary for each business. The most realistic method of estimating working capital is to inquire from established dispensers their needs for working capital. In reality, the expanding business is usually short of working capital; thus the need for support from lending institutions.

BUSINESS RELATIONSHIP WITH THE MANUFACTURER

The largest on-going expense for any hearing aid specialist is payment for hearing aids purchased from the manufacturer or distributor. For an active business, this amount will be several thousand dollars each month. A good business relationship with the manufacturer is important for any successful business. Analyzing buying decisions from previous years is helpful in forecasting projected buying patterns.

Some methods of determining a manufacturer's overall performance are important. The following are factors to consider: shipment policy (Does the manufacturer pay the postage?); credit policy (Are discounts available for cash with order or prompt payment at monthly intervals?); repair rate (Is frequency of repair comparable to other manufacturers?); and repair quality (Is service prompt and reliable?). Although items may seem insignificant when viewed separately, their total value during a given year can be substantial.

BUSINESS RELATIONS WITH THE CONSUMER

Profit for any business results from the payment for product and services. One of the major decisions for business is that of bundling or unbundling the cost of product and services. Bundled strategies incorporate both into one price. In reality, no business is likely to continue its pricing strategy strictly in either category. Historically, most hearing aid specialists have chosen the bundled approach. The primary advantage of this pricing system is fewer discussions are necessary with the customer on this topic. The unbundled approach requires more detail and more explanation for each of the products and services. Most specialists would prefer to keep the number of pricing decisions to a minimum. There are advantages and ardent supporters for each method. Clients will ultimately decide what they prefer. Many hearing aid specialists offer both approaches.

MARKETING

Marketing is the development of products and services and the delivery of these to the consumer, hopefully for a profit. The complexities of marketing a product or service are enormous and strain the ingenuity and management skills of the most talented and enterprising business person. Steiner (1971) lists the following questions for developing a business: Where is the market? What is my company image to my customers? What business do I want to be in five years from now? What are my specific goals for profit improvement? Need I have plans for product improvement? If so, what? What is my greatest strength? Am I using it well? What is my greatest problem? How can I solve it? What share of the market do I want? How can I finance growth? These questions are common to each owner and require definition if a market program is to be developed.

Freiman, (1983, chap. 6) divides the marketing program into six areas. These are:

1. defining the market
2. positioning the product
3. researching consumer needs and wants
4. developing and redeveloping product or service
5. selecting and training personnel
6. developing sales approach and advertising support

1. DEFINING THE MARKET

Who will need your service? Where do they live? What are their needs? What products or services will they require? These questions should be considered and researched in defining the market. Customer requirements are central to a marketing plan because business development mandates good customer information. Business may be developed in related areas such as tinnitis maskers, optical aids, FM equipment in schools, industrial hearing testing, public school hearing testing, audiological evaluations in clinics or hospitals, consulting, teaching, retailing audiometers and other associated testing and fitting equipment. These areas may involve a different marketing approach. Business undertakings in too many areas may jeopardize existing programs. Even in a single business endeavor such as hearing aid dispensing, the owner may wish to develop a market segmentation. Where circumstances permit, a hearing aid specialist may wish to attract only a pediatric or geriatric population. Other considerations could involve geographical areas, socio-economic classes, limited products or service offerings.

Successful hearing aid specialists can provide assistance in defining the market. Additional information can be obtained from census studies, local chambers of commerce, and state and federal agencies. A wealth of information is available from national and state associations for hearing aid specialists, from manufacturers of hearing aids, and various journals such as Audecibel, Hearing Instruments, The Hearing Journal, and other worthwhile publications.

Businesses that prosper do so by planning and not by accident. Whether the plans are brief and concise or detailed and lengthy, they assist the owner in making correct decisions about the business. Hopkins (1981) stated that in management we can potentially control 20 to 30 percent of the factors in business, the other 70 percent is controlled by external factors over which we have no control. Good management will provide the maximum benefit from the factors we can control.

2. POSITIONING THE PRODUCT OR MARKET DEVELOPMENT

For manufacturing companies, positioning involves the development of a product having some special appeal or benefit for specific hearing aid specialists and consumer groups. Selection of a supplier or manufacturer, pricing the product, and determining services offered are major considerations in positioning the product. Brand name has value in attracting customers for the hearing aid specialist. Manufacturers who have developed national advertising programs and who furnish prospective leads provide market support.

Brand name hearing aids are beneficial to the hearing aid specialist, particularly if customers wish to replace their aid with a similar brand instrument. The consumer, by his repeated exposure to national product advertising, may be interested in product identification. Brand name recognition may have negative effects, if previous specialists were disreputable, or if referral sources have a negative attitude toward a particular brand name. Understanding the history of dispensing in a particular area will help minimize poor decisions. In the past several years, there has been a trend toward hearing aid businesses offering products from more than one manufacturer. There are several reasons for this development. These factors are incomplete product line (only ITE), poor quality in certain product offerings, consumer demand for specific products, and specific recommendations from referral sources. The obvious disadvantage of having more than one supplier is a reduction in financial savings because of reduced volume discounts.

Marketing objectives will consider carefully the pricing structure of the product and service. Price structuring is normally based upon 1) an approximate alignment with competitors' prices; 2) manufacturer's suggested retail, if available; 3) percentage of profit; 4) cost of product and service; and 5) consumer demand. The specialist may consider one of these factors as being the most important criteria for pricing. However, several of these strategies may be used to arrive at an overall pricing system.

Where will sales originate? What percentage will be in the office or outside of the office? A business that is highly dependent upon a single source of sales, such as a particular referral agency, is more vulnerable if that referral source is eliminated. A well-rounded source of sales delivers more business security. Methods of increasing sales are numerous. Five general marketing strategies may be considered. First, expanding service or product to existing clients is valuable because most existing clients are satisfied customers and represent an additional source for new products and service. This is an area that receives attention from most specialists. Radcliff and Mahon (1983) state the industry suffers from "the refit syndrome" with as much as 50% to 70% of total sales for a year in this category. Second, identifying market segments which are most likely to be in need of hearing aid services will increase sales. For hearing aid specialists, the senior citizen obviously is known as a highly likely prospect. Radcliff and Mahon (1983) state that a much larger market is available from potential users. Reaching this segment and changing its perception of hearing aid use may be one of the industry's foremost challenges.

Third, increasing personal referral sources by letters of introduction, client follow-up letters, and other methods will help increase business activity. Developing and sustaining referral sources is one of the least expensive sources of sales. However, this area requires attention to detail and in general is time consuming. Many specialists have a form letter that is completed and sent back to the referral source. Personal letters are advisable when time and resources permit because this type of response indicates the specialist's concern and follow-up for client care. The proliferation of letters in the category of "junk mail" has decreased the effectiveness of the form letter.

Fourth, community involvement in service clubs, trade associations, religious and political organizations, and educational institutions will increase the awareness of your business activity. Fifth, specializing in certain products or services not normally found in a given business area is a source of additional business.

3. RESEARCHING CONSUMER NEEDS AND WANTS

Although small business owners cannot approach their marketing tasks as comprehensively as large corporations, many will undertake a casual periodic assessment of the buying habits of their specific market. Many manufacturers have marketing departments that can provide valuable assistance through marketing plans and marketing surveys. The marketing survey provides necessary feedback on client satisfaction and consumer demand. This allows the owner to develop new products and services or fine tune existing ones.

Researching consumer needs and wants is a vital step in marketing. Unless the dispenser understands the buying behavior of the consumer, wasted time and finances are spent in unproductive activities. In today's market a hearing aid specialist who fits only body aid instruments may have completed every facet of business activities correctly. However, sales volume will surely suffer from not understanding consumer demand. The basic need for most customers is better communication skills. They want to participate in social exchange, such as family groups, church activities, and similar groups with greater ease and less embarrassment. Although this need is central to their search for improvement, personality and buying habits create additional wants.

Some want an aid just like their neighbor's or similar comparative shopping. For the hearing aid specialist there is often a discrepancy between what the consumer wants and the acoustic needs. Consumers may want a certain model or style but need something else. Resolving such discrepancies to the client's satisfaction is important. Dictatorial decisions by the hearing aid specialist are likely to result in poor client satisfaction and correspondingly poor financial returns. Understanding these behaviors in marketing a product or service increases customer satisfaction.

Peters and Waterman (1982) list eight attributes that characterize America's most successful companies. Two of these attributes are: concern for the customer; and dedication for providing unparalleled quality, service, and reliability of their product. The dedication for researching consumer wants and needs and providing quality products and services are desirable and necessary attributes of a dispensing business.

Freiman (1983) maintains that the psychographic profile (the study of consumer attitudes) is important in understanding consumer buying patterns. Psychographics consider life style, attitudes, self image, aspirations, goals, and emotional characteristics. Understanding psychographics allows the dispenser to deliver the product or service more effectively and efficiently than the competition. Complete case history information is essential to this step and should be a part of each evaluation.

4. DEVELOPING AND REDEVELOPING PRODUCTS AND SERVICE

Anyone content with the status quo is likely to experience decreasing sales volume and profit. Product design and service is currently a volatile area and must receive constant attention by the specialist. Being sensitive to client complaints and analyzing them to provide better products and services is a good management strategy. Another highly effective method of changing product or service is to be active in national and state trade association meetings. New product development is often introduced at these meetings. Discussion with other similarly motivated specialists is invaluable in modifying service programs. Internal records are another source of information. A record of repair or return for credit can be used to determine if product lines need to be changed or modified.

5. SELECTING AND TRAINING PERSONNEL

Each office is unique, and has the individual thumb print or personality characteristics of the owner. Decisions are made each day of the week that direct and flavor each office. Good management techniques can be practiced or ignored each day. Perhaps, at the most basic level, the office operates and/or reflects the moral, social, and other basic convictions of the owner. The success of each office is dependent upon its purpose. That purpose should be based upon the ultimate welfare of the consumer. Business decisions based upon what is good for the consumer will usually be good decisions. Most hearing aid specialists agree with the statement, "If you take care of the customers, they will take care of you." Financial rewards normally come to those individuals who think first of the client.

Academic training, experience, and attitude are major components to be considered for personnel selection. Each employee's knowledge, attitude, and skills are important to the overall success of the business. Selecting an employee is a highly personal task. Selecting someone who fits into the overall organization is important for continued harmony and productivity in business. A single disagreeable employee can sour the working environment for fellow workers. Creating and maintaining a job description and work manual are effective methods for acclimating new employees to their work experience. In a small business such as hearing aid dispensing, each employee must assume many and varied responsibilities. A job description manual will help eliminate training time and insure coverage in the major areas of responsibility.

An effective manager first starts by determining what types of positions need to be filled. As your business grows, so will your staff. A good manager is ready for that and is ready to create new positions on the basis of need.

Some basic positions are receptionist, secretary, general office person, repair clerk, marketing person, bookkeeper, office manager, personnel manager, computer operator and business manager. Depending on the size of your operation, the same person can probably perform a variety of duties. Because service is important in this industry, you must make a commitment to hiring service-oriented people. Your people must be efficient but they also must care. Many people believe that poor service represents poor quality of product. If you have a staff that treats each customer as a unique individual, they will believe that they have found a genuinely unique dispenser who truly cares about their well being.

Choosing a general office and personnel manager is an important step. A successful office manager should work closely with you and keep in constant communication. The office manager is often a shoulder to cry on as well as a source of office morale. This person has got to be able to function as the "know it all" of the organization. There's never a question of where employees should direct questions. This choice of employee is as important a decision as the choice of receptionist and the choice of secretary.

Perhaps a key to good personnel management is deciding which tasks should be split up. A receptionist should have the sole duty of greeting customers, answering general questions and handling cash. She should be responsible for screening incoming calls, so that your attention is directed toward those calls of utmost importance. The first impression your customers get of you personally is by those you have chosen to represent you.

Since both the receptionist and the secretary interact with clients, a sunny disposition is important. An individual who can be pleasant even on the worst day is the person who is viewed as helpful, pleasant and dependable. Think of times that you reached a secretary that was ambivalent or downright rude. What was your impression of the owner even though you hadn't spoken to him or her?

In searching for a receptionist, the manager must ask several questions: (1) Do they appear to have a "sunny disposition"? Do they smile a lot? Do they have a good sense of humor? (2) Are they able to dress professionally and is their dress appropriate for the type of clientele you serve? (3) What is their attitude toward the hearing impaired? What is their attitude in general? (4) Do they appear to have a long attention span and do they look genuinely interested? (5) Do they have a history of being efficient or do they seem to have the organization skills necessary to run a successful front desk? (6) Do they want to go the extra mile? Asking yourself these questions about any employee can weed out undesirable applicants. Going through this list reduces the probability of hiring a "bad apple."

In choosing a secretary, a few additional questions should be considered. What is their typing ability? Are they able to run high-tech office equipment with ease? Are they able to adapt to new systems easily? Do they have a lot of patience and tolerance? What is the quality of their phone voice? Are they able to sound friendly on the phone at all times? Are they able to handle calls which you would rather avoid? Do they have successful customer relations skills?

Your employees should be mentally challenged. If you have a member of your staff who is not working to his or her full potential, you should inform that person. In-office evaluations are the perfect time for a manager to sit down and review job performance, consider pay increases, and talk to the individual on a more personal level. If an employee is doing badly or making mistakes with no indication of improvement, do not delay your decision to terminate their employment. The longer you wait the harder the decision and the more you doubt your initial feelings. Firing an employee is not a personal attack but a wise business decision that a good manager must make in order to keep his operation running smoothly.

6. DEVELOPING SALES APPROACHES & ADVERTISING SUPPORT

Regardless of how a consumer receives a product whether it is prescribed, dispensed, suggested, recommended, or sold; the legal transfer through a contract is referred to as a sale. Individual specialists may prefer one term over another because of educational background, training experience, or professional affiliation. Regardless of semantic differences, however, the client requires the same assistance in selecting and using a product. Selling is that process whereby the hearing aid specialist assists the consumer in satisfactorily choosing a product or service and in resolving his or her communication needs.

Whiting (1978) lists five steps in the selling process. They are attention, interest, conviction, desire, and close. The hearing aid specialist may not have to go through each step with the client. There is little doubt the client will go through each one in the buying process. All of these steps may not occur at the specialists office. Attention and interest may have been developed previously by advertisements, by discussions with a friend or relative, or by consultation with another professional at a referral agency. The last three steps are usually, but not always, taken at the specialist's office. The conviction step is when the specialist outlines the test results and the benefits to be derived from wearing amplification. If the benefits of amplification are apparent to the client, a positive desire results for the product. The close is the final step. The client is asked to make a decision. Although there is a great deal of common sense to the selling process, information from published books on this subject, from manufacturers of hearing aids and from organizations such as Dale Carnegie and Associates and American Management Association are beneficial. Many consumers put off purchasing a hearing aid and then buy reluctantly. Good sales techniques are helpful in developing well satisfied customers.

The term selling is offensive to some professionals who may prefer counseling, agreements or some other term. Discussion of fees and prices may be equally distasteful. However, by remaining ignorant of the concept and practices which make up a modern marketing program, these individuals are often without the skill to practice their profession or to meet rapidly changing needs. Conaway (1983) stated, "... if you don't know, appreciate, and understand the rules, you simply won't be able to play the game."

ADVERTISING

ADVERTISING CONCEPTS

In the final analysis consumers buy the benefits derived from the product. Hearing impaired consumers buy better hearing, better social communication skills, better family relations, and other benefits. The astute business person understands and accepts the buying logic of the consumers and serves them accordingly.

Hixson (1982) summarized the influence of advertising when she stated "if you think advertising doesn't pay—we understand there are 25 mountains in Colorado higher than Pike's Peak. Can you name one?" Many individuals beginning in the hearing aid business will underestimate the power and usefulness of advertising. In this regard advertising should be thought of not as an expense but as a business investment. Understanding how your products and services can be advertised to the hard of hearing public is important in developing a thriving business. An advertising strategy can be developed around several concepts. Areas to be considered are: 1) environmental factors such as economic changes, social, and cultural behavior, and legal and political restrictions by law; 2) product areas such as product features, intended use of the product, and product comparison, and 3) consumer factors such as attitude and life style. Each business person may concentrate on a particular area, however, most advertising programs should consider several of these concepts.

ADVERTISING BUDGETS

Most advertising specialists recommend budget preparation that will encompass a year's activity. The actual cost of an advertising budget may vary considerably because of location, competition, and the overall business activity desired. If one is to get the most out of advertising dollars, objectives for each program and measurement of the results must be established. The obvious difficulty of setting such objectives and measuring the results are the reasons why so few dealers do. But without objectives and measurements one cannot hope to improve the effectiveness of advertising programs and increase the return on investments. The statement, "If you don't know where you are going, any road will take you there," is an appropriate admonition in wisely choosing and budgeting your advertising program.

Hixson (1981) suggests five potential methods of budgeting for advertising. They are: 1) percentage of sales; 2) unit of sales; 3) competitive; 4) amount judged necessary; and 5) the objective method. The first two methods are fairly self explanatory. A specific amount is simply calculated. Established and successful hearing aid specialists can be helpful in estimating their sales volume. The third approach, competitive, has some similarities to the first two. However, the amount of advertising required for this approach is based upon providing the same advertisement thrust as the competitor. Most hearing aid specialists are sensitive to this system because it is basically a demand approach. If one wants to keep up with the competition, it is necessary to advertise in a corresponding manner. The fourth method, the amount judged necessary, is a goal setting approach. The hearing aid specialist estimates the amount of advertising dollars necessary to achieve a certain sales volume. The fifth method attempts to target a budget to the percentage of sales. This method, according to Hixon, will consider complex economic and competitive information that is probably out of consideration for most small business owners.

The small business person is frequently assailed with different advertising proposals. Most of these will be from individuals or businesses that sell advertising. A well planned advertising program and budget can make the selection or rejection of these offers simpler and more productive.

ADVERTISING IMAGE

Advertising plans should include the overall image for the business. Whether wanted or not, each business has an image in the community or reflects an image through the advertising program it initiates. The obvious objective is to develop the most positive image possible. Zielonko (1983) listed five areas of image advertising. They are product, price, place, people, and promotion image. The selection of brand name, style of aid, pricing, business sign, stationery and business cards, and the quantity of sales people have a powerful affect on the overall image. As Zielonko (1982) stated "... your location and types of facility, the way you present yourself, and what your referral sources say about you, as well as your individual selling style, determine your image, your credibility and your capacity to generate enthusiasm and motivation—strong forces in leading the competition."

President Reagan's decision to use hearing aid amplification and the dramatic increase in hearing aid sales of the canal type is a classic example of the power of image advertising. Regardless of the type of advertising selected, the specialist should choose only those plans which promote and enhance his business.

ADVERTISING MEDIUMS

Several methods of advertisement can be selected. Newspapers, radio, television, office brochures, direct mail, business cards, business signs, displays, exhibits, fairs, home shows, speciality items (key chains, pens, etc.), roadway signs, yellow pages, hand bills, manufacturer informational brochures, holiday greetings, check-up notices, and press releases, or feature articles in newspapers, magazines or special interest publications are typical mediums for advertising. Although normally not labeled as such, letters describing services or products, and letters on client care to other professional or referral agencies, are powerful forms of advertisement. Many hearing aid specialists sponsor hearing clinics, open houses, service clinics, and other promotional special occasions. These events are advertised to the public through various mediums.

Each of these methods provides for a means of increasing office traffic. Most specialists select several for their advertising strategy. The particular medium and the emphasis it receives in the overall advertising program varies according to geographic area, competition, and the individual personality of the owner. A business with no sign, is a sign of no business. This common phrase is applicable to advertising in general. If no attempts are made to advertise, the amount of business activity will surely suffer. Targeting a particular segment of the population is desirable as it is more important to reach the people who count than to count the people you reach. Selecting a desirable advertising medium insures that money is wisely targeted to that population yielding the greatest response.

ADVERTISING STEPS

Wasiak (1983) suggests six steps for advertising. They are: 1) know the product, 2) research the customer, 3) define objectives, strategy, and target audience, 4) develop the advertising concept, 5) develop and execute the advertising plan, and 6) measure and evaluate the results. These steps need not be elaborate and perhaps not even written. However, a written document often is useful for comparison when memory fades. Financial information, time, and effort expenditures are useful in determining future advertising programs and in measuring and evaluating results. The quality of an advertising program is determined by thoroughness, attention to detail, and consistency of programs. Quality programs project into the future. They are not the ones that result from a last desperate attempt to save a failing business.

CHOOSING THE RIGHT WAY TO PRESENT YOUR COMPANY

Successful advertising is the result of good management. Think of advertising as the medium you are using to present your company. In this respect, choose reputable advertising mediums to represent your company.

Begin by asking yourself who you wish to reach and to what mediums they are exposed. For example, one hearing aid dispenser was aware that his elderly customers often looked in the obituaries to see if any of their friends or acquaintances had passed on. He strategically placed his ad in the bottom corner of the obituary page.

Successful managers not only listen to customer needs but also customer conversations. By just plain talking to your customers, you'll find that they often divulge extraneous information such as their preference in radio programs they listen to, newspapers they like to read, and television programs they watch. It is this kind of information that can alert you to where you need to place advertising in order to get their attention.

As a manager of a hearing facility you are aware of the importance of customer relations and you must make telemarketing, direct mail, and promotions a part of your marketing program. A good telemarketer is not selling something but informing the public of a service that his or her business provides. Calling current customers as well as prospective customers is a good way to generate business as well as check on people to see how they are doing.

Using direct mail can be an asset to your organization if the customer is being invited to attend a special event. Invite the customer to join you or call you for more information. Special promotions are a great way to generate questions, not to mention new and repeat business. Keep in mind that the best referral is one made by your own customer.

USE YOURSELF AS A MARKETING TOOL

One of the best tools you have for marketing is yourself. Be an active member of the community. Talk to doctors, nursing home administrators, churches and schools. Let them know what types of services you have available. They cannot refer people to you if they do not know that you are there.

Send out doctors letters and information packets. Keep people informed of progress and technology. Do not be shy about getting your name publicized. When people see it, they will recognize you as a significant part of the community.

Make your company part of the community also by getting involved in community activities. If money allows, sponsor a local team or make a donation in your company's name. One hearing aid dispenser offered to write an editorial column in the senior section of a local newspaper answering questions about hearing loss. You not only get great exposure but most of these types of activities are tax deductible.

OWNER QUALIFICATIONS AND RESPONSIBILITIES

The single most important aspect of a successful business is the choice of a manager. For most small businesses the manager is usually the owner. Allen (1968) sums this up when he states "When it comes to managing a small business, the most difficult of these problems will be faced. There is no magic way to make the management of a small business a simple matter because the management has already been picked. . . . the most important decision a businessman may make is in selecting the president or manager of his business and it is usually himself." Large businesses often use college training, intelligence tests, personality indexes, previous employment records, references, personal interviews, and a host of other information in selecting managers. Most companies will require future management personnel to undergo several months or years of on the job training, to adequately prepare them for management responsibilities. With such attention to selection and training, the company is better assured of a skilled manager. This degree of selection and training is absent or restricted for many small business operations.

A U.S. small business administration pamphlet entitled "Checklist for Going into Business" lists several questions a new owner may ask himself in deciding if he is prepared to go into business. These are:

1. Are you a self starter?
2. How do you feel about other people?
3. Can you lead others?
4. Can you take responsibility?
5. How good an organizer are you?
6. How good a worker are you?
7. Can you make decisions?
8. Can people trust what you say?
9. Can you stick with it?
10. How good is your health?

These questions summarize many of the important considerations a business owner should make in the decision to start a business. Obviously an affirmative answer to each question would imply someone who is ready to begin a business venture. There is a natural tendency for individuals to see greener grass on the other side of the fence. Individuals with no business experience may see the independence, financial reward, and prestige as desirable attributes of a business venture. They may fail to realize the long hours of work necessary to fulfill these expectations. Usually the first three to five years are the most trying and often require 60–70 hours per week of constant diligent work. The financial return during this period is usually growing and may not support the expected life style. The feeling of independence may also fail to meet the new owner's expectations. Radcliff (1982) suggests that business owners are controlled by customers, clients, employees, suppliers, bankers, creditors, landlords, community groups, and the Internal Revenue Service. Each one of these categories can have a powerful effect in reducing your independence.

Economic, environmental, and social conditions will also affect the owner's feeling of independence, especially in adverse times. Dailey (1971) suggests that "the unstressed manager is not a manager at all, only an utopian fiction." Perhaps much of this stress arises from the number of responsibilities the owner assumes in operating a business. It has been said that when the owner goes on vacation, the business loses the services of its chief executive, sales manager, controller, advertising department, personnel director, salesman, head bookkeeper, and janitor.

Consider the following list of activities that are the manager's responsibility: selling and servicing customers; visiting with suppliers; answering technical questions from office personnel; handling customer complaints; planning and controlling work; training; supervision; reading mail; chasing overdue accounts; checking stock items and reordering; management meetings; recruiting; staff problems; personal time; and maintenance activities. Lakin (1973) suggests the efficiency of work production, decision making, and other time consuming activities listed above can be increased by time management. Establishing a priority of work activities in order of importance and in order of completion is the essence of time management.

There is no simple business. A business will be as successful, energetic, complex, insightful, truthful, thoughtful, and service-minded as the owner. The limitations of a business will be the individual and his or her ability to plan and execute business activities. Smith (1984) suggested several skill areas that hearing aid specialists should possess for establishing a successful business. These are 1) to have a friendly, outgoing personality; 2) to manage personnel well; 3) to understand business management; 4) to be creative; 5) to have technical skills for testing,evaluating, and fitting hearing aids; 6) to have sales experience; and 7) to have empathy and compassion for the hard of hearing. Hearing aid dispensing is largely a service business with a heavy emphasis placed upon human relations. Consequently, a business owner must have the ability to understand and work effectively with people. Where do beginning business people get this ability? At the present time on the job training with a successful hearing aid specialist appears to offer the best avenue for acquiring these skills.

Family members are often part of the dispensing business as partners or as hired staff. The inclusion of family members in the business can have both highly desirable advantages and occasionally, potentially adverse consequences. Greater loyalty to the business normally results when hiring a spouse, brother, sister, son, daughter, father, or some other relative. Family members also provide better feedback in decision making. Drucker (1966) says that valid decisions are not available without disagreement. "Yes people" provide little assistance for decision making. Family members will feel more freedom to disagree with a management decision. Staff members who always agree to a decision ("good idea" or "whatever you decide") force the owner to be a slave to his or her opinions. A choice of alternatives is highly desirable in decision making. Loyalty and assistance are highly desirable qualities of any employee and in most circumstances outweigh the disadvantages.

Levinson (1970) lists several potential problems. Firing or disciplining a family member who does not conform to the expected business standards and practices is difficult because of the potential development of poor family relations. The closer the family relationship, the more difficult the decision. If the family member owns a portion of the business, additional complications could be expected. Older family members may create stagnation with a status quo attitude perhaps in direct opposition to younger more progressive members.

Inclusion of family members in a business operation should consider several factors. First, the family member should possess the qualifications for the position and second, pre-employment verbal or written agreements should be discussed in the areas of chain of command, job expectations, and future advances. Third, family members might erroneously expect special treatment for working hours and conditions, vacations, and in other areas that may potentially cause resentment with other office personnel. A clear understanding is obviously important to all concerned.

What provisions should be made for backup assistance to the owner? Generally, if the owner will be gone only a few days, the secretary can simply reschedule appointments. A more serious illness or accident that would require several weeks or months away from the office could be disastrous to the business operation. Owners should seriously consider providing backup employees for themselves, particularly if there is no one else licensed or trained on the office staff. Leaving an office unattended by trained staff for several weeks could be damaging to the vitality of the business.

DECISION MAKING

As a manager, you will be faced with dozens of different decisions on a daily basis. An effective manager analyzes each decision and determines the impact and irreversibility of that decision. Some decisions require complete commitment because they are irreversible. It is these decisions that must be weighed very carefully. Do not jump into an irreversible commitment if you are in doubt.

Reversible decisions can be made more quickly. Be sure to alert those affected that the decision is reversible and will be reversed if certain results are not achieved within an allotted period of time. Your staff is more likely to hold back if you inform them that a change is irreversible.

TIME MANAGEMENT

Time can be your friend as well as your enemy. So use it wisely. Make out a daily schedule of events and a "to do"list of the things that need to be handled in priority order. Allocate specific time in your schedule to handle problems and handle them one at a time. By giving each problem a time frame, you can devote your total attention to find the best solution.

Do not waste your time on matters that have minimal or no return. Spend time on matters that affect your entire business. Managers often avoid problems with which they are not familiar, or that have low-impact on the business. Make a list of decisions your business is facing and number them in order of importance. Then, tackle them one by one.

Do not devote your time to salespeople who will not facilitate the growth of your business. If you do not plan to utilize their services, tell them so. Their time is just as important as yours. If you let them know where they stand, you will not have to deal with the nuisance of trying to get rid of them later or of making an unwanted purchase.

EFFECTIVE CONTROL

Employees should know that any significant decision is not to be made without your knowledge and concurrence. In this sense, you retain control of decisions while also putting yourself in a position to be aware of everything that is going on within your organization. For less significant decisions, a supervisor or business manager can okay decisions but they should keep in constant communication with you.

GROWTH AND IMPROVEMENT

A good manager must know at all times where his business is both professionally and financially. This goal is reached by constant communication with employees and managers. Reports are a good way to get the information that is needed.

A good manager must be aware of inventory, sales, return visits, bad accounts and employee performance. You must keep in constant communication with your bookkeeper to determine profitably. Keeping in touch with your receptionist allows you an inside look at who is coming back and who is not. Your secretary can inform you of frequent questions and comments fielded by phone calls. Your business manager can provide you with stock information and inventory.

Managers cannot rely on numbers alone for all the needed information. When an employee is explaining a financial position, they should make their own determination of whether that report is good or bad in terms of business. Compare your reports monthly and have a due date for them. Allot time in which each employee is to explain each part of your business to you. That way, you are designating duties while also keeping yourself informed.

If you find yourself in a position of having to cut costs, you must ask yourself as well as those working for you what they feel could be eliminated. Work closely with your staff because something might look good on paper that actually works out for the worst when implemented. Look first at what seems to be costing you the most. Talk to employees and determine the actual need of this product or service. Discuss possible solutions such as reduction or elimination of inventory.

IT DOESN'T END WITH SUCCESS

Too often, successful companies become too relaxed and satisfied with performance that they do not grow and aspire to new goals. Many times these companies lose their profitability if they do not have set goals for increasing their success.

New goals must be set and exceeded. One way of achieving these goals is incentives. If your employees are working towards recognition, plaques or monetary rewards, then they compete with each other to reach set goals for themselves and for the company.

BROADEN YOUR SCOPE

As a manager, you must have the ability to keep an open mind. You must not become a victim to tunnel vision. You cannot think of your business as simply a hearing aid dispensing service but as a hearing health care service provider. You do not sell hearing aids alone, you sell solutions to hearing-related problems. If you think in a narrow manner, so will your employees. By thinking in this manner, you can miss serious business opportunities.

The hearing industry is constantly changing and by not trying new things, you are limiting yourself and your company as to what products and services you can provide.

BACKGROUND EDUCATION

The current trend for those entering hearing aid dispensing is to have some college experience, particularly in audiology. Although an audiology background is highly desirable in accumulating technical skills associated with dispensing, business skills are not commonly associated with this type of professional training. Several leading hearing aid specialists were asked to indicate where they would send their successors to seek the necessary skills for the dispensing business. If they could not train the person themselves, they would send them to a respected competitor who would provide the necessary basic training. For centuries one of the most successful training programs in any skilled profession has been on the job training. The apprentice system appears to be, at this time, the most desirable alternative for training the new hearing aid specialist. Generally the novice finds the necessary skills through affiliation with an established dealer.

Currently an AUD (Doctorate in Audiology) degree with emphasis toward clinical audiology is underway in several universities. Whether these future graduates will receive adequate business training is unknown. In the past college training programs were inadequate for those who wanted to enter the dispensing business. Course selection and content did not reflect the needs of the dispenser. In addition many of the instructors were either ignorant of the practical aspects of dispensing or were negatively biased against the profession. Any future training in the area of business will be significantly better than that offered in the past because increasing numbers of college instructors are more favorably inclined towards the dispensing profession.

What specific educational background will be necessary in the future. The current trend of better educated individuals entering the business will continue. At some point, perhaps in the near future, specific education and training requirements will be mandated. The technology and information available to dispensers has dramatically increased in the last five years. How will untrained and uneducated individuals survive in the marketplace. The answer is that probably few will survive unless these individuals can receive on the job training necessary to understand and utilize the new technologies.

CONTINUING EDUCATION

The hearing aid dispensing business is changing dramatically in both product technology and in skills necessary for effective dispensing. Continuing education is mandatory if one is too keep abreast of recent developments in the field. Several national associations provide this needed information. Many states have state laws or regulations which mandate continuing education as a requirement for licensure. State associations have been instrumental in providing continuing education. Colleges and universities have become more sensitive to continuing educational demands and are providing course offerings related to dispensing practices.

There are several state and national organizations serving the hearing aid specialist. Membership in these organizations is beneficial in that they provide a number of business and professional services to the member. Although each organization may provide a slightly different benefit, each exists for the mutual benefit of its membership. Membership in selected organizations can increase individual skills in professional relations, business practices, and product familiarity. Membership in these organizations is beneficial in that they provide a common forum or meeting area where individuals of similar interest can meet and exchange information. Those who are new in hearing aid dispensing will benefit from discussions with other dispensers who have demonstrated superior management practices and subsequent financial success.

PUBLIC AND COMMUNITY RELATIONS

Business is enhanced with good community relations. Promote a professional, trustworthy, and ethical image in your personal appearance and actions, the appearance of your building, and vehicles. Hearing aid dispensing practices are an integral part of the medical as well as the retail business community. Talks to service clubs, churches, schools, and other community groups can increase the public's knowledge of good hearing health care, can create additional exposure for where products and services are available, and enhance your reputation within your community. The end result may be more patients entering your business for products and services.

Your advertising and promotion provide valuable educational material for patients and may be the only source for them to find out what is new, what is available, and what will help them. Public service announcements, talks to groups, booths or screenings at health fairs, and personal information from you are how patients find out about the products, the services available at your business. If they are aware of your business, it can be the place where they can go when they are in need of service.

The community also benefits directly from your business. A good dispensing practice is a source of jobs for not just the hearing aid dispenser. The office manager, receptionist, computer operator and technical assistants all spend and reinvest their pay checks back into the local economy. A business also uses a variety of accounting, legal, retail and banking services which provide local employment. Your business and each of your employees reinvest their money in local stores and services each day. A dispensing practice directly and through their employees becomes a valuable part of the local tax base to support schools, city, township, county, and state government.

OFFICE PERSONNEL

Generally, the attitudes of the office staff reflect the owner's commitment to good hearing health care. Consumers who detect a lack of caring on the part of the office staff would also wisely suspect they might receive the same treatment from the hearing aid specialist. The owner should consider intelligence, personality, and general personal qualifications of this individual. Because the majority of customers fall into a geriatric or senior citizen category, an older, mature employee may have better rapport with the customer. Often the hard of hearing individual needs a kind, patient person to help in resolving his or her problem. The owner should consider developing a job description and training manual for this position. Although the preparation of this document may be detailed and tedious, it provides valuable information in selecting and training an employee. The manual should specify job description, qualifications, working hours, benefits, and salary. Written descriptions of how the telephone is answered, appointments scheduled, fees collected, records kept, and bills paid are representative of some of the material that should be kept in this manual. Providing a detailed description of office procedures will help reduce the owner's time investment in direct supervision.

Knowing and understanding the employment expectations and how each job responsibility is performed, provides a more effective and efficient training program for the employee. Because of the details this person must process, careful consideration should be given to the length of employment expected from this employee.

Generally each owner would not want to replace this person frequently. Consequently, any condition preventing long term employment must be considered carefully. Information concerning the applicant's general health, family planning, job experience, attitude, and future plans is important in selecting an employee. When a replacement employee is hired, supervision or on-the-job training is recommended by the departing employee if they are capable and qualified. Klopp (1984) says this should be considered only if the departing employee has been satisfactory and they have a good relationship with their employer.

Good personnel relationships are essential to a productive and pleasant office. How are good relationships achieved? Lowman (1984) suggests that employees ranked appreciation for work well done as the most important factor in job satisfaction. Other factors in order of importance were: feeling in on things; help with personal problems; job security; good wages; interesting work; possibility of promotion; loyalty of management to workers; good working conditions; and tactful discipline. As each of these factors is under the direct control of the owner, each should be considered in improving job satisfaction. Compliments and employee participation in business decisions are excellent methods for increasing job satisfaction. Blanchard and Johnson (1981) state that too often time is spent in catching an employee doing something wrong. They suggest that a more productive approach would be to catch the employee doing something correct and offer praise.

PART TIME HELP

Part time help is desirable for occasions when there is additional work or when an employee is not available to work because of sickness, vacation, or emergencies. Because of the complexity of the secretarial job a reliable part time person is necessary. The most desirable employee would be the same part time individual. Every owner who has had to experience several days without good secretarial support is acutely aware of the importance of reliable backup employees.

RECORD MANAGEMENT

An efficient system of records, forms, and reports are essential when operating any practice. Good records give an instant picture of the financial health of a business at any time. A good bookkeeping system should be simple to use, easy to understand, reliable, accurate, consistent, and should provide the information you will need to operate your hearing aid business and to meet your tax obligations.

Formalized bookkeeping and accounting systems are available to help you manage the finances of your small hearing aid business. These take several forms; many consist of separate printed and ruled pages for journals, ledgers, receipts, expenses, payroll records, and summaries-all in a convenient, loose-leaf binder. One widely used system available from many office supply stores is manufactured by the Dome Publishing Company Inc., of Warwick, Rhode Island. Other well-planned and comprehensive systems are Data-Rite System, or Alpha System, both are manufactured by Data Management, Inc., of Farmington, Connecticut.

These are minimal records you should keep if you are operating a hearing aid practice.

1. A record of sales made or work performed. A patient's Purchase Agreement can be ordered and customized through a local printer to include specific information about the dispenser; address, license number(s), and the hearing aid and accessories information. Some Purchase Agreements include a waiver to Medical Evaluation paragraph. Generic sales pads and receipts can be bought from local office suppliers; if you prefer a customized statement, receipt, and bill for various services or supplies a local printer would be the source to use.
2. A record of cash receipts listing cash sales and money received from outstanding accounts receivable. Enter each item to show date, name of payer, invoice number, and amount received into a journal of your choice.
3. A record of payments you make to suppliers etc. Make disbursements by check. You should have a business checking

account where you enter in the date, name of payee, check number, amount of each check, and the reason for the payment. This information should then be entered into your journal of records.

4. A petty-cash fund and record. Many small expenses will not be covered by invoices and can be paid in cash. Money used from petty cash should always be replaced with a receipt or a petty cash slip.

OTHER RECORDS

To supplement the four basic records, you'll also want to keep; *AN EQUIPMENT LIST.* It's a good idea to keep individual lists of assets that have a useful life of a year or longer—furniture and fixtures, office machines, buildings, and tools. Show the date the item was purchased, the vendor, a brief description of the item, the check number, and the amount paid. Such lists provide the basis for calculating depreciation and to provide supporting data for fixed-asset accounts. Important to our industry is calibration information on audiometers owned by your practice. The records should include the company, the service technician, the date, and when the next calibration is due. Keeping these records with the audiometer itself makes sense since most State Laws require documentation of calibration. A physical check of the operator's ear may be added to these records.

A RECORD OF BUSINESS AND LIABILITY INSURANCE. A list of each policy showing type and amount of coverage, name of insurance carrier, name of agent or broker, expiration date, and annual premium.

A GENERAL JOURNAL AND LEDGER. An easy way to consolidate useful records is in the form of a journal or book of original entry that records every business transaction chronologically as a debit or credit.

The information for each journal entry can be received from original sources or from the basic records described earlier. In some practices, copies of such transaction records are incorporated into the journal, each record standing as an entry.

A general ledger should also be kept and posted with the dollar amounts of transactions and balances of separately captioned accounts, such as assets, liabilities, capital, receipts (or sales), and expenses. Posting permits the accumulation of all dollar activity for comparison with budget projections.

FINANCIAL STATEMENTS. If you have more than a very small hearing aid business, you'll probably need an outside accountant to prepare these. The most important financial statements: the balance sheet and the profit and loss statement are prepared from the above described basic records. The balance sheet is a view of the business at a given moment. It lists assets, liabilities, and capital. The profit and loss statement can provide an analysis over an extended amount of time. It shows the amount of income received from which expenses and taxes are subtracted, the balance showing profit (or loss).

APPOINTMENT BOOKS that provide control of time and activity are essential. Schedules which provide control of minute, hour, week, month, and year activities are needed. Proper use of an appointment book permits utilization of time and work activity in scheduling evaluations, hearing aid fittings, service work, and administrative time.

REGISTRY BOOKS providing information about instruments ordered, date received, date fitted, repair activity, returned for credit, and related information are mandatory. If records are kept on repair and returns to the manufacturers they can be used to evaluate product quality and success in fittings.

INVENTORY CONTROL RECORDS of some form are necessary. Knowing what supplies to keep, where they can be obtained, at what quantities, at what discounts, at what intervals ordered, and other similar concerns are all important in establishing a good inventory control system. If there are more than one office location, forms for supplies should be used and analyzed frequently.

MISCELLANEOUS FORMS

Many small hearing aid business owners develop their own business system and record management controls. A sampling of various forms used by different Midwestern hearing aid business owners includes: Patient Sign in Sheet, Patient Questionnaires about Hearing Health and Communication History, Loaner Instrument Record, FAX Cover Form, In-Stock Inventory Transfer, Consulting Agreements, Vacation Schedules, Post Card Reminder Cards (Re-test Service), Medical Release Forms, Telephone Marketing Sheets, and Mileage Expense Reports. This list is not exhaustive in scope. Each office will have specific forms for their own purposes. Although information is essential to proper management, a periodic prudent elimination of outdated or nonessential forms should be undertaken on an annual basis.

CLIENT INFORMATION

Good client records are mandatory. These records would normally include the audiometric test results, case history information, fitting requirements, fitting information, and service information. Some of this information is required by state or federal law. Above and beyond the legal requirements, however, is the concern for good client management. Detailed information is essential for good client management.

For economy of form design, printing cost, and client management, the previous information should be kept in one location, the client's file folder. Some manufacturers provide these forms to their purchasers free or at a minimal cost. Whether or not a generic client file information system is suitable for a particular office is dependent upon the intended use. There has been in the past little or no standardization of client information forms except the audiogram. Consequently, each owner will probably be faced with the necessity of designing his or her own forms.

There are several general suggestions that should be considered in the design and selection of this form. First, the paper selected should be of standard size to allow easy filing in a standard filing cabinet. Second, the weight and durability should ensure good maintenance qualities through several years of handling. Third, whenever possible, the majority of the basic information should be printed on the folder itself to eliminate a clutter of loose papers. Preprinting the information on one form also reduces the necessity of having client identification information duplicated on separate sheets. Duplication of effort in this area is a never ending battle. Fourth, do not include on the form information that is used only occasionally. The individual needs of each office will dictate the informational content. However, minimally used information should be excluded. Fifth, the organization of the client information on the form should minimize the need to flip back and forth through the folder to find information. Test information should follow the same principle, and should be located at a convenient location near the fitting information and service history. Sixth, the test information should be restricted to one page so that duplication is convenient when test information must be sent to another office.

OFFICE AND BUSINESS POLICY

The business policy should be clear, concise, and available to the public. Deceptive practices only create ill will and apprehension in the minds of customers. Several areas require definition. First, the payment policy should be posted and clearly visible to the customer. Collection of fees is more comfortable for both the business manager and the client when the terms of payment are known and clearly understood. Second, details of charges for office calls and servicing hearing aids should be clearly understood. Many specialists include some or all service costs in the purchase price of an instrument. The consumer should know what services come with the purchase and which ones will require additional payment. Third, warranty information for the aid should be clearly known and understood. This information is made available by the manufacturer. However, the explanation of warranty is the responsibility of the owner. Fourth, information should be available about the trial period if one is offered. Clients should know the cost of trying the hearing aid and the conditions for return. Finally, other areas that require attention are repair policy before and after warranty expiration, use of loaner hearing aids, and battery purchases. Many specialists have developed a program to supply clients with batteries and other needed supplies. These programs are often detailed in nature and require explanation. Much of the information listed above can be made available on the contract or in an office brochure.

The policies created within your business should never be set in stone; however, your staff should realize that policies are to be followed. Exceptions to the rule only create chaos and can put you in a bad situation. Take the hearing aid dispenser that agreed to go to the home of one of his patients when his manager had dictated that strict office policy prohibited such behavior. After the dispenser did it once, the lady began calling every week demanding that he come to her house every time she needed him. She said that he did not mind doing that because he had done it before. The lady then told her neighbor that he had come to her house and the neighbor wanted the same treatment. Your employees must understand that policies and rules are made for a reason and adherence to those policies is a must.

KEEPING WITHIN THE LAW

Honest and competent lawyers will earn their fee by keeping you out of trouble. Choose a lawyer you respect and trust to advise you. When working with a lawyer, you will want to establish a fee in advance for the work you expect him/her to perform. A lawyer will usually charge you an hourly rate. To save money, you will want to carefully plan in advance the specific questions and information you intend to present to the lawyer. Keep your visiting to a minimum when you know the lawyer's "charge clock" is running.

Your lawyer will advise you on operating as a sole proprietorship, partnership, corporation or Sub S Corporation. Lawyers will also be helpful in determining what permits you will need for your business, zoning regulations for your office, and other areas of legal advice that can keep you out of harm's way.

The most important rule to follow when working with your attorney is to always tell the truth and tell the whole story. You are given a special right when you speak to your lawyer, one that is not available when you talk to your other consultants. This is the "attorney/client privilege" which means that anything you discuss with your lawyer is confidential and cannot be divulged to any other person including law enforcement persons and government officials. Your attorney will advise you that they can only help you on the basis of the information you give them. If you keep some information from them, their advice will be defective.

PHYSICIANS RELATIONS

Lowder (1994) gives the following discussion of physician referral:

> "When my private practice was begun in 1981, I had no patients at all. I assumed that many of my future clients would come from medical referrals. After all I thought, I am an audiologist and am well trained to provide amplification. All I need to do is to inform local physicians that I have opened my office and my waiting room will soon begin to fill. So I began to call on a few doctors to inform them of my new practice."

Lowder further states that:

> "After a while it started to dawn on me that most of my new patients came to me as a result of a patient referral or in response to some form of external marketing, e.g. newspaper ad or direct mail piece. For a while, I sent reports to doctors regardless of whether the patient had been referred to me. At the end of the third year, I concluded that physicians in my area were simply not going to refer their patients to me in any great numbers. Although I had received a few referrals from doctors, most new patients had come from my own marketing efforts. As a result, I discontinued calling on physicians and ended my practice of sending reports to them. I then concentrated my marketing efforts in other areas where I was receiving a greater 'bang for my buck.'"

The preceding experience may be the rule rather than the exception. Other hearing health professionals have also reported difficulty establishing referral relationships with physicians. There are several factors which, added together, make the physician/hearing health professional (HHP) relationship rather tenuous. Physicians and HHP's do not train together. Physicians train in medical schools, HHP's in colleges of liberal arts. The friendships and associations which physicians make with each other (the "good ole boy network") are rarely established between medical students and HHP students. In addition, medical students routinely receive little if any formal training in hearing and hearing loss. Even otolaryngologists, until recently, would frequently advise patients with sensorineural hearing loss that hearing aids would not help them and that nothing could be done to help them with their hearing problem. Hearing loss is a health problem which is difficult for many physicians to identify unless the problem is obvious. Physicians also avoid making recommendations to their patients which, they fear, may be met with resistance. Additionally, doctors may have objections about hearing aids that they have heard from their dissatisfied patients. Doctors also have concerns about the cost of hearing instruments given the complaints they hear from their patients. Is it any wonder that medical professionals "drop the ball" and fail to refer?

Yet, the need for physicians to identify their patients with hearing loss and make appropriate referrals for treatment is enormous. Surveys have repeatedly shown that people first voice their concerns about hearing loss to their family physician. Otolaryngologists and HHP's typically are not consulted first. A personal recommendation and referral by the family physician sends a powerful message to the patient. "I am sending you to a hearing health professional. You can trust this person." As a result, patients who are referred to us by their family physicians tend to be people who will follow our recommendations and use amplification successfully.

There are several barriers involved in forming a good referral relationship with a physician. The basic reason that we hearing health professionals are not receiving more referrals from doctors boils down to a matter of personal trust. Physicians obviously need to be better educated about hearing problems and amplification, but this is a secondary issue. If a physician does not trust you to care for his patient, he/she simply will not refer patients to you. Personal trust is not a matter of professional qualifications. It does not matter so much that you are well-educated with lots of experience and university degrees. What matters most to the referring physician is that he can trust you to care for his patient.

There are a few key factors to consider when attempting to develop a relationship with a physician. First, it will be necessary that you meet with the doctor so that you can get to know each other. Several short meetings may be necessary. Together, you need to specify the doctor's needs with regard to his patients with hearing loss. What specific problem exists that you might be able to solve for this doctor? By doing this, you are placing yourself in the role of problem solver; and ally of the doctor. You are not there as a salesperson. Third, it is important that you ask the physician to refer a specific patient to you. Following your evaluation of that patient, you need to meet with the physician to outline in detail what you did for this patient. By consulting closely with the doctor about his first few referrals, you will begin the process of building trust. It is only after a trusting relationship has been established that the process of educating the doctor can begin.

The fundamental mistake being made by many of us is that we assume education occurs before a personal relationship has been established. Unless a foundation of trust has been established, efforts to educate a doctor typically comes across as a sales pitch. Most physicians have very little interest in another sales pitch.

THIRD PARTY HEARING HEALTH CARE COVERAGE

A common question asked of the audiologist or hearing aid dispenser is whether third party reimbursement will subsidize a new hearing aid. Initially, insurance coverage of hearing tests and hearing aids might sound appealing to the practitioner, but close examination may reveal some pitfalls.

Many third party carriers require that the dispenser sign up as a provider and agree to accept a given rate for their services (audiogram, hearing aid evaluation/selection, dispensing fee). Typically, the reimbursement is less than the established usual and customary cost of services in a given geographic region. If the allowed fees are significantly less than what is judged reasonable to maintain a profitable practice, then the dispenser must reconsider the viability of participating in such a program. If, however, the third party coverage provides a significant client population with minimal competition (reducing the need to market the hearing services), and sufficient reimbursement in a timely manner, then it may be worthwhile to participate in that insurance plan. Better practice management can improve the profitability of insurance-discounted plans and increase the number of discounted patients that can be seen in a given period of time.

To assist in the decision on whether or not to participate as a provider, investigate the payment and denial history of the third party plan. Also, look into the complexity of the filing process and to what types of hearing aids that the insurance company requires the provider to sell. If the resulting net profit is minimal or the patient's hearing aid is compromised because of the maximum allowable cost, then the dispenser might feel it inappropriate to participate in that plan.

In general, third party plans for amplification can be divided into three groups: (A) Government, (B) Insurance Underwriters, and (C) Provider Organizations.

GOVERNMENT-SUBSIDIZED coverage for hearing evaluations and amplification falls under several programs in order to provide for various sectors of the population.

MEDICAID

Medicaid is a cooperative, federal-state medical program that provides hearing aids to needy children in all states and to needy adults in about half the states. Requirements for providing hearing aid services in this program vary markedly from state to state. Additionally, various forms of cost-containment (e.g. minimum hearing loss; binaural limitations; recipient co-payments; pre-approved hearing aid manufacturers and models; prior-authorizations) exist. For specific information, one should contact the state agency that administers Medicaid.

MEDICARE

The largest third party program, Medicare was created to provide medical coverage for the disabled and those over 65 years of age. Under this plan, only an initial diagnostic audiogram under a physician's direction may be covered. However, such tests are NEVER reimbursable when performed for the purpose of prescribing amplification. Additionally, any advertisement that notes Medicare acceptance CANNOT include any information about hearing aids.

CHAMPUS

Civilian Health and Medical Programs for the Uniformed Services (CHAMPUS) provides audiological services and amplification through local professionals if their recipients are not able to obtain the necessary care from a military facility.

VOCATIONAL REHABILITATION

This program provides funds for the evaluation and fitting of hearing aids on individuals who are trying to maintain or obtain a job or an education. Often times the reimbursement rate for fitting hearing aids under this plan is similar to the Medicaid plan in that state.

WORKER'S COMPENSATION

Hearing loss as the result of occupational noise exposure under federal and state regulations can provide for payment of audiology services and hearing aid fittings.

VETERAN'S ADMINISTRATION

Though most veterans with service-related hearing loss are provided with audiological and hearing aid services through a VA facility, special cases (e.g. non-ambulatory veteran, special hearing aid) may result in the provision of services through a local audiological or hearing aid dispenser.

INSURANCE UNDERWRITERS are so new at providing audiology and hearing aid services that they are not sure of the direction to go and are concerned about committing to a program that may end up as non-profitable. As a result, they wait for the employer to request amplification as a benefit, while the employer will tend to wait for the employees to make the request. (The exception would be government mandates on insurance).

As with all third party plans, the potential provider should investigate the company's payment and denial history, their requirements for a provider and prerequisites for fitting a particular person with a hearing aid.

PROVIDER ORGANIZATIONS—Under the guise of Managed Health Care, several plans have evolved in order to deliver quality health care while containing cost. Within this framework, extra benefits, not usually covered by traditional insurance, are provided by offering discounted services through the plan. These benefits (e.g. dental, vision, hearing benefits) often seen as valuable to the enrollee, can be cost-effective to the insurer. This permits the trimming of traditional benefits, while enhancing the insurance package. As a result, there is a growing trend to include the hearing health care professional as a reimbursable provider. Managed Health Care organizations generally consider three criteria in selecting their provider:

A. Multiple distribution points because all their enrollees are not in one location;

B. Standardization to ensure that the enrollees would get the same care at all locations;

C. Quality control to ensure that the enrollees are getting hearing aids and referrals only when they need them.

A necessary part of the managed health care scenario are various quality assurance practices that ensure effective treatment by qualified professionals. These practices include utilization review, quality management, peer review, audits, credentialing and patient satisfaction surveys.

Health Maintenance Organizations and Preferred Provider Organizations

HMO's and PPO's forms of managed health care, offer their services to a given population at discounted rates or a prenegotiated fee. This is done by selectively contracting with only certain primary-care physicians, specialists and allied health care providers.

Provider Networks

Hearing Health Car Provider networks are organized groups of audiologists and hearing aid dispensers in specific geographic regions that provide hearing services and hearing aids at a reduced fee in order to benefit plan members. National Ear Care Plan (NECP), the largest provider organization for hearing health care in the United States, tries to strike a balance between providing its accounts with enough dispensers for convenient access and at the same time protecting its providers from excessive competition. It is their contention that managed care works only if you get more patients into fewer practices in exchange for the discount.

Participation in third party reimbursement plans certainly can increase the hearing aid dispenser's exposure to patients, but there can also be an erosion of profit per unit dispensed. The provider should determine the threshold of deductions that a given business can tolerate and what portion of the practice's patients may be discounted to remain profitable. With this consideration in mind, many practices limit their discounted patient volume to a fraction (20%) of their practice. Of course, the quality of patient service should be the primary concern.

ERRORS IN MANAGEMENT

The errors made by managers may be few and inconsequential or many and devastating. The degree of success or failure will hinge on certain key factors.

First, managers should be well informed about their business. Current up-to-date evaluation of information and ideas are essential for adequate decisions. Business plans for each aspect of a business are as important as road maps are to traveling in unknown territory. Poor information or improper utilization of available data contribute to errors in decisions. There is a delicate balance of knowing how much information to gather and equally important when to act on this information.

Second, decisions should be made in a timely fashion. Every choice in each and every aspect of business can be made decisively, postponed, or ignored. Lack of a decision is itself a decision. Procrastination faces each business owner each day in decisions. Unfortunately, this approach is reactive in nature as the accumulative effect of no decisions may force the manager into a situation where the choices are not under their control any longer. Smith (1994) says that "one of the worst management blunders is the inability to make a plan and stick with it. Most managers make strategic plans for a good reason and swerving from that plan is the easiest way to end up so far off course that it's almost impossible to get back." Smith also suggest a general rule for following your goals. Pick a long term goal and follow it precisely and take immediate action to correct deviations from the goal.

Third, managers must have a value system that incorporates honesty and integrity. Our value system prioritizes information for our decisions. Poor values are a breeding ground for dishonesty, inferior service and other negative factors that affect business. Decisions that affect patients, staff members, and suppliers will be questioned and therefore lack validity without these values. Bait and switch advertising is a classic example of this factor. In the desire to turn a quick buck, short cuts in quality and service will undoubtedly result in dissatisfied customers. Unfortunately, dissatisfied customers tell others and ultimately referral sources and prospective customers are negatively influenced toward the business.

Fourth, there should be zero tolerance for conditions that are detrimental to efficient business operation. Managers should terminate or modify employees who are not peak performers. They also will eliminate products, suppliers, and procedures that restrict or are detrimental to their profit margins. Failure to do so may allow conditions to become acute and irreversible. Shechtman (1994) says that managers often make decisions that mirror those made in the past. These decisions may be comfortable because of tradition or past conditions but they may ignore present and future trends. The philosophy that says "but we always did it this way" ignores the major guiding light of business which is the welfare and profit ability of their business. One of the paradigms in Shechtman's book is "people's ability to change is not a function of capacity but of choice." How true this statement is! Whoever coined the expression "if it is to be, it's up to me" certainly understood commitment. Willpower, determination, resolve and other similar qualities are highly desirable in any manager. These are important qualities in predicting success or failure of a business. We probably all know individuals whose success is compromised by personal problems or personal pleasures. Lack of commitment to a profitable business is certainly a choice but ultimately a negative one.

Although the success of each business is ultimately through the decisions of the manager, it also reflects the quality and effort of his or her staff. The inability to delegate responsibility is a fifth factor. Any manager who does not utilize the creativity and good will of employees is reducing the potential of the business to grow and prosper.

Some anticipate the days events at the office with positive feelings and some with negative feelings. Negative attitudes toward work certainly do not turn into positive feelings towards fellow workers or patients. Many errors can be reduced or eliminated by positive attitudes.

None of us begin our business careers with highly developed managerial skills. For each of us this is where experience and time allow us to become more proficient. Learning from one's mistakes is necessary so that future errors can be reduced. For those individuals that demand good information, make timely decisions, have good value systems and that expect peak performance from themselves and their employees, the path to success will certainly be more assured. These factors are ominous and most certainly personally threatening because the mantle of success or failure rests squarely on the manager's shoulders.

SUMMARY

The role of management strategies, techniques, and procedures will become increasingly important particularly if competition in hearing aid dispensing increases. There is ample evidence that large corporations expend considerable time, money, and effort in establishing good management programs. Although the complexity of small business management procedures are significantly less than large corporations, there is a definite need to provide good management techniques in existing hearing aid businesses. They vary in their complexity, techniques, and success. There is little doubt, however, that among successful practices good management would be a common denominator.

GLOSSARY

American Management Association An organization that offers information in business related areas through lectures, courses and publication. The central office is: American Management Association, 135 West 50th Street, New York, NY 10124-0019.

Dale Carnegie & Associates An organization that offers instruction in the areas of effective speaking and human relations, sales courses, and management throughout the United States. Central offices are: Dale Carnegie and Associates, Inc., 1475 Franklin Avenue, Garden City, NY 11530.

Ratios Gross Profit Margin (GPM): This ratio measures the profitability of the firm relative to sales after deducting the cost of goods sold. This ratio is thought to be an indication of efficiency of the operation and how well your products are priced.

$$\text{GPM} = \frac{\text{Sales—Cost of Goods Sold}}{\text{Sales}}$$

Net Profit Margin (NPM). This ratio measures the efficiency of the business after taxes and expenses.

NPM = Earnings after taxes/Sales.

Average Collection Period (ACP). This ratio measures the effectiveness of how well the account receivables are managed.

ACP = Accounts Receivable/Sales per Day.

Account Payable Turnover (APT). This ratio measures how well your accounts payable are managed or the average amount of time accounts payable are held by the business

APT = Accounts Payable/Purchases per day.

Red flags, as defined by the FDA Regulations 1) Visible congenital or traumatic deformity of the ear. 2) History of active drainage from the ear within the previous 90 days. 3) History of sudden or rapidly progressive hearing loss within the previous 90 days. 4) Acute or chronic dizziness. 5) Unilateral hearing loss of sudden or recent onset within the previous 90 days. 6) Audiometric air-bone gap equal to or greater than 15 decibels at 500 Hz, 1,000 Hz, and 2,000 Hz. 7) Visible evidence of cerumen accumulation or a foreign body in the ear canal. 8) Pain or discomfort in the ear.

REFERENCES

AXELSON, C., "Information System, Management (MIS) Applied," in L. R. Bittel & M. A. Bittel (Eds.), Encyclopedia of Professional Management, New York, McGraw-Hill, 1978.

ALLEN, L. L.,. Starting and Succeeding in Your Own Small Business. New York, Grosset and Dunlap, 1968.

BISGAARD, NIKOLAI; CHRISTIANSEN, CHRISTIAN; and MORRISON, PAUL, Order from Chaos: PC-based Universal Programing interface. Hearing Instruments, Vol. 44, No. 10, October 1993.

BLANCHARD, K. & JOHNSON, J., The One Minute Manager, New York, Berkley Books, 1981.

CONAWAY, J. J., "Your Own Practice: To Buy or Not To Buy," The Hearing Journal, 1983, 36(5), 24–26.

DAILEY, C. A., Entrepreneurial Management, New York, McGraw-Hill, 1971.

DEBOUT, J. M., "Update: The FTC and Hearing Aids," The Hearing Journal, 1984, 37(10), 31; 35–38.

DRUCKER, P. F., The Effective Executive, New York, Harper and Row, 1966.

FOX, H. W., Understanding Your Customer, Fort Worth, U. S. Small Business Administration, No. 4.001, 1983.

FREIMAN, D. J., "Marketing," in William K. Fallon (Ed.) AMA Management Handbook (2nd ed.), New York, American Management Association, 1983.

GOLDSTEIN, ARNOLD., "J. K. Lasser's Operations Forms For Smaller Businesses," 1988 by the J. K. Lasser Tax Institute, a division of Simon & Schuster, Inc.

HIXSON, J., "Five Methods of Budgeting Dispenser Advertising," Hearing Aid Journal, March 1981, 34, 14;26;51.

HIXSON, J., "Marketing: Theory + Practice; = Success," Hearing Instruments, 1982, 33(2) 11–12.

HOPKINS, D. S. The Marketing Plan, New York, The Conference Board, Inc., 1981.

ISSUES AND FACTS '84—Small Business Failures Soar Audecibel, 1984, 33(2), 8.

KLOPP, R., Personal Communication, March, 1984.

LAKIN, A., How to Get Control of Your Time and Life, New York, Signet Book, 1973.

LEVINSON, R. E., Problems in Managing a Family-Owned Business, Fort Worth, U.S. Small Business Administration, No. 2.004, 1970.

LEVITT, T., "Marketing Myopia" in Harvard Business Review, July/August 1960.

LOWDER, K., Personal Correspondence, 1994.

LOWMAN, G., Personal Communication, June 23, 1984.

MCCOLLOM, H. F., and MYNDERS, J. M., Hearing Aid Dispensing Practice. Danville, IL, The Interstate Printers and Publishers Inc., 1984.

MUELLER, J., "Dispensing as a business" in Hearing Instruments, Vol. 41, No. 7, 1990.

NAISBETT, J., Megatrends, New York, Warner Books, 1984.

NATIONAL STEERING COMMITTEE ON COLLABORATIVE MARKETING, "Patient Satisfaction", in Audiology Today, Vol. 5, No. 3, 1993.

NELSON, R. DAVID., "Hearing Instrument Science and Fitting Practices," 1985., National Institute for Hearing Instrument Studies, pp. 559–561.

PETERS, T. J. and WATERMAN, R. H., In Search of Excellence: Lessons from America's Best-Run Companies, New York, Warner Books, 1982.

RADCLIFF, D., "Intrepid Entrepreneurs," Hearing Aid Journal, 1982, 35(2), 4.

RADCLIFF, D. and MAHON, W. J., "Focusing on Consumers," The Hearing Journal, 1983, 36(2), 7–17.

SCOTT, ROBERT., "Office at Home", 1985, Charles Scribner's Sons, New York, pp. 137–140.

SHECHTMAN, MORRIS R. "Working without a Net." Prentice Hall, 1994.

SKAFTE, M. D., "Hearing Health Care Market Potential of the 80's, Part 1: Hearing and Market Analysis," Hearing Instruments, 1984, 35(5), 16–20.

SLOMA, R. S., No-Nonsense Management, New York, Bantam Books, 1977.

SMITH, J., Personal Communication, March, 1984.

SMITH JERRY D., Personal Correspondence, 1994.

STAAB, W., "Excellence in Customer Service" in The Hearing Review, January 1994.

STEINER, G. A., "Approaches to Long-Range Planning for Small Business," in William K. Fallon (Ed.), Managing the Dynamic Small Firm: Readings. Belmont, CA, Wadsworth Publishing Company, 1971.

SWEETOW, ROBERT W., I Love Hearing Aids (Sort of), Hearing Instruments, Vol. 44, No. 8, August 1993.

WASIAK, H., "Marketing Communications," in William K. Fallon (Ed.), AMA Management Handbook, New York, American Management Association, 1983.

WHITING, P. H., The 5 Great Rules of Selling, New York, Dale Carnegie and Associates, 1978.

ZIELONKO, B. K., "Increasing your Hearing Aid Sales, Part 1: Designing Your Market Survey," Hearing Instruments, 1982, 33(9), 14–16.

ZIELONKO, B. K., "Advertising Know-how for the Discriminating Hearing Aid Professional, Part I: Basics Plus Money," Hearing Instruments, 1983, 34(2), 36–38.

ZIELONKO, B. K., "Advertising Know-How for the Discriminating Hearing Aid Profession, Part II, Media, "Hearing Instruments, 1983, 34(4), 8–10.

ZUPKO, K. A., "Creating an Effective Patient Information Booklet," The Hearing Aid Journal, 1982, 35(2), 26–27.

XIV

LEGAL AND ETHICAL ASPECTS OF HEARING INSTRUMENT DISPENSING

MICHAEL J. METZ, Ph.D.

INTRODUCTION

One of the most challenging issues of hearing health care concerns legal and ethical issues. Yet, many dispensers, audiologists and physicians—those involved in dispensing of hearing instruments—may not be able to rationally discuss the issues at the very base of our continuation in the health care field. Most who read this chapter belong to a professional organization. Yet relatively few of these people will have read the Code of Ethics of the organization to which they belong. One Code of Ethics is just like another, right? Further, nobody likes to discuss ethics and morals. It just gets you into trouble, since one cannot agree on what is right, wrong, or ethical. One seldom convinces one's colleagues that one method of professional behavior is correct or ethical. Everyone knows that you can't legislate ethics or morals, so discussing these questions doesn't change anyone's mind. However, frank and open discussions of the issues facing hearing instrument dispensing are essential if continued growth and appropriate professional recognition are to be achieved.

CHAPTER OBJECTIVES

Discussions of ethical issues is necessary because one must understand why ethical principles are required to define the profession in which one works. The clear definition and understanding of ethical stance is necessary, not only to those who belong to a profession, but also to those served by the profession—the consumers of products and services. Those both in and out of any professional field must know where the profession stands. This understanding is part of what is involved in belonging to a "profession". Understanding and consensus is necessary so that members of the profession follow the same rules in monitoring their own behavior and their colleagues. This chapter outlines the legal requirements and ethical objectives in the field of hearing instrument dispensing. Examples are offered in order that those interested in such issues will have a place from which to depart on discussions regarding legal and ethical issues that affect the professional growth of hearing instrument dispensers.

In a litigious society, the issues of what is legal and/or ethical arise more often in the courts as complaints against the practices of a member of the profession. While extreme legal consequences do not happen regularly in the field of hearing instrument dispensing, it is unwise to wait until such legal actions occur before we consider, discuss and arrive at a consensus of what we believe to be a solid ethical and legal foundation.

As any profession evolves, ethical issues related to that specific group generally tend to solidify. It is important that each member of the professional group understand and follow the rules, allowances, methods and limitations of that specific professional group. In the 1970's and 1980's, many professions, including hearing instrument dispensing were besieged with issues of state licensing and federal regulation. The resolution of these issues made hearing instrument dispensing more broadly accepted as a professional activity and tended to solidify methods of operation. This was accomplished despite arguments by various opposing factions within the dispensing community. In the 1990's, the field of hearing instrument dispensing is faced with increased government regulation and control, especially in the context of health care changes. The inclusion of a basic chapter treating legal and ethical issues is a positive indication of increased interest in legal and ethical standards of practice.

A discussion of laws and ethics must start at the level of differentiation between the two areas. There is a significant difference between laws and ethical principles. For example, traffic law requires that you use an automobile turn signal. If you make a turn without using the correct signal, you have broken the law and are subject to legal penalties. Contrast this illegal offense with the concept of driving courtesy, for example, allowing a driver to merge ahead of you, or changing freeway lanes to allow faster drivers to pass you. This courtesy is an example of the difference between legal behavior and ethical, socially conscious behavior. One can think of this responsibility to others as an awareness of the correct thing to do. This courteous behavior is an example of socially ethical behavior.

Both ethics and the law are founded in public policy. While public ethics are concerned with following the socially accepted code of behavior, as determined by that which society considers the polite or right thing to do, professional ethics are founded in the policy of professional organizations. Members of a professional body are expected to hold to a different level of function than would be seen in the behavior of others not in the professional organization. These professional members must not only function in a socially correct manner, they are expected also to function in a manner consistent with other members of the profession. Adherence to these professionally correct behaviors is an inherent part of belonging to the professional group. Indeed, following the professional guidelines of behavior are typically required for membership in the professional organization.

The concept of professional ethics has direct impact on every member of that profession. The behavior of each member of any professional group affects all other members of the group. Even the behavior of others doing the same job as members of the professional group will determine what will be correct for each member and will determine, in large part, the viability and credibility of the whole profession. Since any professional group is composed of its members, it is the behavior of the members that tends to define the group. Insofar as the standard behavior of members in the professional group differs from the expected and socially accepted public behavior, that behavior will define the profession. As a member of that profession, defined by the expected behavior, each member of the professional group will be held to the performance expectations of the others in that profession.

This level of expected professional behavior is generally of a higher level than is expected from a social standpoint. Stated differently, does the public expect a different level of behavior from a professional as compared to a member of the general public? Yes, they do! For example, the public expects the health care professional to place himself or herself in the position of the consumer of that professional service. The public expects the health care professional to perform his or her services on behalf of the consumer. This expectation of professional behavior extends to the point that anyone who provides services related to the profession is expected to perform at the same level of consumer awareness. For example, a nurse or other person working in the office of a physician, and performing services on behalf of the physician, is expected to comply to the same extent with the ethical requirements of the medical field.

If you are a hearing instrument dispenser, you will be held to the ethics of your professional affiliation. Increasingly, you may be held to the standards of other organizations if you perform the same duties, or imply that you perform the same duties, or have represented yourself in any manner as being associated with any other profession. If one attempts to create the impression that his or her duties are similar to another profession such as medicine or law, one may be expected to live up to that standard of practice.

For example, even without formal training, it is fast becoming the responsibility of the hearing instrument dispenser to be aware of ear diseases when fitting a hearing instrument. That is, the hearing instrument dispenser (HID) is expected to recognize many medical problems associated with hearing loss, despite the lack of a universal requirement that the dispensers know specifically about ear diseases. The ability to determine if an ear is infected, diseased or otherwise in need of medical treatment is presumed in the "warning signs" that HIDs must evaluate prior to taking an impression or fitting an instrument. It is presumed that awareness of these signs, and the subsequent appropriate referral, is necessary for the protection of the consumer. Protecting the consumer is becoming a part of the HID's responsibilities, partially because the HID has requested that responsibility. The profession of dispensing has grown to the point that identifying such problems has become the normal standard of practice. Even though it is clinically impossible for the HID to function on the same educational or clinical plane as a physician, the dispenser may be held to the same standards of practice. Obviously, a professional provider who makes claims of possessing skills outside their scope of practice and training assumes the risk of serious legal consequences.

An example of expanding responsibilities involves the prerogative of diagnoses. For example, audiologists do not hold appropriate professional license nor can they assume the privilege or responsibility of making a medical diagnosis. Yet, if the test procedures which the audiologist uses involve tests for the presence or absence of a NVIII tumor, the reporting of tumor-positive results and appropriate follow up for such a test finding may have legal and ethical consequences. It has become the standard of care that the audiologist report these findings as indicative of a serious medical problem. Failure to do so may be viewed as being inconsistent with the generally accepted standard of care rendered by an audiologist. In this situation, the audiologist would face serious legal consequences if appropriate reporting, referral and/or follow-up procedures are not performed. Even though it would be illegal for the audiologist to make a specific diagnosis, the audiologist must function as though such a diagnosis had been made. Functioning in such a manner has become the standard scope of audiological practice. It would be assumed that anyone doing such tests would be capable of correctly interpreting the tests and making judgments proper to the profession of audiology. Therefore, although making a medical diagnosis is illegal, not making decisions about test results may not only have legal consequences, but also may be considered unethical.

We have learned through past experiences that we should be the ones who determine our own professional destiny. Recall the past problems of the United States Food and Drug Administration (FDA) and United States Federal Trade Commission (FTC) hearings of the 1970's which produced such things as mandatory trial periods, instrument guarantees, standard purchase agreements, and the like. More recently, the actions of the FDA and FTC in 1993 dictating to the manufacturers what and how they can advertise is a particularly painful reminder that the government is taking close notice of what we say and do. As members of the profession to which we have elected to belong, we must be involved in the making and changing of the laws that effect our livelihoods. If we do make or change the laws, essentially we will be codifying our standards of practice (our ethics) and allowing for enforcement of these ethical standards in the legal arena. The establishment of these legal standards or laws is often preceded by the embodiment or codifying of our standards of ethical practice.

If one conforms to the laws which govern the business aspects of a dispensing practice, the first criteria of professional business is met. Meeting the ethical requirements will seal the public confidence in the profession. The differences between legalities and ethical considerations involve thoughts suggesting that:

1. One must obey the law, but legal does not equate to ethical and illegal does not equate to unethical.
2. One may violate some ethical principles and still be legal (if the issues arise and warrant, one may be judged unethical by a governing professional organization, but one cannot be prosecuted for violation of any written law).

3. Legal and ethical issues are related, sometimes closely and sometimes distantly.
   a. Sometimes unethical is illegal, but one can conform to all the laws and still be judged unethical.
   b. Most of the time, illegal is unethical, since the ethic standards of organizations do not allow for illegalities.
   c. Ethical behavior is always legal behavior.

We must control situations that threaten our abilities to govern our own ethical development. We must continue to strive to make our ethics equal to or better than other health care providers. If we assume a position in the health care system that is one of a professional provider and not one of ancillary sales of prostheses, we no longer can afford to operate our business solely as a sales oriented entity. We cannot ignore profit, but we must place it in a subservient role—secondary to the well being of the consumers we serve. This level of function is different from the level of salespeople. This level is one of care provider. When we control our own professional and ethical destiny, the laws governing what we do and how we do it will follow.

This laws- follow-ethics progression should teach us that, while we can't legislate ethics, our professional behavior, dictated by the ethical standards of our professional group, can set the stage for the establishment of suitable ethical standards. We can determine the legal posture we will assume as professionals. Establishing a long-term legal position is absolutely necessary if hearing instrument dispensing is to flourish as a full-fledged member of the health care provider profession. The degree to which each of us is involved in these types of ethical decisions, and the degree to which we all agree on what is the "right thing", determine the speed at which the field will progress and the extent to which we will be included in the health care plans.

If we are concerned only with the technicalities of instrument dispensing and the business aspects, legal and ethical behaviors may not take a prime position. We get involved only when a legal or ethical issue threatens our business. Some misconceptions concerning ethics may be more easily understood in considering the following rather obvious rules.

Rule 1

Everyone functions in what he/she perceives to be his/her own best interest. This is a basic rule of human behavior. The rule is based in human nature and is inherently good . . . so far as it goes.

Rule 2

Your don't need anyone to tell you when you are illegal and/or unethical. This rule is inherently not true except on the level of personal standards of behavior. What is legal is determined by the laws and the courts. You establish moral rules for yourself. All professions must adhere to laws governing their practice or functioning. Ethical issues are different. Ethical behavior is not situational, nor is it up to the person to determine. Personal ethics may be called morals. Morals, dependent upon the individual, are subject to some degree of personal interpretation, and can be influenced heavily by religious beliefs. Ethics are always based on what a group decides is right or correct. Sometimes, individual interpretations of what the group would likely consider correct is allowed, but generally the member of the group depends upon the group to determine what is correct. It is the responsibility of the group to determine appropriate behavior and to communicate this standard to other members of the group. It is the responsibility of the individual member of the group to function in the manner proscribed by the group.

Rule 3

Everyone who does not act as you do is either illegal, unethical, or both. See the above discussion—this rule is obviously not true. There are many things wrong with this rule.

The legal stance of any profession is determined in the educational and licensing requirements of the state in which the provider practices. There is no apparent argument here. Everyone would agree with this statement. The ethical stance of a profession, especially a health care profession, depends upon the degree to which the provider of health care places the benefits to the other party ahead of the benefits to him/her self. On the surface, this statement of patient-before-provider would appear clear and obvious to most health care providers. However, it is in this area an emerging professional field struggles to rise to a level perceived by the public to be acceptable. This raising of ethical standards and the relationship of ethics to the legal requirements are best illustrated with examples.

Example 1. A business person is expected to provide information to the customer. The customer may expect this information to be somewhat biased towards that particular product. An additional expectation is that the business person charge a "fair market" price for his/her goods and services. Profit is the motive of business and the consumer usually realizes that fact. Deliberate ignorance of the truth by the business person will not be tolerated, but the salesperson may be expected to proclaim the benefits of the product perhaps to the exclusion of the problems. The consumer usually takes this sales pitch with "a grain of salt". The business person is expected to take only a reasonable profit. The ethics of the salesperson in this situation are set by the group to which the salesperson belongs—the business community. There is also a hierarchy of business practices within the business community. Some business people may take more liberty with the exact facts than do others. A typical and common example of these different expectations may be found in selling automobiles. What is the typical impression of an automobile salesperson held by the general public? Is this impression different than that held for an insurance salesperson or a department store manager? Where does the leniency of the sales pitch become "failure to disclose"? Inspection of the generally held values to which we hold these and other members of the business world will reveal that, while we expect honesty for the most part, we seldom expect such individuals to function in our best interest to the exclusion of their primary motive.

Example 2. A friend with whom a person does business typically is expected to act with more integrity, a higher standard, or with unquestioned honesty. That is, when the consumer deals with the business person who is a friend, it is typical that a higher level of disclosure is expected in the transaction. A higher level of honesty is assumed by the buyer. This business person/friend is expected to function less in the interest of profit and more in the interest of the friend. That is why many people seek out a personal friend with whom to do business. The social ethic dictates against telling untruths to friends and tempers the business sales pitch.

Example 3. A physician is expected to function in the best interest of the patient. Profit is still a motive for the physician, as it is for all those who are required to make a living. However, the profit motive is placed in a different perspective in that the public expects the physician will serve the needs of the patient. This patient service takes a primary position in the physician's standards of practice. It is so stated in the physician's code of ethical behavior and historically has been practiced by all members of the physician's profession. The public expects the physician to perform in this more selfless manner. The professional image of the physician requires this level of performance.

Many other health care profession members are placed in the same category as other medical health professionals by most of the general public. Most of these health care professionals have made great efforts to place themselves in that position in order to inspire public trust. The expectations of the public are that, as licensed professional, dealing with health related issues, "You will put my needs ahead of your own."

This higher level of professional function or ethical behavior is what helps to define a profession as a profession. Professional behavior in the health care field requires that the person providing service function on behalf of another individual. The degree to which the professional functions for the benefit of the other party, as well as the level of the benefit to the other party, determines the level of ethics to which that professional is held. The converse of this statement is also true: the level of ethics held by the professional field determines the expected altruistic behavior of the person providing the care.

One may see the irony of statements such as Professional Salesman, or Professional Carpet Layer or any profession that doesn't act to protect the other person. Such individuals may belong to a profession in the sense of a trade group, and they may even have codified Code of Ethics or Behavior. However, they are not subject to professional standards and ethical levels of function other than those that apply to the correctness of their business practices. One should be aware at this point of the direction of evolution of the field of hearing instrument dispensing. In the emerging and recognized **professional** field of hearing instrument dispensing, the level of provision of goods and services to the public may no longer be sufficient to avoid reprisals on ethical or legal levels. A higher level of functioning may be necessary not only because of the educational and technical advances of the dispensing field, but also because of the level of service provision by others who also provide similar goods and services. Over the past decades, hearing instrument dispensing has made significant progress in presenting a professional image to the consuming public. A part of this changing professional image involves a change in ethical behavior. Ethics cannot be taught but ethics and ethical standards can be explained. Behavior can be changed. And the better understood the ethical questions and the more all hearing instrument dispensers function in the best interest of the hearing impaired, the better prepared we will be to meet the needs of the consumers we intend to serve.

LEGAL CONSIDERATIONS

Those practicing hearing instrument dispensing will make every effort to be legal. Legal behavior in the field consists primarily of two areas of function—advertising and contracts. There are other legal considerations that arise from time to time, such as sales approaches, descriptions and predictions of benefits, pricing of the products and accompanying services, disclosures and required legal statements, but these legal issues involving contracts and advertising constitute the baseline. Contracts and advertising, to a large extent, set the tone for the professional dispensing practice.

CONTRACTS

Hearing instrument sales contacts should outline exactly what is expected from each party involved in the contract. From a legal standpoint, a contract should limit the liability of all parties to the contract, and should specify each party's responsibilities to every other party in the contract. Usually, contracts relating to hearing instrument sales and services involve only the buyer of the instrument and the dispenser. There is, however, a large variation in contracts and many lack the basic fundamentals of what is legally required.

The minimum legal requirements for the delivery of a hearing instrument will vary slightly by state. The basics of the contract will however remain essentially the same. In return for the charges relating to the instrument and associated services, the consumer expects to find considerable information specified on the contract. A simple bill of sale is usually not sufficient for such transactions. Instrument cost, dispensing services, earmolds, batteries, and all other supplies given to the consumer should be detailed on the contract. This protects not only the consumer, but also the dispenser. Terms of the guarantees, if any, should also be clearly stated, as should any fees or costs that are not refundable to the consumer. Both the name of the consumer and the hearing instrument dispenser should appear on the contract and it is typical that addresses and phone numbers of both parties also are incorporated into the identifying information. It is also required that the manufacturer, instrument model number(s) and serial number(s) of the instrument(s) appear on the agreement. These items are basic and should appear on all contracts despite the state in which the hearing instrument dispenser practices.

The return policy, as specified by the state in which the transaction in consummated, must be outlined on the contract. Some states, such as California, require specific language and type size in the outlining of such return policies. The standard and required length of a trial period is 30 calendar days from the date the contract is signed. This time period may be extended but cannot be shortened. The dispenser expects the instrument to be returned by the end of the trial period if the consumer wants a refund. The dispenser expects the instrument to be returned in normal, working condition. It is generally accepted, if the consumer damages or loses the instrument within the trial period, he/she cannot have money returned. Without specifically stating such on the contract, this return for credit policy may not be enforceable.

The consumer expects the hearing instrument(s) to be delivered in good working order. He or she expects that the dispenser will provide the services related to the fitting of the instrument and the earmold. The consumer expects the instrument to be warranted against defects. In brief, the contract should be clear and unquestionable with respect to such items as:

1) Make, model and serial number(s) of the instrument(s) being sold,
2) Names and addresses of the buyer and the seller,
3) Exact costs (these should be itemized to separate products from services),
4) A statement concerning instrument condition, such as new, reconditioned, as-is, etc.,
5) Pertinent hearing instrument dispenser license or certification information,
6) Specifics of instrument warranty or guarantee,
7) Return policies, specific lengths of time and exact specification of expiration date(s),
8) Fees that are or are not refundable (these should be itemized in exact detail),
9) Follow-up services and tangible goods that are included in the agreement,
10) The sources of **any** additional charges made to parties of the contract,
12) The date the contract was signed by both parties, and
13) The signatures of all parties involved in the contract.

Some states may require additional contract information. For example, California **requires** the Assistive Device Warranty Act (the Song-Beverly Consumer Warranty Act) wording, in 10 point sized type. Such wording must appear an all sales contracts. Some states may require additional information. Cooling off periods and notification of such time periods may be required on out-of-office sales. Should the instrument be used or re-conditioned, or should it be sold with less than the standard warranty, the contract should be clear in defining these limitations.

Modifications of contracts, as determined by the dispenser, should be carefully considered. For example, if the dispenser adds that batteries are included with the hearing instrument without specifying how many batteries and for how long, the contract may be interpreted that batteries are included for the length of the warranty. Another example concerns the one year loss and damage policy provided for most hearing instruments. Most contracts fail to tell the buyer that, once the instrument is replaced during the coverage period for loss and damage, the manufacturer considers the loss policy filled and complete. That is, the manufacturer will not replace the lost instrument if it is lost a second time. Some dispensers have found out the hard way that, if the contract does not specifically state the terms of the loss and damage policy, the dispenser, and not the manufacturer, is the one to whom the consumer turns for resolution.

Additions to contracts that support or clarify the dispenser's business practices may appear appropriate but may lead to future trouble. One should consider the following.

1) Does the contract promise things that cannot or will not be delivered?
2) Do contract modifications imply benefits that are impossible?
3) Do the modifications make things more or less clear?

Federal Trade Commission regulations are presented here in a summarized form (courtesy of the Hearing Aid Dispensers Examining Committee, State of California). These regulations require the following information appear on any hearing instrument sales contract:

1) Warrantor's name and mailing address;
2) Who is protected by the warranty, including limitations;
3) Precisely what parts, components or characteristics and properties the warranty covers and what it excludes;
4) What items or services the warrantor will pay for, and those, if any, for which the buyer must pay;
5) When the warranty term begins (if other than the date of purchase);
6) The warranty's duration;
7) Whom to contact to obtain warranty service (including names, addresses, and telephone numbers;

8) Step-by-step instructions to follow to obtain service;
9) Any expenses the buyer may be required to pay.

It is important to have contracts checked by an attorney. No one would ask an attorney's advice on how to fit a hearing instrument, but it would seem reasonable to ask the attorney's advice relative to legal contract issues. Although most contract attorneys cannot be legally bound to insure that your contracts conform to existing laws, they will find the obvious errors in almost all contracts.

Regarding contracts, a dispenser gets little assistance from most hearing instrument manufacturers. One presumes that providing customers with legal advice involves a more visible legal profile than is necessary for their functioning. The manufacturers appear not to take legal responsibility when they don't have to assume it. If the manufacturers gave legal advice, their attorneys would probably advise that they charge for it since it certainly increases their legal liability. No one should increase their legal exposure without being adequately compensated for such exposure. More importantly, manufacturers may not know much about local or state requirements beyond those that are required in their manufacturing procedures.

There is no such thing as a perfect contract, although there are basic materials that will help you to draw up a basic agreement. Most libraries have reference books on basic business agreements. These basic forms may need modification, but they provide a reasonable starting point. It may be more cost effective for a dispensing group to produce a standard contract and then share the cost of an attorney. If you're in doubt, the attorney cost is usually significantly less that the cost of being sued by a patient/consumer.

A few thoughts are in order concerning spoken and unspoken agreements. There are other expectations, by the consumer and the dispenser, which do not appear on the contract. These expectations, when they are not expressively covered in written form on the contract, can be viewed as legally binding on both parties to the contract. For example, most dispensers expect the consumer will be cooperative in the dispensing environment. This cooperation is essential to the correct fitting of an instrument but required cooperation is subjective and is typically not mentioned in the contract. The contract usually does not mention that the consumer will not use the instrument in a damaging manner and will try to the best of his/her abilities to use the instrument effectively. If the consumer does not try to use the instrument correctly, or damages the instrument during the course of normal use, there can be no penalties unless stated in the contract. The consumer may have some responsibility for misuse even if it is not stated in the contract as it is difficult to outline such expectations in a contract. When failures of the hearing instrument fitting occurs due to such factors, it is more likely than not that the dispenser will return the instrument and refund money to the consumer, even though it may be judged that the consumer failed materially in the performance of what the instrument dispenser expected from the user.

Attorneys who have dealt with dispenser versus consumer complaints and subsequent legal actions state that many of these actions arise out of issues promised, implied, or otherwise incorrectly alluded to by the dispenser. The consumer-turned-plaintiff alleges that the dispenser-turned-defendant promised that the instruments would eliminate background noise, or be invisible in the ear, or never need batteries, etc. The dispenser replies that these promises were never made and that the consumer-plaintiff simply didn't understand what was truly stated. Too many sales have been made with these types of misunderstandings as an implied part of the agreement entered into by the buyer and the dispenser. The buyer expects things that are unrealistic and the dispenser fails to clarify these misconceptions. The question is "Where is the responsibility?" The answer, of course, has considerable legal precedent in the concept of complete disclosure.

What the dispenser agrees to deliver is obvious in the exact terms of the contract. What is delivered may not be so obvious. Failure to communicate specific information means the buyer may assume more than intended or expects less difficulty than is reasonable. The medical profession has learned, via large monetary settlements, the consequences of failure to completely disclose all aspects of surgery, care, or treatment. The hearing instrument professional may expect similar, though not so serious, consequences of failure to disclose or failure to adequately explain. These behaviors may be judged illegal. Recall that all illegal actions most likely also will be judged as unethical.

Here is a suggestion to help set the atmosphere in which consumers are treated in a legal manner. How one deals with a patient/client/customer may help one to make differentiations, i.e. the way one thinks about patients/clients may help to determine how they are to be treated. Thinking of the consumer as a person needing service, expertise, sophisticated clinical help, and other abilities the field of HID possesses, may aid in placing of the needs of this consumer in the appropriate primary position. One may begin to think of the consumer as more of a patient and less of a cash source. Set the parameters of the dispensing practice according to good business principles—location, advertising and promotion, necessary clinical tools and skills, appropriate accounting practices, and reasonable and profitable prices. Then, proceed dispensing clinical services to the hearing impaired. This approach assures legality and also puts one well on the road to functioning legally and ethically.

Make sure that sales contracts are in order. Make sure they contain all the required information and protect not only the dispenser but also the consumer. If the contract doesn't protect both parties, it generally will be held invalid. Assure that all necessary contracts are in place before proceeding. Sales contracts, rental contracts, contracts for loaner instruments, additional services, insurance, etc. are apart of the required paperwork. Be sure that everybody involved in the contract gets a complete copy of the agreement. No-carbon-required (NCR) copies assure that all parties to the contract get identical information. Copies are less expensive than legal expenses.

Specify exactly what is to be delivered for an exact price, not only on sales contracts but also on any price quotes. Estimates of the cost of goods and services are acceptable if they are specified as estimates. It would be prudent to specify the expiration date of the estimate. One would be hard pressed to honor an estimate for the purchase of a hearing instrument that was two, three or more years old!

Hearing instrument repair contracts are another source of problems. Repair contracts are simple to devise. What happens when the consumer is quoted the usual price for repair and warranty and the factory cost is twice what was expected? A well worded repair contract not only limits the dispenser's liability in assuming more of the cost than good accounting practices would dictate as normal, but makes the repairs understandable to the consumer. A good contract for repair will protect both parties and eliminate arguments when the higher-than-normal repair charges are received.

Loaner contracts are essential if one provides this service to the consumer. Otherwise, one may loan and subsequently lose instruments that are better than those being repaired. How will one enforce the replacement cost of lost loaner instruments? What happens if the consumer breaks the loaner instrument? All these things must be stated in the loaner contract to provide this service in a legal manner. What if the consumer likes the loaner so well that he/she doesn't return to the office? Without a valid loaner contract, one has no legal recourse to be compensated for the "lost" instrument.

Suppose one fails to write all these things down as a standard contract? Where do consumers go when the dispensing situation deteriorates and specifics are not in writing? If the hearing instrument specialist does not satisfy the consumer, they will generally file a complaint with the Better Business Bureau, the State licensing board, the local or state professional organization. The Better Business Bureau will generally call or write asking for the dispenser's side of the disagreement. The Bureau generally keeps a list of companies that have complaints lodged with them. They have no power to enforce but do communicate with law enforcement agencies when the situation or circumstance demand such action.

Trade, local, or state organizations or groups also have no legal authority but can help solve the consumer's problem before a government agency intervenes. Generally these organizations conduct a superficial investigation by talking to both parties and attempting to arrive at a compromise at best, and full restitution to either party at worst. A good example of the interceding activities of a typical organization is the ethics committee of many state dispensing organizations.

If the consumer lives in a state having an enforceable licensing law, there is usually a state licensing board. This board will seek information about the supposed wrong doing and take one of several available courses of action. This board may abandon the complaint due to a misunderstanding by the consumer. If the complaint has merit, the board may issue warnings or impose censure upon the dispenser. The board may remand the case to local law enforcement authorities for further investigation, arrest, detainment, or other legal action if the complaints are sufficient in degree or number to warrant such action.

ADVERTISING

It is tempting to manage this topic with only two words of advice—Don't Advertise. The rationale for this approach involves the wide spread aversion to any type of public or media advertising maintained by many professional people. This professional, no-advertising stance still represents the standard of practice by many clinicians in other professions. It is neither illegal nor unethical to advertise. The law allows truthful advertising as a protection to the consumer and it has been decided in legal cases that professional groups and ethical boards of professional organizations cannot prohibit advertising.

The issue of professional advertising was highlighted by a legal decision in 1978 (National Society of Professional Engineers versus United States, 1978) involving a professional engineering association that ruled the advertising by one professional engineer violated the Code of Ethics of his profession. The engineer brought legal action against the association and prevailed in the appellate courts. The legal logic was that the organization may not censure an individual's attempt to place his name before the public in the form of advertising. It was ruled that such action constituted a restraint of trade and a violation of an individual's right to free speech. This legal decision has been construed to allow members of all professional organizations to advertise their services. Prior to this decision, all media advertising by members of the medical and dental professions, hospitals, and all suppliers of professional goods and services had not been allowed on ethical grounds.

This decision changed the way professions looked at advertising. It has influenced current methods of advertising which many dispensers employ. Prior to this decision, HIDs commonly advertised price, products and services. Many dispensers continue to advertise in this manner. The effect of professional advertising is also evident in the deliberations of the Food and Drug Administration and the Federal Trade Commission (1993).

Federal government agencies have stated, and supported their statements with definitive actions, that manufacturing claims and those of the dispensing community that cannot be documented by peer-reviewed research will not be tolerated. For example, claims of noise reduction capabilities of circuits, based upon anecdotal information only, have been disallowed by these government agencies. Following the decision by the FDA and the FTC, considerable discussion occurred regarding questions of what constitutes legitimate advertising and appropriate substantiating research for claims of instruments. It may be some years before these issues are completely resolved.

The issues themselves, however, indicate the gradual change from a strictly business approach in advertising to an approach based upon the professional changes. That is, it may have been considered only borderline to make claims of instrument performance in the past. Now, federal and state government agencies, as well as the ethical committees of professional organizations, are monitoring the advertising practices of their constituents.

In a larger sense, it behooves all dispensers to adhere to a level of advertising that places an increased emphasis on the professional aspect of the dispensing field. If the profession is to be judged publicly, the appearance of advertising and the gradual movement of the dispensing community into the area of "professionalism" requires this constraint. Although some dispensers adhere to old advertising patterns, over time these methods may be judged unethical.

It is possible that unethical advertisement may never be judged illegal. These issues have been ruled upon by various courts, including the United States Supreme Court. For specific discussions regarding advertising, the reader is referred to the following cases:

American Medical Association versus Federal Trade Commission, 638 f.2d 433, 449 (2d Cir.), 1980.

Arizona versus Maricopa County Medical Society, 457 U.S. 332, 348–49, 1982.

Brunswick Corporation versus Pueblo Bowl-O-Mat, Inc., 429 U.S. 477, 488, 1977.

Goldfarb versus Virginia State Bar, 421 U.S. 773, 1975.

National Society of Mechanical Engineers versus United States, op.cit.

In short, these cases made clear that many types of professional regulation or limitation of advertising violate the laws governing restriction of trade. As such, there are no legal limitations on the type, quality, quantity and direction of advertisement other than what would violate the truth. And these violations of truth are typically defined by the Business Codes or the Business and Professions Codes of all states. As frightening as this concept may be, there are complex and confusing legal principles involved. The more true course is that the nature and extent of advertising should be determined by a peer group of professional associations affected. Recall that people who perform the same professional duties are essentially members of the same professional group whether they elect to join the group or not.

Universally, state and federal business codes prohibit advertisement that is false, misleading or deceptive. The codes prevent the advertiser from stating things are false or misleading. They prevent implying things that are deceptive. A reasonable model for legal advertising has been determined in California. The following are requirements under California Business and Professions Codes:

Price advertising must be exact, without the use of phrases like "as low as", "and up", lowest prices"., or words or phrases of similar import. (Advertising a discount is not illegal unless it is misleading or false.)

Any advertisement using words of comparison must be based on verifiable data substantiating the comparison.

In price advertising, the price for each product or service must be clearly identifiable.

The price advertised for a product must include charges for related professional services, including dispensing and fitting services, unless the advertisement clearly states otherwise.

The dispenser may not compensate or give anything of value to a representative of the press, radio, television, or other communication medium for professional publicity unless the fact of compensation is made known in the publicity.

Business names should not be so broad as to connote comprehensive and diagnostic hearing services, unless the dispenser is also licensed as a physician or audiologist. (for example it would be considered incorrect to advertise the "XYZ Hearing Aid Center" as the "XYZ Hearing Center".)

Dispensers should not advertise "free hearing test" or hearing tests without further qualification, since the statement connotes comprehensive, diagnostic testing not within a hearing instrument dispenser's scope of practice. It is acceptable to advertise "free test to determine if you could be helped by a hearing aid" or to use words of similar import to clarify the nature of the testing performed by a hearing instrument dispenser.

Sending consumers preset appointment information as part of a direct mail solicitation is prohibited because it is deceptive and misleading and thus constitutes a violation of the code.

Hearing Instrument dispensers should not utilize anonymous or blind advertising, but should disclose the name of the business or dispenser in each ad. For example, it is incorrect in the context of an ad to state "If you have a hearing problem, call 123-4567. Instead, it could be stated "For information on how you can be helped by a hearing instrument, call Mr. Dispenser, a licensed hearing instrument dispenser, at the XYZ Hearing Aid Center."

If an ad refers to a dispenser's board certification, the ad should indicate specifics, written in a manner that is easily understood by consumers. Also, the California licensing law provides for licensing dispensers, not specialists.

Correct:	*John Doe, Hearing Aid Dispenser*
	Jane Doe, Board Certified Hearing Instrument Specialist
Incorrect:	*Jack Doe, BC-HIS*
	Jill Doe, Hearing Aid Specialist

Laws and regulations regarding correct advertising may vary depending upon the state in which the dispenser practices. However, the rather strict and prohibitive California law represents the direction which the regulations concerning advertising are moving. It would appear that such movement is necessary to enable the consuming public to differentiate between more simple business entities and those of professional entities.

ETHICAL ISSUES

We have come full circle with regard to that which constitutes ethics and ethical behavior. Recall that ethical behavior is that which is considered the right thing to do. Stated another way, ethics are a "a consensus of social norms and behavior", founded in public policy and based upon public opinion. Ethical behavior involves the concept of what would be considered "correct" group behavior.

Professional ethics are defined by the professional group and ethical professional behavior is defined by comparison of individual behavior to that of the average peer member of the group. Twenty years ago, virtually all hearing instruments dispensed in the United Sates were dispensed by members of a group which did not hold a professional license. This group was composed of people who dealt with the retail aspects of hearing aids. In the past twenty years, retail instrument sales have changed. In the mid 1990's, over 50% of all hearing instruments dispensed are fit by audiologists and/or physicians.

The modern hearing instrument dispenser, compared to that of twenty years age, has more education, more clinical skills, and access to more technology. Since the composition of the peer group has changed, comparisons to the average dispenser have changed. Those things considered correct, ethical, and legal twenty years ago, may not be correct, ethical, or legal today. Dispensers who behaved in a certain manner in times past, may not do so now since certain aspects of that past behavior may be judged unethical or illegal.

The privileges and, correspondingly, the expanding responsibilities of a dispensing professional may be of more concern to those who have been dispensing for a long time rather than those dispensers just entering the field. This expanding responsibility is evident in the requirement to refer consumers who demonstrate ear and hearing problems beyond the clinical skills of the dispenser. Not meeting this particular responsibility may lead to ethical censure and to legal difficulties. This aspect of responsibility for referral without privilege of diagnosis may be difficult for some to accept. An argument that experience in practicing will suffice for academic training is not sufficient for reasons that ought to be obvious to any who gives more than cursory thought to the problem. Caring for ill people for any number of years will not teach the care giver the practice of medicine. Although the dispenser may have a high success rate of fitting instruments, the treatment of hearing loss encompasses more than the fitting of hearing instruments. Successful fittings are not the measure of clinical prowess any more than bandaging a wound is the measure of medical expertise.

The professional practice of instrument dispensing, in the process of moving from a retail business to a more science related discipline, is changing dramatically. In this change, those factors which define ethical behavior are also evolving, since the "peer group" is changing and growing. The ethical behavior required by the group is reflective of the time in which the behavior occurs. This does not mean that unethical behavior is situational, it simply means that when the act or action was committed, the judgment of ethics must take place in that time. For example, prior to the 1980s, it was considered unethical for audiologists to dispense hearing instruments. Those audiologists who did dispense prior to those years were judged to be unethical by the audiology profession. An audiologist who dispensed hearing instruments before approximately 1979 was considered unethical by the peer group to which that individual belonged. In 1994, the same action could be judged as ethical by the group because attitudes and regulations have changed. Stated another way, ethics change with respect to amounts, degrees, who they include, what is good and bad, what actions are accepted, how they used to be, what they may become, etc. Professionalism through ethical stance has to do with the relationship the individual has with the group at that time. One cannot persist in methods which were correct in time past without risk of being judged unethical.

While ethics cannot be legislated in the typical sense, they can be defined and enforced in the legal and the professional arena. Ethical matters should be judged by the group to whom the ethics apply. If they are not judged by this group, but judged by the general public or political bodies, the interpretation of a supposed ethical violation may be considerably different than that which the associated group would have interpreted. Consider the following examples.

Example 1

As hearing instrument dispensers, we believe that any hearing loss detracts from the pleasures of life determined by adequate communication. We believe that hearing better is a positive contribution to living a better life. We think that being able to hear more is good. However, when the FDA ruled on this very matter, they concluded that equating better hearing with better life could be construed by the consumer differently than what was meant by the manufacturer. Therefore this statement constituted illegal advertising. Having the FDA judge this matter was not in the best interest of HIDs. How could this situation have been avoided? Who should make the decisions concerning how and what to advertise? What sanctions should be carried out when rules of advertising are violated?

Example 2

In one state, a legal opinion was offered by an attorney employed by that state board of licensing. This attorney stated that the removal of cerumen by an audiologist constituted "the invasion of a bodily orifice" and thus was not within the audiologist's scope of practice within that state. This ruling, while not constituting a legal interpretation of the licensing law of that state (only the attorney general or the legislature of the state can so bind the interpretation of the law), precluded audiologists from the management of ear wax. (It really does not prevent an audiologist from managing cerumen, it just precludes his or her malpractice insurance from covering problems arising from such management.) It becomes, in a practical sense, "illegal" to do such management. This illegality makes the management of cerumen risky in that state, but legal as well as ethical in other states of the country. Clearly, this is an example of someone not well versed in the professional training, abilities, and scope of the profession making a judgement about the legalities and ethical behaviors of that profession. This judgement is not considered to be in the best interest of audiologists or HIDs, and it would have been better if the decision about what lies within the scope of professional practice had been left to the professional people affected by such a decision. How does this decision or situation affect the ability of the hearing instrument dispenser to expand the scope of practice? Would the removal of cerumen by an audiologist be considered illegal, unethical, both, or neither?

This first example is illustrative of the fact that actions that seem right may be judged wrong. The second example illustrates that actions may be illegal but may not be unethical. In general, we have decided that most illegal actions are also unethical. However, we can see this seemingly obvious statement may not always be held correct.

It is always interesting to pose some examples of ethical dilemmas. Discussion of or thought directed to these examples may help clarify thinking about ethical issues. Recall that ethical decisions cannot be made without judging how the professional group would agree or disagree with the decision. The behavior and the group go together.

ETHICAL DILEMMA NO. 1

What happens when what you think is good for your business profits conflicts with what is best for the customer or the patient? (Does your choice of descriptor for the consumer define the situation as primarily being one of a business or professional relationship?) The way you think about patient versus customer may determine your answer to this conflict. Professionals, trained in the fields of medicine, audiology and instrument dispensing have patients and perhaps the expected behavior in treating that consumer will be different than if this consumer is treated as a customer. If you are professional, you ought to be held to a higher standard with respect to the manner in which the consumer is treated. This professional treatment also holds with respect to profits. That is, if you act as a professional, you will be expected to place the benefits to the consumer (patient) in the foremost position. You can be concerned with profits, but only in a secondary position. This difference defines a professional relationship in comparison to business relationship.

ETHICAL DILEMMA NO. 2

Is it best for your business to maximize profits by charging the most for your products and services? Is this ever in conflict with your professional ethics or the professional ethics of persons in the same or similar situations? Of course it conflicts! It always conflicts when that which is appropriate interferes with the maximum profits that can be generated in the relationship between you and the consumer. If it didn't conflict, there would be no dilemma and everyone would always do the correct thing. The resolution of this conflict is the key issue. The manner in which you approach the situation determines whether the resolution is ethical. Unfortunately, you may decide to manage the situation in a manner that significantly differs from the way in which other members of the profession would resolve the problem. If your decision differs from that which would come from the group, your resolution of the situation may be judged as unethical.

ETHICAL DILEMMA NO. 3

There is a classic story of a student in a college class of Business Ethics who told the instructor he understood the concepts of business ethics, but could the instructor give examples of what constituted good business ethics. The instructor replied that the student really didn't understand and the question he asked was a demonstration of this lack of understanding. Some people don't understand this example. Do you?

ETHICAL DILEMMA NO. 4

If the consumer can be helped equally with hearing instruments that are appropriate but less expensive, are you unethical if you recommend the more expensive instruments? (Is an auto salesman unethical by recommending all the options?) What if you believe the more expensive instruments may be better, they just haven't been proven yet? What are your responsibilities for knowing what constitutes the newest technologies and applications? What are your responsibilities for being well-versed in the literature and research involved in instrument dispensing? How could you ever fit a hearing loss patient with instruments that have not been verified in terms of benefits?

ETHICAL DILEMMA NO. 5

It is argued that "I must make a reasonable profit so I can stay in business and my consumer can be given continued (or correct, best, or appropriate) services from me. That profit mandate enables me to charge reasonably (or more than the guy down the street who doesn't know as much as I do, whatever the market will allow, the same as anyone else, less, etc.). This could be a "closer call" than the prior example, since higher levels of training, more experience, etc. ought to be worth more than inexperience and/or no training. But again, the answer lies in how the other members of the professional group to which the clinician belongs, aspires to belong, makes appearances of belonging to, etc. would judge this situation. If that professional group thinks those costs are right, then they are right, by definition. The difficulty is that you don't get to belong to two different groups depending upon the decision you want at the time. A correct professional decision may not be the same as the correct business decision. If the decisions were the same, the answer would be obvious and no dilemma would exist.

ETHICAL DILEMMA NO. 6

What's wrong with this statement. "An ethical act is any act after which you feel good" Answer: "Nothing", if it applies to a personal ethical system. What does this statement say about everyone establishing their own ethical standards? (Recall that professional ethics are the standards of a group.) Stated more appropriately, "A professional ethical act is any act after which the group would feel good".

Clearly, it is easier to define legal than it is to define ethical. If it's legal, it's in the book and can be readily referenced. If it's ethical, it's only written down in general terms in a Code of Ethics. Further, the decision of "correct" must always be representative of the consensus thinking of the group at that time. As the group opinions or right and wrong change, so does the ethical judgement of correctness. That's one reason why ethics (and, on a personal basis, morals) are not legislated in the standard manner—the legislation would need to change too often. This changing concept of correctness makes it harder for us, the professional field, to define ourselves. Recall that the extent to which we are professional is determined, at least to some degree, by the altruistic level of these concepts of the right way to treat our consumers. We define ourselves by our actions. That's why, although one must discuss legalities, ethics are a more interesting topic and lead to a lot more argument.

SUMMARY AND CONCLUSIONS

We have discussed the fact that people expect more from doctors, lawyers, and other recognized professionals than they do from most business people. When the public believes that they are not being served on a professional level, their reactions are ones of betrayal, disbelief and skepticism. Why do you suppose that is true? Stromberg (1990), in a paper presented to the American Speech-Language Hearing Association, speculated on the skepticism in the minds of both the public and the profession itself.

> One reason (for the skepticism) is that most fields have experienced an *erosion of professional sovereignty* in the face of demands that professionals be more "accountable" to the public. In past eras, doctors, lawyers, engineers, and other professionals were viewed with awe and treated with deference. This is far less so today. Instead, there is a common perception, as George Bernard Shaw said, that "Every profession is a conspiracy against the laity [the public]." The remoteness and paternalism of many professions are no longer acceptable. Consumerism and the proliferation of information have reduced people's willingness to defer to professional's judgements. Today, people want to feel empowered. they demand to know what lies behind the professional's decisions. And when clients or patients second-guess the professionals, they are willing to question not only their competence but also their ethics.

This public skepticism, which gives rise to professional acountability, is a major driving force in the rising expectations the public (and other professionals) place on hearing instrument dispensing. Recall that we have asked and worked hard for this recognition and concomitant responsibility. When the public we serve experiences products, product claims, or services that are less than we proclaim, the skepticism may be warranted. We must not allow this to happen.

What each of us does adds, detracts, or maintains our ethical position. If more of us detract from that which is expected, the field of hearing instrument dispensing may not rise to the professional level that we wish. Stated another way, as we establish ourselves as professional, the more the altruistic interests of the patient become the guiding principle of our behavior. Our fixation on the profit motive to the exclusion of the patient's best interests tends to keep our professional goals at the level of business only ethics. The alternative is to stay the same and remain only a business, forfeiting the professional status afforded by many states and the ability to bill insurance, avoid business and sales taxes, and engage in the health care field on a professional level.

Does our current position place us in a position that requires, demands, or expects more public trust? In the past 10–20 years, federal and state regulations have changed. As licensing, educational requirements, advertising, fitting appliances and methods have changed, we have become more professional and, the public does expect more from us. When one observes the government (FDA, FTC) involvement in the field, it is reasonable to expect that our position in the hearing health care arena will be more defined and that higher ethical standards will be demanded in the future.

In a sense, we are asking the public to place more demands upon us as we gain sophistication and expertise in our field. We ask for an elevated position when we request to become the entry point for hearing health care. We seek this level of responsibility when we expect to bill third party carriers for our products and services. We invite closer public scrutiny of our standards when we license ourselves and move beyond a simple sales approach to our products and services.

The ethical standards to which we must adhere can be summarized very simply: Do the right thing, as determined by the group. That's the essence of all professional ethics.

Where can you learn more of the ethical issues that face us now and in the future? Look in the references and read the few sources that pertain directly to our field. Become involved in the issues that face your profession. Demand of your self and others that all "do the right thing" at all times. Why should we be concerned with the ethical behavior of others in ***OUR*** field? If we don't, who will? Perhaps our methods of dealing with these ethical issues are the indicators or the true measure of our emergence as a genuine consumer-related professional group. We should not tolerate persons who do not perform at a level directed by our **professional** standards. Our professional standards must evolve, not by mandate, but by each member of the profession practicing the way it should be done.

GLOSSARY

Audiologist An individual practicing in the field of Audiology who is duly licensed by the state in which he/she practices, and/or is certified as clinically competent (CCC-A) by the American Speech-Language-Hearing Association.

Ethics The system or code of morals of a particular person, group, profession, etc.

Ethical behavior Behavior which conforms to the standards of conduct of a given profession or group. Conduct which a peer group deems correct by way of a Code of Ethics and/or the standards of practice of that particular group.

Federal Trade Commission A Federal agency whose duty is to investigate unfair methods of competition in business, fraudulent advertising, etc., and to prosecute those guilty of such practices.

Food and Drug Administration A Federal agency whose duty is to approve, investigate, and monitor, the food, food additives, medications, prostheses including hearing instruments, and other medical devices in the public domain.

Hearing Instrument Dispenser (HID) An individual practicing in the field of hearing instrument dispensing who is duly licensed to do so in the state such practice is performed.

Legal behavior Behavior which conforms to all legal requirements. Legal behavior is not necessarily moral or ethical.

Moral behavior Behavior which conforms to personal or religious beliefs of being correct. Moral behavior may be illegal and/or unethical.

Professional behavior Behavior which conforms to all legal requirements and ethical standards of the group to which the professional belongs.

REFERENCES

AMERICAN MEDICAL ASSOCIATION VERSUS FEDERAL TRADE COMMISSION, 638 f.2d 433, 449 (2d Cir.), 1980.

ARIZONA VERSUS MARICOPA COUNTY MEDICAL SOCIETY, 457 U.S. 332, 348–49, 1982.

BRUNSWICK CORPORATION VERSUS PUEBLO BOWL-O-MAT, INC., 429 U.S. 477, 488, 1977.

CALIFORNIA, STATE OF HEARING AID DISPENSERS EXAMINING COMMITTEE, Personal Communication, 1994.

CALIFORNIA BUSINESS AND PROFESSIONS CODE, Sections 651, 3301, 3401(f), and 3428.

GOLDFARB VERSUS VIRGINIA STATE BAR, 421 U.S. 773, 1975.

NATIONAL SOCIETY OF PROFESSIONAL ENGINEERS V. UNITED STATES, 435 U.S. 679, 697–98, (1978).

RESNICK, DAVID M., *Professional Ethics for Audiologists and Speech-Language Pathologists,* Singular Publishing Group, Inc., San Diego, CA, 1993.

STROMBERG, C. et al., *The Psychologist's Legal Handbook,* Washington, D.C.: Council for the National Register, 1988.

STROMBERG, C., Key Legal Issues in Professional Ethics, in *Reflection on Ethics: A Compilation of Articles Inspired by the May, 1990 ASHA Ethics Colloquium,* American Speech-Language & Hearing Assoc., Rockville, MD, 1990.

Index

Numbers in **bold** refer to figures

A

B

I

Q

R

T

U

V

W

Y

Z